Essential Neuropharmacology

The Prescriber's Guide

Second edition

T0201657

Essential Neuropharmacology
The Prescriber's Guide

Second edition

Stephen D. Silberstein

Professor Jefferson Medical College, Thomas Jefferson University and Director, Jefferson Headache Center, Thomas Jefferson University Hospital, Philadelphia, PA, USA

Michael J. Marmura

Assistant Professor, Department of Neurology, Jefferson Headache Center, Thomas Jefferson University Hospital, Philadelphia, PA, USA

Hsiangkuo Yuan

Visiting Scholar, Thomas Jefferson University Hospital, Department of Neurology, Philadelphia, PA, USA

Consultant Editor

Stephen M. Stahl

Adjunct Professor of Psychiatry, University of California, San Diego, CA, USA and Honorary Visiting Senior Fellow at the University of Cambridge, Cambridge, UK

With illustrations by

Nancy Muntner

Neuroscience Education Institute

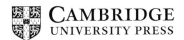

CAMBRIDGE
UNIVERSITY PRESS

CAMBRIDGE
UNIVERSITY PRESS

University Printing House, Cambridge CB2 8BS, United Kingdom

Cambridge University Press is part of the University of Cambridge.

It furthers the University's mission by disseminating knowledge in the pursuit of education, learning and research at the highest international levels of excellence.

www.cambridge.org
Information on this title: www.cambridge.org/9781107485549

© S.D. Silberstein, M.J. Mamura and H. Yuan (2010) 2015

First published 2010
Second edition 2015
Reprinted 2017

Printed in the United Kingdom by Bell and Bain Ltd, Glasgow

A catalog record for this publication is available from the British Library

Library of Congress Cataloging in Publication data
Silberstein, Stephen D., author.
Essential neuropharmacology : the prescriber's guide / Stephen D. Silberstein, Michael J. Marmura, Hsiangkuo Yuan ; consultant editor, Stephen M. Stahl ; with illustrations by Nancy Muntner. – Second edition.
    p. ; cm.
Includes bibliographical references and index.
ISBN 978-1-107-48554-9 (Paperback)
I. Marmura, Michael James, author. II. Yuan, Hsiangkuo, author. III. Title.
[DNLM: 1. Central Nervous System Agents–pharmacology–Handbooks. 2. Central Nervous System Agents–therapeutic use–Handbooks. 3. Central Nervous System Diseases–drug therapy–Handbooks.
QV 39]
RM315
615′.78–dc23   2015012669

ISBN 978-1-107-48554-9 Paperback

Every effort has been made in preparing this book to provide accurate and up-to-date information which is in accord with accepted standards and practice at the time of publication. Although case histories are drawn from actual cases, every effort has been made to disguise the identities of the individuals involved. Nevertheless, the authors, editors and publishers can make no warranties that the information contained herein is totally free from error, not least because clinical standards are constantly changing through research and regulation. The authors, editors and publishers therefore disclaim all liability for direct or consequential damages resulting from the use of material contained in this book. Readers are strongly advised to pay careful attention to information provided by the manufacturer of any drugs or equipment that they plan to use.

Contents

Icons

 α_2-adrenergic agonist

 antiarrhythmic

 anticholinergic

 anticoagulant

 antiemetic

 antiepileptic drug

 antihistamine

 antineoplastic agent

 antiparkinson agent

 antiplatelet agent

 antipsychotic

 atypical antidepressant

 benzodiazepine

 β-blocker

calcium channel blocker

 cannabinoid

 catecholamine analog

 chelating agent

 cholinesterase inhibitor

 corticosteroid

 ergot

 immunomodulator

 immunosuppressant

 melatonin receptor agonist

 monoamine-depleting agent

 mood stabilizer

 muscle relaxant

 neuromuscular drug

 neurotoxin

NMDA receptor antagonist

 non-steroidal anti-inflammatory drug (NSAID)

 orexin receptor antagonist

 osmotic diuretic

 potassium channel blocker

 psychostimulant

 selective serotonin reuptake inhibitor

 serotonin and norepinephrine reuptake inhibitor

 thrombolytic agent

 tricyclic/tetracyclic antidepressant

 triptan

 How the drug works, mechanism of action

 Best augmenting agents to add for partial response or treatment-resistance

 Life-threatening or dangerous adverse effects

Weight Gain: Degrees of weight gain associated with the drug, with unusual signifying that weight gain is not expected; not unusual signifying that weight gain occurs in a significant minority; common signifying that many experience weight gain and/or it can be significant in amount; and problematic signifying that weight gain occurs frequently, can be significant in amount, and may be a health problem in some patients

Sedation: Degrees of sedation associated with the drug, with unusual signifying that sedation is not expected; not unusual signifying that sedation occurs in a significant minority; common signifying that many experience sedation and/or it can be significant in amount; and problematic signifying that sedation occurs frequently, can be significant in amount, and may be a health problem in some patients

Tips for dosing based on the clinical expertise of the author

Drug interactions that may occur

Warnings and precautions regarding use of the drug

Information regarding use of the drug during pregnancy

Clinical pearls of information based on the clinical expertise of the author

Suggested reading

Preface

The past few years have been extremely exciting for both neuroscientists and clinicians. We are unlocking the mysteries of the human mind and applying these discoveries to create better treatment for those affected with neurological disorders, leading to more effective therapies. A new patient-centered medicine approach will hopefully lead to fewer side effects and increased efficacy.

This edition of *Essential Neuropharmacology* focuses on pharmacological treatment; however, substantial improvements in surgical and medical device treatments for neurological disorders have occurred. These include surgical treatments for epilepsy, deep brain stimulation, transcranial magnetic stimulation, vagal nerve stimulation, and occipital and other nerve stimulators for pain. Due to improvements in safety and proven efficacy, some of these procedures may now be considered earlier, rather than as a last resort.

Given the expanding role of neurologists, we also decided to widen the focus of the textbook to include areas such as sleep and neuro-oncology. The practice of sleep medicine has expanded and chemotherapy has been established as effective when combined with other treatments for the treatment of some brain cancers, such as glioblastoma and CNS lymphoma, and neurologists increasingly are working with neurosurgeons and radiation oncologists to manage these challenging disorders.

Like most neurologists, we became interested in neurology due to our fascination with the nervous system and by the fact that there is so much more to learn. The scope of neurological practice continues to expand, with increasing degrees of specialization. Although we practice based on available evidence, often we must revert to trial and error for our difficult cases. Keeping track of the newest medications and developments in our expanding field is a challenge. We have all had the experience of running into a complicated patient, and we know how important it is to discuss the case with an expert. We hope that this text will help those who don't have immediate access to such expertise and will lead to better care for patients with neurological disorders.

Acknowledgements

The authors wish to thank Thomas Leist MD, Jon Glass MD, Maya Carter MD, Daniel Hexter MD, Tso-wei Liang MD, Daniel Kremmens MD, and Alex Papangelou MD for their subspecialty advice as well as Larry Charleston IV MD who assisted with the first edition.

Michael Marmura would like to thank his wife Stacey and son Alec for their love and support. He would like to dedicate this edition to the memory of his father William who passed away earlier this year.

Stephen Silberstein would like to thank his wife Marsha, sons Aaron and Joshua, daughters-in-law Miriam and Stephanie, and grandchildren Molly and Jake for their love and excitement.

Hsiangkuo Yuan would like to thank his parents Grace and John, brother Sean, wife Jie Ren, and daughters Deanna and Adelyn for their love and support.

ACETAZOLAMIDE

THERAPEUTICS

Brands
- Diamox, Diamox-Sequels, Azomid, AZM, Dazamide, Novo-Zolamide

Generic?
- Yes

Class
- Antiepileptic drug (AED)

Commonly Prescribed for
(FDA approved in bold)
- **Adjunctive treatment for centrencephalic epilepsies (petit mal, unlocalized)**
- **Acute mountain sickness**
- **Edema due to congestive heart failure or medication**
- **Glaucoma**
- Adjunctive treatment for generalized tonic-clonic and partial seizures
- Idiopathic intracranial hypertension (IIH) (pseudotumor cerebrii)
- Episodic ataxias type 1 and 2
- Hemiplegic migraine
- Mitochondrial encephalopathy with lactic acidosis and stroke-like episodes (MELAS)
- Marfan syndrome
- Sleep apnea

How the Drug Works
- Blocks the carbonic anhydrase enzyme, which is responsible for converting carbon dioxide and water to bicarbonate. This increases excretion of sodium, potassium, bicarbonate, and water, producing alkaline diuresis. In epilepsy, it decreases excessive neuronal discharge in CNS due to either slight degree of acidosis or perhaps reduction of extracellular calcium. It also reduces production of CSF and aqueous humor

How Long Until It Works
- Seizures: within a few days
- IIH: maximum benefit in 4–6 weeks

If It Works
- Seizures: goal is the remission of seizures. Continue as long as effective and well tolerated. Consider tapering and slowly stopping after 2 years seizure-free, depending on the type of epilepsy
- IIH: monitor visual fields and papilledema and symptoms such as visual obscurations and headache

If It Doesn't Work
- Increase to highest tolerated dose
- Seizures: consider changing to another agent, adding a second agent, using a medical device, or a referral for epilepsy surgery evaluation. When adding a second agent, keep drug interactions in mind
- IIH: eliminate symptomatic causes such as drugs or toxins, encourage weight loss if patient is obese, consider loop diuretics or topiramate. Lumbar puncture often provides short-term relief of symptoms. For visual loss, optic nerve defenestration or CSF shunting (lumboperitoneal or ventriculoperitoneal) may be needed

Best Augmenting Combos for Partial Response or Treatment-Resistance
- Epilepsy: acetazolamide itself is usually an augmenting agent. Relatively few interactions with other AEDs. Topiramate and zonisamide have similar mechanisms of action, so acetazolamide is not usually combined with these agents
- IIH: furosemide and topiramate may be helpful. Combine with caution due to risk of kidney stone formation

Tests
- Obtain a CBC when starting drug and during therapy. Check bicarbonate, potassium, and sodium levels if symptoms of metabolic acidosis develop

ADVERSE EFFECTS (AEs)

How the Drug Causes AEs
- Related to carbonic anhydrase inhibition, which can cause metabolic acidosis and electrolyte imbalances

Notable AEs
- Paresthesias, tinnitus, sedation, GI disturbance (anorexia, nausea/vomiting, diarrhea, taste alteration, appetite suppression, weight loss), myopia

(transient), renal calculi, frequent urination, and photosensitivity

 ## Life-Threatening or Dangerous AEs

- Blood dyscrasias (agranulocytosis, hemolytic anemia, leukopenia, thrombocytopenia). Hypokalemia. Rash including Stevens-Johnson syndrome. Fulminant hepatic necrosis

Weight Gain
- Unusual

unusual   not unusual   common   problematic

Sedation
- Not unusual

unusual   not unusual   common   problematic

What to Do About AEs
- Lower dose when used for epilepsy or IIH. If AEs are significant, discontinue and change to another agent. Paresthesias may respond to high-potassium diets or potassium supplements

Best Augmenting Agents to Reduce AEs
- Concomitant topiramate, zonisamide, ketogenic diet predisposes to metabolic acidosis and kidney stones. Metformin may also promote acidosis

DOSING AND USE

Usual Dosage Range
- Epilepsy: age > 12: 375–1000 mg daily. Age < 12: 10–20 mg/kg/day. catamenial: 8~30 mg/kg/day
- IIH: 250–2000 mg daily
- Edema: 250–375 mg every other day
- Mountain sickness: 500–1000 mg daily

Dosage Forms
- Tablets: 125, 250 mg. Sustained release 500 mg
- Injection: 500 mg vials

How to Dose
- Epilepsy: start at 125–250 mg twice daily, with a lower starting dose (250 mg daily) for patients already on other AEDs. Occasionally used at higher doses, but not necessarily more effective
- IIH: start at 250–500 mg/day in 2 divided doses. Increase as tolerated to 1000 mg/day. Occasionally used at higher doses, depending on tolerability and effect on visual symptoms
- Acute mountain sickness: start 24–48 hours before ascent and continue for 48 hours or as long as needed to control symptoms. Usual dose 250–1000 mg/day
- Congestive heart failure: 250–375 mg daily, skipping doses every 2–3 days to maintain effect

 ## Dosing Tips
- Citrus juice and fluids may help decrease risk of kidney stone formation. Taking with food can decrease AEs

Overdose
- Ataxia, anorexia, nausea, paresthesias, vomiting, tremor, and tinnitus. Induce emesis or gastric lavage. Supplement with bicarbonate or potassium as necessary

Long-Term Use
- Safe for long-term use. Tolerance due to increased carbonic anhydrase production in glial cells

Habit Forming
- No

How to Stop
- Taper slowly
- Abrupt withdrawal can lead to seizures in patients with epilepsy
- Papilledema or headaches may recur within days to months of stopping

Pharmacokinetics
- Tablets have peak effect at 2–4 hours, with 8–12 hours duration of action. Sustained-release tablets have peak effect at 3–6 hours and duration of 18–24 hours. 70–90% protein bound. Not metabolized and excreted unchanged by kidneys

Drug Interactions

- Not affected by other AEDs
- Decreases levels of primidone, lithium
- Increases levels of cyclosporine, carbamazepine, phenytoin, phenobarbital
- Concurrent use with salicylates can increase AEs of both
- Prolongs effects of amphetamines, quinidine

Do Not Use

- Known hypersensitivity to the drug. Depressed potassium or sodium levels, significant kidney or hepatic disease, hyperchloremic acidosis, adrenocortical insufficiency, and suprarenal gland dysfunction

 Other Warnings/ Precautions

- Carbonic anhydrase inhibitors are sulfonamides. There may be cross-sensitivity with antibacterial sulfonamides. Increased risk of hyponatremia when combined with carbamazepine or oxcarbazepine

SPECIAL POPULATIONS

Renal Impairment

- Renal insufficiency can lead to increased toxicity. Use with caution

Hepatic Impairment

- Use with caution. Patients with severe disease have an increased risk of hyperammonemia or bleeding complications

Cardiac Impairment

- Severe hypokalemia causes cardiac arrhythmias. Chronic metabolic acidosis may lead to hyperventilation and decreases left ventricular function – use with caution in patients on β-blocker or calcium channel therapy

Elderly

- Use with caution

 Children and Adolescents

- Safety and effectiveness in the pediatric population is unknown. Suggested daily dose is 8–30 mg/kg

 Pregnancy

- Category C. Risks of stopping medication must outweigh risk to fetus for patients with epilepsy. Seizures and potential status epilepticus place the woman and fetus at risk and can cause reduced oxygen and blood supply to the womb
- In IIH, consider lumbar puncture as an alternative to medication, especially in the first few months of pregnancy, and monitor closely for visual changes
- Supplementation with 0.4 mg of folic acid before and during pregnancy is recommended

Breast Feeding

- A small percentage is excreted in breast milk. Monitor infant for sedation, poor feeding, or irritability

THE ART OF NEUROPHARMACOLOGY

Potential Advantages

- Inexpensive adjunctive medication for epilepsy and useful in the treatment of IIH and episodic ataxias. Rapid onset of action

Potential Disadvantages

- Not a first-line drug in epilepsy or migraine due to ineffectiveness and AEs. Tolerance

Primary Target Symptoms

- Seizure frequency and severity; headache or papilledema in IIH

Pearls

- In epilepsy, appears most effective in children with petit mal epilepsy, but may be effective in patients with grand mal, mixed, or myoclonic seizures
- Acetazolamide was used for migraine aura status in case reports

- Acetazolamide is occasionally used for treatment of migraine. Large, double-blind, placebo-controlled trials did not indicate effectiveness
- First-line for IIH by lowering the CSF production. In a recent trial comparing 6 months of acetazolamide (up to 4 g/day) to placebo, significant improvements were found in visual field function and papilledema but with 19% dropout. It did not appear to reduce associated headache
- In an open-label study on IIH, topiramate was as effective as acetazolamide but with prominent weight loss, which is beneficial for treating IIH
- In patients under topiramate or metformin, spironolactone can be an alternative
- First-line agent for treatment of episodic ataxias at an average dose of 500–750 mg/day. Type 2 responds better than type 1 in most cases
- Similar to episodic ataxia type 2, familial hemiplegic migraine type 1 is a channelopathy caused by a mutation of the *CACNA1A* gene. Case reports suggest acetazolamide can be used to treat hemiplegic migraine
- Found to be dramatically effective in a subset of MELAS patients with episodic weakness associated with specific mitochondrial DNA mutations
- As a diuretic, increased doses do not increase effect. Results are often improved with alternating days of treatment
- The acetazolamide challenge test is used to decide indications for CSF shunting
- Good for intermittent use, such as in catamenial epilepsy

Suggested Reading

Auré K, Dubourg O, Jardel C, Clarysse L, Sternberg D, et al. Episodic weakness due to mitochondrial DNA MT-ATP6/8 mutations. *Neurology.* 2013;81(21):1810–18.

Biousse V, Bruce BB, Newman NJ. Update on the pathophysiology and management of idiopathic intracranial hypertension. *J Neurol Neurosurg Psychiatry.* 2012;83(5):488–94.

Kayser B, Dumont L, Lysakowski C, Combescure C, Haller G, Tramèr MR. Reappraisal of acetazolamide for the prevention of acute mountain sickness: a systematic review and meta-analysis. *High Alt Med Biol.* 2012;13 (2):82–92.

Kossoff EH, Pyzik PL, Furth SL, Hladky HD, Freeman JM, Vining EP. Kidney stones, carbonic anhydrase inhibitors, and the ketogenic diet. *Epilepsia.* 2002;43(10):1168–71.

Reiss WG, Oles KS. Acetazolamide in the treatment of seizures. *Ann Pharmacother.* 1996;30(5):514–19.

Robbins MS, Lipton RB, Laureta EC, Grosberg BM. CACNA1A nonsense mutation is associated with basilar-type migraine and episodic ataxia type 2. *Headache.* 2009;49(7):1042–6.

Wall M, McDermott MP, Kieburtz KD, Corbett JJ, Feldon SE, et al. Effect of acetazolamide on visual function in patients with idiopathic intracranial hypertension and mild visual loss: the idiopathic intracranial hypertension treatment trial. *JAMA.* 2014;311(16):1641–51.

ALEMTUZUMAB

THERAPEUTICS

Brands
- Lemtrada, Campath, MabCampath, Campath-1H

Generic?
- No

Class
- Immunosuppressant

Commonly Prescribed for
(FDA approved in bold)
- **Relapsing forms of multiple sclerosis (MS)**
- **B-cell chronic lymphocytic leukemia (B-CLL)**
- Induction therapy in organ transplantation
- Sporadic inclusion body myositis (sIBM)

How the Drug Works
- It is a humanized IgG$_1$ kappa antibody that targets cell-surface glycoprotein CD52, which is expressed at a high level on T and B lymphocytes. Upon binding, it induces antibody-dependent cellular cytolysis and complement-mediated lysis of T and B lymphocytes. It particularly targets CD4+ naïve and CD8+ naïve T cells, and mature naïve B cells with proportional increase in regulatory T cells and memory T/B cells. Lymphocyte counts decrease after each course of treatment. Cells that escaped depletion may cause secondary autoimmunity. It also has prolonged decrease in the secretion of proinflammatory cytokines (interleukin [IL]-17, IL-22)

How Long Until It Works
- Months to years. In trials, treated patients had fewer relapses up to 2–5 years

If It Works
- Continue to use until ineffective. Screen for AEs

If It Doesn't Work
- It is the third-line treatment for relapsing forms of MS. If it fails, consider combination therapy with other disease-modifying agents

 Best Augmenting Combos for Partial Response or Treatment-Resistance
- Acute MS attacks are often treated with glucocorticoids, especially if there is functional impairment due to vision loss, weakness, or cerebellar symptoms
- Treat common clinical symptoms with appropriate medication for spasticity (baclofen, tizanidine), neuropathic pain, and fatigue (modafinil)
- It is uncertain whether combined use of 2 types of antibodies or adding another disease-modifying agent is beneficial to MS

Tests
- CBC and platelet counts (monthly), thyroid function tests (every 3 months), and renal function (regularly) until 4 years after the last infusion. Yearly skin exams

ADVERSE EFFECTS (AEs)

How the Drug Causes AEs
- Most AEs are likely related to immunosuppression or hypersensitivity

Notable AEs
- Rash, headache, pyrexia, nasopharyngitis, nausea, urinary tract infection, fatigue, insomnia, upper respiratory tract infection, herpes infection, thyroid gland disorder, fungal infection, arthralgia, back pain, diarrhea, paresthesia, dizziness, abdominal pain, flushing, vomiting

 Life-Threatening or Dangerous AEs
- Thyroid disorders (20%)
- Immune thrombocytopenic purpura
- Anti-glomerular basement membrane disease
- Leukopenia, pancytopenia
- Severe infection
- Anaphylaxis
- Increased risk of malignancy (thyroid cancer, melanoma, lymphoproliferative disorder)

Weight Gain
- Unusual

unusual — not unusual — common — problematic

Sedation
- Unusual

unusual | not unusual | common | problematic

What to Do About AEs
- Control infection. Supportive treatment

Best Augmenting Agents to Reduce AEs
- Most AEs will not respond to augmenting agents

DOSING AND USE

Usual Dosage Range
- A total of 96 mg is the standard dose for MS

Dosage Forms
- Injection: 12 mg/1.2 mL, 30 mg/1 mL in a single-use vial

How to Dose
Lemtrada (for MS)
- First course: 12 mg/day on 5 consecutive days. IV infusion over 4 hours
- Second course (1 year after): 12 mg/day on 3 consecutive days
- It is available only through a restricted distribution program called the Lemtrada Risk Evaluation and Mitigation Strategy (REMS) Program
- Premedicate with corticosteroid for the first 3 days of each course
- Herpes prophylaxis for a minimum of 2 months after each course or until CD4+ lymphocyte count is > 200/mm^3, whichever occurs later

Campath (for B-CLL)
- Escalate to recommended dose of 30 mg/day 3 times per week for 12 weeks. IV infusion over 2 hours
- Premedicate with oral antihistamine and acetaminophen prior to dosing
- Administer prophylaxis against *Pneumocystis jiroveci* pneumonia (PCP) and herpes virus infections

Overdose
- Doses greater than those recommended may increase the intensity and/or duration of infusion reactions or its immune effects. There is no known antidote for alemtuzumab overdosage

Long-Term Use
- Risk of infection, autoimmunity, and malignancy. Use beyond the approved dose or term is not recommended

Habit Forming
- No

How to Stop
- No need to taper

Pharmacokinetics
- Alemtuzumab serum concentrations reach maximum at the last day of infusion. It is largely confined to the blood and interstitial space. It is degraded by widely distributed proteolytic enzymes. Half-life 2 weeks

 Drug Interactions
- No formal drug interaction studies have been conducted. Increases risk of serious infection when used with other immunosuppressants (e.g., azathioprine, cyclosporine, methotrexate, and 6-mercaptopurine) or inhibitors of tumor necrosis factor-α (TNF-α)

 Other Warnings/Precautions
- Infusion reactions usually occur within 2 hours but some reactions were reported after 24 hours
- Because of risk of autoimmunity, infusion reactions, and the risk of some kinds of cancers, Lemtrada is only available through the Lemtrada REMS Program

Do Not Use
- Hypersensitivity to drug. Severe infection. HIV

SPECIAL POPULATIONS

Renal Impairment
- May cause anti-glomerular basement membrane disease

Hepatic Impairment
- Not studied

Cardiac Impairment
- Does not prolong QTc interval

Elderly
- Not studied

Children and Adolescents
- It is not known if it is safe and effective for use in children under 17 years of age

Pregnancy
- Category C. Placental transfer of antithyroid antibodies resulting in neonatal Graves' disease has been reported. Use only if benefit of preventing MS relapse outweighs risk. Women of childbearing potential should use effective contraceptive measures when receiving a course of treatment with alemtuzumab and for 4 months following that course of treatment

Breast Feeding
- It is excreted in breast milk. Do not breast feed on drug

THE ART OF NEUROPHARMACOLOGY

Potential Advantages
- Effective treatment for some of the most disabled MS patients including those failing first-line agents. Efficacy may be superior to other disease-modifying agents

Potential Disadvantages
- Rare but potentially fatal AEs of autoimmunity, opportunistic infection, and malignancy. Only available through specific infusion centers as IV infusion. Need for long-term monitoring

Primary Target Symptoms
- Decrease in relapse rate, prevention of disability, and slower accumulation of lesions on MRI

Pearls
- At this point, due to potentially severe AEs, it is usually reserved for patients with a very severe form of relapsing MS who have failed 2 types of disease-modifying treatments and are not candidates for natalizumab
- May be an alternative to natalizumab in patients with JC virus antibodies
- In clinical trials, the lowest cell counts occurred 1 month after a course of treatment at the time of the first post-treatment blood count. Lymphocyte counts then increased over time: B-cell counts usually recovered within 6 months; T-cell counts increased more slowly and usually remained below baseline 12 months after treatment. Approximately 60% of patients had total lymphocyte counts below the lower limit of normal 6 months after each treatment course and 20% had counts below the lower limit of normal after 12 months
- It is also approved for relapsing-remitting MS with superior 2-year relapse-free rate and reduced disability progression than interferon-β (INFβ)-1a in previously treated patients; superior 2-year relapse-free rate than INFβ-1a in treatment-naïve patients. The efficacy appears to continue beyond treatment period. However, it was associated with greater side effects (infection, malignancy, thyroid disorder, autoimmunity, thrombocytopenic purpura)
- Given higher rates of remission compared to INFβ-1a and -1b, might eventually have a place as an induction therapy prior to initiation of other agents
- In successfully treated patients consider initiating other treatment only after lymphocyte counts have normalized
- CAMMS223: alemtuzumab remained significantly more efficacious than INFβ-1a up to 5 years of study period
- In a small trial of 13 sIBM patients, alemtuzumab 0.3 mg/kg/day for 4 days slows the disease progression up to 6 months, improves the strength of some patients, and reduces endomysial inflammation and stressor molecules. Bimagrumab (activin receptor II antibody) is another investigational drug showing promising results on increasing muscle mass and function

ALEMTUZUMAB (continued)

 Suggested Reading

Coles AJ, Fox E, Vladic A, Gazda SK, Brinar V, Selmaj KW, et al. Alemtuzumab more effective than interferon β-1a at 5-year follow-up of CAMMS223 Clinical Trial. *Neurology.* 2012;78(14):1069–78.

Cossburn M, Pace AA, Jones J, Ali R, Ingram G, Baker K, et al. Autoimmune disease after alemtuzumab treatment for multiple sclerosis in a multicenter cohort. *Neurology.* 2011;77(6):573–9.

Dalakas MC, Rakocevic G, Schmidt J, Salajegheh M, McElroy B, Harris-Love MO, et al. Effect of Alemtuzumab (CAMPATH 1-H) in patients with inclusion-body myositis. *Brain.* 2009;132(6):1536–44.

Garnock-Jones KP. Alemtuzumab: a review of its use in patients with relapsing multiple sclerosis. *Drugs.* 2014;74(4):489–504.

Zhang X, Huang H, Han S, Fu S, Wang L. Alemtuzumab induction in renal transplantation: a meta-analysis and systemic review. *Transpl Immunol.* 2012;27(2-3):63–8.

ALMOTRIPTAN

THERAPEUTICS

Brands
- Axert, Almogran

Generic?
- Yes

 Class
- Triptan

Commonly Prescribed for
(FDA approved in bold)
- **Acute treatment of migraine in adults and adolescents (> 12 years old)**
- Menstrual migraine

 How the Drug Works:
- Selective 5-HT$_{1B/1D/1F}$ receptor agonist. In addition to vasoconstriction on meningeal vessels, its antinociceptive effect is likely due to blocking the transmission of pain signals at trigeminal nerve terminals (preventing the release of inflammatory neuropeptides) and synapses of second-order neurons in trigeminal nucleus caudalis. Although it generally does not penetrate BBB, it has been postulated that transient permeability may occur during a migraine attack

How Long Until It Works
- 1–2 hours or less

If It Works
- Continue to take as needed. Patients taking acute treatment more than 2 days/week are at risk for medication-overuse headache, especially if they have migraine

If It Doesn't Work
- Treat early in the attack – triptans are less likely to work after the headache becomes moderate or severe, regardless of cutaneous allodynia, which is a marker of central sensitization
- Address life style issues (e.g., stress, sleep hygiene), medication use issues (e.g., compliance, overuse), and other underlying medical conditions
- Change to higher dosage, another triptan, another administration route, or

combination of other medications. Add preventive medication when needed
- For patients with partial response or reoccurrence, other rescue medications include NSAIDs (e.g., ketorolac, naproxen), antiemetic (e.g., prochlorperazine, metoclopramide), neuroleptics (e.g., haloperidol, chlorpromazine), ergots, antihistamine, or corticosteroid

 Best Augmenting Combos for Partial Response or Treatment-Resistance
- NSAIDs or antiemetics/neuroleptics are often used to augment response

Tests
- None required

ADVERSE EFFECTS (AEs)

How the Drug Causes AEs
- Direct effect on systemic serotonin receptors (e.g., 5-HT$_{1B}$ agonism on vasoconstriction)

Notable AEs
- Tingling, flushing, sensation of burning, vertigo, sensation of pressure, heaviness, nausea

 Life-Threatening or Dangerous AEs
- Serotonin syndrome. Rare cardiac events including acute myocardial infarction and vasospasm have been reported with almotriptan. Life-threatening cardiac arrhythmias have been reported with other triptans

Weight Gain
- Unusual

unusual · not unusual · common · problematic

Sedation
- Unusual

unusual · not unusual · common · problematic

What to Do About AEs
- In most cases, only reassurance is needed. Lower dose, change to another

triptan, or use an alternative headache treatment

Best Augmenting Agents to Reduce AEs

- Treatment of nausea with antiemetics is acceptable. Other AEs decrease with time

DOSING AND USE

Usual Dosage Range

- 6.25–12.5 mg

Dosage Forms

- Tablets: 6.25 and 12.5 mg

How to Dose

- Most adult patients respond best at 12.5 mg oral dose and 6.25 mg for adolescents. Give 1 pill at the onset of an attack and repeat in 2 hours for a partial response or if the headache returns. Maximum 25 mg/day. The safety of treating > 4 migraine in a 30-day period has not been studied. Limit 10 days/month

Dosing Tips

- Treat early in attack

Overdose

- May cause hypertension, cardiovascular symptoms. Other possible symptoms include seizure, tremor, extremity erythema, cyanosis, or ataxia. For patients with angina, perform ECG and monitor for ischemia for at least 20 hours

Long-Term Use

- Monitor for cardiac risk factors with continued use

Habit Forming

- No

How to Stop

- No need to taper. Patients who overuse triptans often experience withdrawal headaches lasting up to several days

Pharmacokinetics

- Half-life about 3–4 hours. T_{max} orally 1–4 hours. Bioavailability is 80%. Metabolized by monoamine oxidase (MAO)-A (27%; inactive indoleacetic acid metabolites) and CYP3A4/2D6 (12%; inactive GABA derivatives). 35% protein binding. Eliminated primarily by renal excretion (75%)

Drug Interactions

- MAO-A inhibitors may make it difficult for drug to be metabolized
- Minimal increase in concentration with CYP3A4 inhibitors – no need for dose adjustment

Do Not Use

- Patients with proven hypersensitivity
- Within 2 weeks of MAO-A inhibitors, or within 24 hours of ergot-containing medications such as dihydroergotamine
- History of stroke, transient ischemic attack, hemiplegic/basilar migraine, Wolff-Parkinson-White syndrome, peripheral vascular disease, ischemic heart disease, coronary artery vasospasm, ischemic bowel disease, and uncontrolled hypertension

SPECIAL POPULATIONS

Renal Impairment

- Start at 6.25 mg in those with moderate to severe renal impairment (CrCl < 30 mL/min). May be at increased cardiovascular risk. Avoid concomitant use of CYP3A4 inhibitors in patients with renal impairment

Hepatic Impairment

- Drug metabolism may be decreased. Do not use with severe hepatic impairment. Avoid concomitant use of CYP3A4 inhibitors in patients with hepatic impairment

Cardiac Impairment

- Do not use in patients with known cardiovascular or peripheral vascular disease. May have increased risk for vascular event

Elderly

- At an increased risk for cardiovascular incident. Most studies were done in patients

< 65 years old. In elderly with no other coronary artery disease risk factors beside age (male > 45, female > 55), it is generally safe

Children and Adolescents

- Safety and efficacy have not been established in children. Among triptans, almotriptan has the highest response rate in adolescents. Triptan trials in children were negative, due to higher placebo response

Pregnancy

- Category C. Use only if potential benefit outweighs risk to the fetus. Migraine often improves in pregnancy, and other acute agents (opioids, neuroleptics, prednisone) have more proven safety

Breast Feeding

- Almotriptan is found in breast milk. Use with caution

THE ART OF NEUROPHARMACOLOGY

Potential Advantages

- Effective with good consistency and excellent tolerability, even compared to other oral triptans. Less risk of overuse than opioids or barbiturate-containing treatments

Potential Disadvantages

- Cost, and the potential for medication-overuse headache. May not be as effective as other triptans

Primary Target Symptoms

- Headache pain, nausea, photo- and phonophobia

 Pearls

- Early treatment of migraine is most effective
- Lower AEs compared to other triptans. Good consistency and pain-free response, making it a good choice for patients with anxiety prone to medication side effects
- May not be effective when taken during the aura, or once headache begins
- In patients with "status migrainosus" (migraine lasting more than 72 hours) neuroleptics and dihydroergotamine are more effective
- Triptans were not originally studied for use in the treatment of basilar or hemiplegic migraine
- Triptans can be used to treat tension-type headache in migraineurs but not in patients with pure tension-type headache
- Patients taking triptans more than 10 days/month are at increased risk of medication-overuse headache, which is less responsive to treatment
- Chest and throat tightness are usually benign and may be related to esophageal spasm rather than cardiac ischemia. These symptoms occur more commonly in patients without cardiac risk factors
- Combination use of SNRI and triptans does not lead to serotonin syndrome, which requires activation of 5-HT_{2A} receptors and a possible limited role of 5-HT_{1A}. However, triptans are agonists at the 5-$HT_{1B/1D/1F}$ receptor subtypes, with weak affinity for 5-HT_{1A} receptors and no activity at the 5-HT_2 receptors. Given the seriousness of serotonin syndrome, caution is certainly warranted and clinicians should be vigilant for serotonin toxicity symptoms and signs to insure prompt treatment

Suggested Reading

Diener HC, Gendolla A, Gebert I, Beneke M. Almotriptan in migraine patients who respond poorly to oral sumatriptan: a double-blind, randomized trial. *Eur Neurol.* 2005;53 Suppl 1:41–8.

Dodick D, Lipton RB, Martin V, Papademetriou V, Rosamond W, MaassenVanDenBrink A, et al. Consensus statement: cardiovascular safety profile of triptans (5-HT agonists) in the acute treatment of migraine. *Headache.* 2004;44 (5):414–25.

Evans RW, Tepper SJ, Shapiro RE, Sun-Edelstein C, Tietjen GE. The FDA alert on serotonin syndrome with use of triptans combined with selective serotonin reuptake inhibitors or selective serotonin-norepinephrine reuptake inhibitors: American Headache Society position paper. *Headache.* 2010;50(6):1089–99.

Ferrari MD, Roon KI, Lipton RB, Goadsby PJ. Oral triptans (serotonin 5-HT (1B/1D) agonists) in acute migraine treatment: a meta-analysis of 53 trials. *Lancet.* 2001;358(9294):1668–75.

Gladstone JP, Gawel M. Newer formulations of the triptans: advances in migraine management. *Drugs.* 2003;63(21):2285–305.

Mathew NT, Finlayson G, Smith TR, Cady RK, Adelman J, Mao L, Wright P, Greenberg SJ; AEGIS Investigator Study Group. Early intervention with almotriptan: results of the AEGIS trial (AXERT Early Migraine Intervention Study). *Headache.* 2007;47(2):189–98.

ALTEPLASE

THERAPEUTICS

Brands
- Activase, Cathflo Activase

Generic?
- Yes

Class
- Thrombolytic agent

Commonly Prescribed for
(FDA approved in bold)
- **Acute ischemic stroke (AIS)**
- **Acute myocardial infarction (AMI)**
- **Pulmonary embolism (PE)**
- **Restoration of function to central venous access device**

How the Drug Works
- Alteplase is a tissue plasminogen activator (tPA). It binds to fibrin in a thrombus and converts the entrapped plasminogen to plasmin, initiating a local fibrinolysis with little systemic effect

How Long Until It Works
- Less than 1 hour, often earlier

If It Works
- After administration, monitor in intensive care – preferably in an acute stroke or cardiac unit

If It Doesn't Work
- Alteplase is not always effective and has risks. After initial monitoring period in intensive care, continue standard AIS, AMI, or PE care

Best Augmenting Combos for Partial Response or Treatment-Resistance
- Alteplase with heparin may improve the clinical course of PE

Tests
- Ensure no contraindications are present before administering drug. For all patients with suspected AIS with onset less than 3 hours prior, immediately type and screen, obtain CBC, glucose, coagulation tests, and ensure no intracranial bleeding (usually with head CT)

ADVERSE EFFECTS (AEs)

How the Drug Causes AEs
- Activating plasminogen increases bleeding risk

Notable AEs
- Superficial bleeding (e.g., at puncture sites), fever, hypotension, dyspnea, nausea, urticaria, and flushing

Life-Threatening or Dangerous AEs
- Internal bleeding (intracranial, GI, GU, or retroperitoneal), anaphylactic reaction, reperfusion arrhythmias, and thrombocytopenia

Weight Gain
- Unusual

Sedation
- Unusual

What to Do About AEs
- Stop infusion for any serious bleeding. Can use fresh frozen plasma if needed

Best Augmenting Agents to Reduce AEs
- Most AEs cannot be reduced by an augmenting agent

DOSING AND USE

Usual Dosage Range
- 90 mg or less for AIS, 100 mg or less for AMI or PE

Dosage Forms
- Lyophilized powder for injection: 2 mg in 2 mL, 50 mg in 50 mL, 100 mg in 100 mL

How to Dose

- AIS: give 0.9 mg/kg (not to exceed 90 mg) in 1 hour, with 10% of the dose given in the first 1 minute
- AMI: give 15 mg as a bolus for all patients. For patients weighing more than 67 kg, then give another 50 mg over 30 minutes and then 35 mg over the next 60 minutes. For patients less than 67 kg, give 0.75 mg/kg over the 30 minutes after the bolus and then 0.50 mg/kg over the next 60 minutes
- PE: 100 mg over 2 hours and restart heparin once partial thromboplastin or thrombin time is less than twice normal
- Central venous access restoration: instill 2 mg into catheter

 Dosing Tips

- Give alteplase as soon after AIS as possible (< 3–4.5 hours) to achieve best functional outcome once it has been determined that there are no contraindications

Overdose

- Bleeding complications are common. Treat, if needed, with fresh frozen plasma. Bradycardia, flushing, dyspnea, or hypotension can occur

Long-Term Use

- May be repeated after weeks of previous use if indicated. Not used for prophylaxis

Habit Forming

- No

How to Stop

- Not applicable

Pharmacokinetics

- Rapid hepatic metabolism by hydrolysis in liver. 80% of drug is cleared within 10 minutes after ending infusion

 Drug Interactions

- Anticoagulants such as heparin, vitamin K antagonists increase bleeding risk
- Antiplatelet agents such as aspirin, dipyridamole, clopidogrel, and abciximab may increase bleeding risk when given prior to or soon after alteplase therapy
- NSAIDs may increase risk of GI bleed

- Nitroglycerin decreases alteplase concentrations. Avoid using
- Valproate may increase concentrations
- Dopamine may reduce activity and cause particulate formation

 Other Warnings/ Precautions

- Cholesterol embolism causing renal failure, pancreatitis, bowel infarction, gangrenous digits, or AMI is a rare complication of thrombolysis

Do Not Use

- Evidence of intracranial hemorrhage or suspected subarachnoid hemorrhage
- Serious head trauma
- History of intracranial bleeding, neoplasm, or arteriovenous malformation
- Active internal bleeding
- Recent intracranial or intraspinal surgery
- Seizure at the onset of stroke
- Bleeding diathesis (PT INR > 1.7, heparin within 48 hours [aPTT < 40], platelet count < 100 000/mm^3)
- Uncontrolled hypertension at the time of treatment (greater than 185 systolic or 110 diastolic)

SPECIAL POPULATIONS

Renal Impairment

- Reduce dose and use with caution with severe renal disease

Hepatic Impairment

- Reduce dose and use with caution with severe hepatic disease

Cardiac Impairment

- No known effects

Elderly

- Patients over 75 are more likely to have bleeding complications

 Children and Adolescents

- Not studied in children

Pregnancy

- Category C. Use if potential benefit outweighs risks. Increased risk of hemorrhage when given less than 10 days post-partum

Breast Feeding

- Unknown if present in breast milk, use with caution

THE ART OF NEUROPHARMACOLOGY

Potential Advantages

- Proven treatment for acute stroke in adults

Potential Disadvantages

- Must be used within the acute window. Multiple potential complications (intracranial hemorrhage 5.8–6.8% within 7 days)

Primary Target Symptoms

- Improving neurological function and reducing disability resulting from ischemic stroke

Pearls

- Must meet National Institute of Neurological Disorders and Stroke (NINDS) inclusion/exclusion criteria
- NINDS (1995) found IV tPA effective for AIS within 3 hours. ECASS-3 trial (2009) demonstrated IV tPA effective within 4.5 hours in appropriate patients. In IST-3 trial (2014), IV tPA within 3–6 hours had excess 7-day mortality over control (3.5%) and did not improve 18-month mortality over control. MR CLEAN trial (2014) suggested intra-arterial therapy (tPA or mechanical, with or without prior IV tPA) within 6 hours for AIS due to proximal intracranial (A1, A2, M1, M2) occlusion. Overall mortality rate (90th day) is around 20–30%
- Effective in improving disability when given in 4.5–6-hour window. The benefit is greatest when given within 3 hours. Later treatment is less beneficial due to less tissue to salvage, rather than more hazards
- If treated within 3 hours, 9% reach independence (modified Rankin score 0–2)
- The relative and absolute benefits of tPA are at least as large in older as in younger people but overall severe IS morbidity is still very high in elderly patients with large strokes
- Pediatric studies using alteplase for pediatric stroke are lacking. The appropriate dose may be 0.75 mg/kg rather than the 0.9 mg/kg used in adults. There is no evidence for intra-arterial thrombolysis in children with IS
- No coadministration of heparin and aspirin during the first 24 hours
- Control blood pressure and maintain below 185/110 mm Hg during treatment. Blood pressures are often elevated in AIS
- Less likely to be effective for larger artery AIS (i.e., carotid occlusion)
- Recent studies suggest that alteplase is likely safe when given for "stroke mimics" such as seizure or migraine. Given that alteplase is less likely to work when delayed, giving alteplase after ruling out hemorrhage is probably better than waiting for imaging to confirm the diagnosis (i.e., MRI)

Suggested Reading

American College of Emergency Physicians, American Academy of Neurology. Clinical Policy: Use of intravenous tPA for the management of acute ischemic stroke in the emergency department. *Ann Emerg Med.* 2013;61(2):225–43.

Berkhemer OA, Fransen PSS, Beumer D, van den Berg LA, Lingsma HF, Yoo AJ, et al. A randomized trial of intraarterial treatment for acute ischemic stroke. *N Engl J Med.* 2014;372(1):11–20.

Jordan LC. Thrombolytics for acute stroke in children: eligibility, practice variability, and pediatric stroke centers. *Dev Med Child Neurol.* 2015;57(2):115–16.

Wardlaw JM, Murray V, Berge E, del Zoppo G, Sandercock P, Lindley RL, et al. Recombinant tissue plasminogen activator for acute ischaemic stroke: an updated systematic review and meta-analysis. *Lancet.* 2012;379(9834):2364–72.

Whiteley WN, Thompson D, Murray G, Cohen G, Lindley RI, Wardlaw J, Sandercock P; IST-3 Collaborative Group. Effect of alteplase within 6 hours of acute ischemic stroke on all-cause mortality (third International Stroke Trial). *Stroke.* 2014;45:3612–17.

Zinkstok SM, Engelter ST, Gensicke H, et al. Safety of thrombolysis in stroke mimics: results from a multicenter cohort study. *Stroke.* 2013;44(4):1080–4.

AMANTADINE

THERAPEUTICS

Brands
- Symmetrel, Symadine

Generic?
- Yes

Class
- Antiparkinson agent

Commonly Prescribed for
(FDA approved in bold)
- **Parkinson's disease (PD)**
- **Drug-induced extrapyramidal reactions**
- **Influenza-A prophylaxis/treatment**
- Post-encephalitic parkinsonism
- Vascular parkinsonism
- Fatigue in multiple sclerosis (MS)
- Accelerate recovery after traumatic brain injury
- Attention deficit hyperactivity disorder
- SSRI-related sexual dysfunction
- Tardive dyskinesia

How the Drug Works
- The mechanism of action in PD is poorly understood but animal studies suggest either that it induces release or decreases reuptake of dopamine. Also is a weak NMDA receptor antagonist that in animals decreases release of acetylcholine from the striatum. Treats and prevents influenza-A by preventing the release of viral nucleic acid into the host cell by interfering with the function of a viral M2 protein. It may also prevent virus assembly during replication

How Long Until It Works
- PD: 48 hours or less

If It Works
- PD: most patients require dose adjustment over time and will need to take other agents, such as levodopa

If It Doesn't Work
- PD: motor symptoms, such as bradykinesia, gait, and tremor should improve. Reduces extrapyramidal reactions, such as dyskinesias, and can allow reduction of carbidopa-levodopa doses. Non-motor

symptoms, including autonomic symptoms such as postural hypotension, depression, and bladder dysfunction, do not improve. If the patient has significantly impaired functioning, add levodopa or a dopamine agonist
- Fatigue: MS-related fatigue may respond to stimulants or modafinil

Best Augmenting Combos for Partial Response or Treatment-Resistance
- For suboptimal effectiveness add carbidopa-levodopa with or without a catechol-*O*-methyltransferase (COMT) inhibitor or dopamine agonist depending on disease severity. Monoamine oxidase (MAO)-B inhibitors may also be beneficial
- For younger patients with bothersome tremor anticholinergics may help
- For severe motor fluctuations and/or dyskinesias with good "on" time, functional neurosurgery is an option
- Depression is common in PD and may respond to low-dose SSRIs
- Cognitive impairment/dementia is common in mid- to late-stage PD and may improve with acetylcholinesterase inhibitors
- For patients with late-stage PD experiencing hallucinations or delusions, withdraw amantadine and consider oral atypical neuroleptics (quetiapine, olanzapine, clozapine). Acute psychosis is a medical emergency that may require hospitalization

Tests
- None required

ADVERSE EFFECTS (AEs)

How the Drug Causes AEs
- Effects on dopamine concentrations and possible anticholinergic effects

Notable AEs
- Nausea, dizziness, insomnia, and blurry vision most common. Depression, anxiety, confusion, livedo reticularis, dry mouth, constipation, peripheral edema, orthostatic hypotension, nervousness, and headache can occur. Can exacerbate preexisting seizure disorders

Life-Threatening or Dangerous AEs

- Abrupt discontinuation has been associated with the development of neuroleptic malignant syndrome
- Rare suicide attempts or ideation, even in those with no history of psychiatric disorders

Weight Gain

- Unusual

unusual not unusual common problematic

Sedation

- Common

unusual not unusual common problematic

What to Do About AEs

- Titrate slowly to avoid GI side effects. Most AEs require reducing dose or stopping medication

Best Augmenting Agents to Reduce AEs

- Most AEs cannot be reduced by use of an augmenting agent

DOSING AND USE

Usual Dosage Range

- PD: 100–200 mg in divided doses. Occasionally up to 400 mg/day

Dosage Forms

- Tablets/capsules: 100 mg
- Syrup: 50 mg/5 mL

How to Dose

- Start at 100 mg daily or 100 mg twice daily in patients on no other PD medications with no other major medical problems. In 1 week or more can increase by 100 mg
- Occasionally patients will require doses of 300 mg or 400 mg in divided doses to achieve optimal clinical effect

 ### Dosing Tips

- Initial sedation may improve with time or dividing doses

Overdose

- Symptoms relate to anticholinergic effects. May include renal, respiratory, or CNS AEs or cardiac effects, including arrhythmia, tachycardia, or hypertension. Deaths have been reported with as little as 1 g

Long-Term Use

- Safe for long-term use. Effectiveness may decrease over time

Habit Forming

- No

How to Stop

- Taper slowly and monitor for parkinsonian crisis. Abrupt withdrawal may also precipitate delirium, hallucinations, agitation, depression, pressured speech, anxiety, stupor, or paranoia

Pharmacokinetics

- Most drug is excreted unchanged in the urine. Peak effect is at 1.5–8 hours and half-life an average of 17 hours. Doses over 200 mg may cause greater than proportional increases in levels

 ## Drug Interactions

- Anticholinergics can increase the mild anticholinergic effects of amantadine
- Quinidine, triamterene, thiazide diuretics, and trimethoprim/sulfamethoxazole impair renal clearance of amantadine and can increase plasma concentrations
- Thioridazine with amantadine can increase PD tremor

 ## Other Warning/ Precautions

- May cause mydriasis due to anticholinergic AEs. Do not give to patients with untreated angle-closure glaucoma

Do Not Use

- Known hypersensitivity to the drug

SPECIAL POPULATIONS

Renal Impairment

- Decrease dose for impaired function. CrCl 30–50 mL/min: 200 mg day 1 then 100 mg daily. 15–29 mL/min: 200 mg day 1 then

100 mg every other day. $<$ 15 mL/min or hemodialysis: 200 mg every 7 days

Hepatic Impairment
- May cause elevation of liver enzymes. Use with caution

Cardiac Impairment
- Infrequently causes congestive heart failure or peripheral edema. Use with caution

Elderly
- There is reduced drug clearance, but no dose adjustment needed as the dose used is the lowest that provides clinical improvement

 Children and Adolescents
- Use for influenza treatment in children aged 1 or greater (PD is rare in pediatrics)

 Pregnancy
- Category C. Teratogenic in some animal studies. Risks may include cardiovascular maldevelopment. Use only if benefits of medication outweigh risks

Breast Feeding
- Excreted in breast milk. Do not use

THE ART OF NEUROPHARMACOLOGY

Potential Advantages
- Relief of dyskinesias in PD. Relatively quick-acting and less sedation than other

treatments. Useful in some patients for fatigue

Potential Disadvantages
- Usually not a first-line treatment for PD. No evidence of neuroprotection against PD. Generally less effective than levodopa and risks significant CNS AEs including hallucinations

Primary Target Symptoms
- PD: motor dysfunction and dyskinesias

 Pearls
- Useful for PD patients with dyskinesias. Level C evidence for its use in tardive dyskinesia
- Can cause anticholinergic AEs (dry mouth, urinary retention) despite no known action on receptors. This and hallucinations may limit treatment
- Use with caution in patients with heart failure, arrhythmia, and seizure
- Used for the treatment of MS-related fatigue at doses of 200–400 mg/day. However, its use was not substantiated by a Cochrane review
- May be useful in the treatment of traumatic brain injury, including children, at doses of 200–400 mg/day
- Amantadine accelerated the pace of functional recovery during active treatment in patients with post-traumatic disorders of consciousness. In theory, may be effective for chronic pain disorders such as migraine, but not studied in large placebo-controlled trials

Suggested Reading

Abdel-Salam OM. Drugs used to treat Parkinson's disease, present status and future directions. *CNS Neurol Disord Drug Targets.* 2008;7(4):321–42.

Bhidayasiri R, Fahn S, Weiner WJ, Gronseth GS, Sullivan KL, Zesiewicz TA, et al. Evidence-based guideline: treatment of tardive syndromes: report of the Guideline Development Subcommittee of the American Academy of Neurology. *Neurology.* 2013;81(5):463–9.

Chen JJ, Swope DM. Pharmacotherapy for Parkinson's disease. *Pharmacotherapy.* 2007;27(12 Pt 2):161S–73S.

Giacino JT, Whyte J, Bagiella E, Kalmar K, Childs N, Khademi A, et al. Placebo-controlled trial of amantadine for severe traumatic brain injury. *N Engl J Med.* 2012;366(9):819–26.

Pucci E, Branãs P, D'Amico R, Giuliani G, Solari A, Taus C. Amantadine for fatigue in multiple sclerosis. *Cochrane Database Syst Rev.* 2007; (1):CD002818.

AMIFAMPRIDINE

THERAPEUTICS

Brands
- 3,4-diaminopyridine, Firdapse, Zenas

Generic?
- Yes

Class
- Potassium channel blocker

Commonly Prescribed for
(FDA approved in bold)
- Lambert-Eaton myasthenic syndrome (LEMS)
- Congenital myasthenia gravis (CMG)
- Multiple sclerosis (MS)
- Downbeat nystagmus, cerebellar gait disorder

How the Drug Works
- Potassium channel blocker. Reduces flow of potassium across nerve terminal membranes and increases calcium influx with prolongation of action potential. This promotes presynaptic release of acetylcholine and may improve weakness and autonomic dysfunction

How Long Until It Works
- About 20 minutes, but maximum effect might take a few days

If It Works
- Continue to use to reduce symptoms of LEMS or CMG at lowest required dose. In LEMS, disease-modifying treatments, such as plasma exchange, IV immune globulin, corticosteroids, and immunosuppressives such as azathioprine are useful. Identifying malignancy such as small-cell lung cancer is essential

If It Doesn't Work
- LEMS: treat with immunological therapy. Removal of neoplasm may improve symptoms
- CMG: establish the type. Presynaptic forms may respond to 3,4-diaminopyridine. Acetylcholinesterase inhibitors may improve or worsen symptoms, depending on the disorder

 ### Best Augmenting Combos for Partial Response or Treatment-Resistance
- May be combined with pyridostigmine, which increases the available amount of acetylcholine for receptor binding and may allow reduction of dose

Tests
- Obtain baseline CBC, electrolytes, glucose, blood urea nitrogen, creatinine, liver function tests. Repeat monthly for 3 months, then every 6 months while on treatment

ADVERSE EFFECTS (AEs)

How the Drug Causes AEs
- Some AEs are related to acetylcholine release, others are unknown

Notable AEs
- Paresthesias, perioral numbness, insomnia, abdominal pain

Life-Threatening or Dangerous AEs
- Seizures, delirium: most common at doses of 100 mg or greater

Weight Gain
- Unusual

unusual   not unusual   common   problematic

Sedation
- Unusual

unusual   not unusual   common   problematic

What to Do About AEs
- Lower dose, supplement with pyridostigmine in LEMS. For first seizure, lower dose or discontinue and evaluate for metastatic brain tumor. For recurrent seizure, discontinue

Best Augmenting Agents to Reduce AEs
- Cannot be reduced with augmenting agents

DOSING AND USE

Usual Dosage Range
- 15–80 g/day

Dosage Forms
- Tablets: 5 mg

How to Dose
- Start at 10 mg orally 3–4 times daily or as tolerated. Increase every 1–2 weeks by 5 mg until maximum benefit, up to 80 mg/day. For suboptimal benefit in LEMS, add pyridostigmine

Dosing Tips
- Dose requirements may change over time. Periodically attempt to lower dose

Overdose
- Seizures and encephalopathy have been reported

Long-Term Use
- Requires frequent monitoring for hematological or renal complications

Habit Forming
- No

How to Stop
- No need to taper, but LEMS symptoms may worsen

Pharmacokinetics
- Bioavailability 30%. The pharmacokinetics and systemic exposure to amifampridine are notably influenced by the overall metabolic acetylation activity of *N*-acetyl transferase (NAT) enzymes and NAT2 genotype, which is subject to genetic variation. The plasma elimination half-life is approximately 2.5 hours for the amifampridine and 4 hours for the 3-*N*-acetylated amifampridine metabolite

Drug Interactions
- No significant drug interactions via CYP450 due to lack of metabolism
- The concomitant use of amifampridine and a cholinergic drug may increase the effect of both products. Do not combine with acetylcholinesterase inhibitors other than pyridostigmine

Other Warnings/Precautions
- The use of amifampridine in pateints with the non-paraneoplastic form of LEMS should only be commenced following a thorough assessment of the risk–benefit to the patient. Asthma patients should be monitored

Do Not Use
- Hypersensitivity to drug

SPECIAL POPULATIONS

Renal Impairment
- No known effects. Upward dose titration should be discontinued if any adverse reaction occurs

Hepatic Impairment
- No known effects. Upward dose titration should be discontinued if any adverse reaction occurs

Cardiac Impairment
- May prolong QTc. Clinical and ECG monitoring are indicated at the initiation of the treatment and yearly thereafter

Elderly
- Unknown

Children and Adolescents
- Unknown

Pregnancy
- Unknown. Use only if benefits of medication outweigh risks

Breast Feeding
- Unknown if excreted in breast milk. Do not use

THE ART OF NEUROPHARMACOLOGY

Potential Advantages
- Fewer AEs than other symptomatic agents for LEMS

Potential Disadvantages

• Does not alter disease outcome in LEMS.
  Limited availability

Primary Target Symptoms

• Weakness associated with LEMS, CMG,
  or MG

 Pearls

• Unlike MG, LEMS is a presynaptic disorder
  of neuromuscular transmission. LEMS is an
  autoimmune disease with antibodies
  directed against the voltage-gated calcium
  channels. LEMS is usually associated with
  small-cell lung cancer
• Not approved in the US but available on a
  compassionate-use basis
• Effective in the majority of LEMS patients,
  with or without malignancy
• In studies improved both strength and
  resting compound muscle amplitude

• Pyridostigmine or other
  acetylcholinesterase inhibitors alone are
  usually not effective in LEMS
• CMG is a group of disorders that are
  genetic – immunotherapy is not effective,
  so symptomatic treatment is the rule.
  Ptosis and ophthalmoplegia are common
  and age of presentation is variable. Some
  variants may respond to
  acetylcholinesterase inhibitors
• In small clinical trials, effective for
  improving motor symptoms and fatigue in
  MS. Experimental studies suggest
  enhancement of excitatory synaptic
  transmission
• Compared to 4-aminopyridine, more
  effective with fewer AEs in LEMS because
  of lack of CNS penetration, but
  4-aminopyridine is likely superior for
  treating MS symptoms and is FDA approved
  to improve walking speed in MS

 Suggested Reading

Bever CT Jr, Anderson PA, Leslie J, Panitch HS, Dhib-Jalbut S, Khan OA, Milo R, Hebel JR, Conway KL, Katz E, Johnson KP. Treatment with oral 3,4 diaminopyridine improves leg strength in multiple sclerosis patients: results of a randomized, double-blind, placebo-controlled, crossover trial. *Neurology.* 1996;47(6):1457–62.

Engel AG. The therapy of congenital myasthenic syndromes. *Neurotherapeutics.* 2007;4(2):252–7.

Lindquist S, Stangel M. Update on treatment options for Lambert-Eaton myasthenic syndrome: focus on use of amifampridine. *Neuropsychiatr Dis Treat* 2011;7:341–9.

Maddison P, Newsom-Davis J. Treatment for Lambert-Eaton myasthenic syndrome. *Cochrane Database Syst Rev.* 2005;(2):CD003279.

Oh SJ, Claussen GG, Hatanaka Y, Morgan MB. 3,4-Diaminopyridine is more effective than placebo in a randomized, double-blind, cross-over drug study in LEMS. *Muscle Nerve.* 2009;40(5):795–800.

Polman CH, Bertelsmann FW, de Waal R, van Diemen HA, Uitdehaag BM, van Loenen AC, Koetsier JC. 4-Aminopyridine is superior to 3,4-diaminopyridine in the treatment of patients with multiple sclerosis. *Arch Neurol.* 1994;51(11):1136–9.

Sedehizadeh S, Keogh M, Maddison P. The use of aminopyridines in neurological disorders. *Clin Neuropharmacol.* 2012;35:191–200.

THERAPEUTICS

Brands
- Elavil, Amitid, Amitril, Endep, Elatrol, Laroxyl, Saroten, Redomex, Triptafen, Tryptanol, Tryptizol, Trepiline, Triptyl

Generic?
- Yes

Class
- **Tricyclic** antidepressant (TCA)

Commonly Prescribed for
(FDA approved in bold)
- **Depression**
- Migraine prophylaxis
- Tension-type headache prophylaxis
- Fibromyalgia
- Neuropathic pain
- Post-herpetic neuralgia
- Bulimia nervosa
- Insomnia
- Anxiety
- Nocturnal enuresis
- Pseudobulbar affect
- Arthritic pain

How the Drug Works
- The mechanism of action of amitriptyline and its active metabolite (nortriptyline) is probably related to reuptake inhibition of serotonin and norepinephrine at the synaptic clefts of brain and spinal cord
- It also exhibits antagonism on 5-HT$_{2A}$, 5-HT$_{2C}$, 5-HT$_6$, 5-HT$_7$, α_1-adrenergic, muscarinic, H$_1$, and NMDA receptors, and agonism on opioid (σ_1, σ_2) receptors
- Antinociceptive and antidepressive effects are more likely related to adaptive changes in serotonin and norepinephrine receptor systems over time

How Long Until It Works
- Migraines: effective in as little as 2 weeks, but can take up to 3 months on a stable dose to see full effect
- Neuropathic pain: usually some effect within 4 weeks
- Insomnia, anxiety, depression: may be effective immediately, but full effects often delayed 2–4 weeks

If It Works
- Migraine: goal is a 50% or greater reduction in migraine frequency or severity. Consider tapering or stopping if headaches remit for more than 6 months or if considering pregnancy
- Neuropathic pain: the goal is to reduce pain intensity and symptoms, but usually does not produce remission
- Insomnia: continue to use if tolerated and encourage good sleep hygiene

If It Doesn't Work
- Increase to highest tolerated dose
- Migraine: address other issues, such as medication overuse, other coexisting medical disorders, such as anxiety, and consider changing to another agent or adding a second agent
- Neuropathic pain: either change to another agent or add a second agent
- Insomnia: if no sedation occurs despite adequate dosing, stop and change to another agent

Best Augmenting Combos for Partial Response or Treatment-Resistance
- Migraine: for some patients, low-dose polytherapy with 2 or more drugs may be better tolerated and more effective than high-dose monotherapy. May use in combination with AEDs, antihypertensives, natural products, and non-medication treatments, such as biofeedback, to improve headache control
- Neuropathic pain: TCAs, AEDs (gabapentin, pregabalin, carbamazepine, lamotrigine), SNRIs (duloxetine, venlafaxine, milnacipran, mirtazapine, bupropion), capsaicin, and mexiletine are agents used for neuropathic pain. Opioids (morphine, tramadol) may be appropriate for long-term use in some cases but require careful monitoring

Tests
- Check ECG for QTc prolongation at baseline and when increasing dose, especially in those with a personal or family history of QTc prolongation, cardiac arrhythmia, heart failure, or recent myocardial infarction. If patient is on diuretics, measure calcium, potassium, and magnesium at baseline and periodically

ADVERSE EFFECTS (AEs)

How the Drug Causes AEs

- Anticholinergic and antihistaminic properties are causes of most common AEs. Blockade of α_1-adrenergic receptors may cause orthostatic hypotension and sedation

Notable AEs

- Constipation, dry mouth, blurry vision, increased appetite, nausea, diarrhea, heartburn, weight gain, urinary retention, sexual dysfunction, sweating, itching, rash, fatigue, weakness, sedation, nervousness, restlessness

 Life-Threatening or Dangerous AEs

- Orthostatic hypotension, tachycardia, QTc prolongation, and rarely death
- Increased intraocular pressure
- Paralytic ileus, hyperthermia
- Rare activation of mania or suicidal ideation
- Rare worsening of existing seizure disorder

Weight Gain

- Problematic

unusual   not unusual   common   problematic

Sedation

- Common

unusual   not unusual   common   problematic

What to Do About AEs

- For minor AEs, lower dose or switch to another agent. If tiredness/sedation are bothersome, change to a secondary amine (i.e., nortriptyline, desipramine). For serious AEs, lower dose and consider stopping

Best Augmenting Agents to Reduce AEs

- Try magnesium for constipation. For migraine, consider using with agents that cause weight loss (i.e., topiramate)

DOSING AND USE

Usual Dosage Range

- Depression, anxiety: 50–150 mg/day
- Migraine/pain: 10–100 mg/day

- Tension-type headache: 35–75 mg/day

Dosage Forms

- Tablets: 10, 25, 50, 75, 100, and 150 mg

How to Dose

- Initial dose 10–25 mg/day taken about 1 hour before sleep. Effective range from 10 to 400 mg but typically 150 mg or less

 Dosing Tips

- Start at a low dose, usually 10 mg, and titrate up every few days as tolerated. Low doses are often effective for pain even though they are below the usual effective antidepressant dose

Overdose

- Cardiac arrhythmias and ECG changes; death can occur. CNS depression, convulsions, severe hypotension, and coma are not rare. Patients should be hospitalized. Sodium bicarbonate can treat arrhythmia and hypotension. Treat shock with vasopressors, oxygen, or corticosteroids

Long-Term Use

- Safe for long-term use

Habit Forming

- No

How to Stop

- Taper slowly to avoid withdrawal symptoms, including headache, nausea, and rebound insomnia. Withdrawal symptoms usually last less than 2 weeks. For patients with well-controlled pain disorders, taper very slowly (over months) and monitor for recurrence of symptoms

Pharmacokinetics

- Metabolized primarily by CYP2D6 and CYP1A2. Half-life 10–28 hours and metabolized to nortriptyline. 90–95% protein bound. Steady state typically reached in 1–3 weeks (slow hydroxylators may take longer period)

 Drug Interactions

- CYP2D6 inhibitors (e.g., duloxetine, paroxetine, fluoxetine, bupropion, cimetidine, quinidine, phenothiazines,

propafenone), CYP1A2 inhibitors (e.g., fluvoxamine, ciprofloxacin), and valproic acid can prevent its metabolism to nortriptyline and increase amitriptyline concentrations
- Phenothiazines (e.g., chlorpromazine, prochlorperazine, promethazine) increase TCA levels
- Enzyme inducers (e.g., rifampin, smoking, dexamethasone) can lower levels
- Tertiary amine TCAs (amitriptyline, imipramine) inhibit drugs that are metabolized by CYP2C19 (e.g., proton pump inhibitors, phenytoin, citalopram, clopidogrel) and CYP2D6 (e.g., β-blockers, antidepressants, antipsychotics, tramadol)
- Tramadol increases risk of seizures in patients taking TCAs
- Use with clonidine has been associated with increases in blood pressure and hypertensive crisis
- May reduce absorption and bioavailability of levodopa
- May alter effects of antihypertensive medications and cause prolongation of QTc, especially problematic in patients taking drugs that induce bradycardia
- Use together with anticholinergics can increase AEs (e.g., risk of ileus)
- Methylphenidate may inhibit metabolism and increase AEs
- Use within 2 weeks of MAOIs may risk serotonin syndrome

Other Warnings/Precautions
- May increase risk of seizure

Do Not Use
- Proven hypersensitivity to drug or other TCAs
- Concomitant use of MAOIs
- In acute recovery after myocardial infarction or uncompensated heart failure
- In conjunction with antiarrhythmics that prolong QTc interval
- In conjunction with medications that inhibit CYP2D6

Renal Impairment
- Use with caution. May need to lower dose

Hepatic Impairment
- Use with caution. May need to lower dose

Cardiac Impairment
- Do not use in patients with recent myocardial infarction, severe heart failure, history of QTc prolongation, orthostatic hypotension, or electrolyte imbalance (hypocalcemia, hypokalemia, hypomagnesemia)

Elderly
- More sensitive to AEs, such as sedation, hypotension. At risk for anticholinergic crisis. Start with lower doses

 ## Children and Adolescents
- Some data for children over 12 and an appropriate treatment for adolescents with migraine, especially children with insomnia who are not overweight. In children less than 12, most commonly used at low dose for treatment of enuresis

 ## Pregnancy
- Category C. Crosses the placenta and may cause fetal malformations or withdrawal symptoms. Generally not recommended for the treatment of pain or insomnia during pregnancy. For patients with depression or anxiety, SSRIs may be safer than TCAs

Breast Feeding
- Some drug is found in breast milk and use while breast feeding is not recommended

THE ART OF NEUROPHARMACOLOGY
Potential Advantages
- Proven effectiveness in multiple pain disorders. Can treat insomnia and depression, which are common in patients with chronic pain

Potential Disadvantages
- AEs are often greater than with SSRIs or SNRIs and many AEDs. More anticholinergic AEs than other TCAs. Weight gain and sedation can be problematic

Primary Target Symptoms
- Headache frequency and severity
- Reduction in neuropathic pain

Pearls
- Level A recommendation for use in prophylaxis of tension-type headache, and treatment of fibromyalgia
- Level B recommendation for efficacy in migraine prophylaxis, post-traumatic neuropathic pain, and cancer neuropathic pain but inefficacy in HIV neuropathic pain and phantom limb pain
- Based on a Cochrane review on TCA and phantom limb pain, morphine, gabapentin, and ketamine demonstrate trends towards short-term analgesic efficacy. Memantine and amitriptyline were ineffective for phantom limb pain. Results, however, are to be interpreted with caution as these were based mostly on a small number of studies with limited sample sizes that varied considerably and also lacked long-term efficacy and safety outcomes
- In patients with neuropathic pain or headache, offers relief at doses below usual antidepressant doses, and can treat coexisting insomnia
- The number of patients needed to treat is 3.6 with relative risk of 2.1 for achieving at least moderate pain relief
- Based on a recent Cochrane review on amitriptyline and neuropathic pain, amitriptyline should continue to be used as part of the treatment of neuropathic pain or fibromyalgia, but only a minority of patients will achieve satisfactory pain relief
- For patients with significant anxiety or depressive disorders, not as effective as newer drugs but with more AEs. Consider treatment of depression or anxiety with another agent together with a low dose of amitriptyline or other TCA for pain
- Norepinephrine:serotonin transporter binding ratio = 1.5:1
- TCAs can often precipitate mania in patients with bipolar disorder. Use with caution
- Despite interactions, expert psychiatrists may use with MAOIs for refractory depression
- Increases non-REM sleep time and decreases sleep latency
- Effective for nocturnal enuresis in children. Usual dose is 25 mg for children 6–10 and 50 mg for those 11 and older
- May be used to treat pathological laughing or crying due to forebrain disease at doses of 30–75 mg/day
- Previously used for ADHD before new treatments became available. May be useful as an adjunct for patients with pain and coexisting ADHD
- From a recent Cochrane review on TCAs and ADHD, most evidence on TCAs relates to desipramine. Findings suggest that, in the short term, desipramine improves the core symptoms of ADHD, but its effect on the cardiovascular system remains an important clinical concern. Thus, evidence supporting the clinical use of desipramine for the treatment of children with ADHD is low

---

Suggested Reading

Alviar MJM, Hale T, Dungca M. Pharmacologic interventions for treating phantom limb pain. *Cochrane Database Syst Rev.* 2011;12: CD006380.

Attal N, Cruccu G, Baron R, Haanpää M, Hansson P, Jensen TS, et al. EFNS guidelines on the pharmacological treatment of neuropathic pain: 2010 revision. *Eur J Neurol.* 2010;17(9):1113–88.

Bendtsen L, Evers S, Linde M, Mitsikostas DD, Sandrini G, Schoenen J, et al. EFNS guideline on the treatment of tension-type headache – report of an EFNS task force. *Eur J Neurol.* 2010;17(11):1318–25.

Häuser W, Thieme K, Turk DC. Guidelines on the management of fibromyalgia syndrome – a systematic review. *Eur J Pain.* 2010 Jan;14(1):5–10.

Moore RA, Derry S, Aldington D, Cole P, Wiffen PJ. Amitriptyline for neuropathic pain and fibromyalgia in adults. *Cochrane Database Syst Rev.* 2012;12:CD008242.

Otasowie J, Castells X, Ehimare UP, Smith CH. Tricyclic antidepressants for attention deficit hyperactivity disorder (ADHD) in children and adolescents. *Cochrane Database Syst Rev.* 2014;9:CD006997.

Silberstein SD, Goadsby PJ. Migraine: preventive treatment. *Cephalalgia.* 2002;22(7):491–512.

Solomon CG, Johnson RW, Rice ASC. Postherpetic neuralgia. *N Engl J Med.* 2014;371(16):1526–33.

Verdu B, Decosterd I, Buclin T, Stiefel F, Berney A. Antidepressants for the treatment of chronic pain. *Drugs.* 2008;68(18):2611–32.

Zin CS, Nissen LM, Smith MT, O'Callaghan JP, Moore BJ. An update on the pharmacological management of post-herpetic neuralgia and painful diabetic neuropathy. *CNS Drugs.* 2008;22(5):417–42.

APIXABAN

THERAPEUTICS

Brands
- Eliquis

Generic?
- No

Class
- Anticoagulant

Commonly Prescribed for
(FDA approved in bold)
- **Prevention of stroke and systemic embolism in adult patients with non-valvular atrial fibrillation (NVAF)**
- **Primary prevention of venous thromboembolic (VTE) events in adult patients who have undergone elective total hip arthroplasty (THA) or total knee arthroplasty (TKA)**
- Treatment of cerebral venous thromboembolism

How the Drug Works
- Apixaban is a selective reversible inhibitor of both free and clot-bound factor Xa, and prothrombinase activity, thereby reducing the conversion of prothrombin to thrombin and thrombus formation. Thrombin-induced platelet aggregation is also inhibited

How Long Until It Works
- Peak concentration in 3–4 hours

If It Works
- Monitor for signs of bleeding. Assess liver function periodically as clinically indicated

If It Doesn't Work
- Correct the underlying disorder. Use a higher dose or switch to different anticoagulant

Best Augmenting Combos for Partial Response or Treatment-Resistance
- None

Tests
- The degree of anticoagulation does not need to be assessed

ADVERSE EFFECTS (AEs)

How the Drug Causes AEs
- Reduced coagulation due to inhibited thrombin formation

Notable AEs
- Bleeding, nausea/vomiting, constipation

Life-Threatening or Dangerous AEs
- The yearly incidence of life-threatening bleed is 0.11 %, intracranial hemorrhage 0.3 %, and major GI bleed 0.83 %

Weight Gain
- Unusual

unusual   not unusual   common   problematic

Sedation
- Unusual

unusual   not unusual   common   problematic

What to Do About AEs
- Discontinue treatment, supportive care. Active charcoal reduces absorption. Not effective: vitamin K, protamine sulfate, hemodialysis

Best Augmenting Agents to Reduce AEs
- In most cases discontinuation and changing to another medication is more practical than trying to reduce AEs with another medication

DOSING AND USE

Usual Dosage Range
- 2.5–5 mg twice daily

Dosage Forms
- Tablet. 2.5 and 5 mg

How to Dose
For NVAF
- 2.5 mg twice daily for patients with any 2 of the following 3 factors: > 80 years old, body weight < 60 kg, serum Cr > 1.5 mg/dL

- If 1 or fewer of the above factors is present, use 5 mg twice daily for stroke prevention
- 2.5 mg twice daily if used with strong CYP3A4 and P-glycoprotein (P-gp) inhibitor

For deep vein thrombosis prophylaxis
- 2.5 mg twice daily

Conversion between other anticoagulants
- Converting from warfarin: discontinue warfarin and start apixaban when INR < 2
- Converting to warfarin: discontinue apixaban and bridge with parenteral anticoagulant until INR 2–3
- Converting from heparin/low molecular weight heparin (LMWH): start at the time of discontinuation (heparin) or 2 hours before the next scheduled time (LMWH)
- Converting to heparin/LMWH: add heparin at the time of next dose of apixaban

Dosing Tips
- Crushed or single tablet have similar effects

Overdose
- May lead to hemorrhagic complications.

Long-Term Use
- Safe for long-term use

Habit Forming
- No

How to Stop
- A specific antidote for apixaban is not available. It is not dialyzable due to high protein binding. Investigational antidotes include aripazine and andexanet

Pharmacokinetics
- Metabolized mainly via CYP3A4. Eliminated in urine (27%) and feces (63%). Half-life 10–14 hours

Drug Interactions
- Anticoagulants such as heparin, vitamin K antagonists increase bleeding risk. Concomitant usage of apixaban and enoxaparin resulted in ~50% increase in peak anti-Xa activity
- Antiplatelet agents such as aspirin, dipyridamole, clopidogrel, and abciximab may increase bleeding risk

- Long-term NSAIDs may increase risk of GI bleed
- CYP3A4 or P-gp inhibitors (e.g., amiodarone, ketoconazole, clarithromycin, fluoxetine, naproxen) increase drug concentration
- CYP3A4 or P-gp inducers (rifamycin, carbamazepine, phenytoin, St. John's wort) lower drug concentration

Other Warnings/ Precautions
- Procedure with minor bleeding risk: stop 1 day before procedure and start 12~24 hours after procedure. If CrCl < 50 mL/min stop 2 days before
- Procedure with major bleeding risk: stop 2 days before procedure and start 2–3 days after procedure. If CrCl < 50 mL/min stop 3 days before

Do Not Use
- History of mechanical heart valve replacement
- Hypersensitivity to the drug
- Evidence of major bleeding (e.g., intracranial, intra-abdominal, retroperitoneal, intra-articular, etc.)
- Serious trauma
- Prior to major surgery

SPECIAL POPULATIONS

Renal Impairment
- Patients with end-stage renal disease maintained on stable hemodialysis with the recommended dose of 5 mg twice daily
- Reduction in dose to 2.5 mg twice daily for either ≥ 80 years of age or body weight ≤ 60 kg

Hepatic Impairment
- No adjustment needed in mild impairment. No information on moderate impairment. Contraindicated in severe hepatic impairment

Cardiac Impairment
- Safety information is lacking for use in patients with mechanical valve. Use is not recommended

Elderly

- 2.5 mg twice daily for either ≥ 80 years of age or body weight ≤ 60 kg or serum Cr ≥ 1.5 mg/dL

Children and Adolescents

- Not studied in children

Pregnancy

- Category B. May increase hemorrhage during pregnancy and delivery

Breast Feeding

- Unknown if present in breast milk. Discontinue use

THE ART OF NEUROPHARMACOLOGY

Potential Advantages

- Proven treatment for stroke and systemic embolism prevention in adults with AF
- Better than aspirin, non-inferior to warfarin in reducing rate of stroke and systemic embolism from AF
- Has a lower risk than warfarin for hemorrhagic stroke and major bleeding, and marginally lower risk of death from any cause

Potential Disadvantages

- Increased risk of bleeding although less than warfarin. Lack of antidote or monitoring lab test. Not dialyzable

Primary Target Symptoms

- Reduce recurrent attacks of cerebral embolism caused by cardiogenic thrombi due to AF. Reduce venothromboembolism following TKA or THA

Pearls

- Effective in patients with NVAF with prior stroke, transient ischemic attack (TIA), or a CHA2DS2-VASc score of 2 or greater (Level of Evidence B)
- Compared to warfarin, fewer serious AEs and equal effectiveness in preventing ischemic stroke
- No large head-to-head comparisons with other newer agents in clinical trials
- Recommended in patients with NVAF unable to maintain a therapeutic INR level with warfarin. (Level of Evidence C)
- Has the lowest bleeding risk among the 3 new anticoagulants
- Compared to enoxaparin 40 mg/day has a lower incidence of all-cause death and major venothromboembolism
- For cerebral venous thrombosis, despite a lack of evidence, it is often recommended to use vitamin K antagonist for 3–12 months. Longer duration is reserved for those with severe coagulopathies or recurrent VTE. For newer anticoagulants, although no evidence available, their lower intracranial bleeding rate might offer them a potential role for cerebral venous thrombosis

Suggested Reading

Alexander JH, Lopes RD, James S, Kilaru R, He Y, Mohan P, et al. Apixaban with antiplatelet therapy after acute coronary syndrome. *N Engl J Med.* 2011;365(8):699–708.

Deedwania P, Huang GW. An evidence-based review of apixaban and its potential in the prevention of stroke in patients with atrial fibrillation. *Core Evid.* 2012;7:49–59.

January CT, Wann LS, Alpert JS, Calkins H, Cleveland JC, Cigarroa JE, et al. 2014 AHA/ACC/HRS guideline for the management of patients with atrial fibrillation: a report of the American College of Cardiology/American Heart Association Task Force on practice guidelines and the Heart Rhythm Society. *Circulation.* 2014;130(23):e199–267. Erratum in *Circulation.* 2014;130(23):e272–4.

Weimar C. Diagnosis and treatment of cerebral venous and sinus thrombosis. *Curr Neurol Neurosci Rep.* 2014;14(1):417.

THERAPEUTICS

Brands
- Apokyn, Apo-go, Uprima

Generic?
- No

Class
- Antiparkinson agent

Commonly Prescribed for
(FDA approved in bold)
- **Parkinson's disease (PD): acute intermittent treatment of "off" episodes**

How the Drug Works
- It is a dopamine partial agonist to D_{2-4} receptors. D_2 agonism is likely the main reason for effectiveness in PD. Despite its name, does not actually contain morphine or act on morphine receptors

How Long Until It Works
- PD: 10–60 minutes

If It Works
- PD: this is an adjunctive medication designed for use with other PD treatments. Continue to adjust other PD treatments to achieve maximum functionality

If It Doesn't Work
- PD: adjust PD medication regimen, determine compliance with medications, and reconsider the diagnosis

Best Augmenting Combos for Partial Response or Treatment-Resistance
- Patients requiring frequent injections will need an improved treatment plan to avoid severe "off" periods. Strategies include shortening the interval of levodopa dosing, adding catechol-*O*-methyltransferase (COMT) inhibitors, or adding longer-acting dopamine agonists

Tests
- None required

ADVERSE EFFECTS (AEs)

How the Drug Causes AEs
- Direct effect on dopamine receptors

Notable AEs
- Injection site reactions, drowsiness, nausea or vomiting, dizziness, postural hypotension, hallucinations, edema. Less common hypersexuality or erections

Life-Threatening or Dangerous AEs
- May cause somnolence or sudden-onset sleep. Severe orthostatic hypotension and nausea/vomiting, even when compared to other PD treatments

Weight Gain
- Unusual

unusual | not unusual | common | problematic

Sedation
- Common

unusual | not unusual | common | problematic

What to Do About AEs
- Orthostatic hypotension: the first dose should be given in a monitored setting (such as a physician's office). Check supine and standing blood pressure predose and 20, 40, and 60 minutes after injection. If there is no clinical improvement and no AEs, a dose of 4 mg can be given, no earlier than 2 hours after the initial dose

Best Augmenting Agents to Reduce AEs
- Nausea/vomiting: at least 3 days before initiating therapy, start trimethobenzamide 300 mg 3 times a day and continue this for at least 2 months. When given alone, apomorphine causes severe nausea and vomiting. Domperidone, an antidopaminergic drug that does not cross the BBB, is an alternative treatment for nausea – typically starting at 10 mg 3–4 times a day

DOSING AND USE

Usual Dosage Range
- PD: 2–6 mg per dose, up to 20 mg/day

Dosage Forms
- SC injection: 10 mg/mL in 3 mL cartridges

How to Dose
- PD: before starting therapy, monitor for orthostatic hypotension
- The usual starting dose for acute "off" episodes is 1 mg less than the tolerated test dose. If the patient tolerates the 4 mg test dose, start at 3 mg. If the patient tolerates 3 mg, start at 2 mg and so on

 Dosing Tips
- Start with low dose and increase as needed and based on response and side effects
- For patients resuming therapy after an interruption of 1 week or more, start at the 2 mg dose. The dose may then be increased by 1 mg every few days as an outpatient to a maximum of 6 mg per dose and total daily dose of 20 mg/day. The average number of daily doses in clinical trials was 3 per patient

Overdose
- Symptoms include severe orthostatic hypotension, nausea, and vomiting. Somnolence, agitation, chest and abdominal pain, or dyskinesias can occur

Long-Term Use
- Safe for long-term use

Habit Forming
- No

How to Stop
- Designed for acute use only

Pharmacokinetics
- Peak plasma levels in 10–60 minutes

 Drug Interactions
- Serotonin 5-HT₃ antagonists used to treat nausea such as ondansetron, dolasetron can cause profound hypotension and loss of consciousness
- Use with caution with antihypertensives (due to risk of orthostatic hypotension) or QTc prolonging medications

- Dopamine antagonists reduce drug effectiveness

 Other Warnings/ Precautions
- Sodium metabisulfite is a metabolite and can cause reactions in patients allergic to sulfites

Do Not Use
- Hypersensitivity to the drug
- Concomitant use with 5-HT₃ antagonists

SPECIAL POPULATIONS

Renal Impairment
- Mild to moderate impairment: start at 1 instead of 2 mg

Hepatic Impairment
- Increased concentrations can occur with mild to moderate impairment. Use with caution

Cardiac Impairment
- No known effects

Elderly
- No dose adjustment needed with normal renal function. The dose used is the lowest that provides clinical improvement

 Children and Adolescents
- Not studied in children (PD is rare in pediatrics)

 Pregnancy
- Category C. Use only if benefits of medication outweigh risks

Breast Feeding
- Unknown if excreted in breast milk

THE ART OF NEUROPHARMACOLOGY

Potential Advantages
- The only drug approved for emergency treatment of "off" episodes in PD. Rapid onset of action

Potential Disadvantages
- Severe nausea. Cost. Advanced PD patients often have difficulty using SC injection during "off" periods and a caregiver may be needed to administer

Primary Target Symptoms
- PD: acute freezing and "off episodes" with markedly impaired motor dysfunction including bradykinesia, hand function, gait and resting tremor

 Pearls
- Efficacious for treatment of motor fluctuation and as symptomatic adjunct to levodopa
- For patients with advanced PD, make sure to ask about "off" periods: how often they occur, severity, and how the patient or caregiver manages them
- In advanced PD, "freezing" becomes more unpredictable over time despite well-designed medication regimens, and apomorphine can be a useful adjunct

- May be particularly helpful for nighttime symptoms, including pain and restless leg syndrome
- Daytime apomorphine continuous infusion (12–16 hours/day) has been used to avoid pulsatile medication and reduce oral medication. It also improves non-motor symptoms (e.g., hyperhidrosis, nocturia, urgency of micturition, and fatigue) but with visual hallucination and paranoid ideations
- Both apomorphine and deep brain stimulation (DBS) decrease daily off time. Only DBS reduces dyskinesia duration and severity but with more neuropsychiatric side effects
- Previously used off-label for erectile dysfunction but now being replaced by sildenafil and others. It may exert anti-Alzheimer's disease effect by enhancing the degradation of intracellular amyloid β (activation of proteasome and insulin-degrading enzyme) or antioxidation (upregulated glutathione peroxidase). Both are independent from dopamine signaling pathway

 Suggested Reading

Antonini A, Isaias IU, Rodolfi G, Landi A, Natuzzi F, Siri C, et al. A 5-year prospective assessment of advanced Parkinson disease patients treated with subcutaneous apomorphine infusion or deep brain stimulation. *J Neurol.* 2011;258(4):579–85.

Fox SH, Katzenschlager R, Lim S-Y, Ravina B, Seppi K, Coelho M, et al. The Movement Disorder Society Evidence-Based Medicine Review Update: Treatments for the motor symptoms of Parkinson's disease. *Mov Disord.* 2011;26 Suppl 3:S2–41.

Gunzler SA. Apomorphine in the treatment of Parkinson disease and other movement disorders. *Expert Opin Pharmacother.* 2009;10(6):1027–38.

Kolls BJ, Stacy M. Apomorphine: a rapid rescue agent for the management of motor fluctuations in advanced Parkinson disease. *Clin Neuropharmacol.* 2006;29(5):292–301.

Kvernmo T, Houben J, Sylte I. Receptor-binding and pharmacokinetic properties of dopaminergic agonists. *Curr Top Med Chem.* 2008;8(12):1049–67.

Martinez-Martin P, Reddy P, Antonini A, Henriksen T, Katzenschlager R, Odin P, et al. Chronic subcutaneous infusion therapy with apomorphine in advanced Parkinson's disease compared to conventional therapy: a real life study of non motor effect. *J Parkinsons Dis.* 2011;1(2):197–203.

Ohyagi Y. Apomorphine: a novel efficacy for Alzheimer's disease and its mechanisms. *J Alzheimers Dis Parkinsonism.* 2012;2(4):1000e122.

Stacy M, Silver D. Apomorphine for the acute treatment of "off" episodes in Parkinson's disease. *Parkinsonism Relat Disord.* 2008;14(2):85–92.

THERAPEUTICS

Brands
- Emend

Generic?
- No

 Class
- Antiemetic

Commonly Prescribed for
(FDA approved in bold)
- **Prevention of nausea and vomiting (chemotherapy, postoperative)**
- Nausea and vomiting (gastroenteritis, pregnancy)
- Pruritus

 How the Drug Works
- Selective blocking agent of substance P/ neurokinin 1 (NK$_1$) receptors. No affinity for 5-HT$_3$, dopamine, and corticosteroid receptors. It augments the antiemetic activity of the 5-HT$_3$ antagonist ondansetron and corticosteroid dexamethasone

How Long Until It Works
- Less than an hour

If It Works
- Use at lowest effective dose

If It Doesn't Work
- Increase dose, or discontinue and change to another agent

 Best Augmenting Combos for Partial Response or Treatment-Resistance
- May add D$_2$ antagonist, 5-HT$_3$ antagonist, antihistamine, benzodiazepine, or corticosteroid

Tests
- None required

ADVERSE EFFECTS (AEs)

How the Drug Causes AEs
- Not known

Notable AEs
- Asthenia, diarrhea, hiccup, pruritus, hair loss

 Life-Threatening or Dangerous AEs
- Hypersensitivity reactions such as angioedema and Stevens-Johnson syndrome have been reported

Weight Gain
- Unusual

unusual   not unusual   common   problematic

Sedation
- Unusual

unusual   not unusual   common   problematic

What to Do About AEs
- Reduce dose or discontinuation

Best Augmenting Agents to Reduce AEs
- Symptomatic management

DOSING AND USE

Usual Dosage Range
- 40–150 mg

Dosage Forms
- Capsule: 40, 80, 125 mg
- Injection (fosaprepitant dimeglumine): 115, 150 mg

How to Dose
- For chemotherapy-induced nausea/ vomiting: 125 mg 1 hour prior to chemotherapy (day 1) and 80 mg daily (day 2–3), with or without 5-HT$_3$ antagonist and corticosteroid
- For postoperative nausea/vomiting: 40 mg within 3 hours prior to anesthesia induction

 Dosing Tips
- Can be taken with or without food. Only for short-term use

Overdose
- May develop drowsiness or headache

Long-Term Use
- Not been studied

Habit Forming
- No

How to Stop
- No need to taper

Pharmacokinetics
- Bioavailability 60–65%. > 95% protein bound. Metabolized predominantly by CYP3A4. Not renally excreted. Half-life 9–12 hours

 Drug Interactions
- Increased level by CYP3A4 inhibitor (ketoconazole, clarithromycin, antiviral, diltiazem, cisapride, etc.)
- Decreased level by CYP3A4 inducer (rifampin, carbamazepine, phenytoin, etc.)
- As a CYP2C9 inducer, lowers the concentration of warfarin, naproxen, fluoxetine, etc.
- As a CYP3A4 inhibitor, increases the concentration of many drugs
- May reduce the efficacy of hormonal contraceptives

 Other Warnings/ Precautions
- May mask a progressive ileus or gastric obstruction

Do Not Use
- Known hypersensitivity

Renal Impairment
- No adjustment necessary

Hepatic Impairment
- No dose adjustment needed for mild to moderate impairment

Cardiac Impairment
- Typically needs no adjustment

Elderly
- Typically needs no adjustment

 Children and Adolescents
- Safety and effectiveness have not been established

 Pregnancy
- Category B. Use for significant migraine or nausea during pregnancy if needed

Breast Feeding
- Found in breast milk. Little information is available. Bottle feed if possible

THE ART OF NEUROPHARMACOLOGY

Potential Advantages
- Novel mechanism

Potential Disadvantages
- Drug interaction with CYP3A4 inhibitor/ inducer

Primary Target Symptoms
- Nausea and vomiting

 Pearls
- Commonly used in combination with dexamethasone and ondansetron for chemotherapy-induced nausea and vomiting
- May be effective for patients with chronic pruritus
- Not effective in major depressive disorder or generalized anxiety disorder
- Theoretically useful in treatment of chronic pain and inflammation but not established in human trials

Suggested Reading

Aapro MS, Schmoll HJ, Jahn F, Carides AD, Webb RT. Review of the efficacy of aprepitant for the prevention of chemotherapy-induced nausea and vomiting in a range of tumor types. *Cancer Treat Rev.* 2013;39(1):113–17.

Basch E, Prestrud AA, Hesketh PJ, Kris MG, Feyer PC, Somerfield MR, et al. Antiemetics: American Society of Clinical Oncology clinical practice guideline update. *J Clin Oncol.* 2011;29 (31):4189–98.

Gan TJ, Apfel CC, Kovac A, Philip BK, Singla N, Minkowitz H, et al. A randomized, double-blind comparison of the NK1 antagonist, aprepitant, versus ondansetron for the prevention of postoperative nausea and vomiting. *Anesth Analg.* 2007;104(5):1082–9.

Hafizi S, Chandra P, Cowen J. Neurokinin-1 receptor antagonists as novel antidepressants: trials and tribulations. *Br J Psychiatry.* 2007;191:282–4.

Ständer S, Siepmann D, Herrgott I, Sunderkötter C, Luger TA. Targeting the neurokinin receptor 1 with aprepitant: a novel antipruritic strategy. *PLoS One.* 2010;5(6):e10968.

ARIPIPRAZOLE

Brands
- Abilify, Abilify Discmelt, Abilify Maintena

Generic?
- No

Class
- Atypical antipsychotic

Commonly Prescribed for
(FDA approved in bold)
- **Schizophrenia in adults and adolescents**
- **Bipolar I disorder (mixed and manic episodes) as monotherapy or adjunct to lithium or valproate**
- **Irritability associated with autistic disorder**
- **Adjunctive therapy for major depressive disorder**
- **Gilles de la Tourette syndrome (GTS; 6–18 years old)**
- Agitation in patients with Alzheimer's dementia (AD)
- Augmentation for refractory obsessive-compulsive disorder
- Anxiety disorder
- Insomnia

How the Drug Works
- It is a phenylpiperazine derivative that acts as partial agonist with high affinity towards 5-HT$_{1A}$, 5-HT$_7$, and D$_{2-3}$ receptors, and moderate affinity towards 5-HT$_{1D}$, 5-HT$_{2C}$, and D$_4$ receptors. As a partial agonist, it blocks receptors at high dopamine and serotonin levels, but activates receptors at low levels. It also exerts moderate antagonism on 5-HT$_{2A/2B}$, H$_1$, and $\alpha_{1,2}$-adrenergic receptors but with no effect on muscarinic receptors. Antagonism on D$_2$ receptors relieves positive symptoms; antagonism on 5-HT$_{2A}$ relieves negative symptoms

How Long Until It Works
- Schizophrenia/bipolar: may be effective in days, more commonly takes weeks or months to determine best dose and achieve best clinical effect. Usually 4–6 weeks

- Agitation/insomnia: may be effective immediately

If It Works
- Continue to use at lowest required dose. Most patients with schizophrenia see a reduction in psychosis with neuroleptics. However, it may worsen psychosis in patients with Parkinson's disease (PD) or dementia with Lewy bodies (DLB)

If It Doesn't Work
- Increase dose
- Psychosis related to PD or DLB: clozapine is more efficacious for acute treatment only
- Insomnia: if no sedation occurs despite adequate dosing, change to another agent

 Best Augmenting Combos for Partial Response or Treatment-Resistance
- Patients with affective disorders, such as bipolar disorder, may respond to mood-stabilizing AEDs, lithium, or benzodiazepines

Tests
- Prior to starting treatment and periodically during treatment, monitor weight, blood pressure, lipids, and fasting glucose due to risk of metabolic syndrome

How the Drug Causes AEs
- Antagonism on H$_1$, 5-HT$_{2C}$, and D$_2$ may cause weight gain; antagonism on α_1 can cause orthostatic hypotension; antagonism on H$_1$ and 5-HT$_{2A}$ can cause sedation

Notable AEs
- CNS: dizziness, personality disorder, akathisia, sedation, fatigue, asthenia, tremor, insomnia
- Autonomic: dry mouth, postural hypotension, blurred vision
- Gastrointestinal: constipation, drooling, decreased appetite, nausea

 Life-Threatening or Dangerous AEs
- Tardive dyskinesia (lower risk than conventional neuroleptics)
- Metabolic syndrome

- Neuroleptic malignant syndrome (rare compared with conventional antipsychotics)
- Agranulocytosis (very rare)
- Seizure

Weight Gain
- Not unusual

unusual   not unusual   common   problematic

Sedation
- Common

unusual   not unusual   common   problematic

What to Do About AEs
- Take at night: for many disorders there is no need for daytime dosing

Best Augmenting Agents to Reduce AEs
- Most AEs cannot be reduced with an augmenting agent

DOSING AND USE

Usual Dosage Range
- Bipolar disorder/schizophrenia: 10–15 mg/day

Dosage Forms
- Tablets: 2, 5, 10, 15, 20 mg
- Tablet, orally disintegrating: 10, 15 mg
- Solution, oral: 1 mg/mL
- Injection: 9.75 mg/1.3 mL
- Injection (extended release): 300, 400 mg/ syringe

How to Dose
- Schizophrenia/bipolar I: 10–15 mg/day. May increase to 30 mg/day
- Adjunct for depression: 2–15 mg/day. Titrate 2–5 mg/day every week
- Agitation: 5.25–15 mg IM every 2 hours, up to 30 mg/day
- GTS: 2 mg/day. Titrate every 2 days to 5 mg/ day (< 50 kg) or 10 mg/day (≥ 50 kg)

 Dosing Tips
- For injection, do not administer IV or SC. For oral form, can be taken with food. Use at night if sedation is a problem. Elderly and children often need lower doses

Overdose
- Vomiting, somnolence, tremor. Standard management with activated charcoal. Hemodialysis not effective

Long-Term Use
- Safe for long-term use with appropriate monitoring

Habit Forming
- No

How to Stop
- Gradual withdrawal is advised

Pharmacokinetics
- T_{max} 3–5 hours (oral) and 1–3 hours (IM). Hepatic metabolism to active metabolites via CYP2D6 and CYP3A4. Half-life 75–94 hours. > 99% protein bound. Reach steady state in 2 weeks

 Drug Interactions
- Strong CYP3A4 inhibitor (e.g., protease inhibitor, macrolide, azole antifungals, nefazodone) and moderate CYP3A4 inhibitor (e.g., aprepitant, verapamil, grapefruit juice) can increase drug levels; reduce aripiprazole dose
- Strong CYP2D6 inhibitor (e.g., fluoxetine, paroxetine, bupropion, quinidine, ritonavir) and moderate CYP2D6 inhibitor (e.g., sertraline, duloxetine) can increase drug levels; reduce aripiprazole dose
- CYP enzyme inducer (e.g., dexamethasone, rifampin, carbamazepine, phenytoin, barbiturate, St. John's wort) can lower drug level
- It does not affect the level of valproate, lithium, lamotrigine, warfarin, lorazapem, and most SSRIs

 Other Warnings/ Precautions
- Increased mortality from aripiprazole use in elderly patients with dementia-related psychosis

Do Not Use
- Proven hypersensitivity to aripiprazole

Renal Impairment
- No dose adjustment needed

Hepatic Impairment
- No dose adjustment needed

Cardiac Impairment
- May worsen orthostatic hypotension. Use with caution. No known risk of QTc prolongation

Elderly
- Start with lower doses. Greater risk for infection, stroke, and other AEs in those with dementia-related psychosis

Children and Adolescents
- Schizophrenia (13–17 years): start at 2 mg/day. Titrate to 5 and 10 mg/day every 2 days. Long-term efficacy unknown
- Irritability associated with autism (6–17 years): start at 2 mg/day. Titrate 5 mg/day every week until 10–15 mg/day. Long-term efficacy unknown
- Bipolar I (10–17 years): start at 2 mg/day. Titrate to 5 and 10 mg/day every 2 days

Pregnancy
- Category C. Probably safer than AEDs during pregnancy for bipolar disorder. Use only if benefit outweighs risks

Breast Feeding
- It is found in breast milk. Use while breast feeding is generally not recommended

Potential Advantages
- Partial agonist effect with lower risk of dyskinesia. No known risk of QTc prolongation. More weight neutral than other atypical antipsychotics. Proven efficacy for depression

Potential Disadvantages
- Probably less effective than clozapine. Drug interaction by CYP450

Primary Target Symptoms
- Psychosis, depression, mania, and insomnia

Pearls
- May be useful for migraine refractory to standard treatment
- May improve psychosis in treating vascular parkinsonism
- Risperidone, olanzapine, and aripiprazole are recommended for treating agitation associated with dementia, although with potential harms (e.g., infection, cardiovascular event). Quetiapine, SSRIs, and trazodone remain investigational. Valproate is not advised. Olanzapine 10 mg IM (number needed to treat [NNT] 3), aripiprazole 9.75 mg IM (NNT 5), ziprasidone 10–20 mg IM (NNT 3)
- Aripiprazole can worsen parkinsonian symptoms in treating psychosis associated with PD or DLB. Only clozapine has A-level support. Quetiapine may also be considered
- From a Cochrane review on antipsychotics for schizophrenia, aripiprazole is less effective than olanzapine but has fewer side effects. It is similar to risperidone and may be better than ziprasidone. It has fewer side effects than olanzapine and risperidone
- Patients with BMI < 23 kg/m^2 are likely to gain weight; those with BMI > 27 kg/m^2 are likely to lose weight
- Less weight gain than risperidone and olanzapine. May lower the metabolic effect from clozapine
- For GTS requiring medication, consider α agonist (clonidine, guanfacine), antipsychotics (haloperidol, pimozide, risperidone), dopamine depletor (tetrabenazine). FDA currently approves haloperidol, pimozide, and aripiprazole

Suggested Reading

Citrome L. Comparison of intramuscular ziprasidone, olanzapine, or aripiprazole for agitation. *J Clin Psychiatry.* 2007;68(12):1876–85.

Friedman JH. Parkinson disease psychosis: update. *Behav Neurol.* 2013;27(4):469–77.

Herrmann N, Lanctôt KL, Hogan DB. Pharmacological recommendations for the symptomatic treatment of dementia: the Canadian Consensus Conference on the Diagnosis and Treatment of Dementia 2012. *Alzheimers Res Ther.* 2013;5(Suppl 1):S5.

Khanna P, Suo T, Komossa K, Ma H, Rummel-Kluge C, El-Sayeh HG, et al. Aripiprazole versus other atypical antipsychotics for schizophrenia. *Cochrane Database Syst Rev.* 2014;1: CD006569.

LaPorta LD. Relief from migraine headache with aripiprazole treatment. *Headache.* 2007;47(6):922–6.

Pae C-U, Serretti A, Patkar AA, Masand PS. Aripiprazole in the treatment of depressive and anxiety disorders: a review of current evidence. *CNS Drugs.* 2008;22(5):367–88.

Wenzel-Seifert K, Wittmann M, Haen E. QTc prolongation by psychotropic drugs and the risk of torsade de pointes. *Dtsch Arztebl Int.* 2011;108(41):687–93.

ARMODAFINIL

THERAPEUTICS

Brands
- Nuvigil

Generic?
- No

Class
- Psychostimulant

Commonly Prescribed for
(FDA approved in bold)
- **Reducing excessive sleepiness in patients with narcolepsy or shift work disorder**
- **Reducing excessive sleepiness in patients with obstructive sleep apnea (OSA)/ hypopnea syndrome**
- Attention deficit hyperactivity disorder
- Fatigue in multiple sclerosis (MS), depression, cancer, HIV, fibromyalgia, or post-stroke patients
- Bipolar depression

How the Drug Works
- Armodafinil is the R-enantiomer of modafinil (a mixture of R- and S-enantiomers). R-modafinil binds to the dopamine transporter (DAT) with 3-fold higher affinity than S-modafinil
- No binding to serotonin transporter or norepinephrine transporter
- It may act on the hypothalamus by stimulating wake-promoting areas, or inhibiting sleep-promoting areas. Increases neuronal activity selectively in the hypothalamus and activates tuberomammillary nucleus neurons that release histamine
- It also activates hypothalamic neurons that release orexin/hypocretin

How Long Until It Works
- Typically 2 hours, although maximal benefit may take days to weeks

If It Works
- Continue to use indefinitely as long as symptoms persist. Complete resolution of symptoms is unusual. Does not cause insomnia when dosed correctly

If It Doesn't Work
- Change to most effective dose or alternative agent. Re-evaluate treatment of underlying cause (e.g., OSA) of fatigue. Consider other causes of fatigue (e.g., anemia, heart disease) as appropriate. Screen for use of CNS depressants that can interfere with sleep (e.g., opioids or alcohol)

Best Augmenting Combos for Partial Response or Treatment-Resistance
- In treating OSA, armodafinil is an adjunct to standard treatments such as continuous positive airway pressure (CPAP), weight loss, and treatment of obstruction when possible
- In narcolepsy with cataplexy, TCAs or SNRIs may be of some help on cataplexy. Sleep hygiene is also important. As a last resort, sodium oxybate can be used for both narcolepsy and cataplexy

Tests
- None required

ADVERSE EFFECTS (AEs)

How the Drug Causes AEs
- AEs are probably related to drug actions on CNS neurotransmitters

Notable AEs
- Nervousness, insomnia, headache, nausea, anorexia, palpitations, dry mouth, diarrhea, hypertension

Life-Threatening or Dangerous AEs
- Transient ECG changes have been reported in patients with preexisting heart disease (left ventricular hypertrophy, mitral valve prolapse)
- Rare psychiatric reactions (activation of mania, anxiety)
- Rare severe dermatological reactions

Weight Gain
- Unusual

unusual   not unusual   common   problematic

Sedation

- Unusual

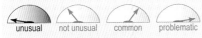

What to Do About AEs

- Try lowering the dose. If insomnia, do not take later in the day

Best Augmenting Agents to Reduce AEs

- Most AEs do not respond to adding other medications

DOSING AND USE

Usual Dosage Range

- 50–250 mg daily

Dosage Forms

- Tablets: 50, 150, 200, 250 mg

How to Dose

- Start at 150 mg in the morning
- Patients with narcolepsy are more likely to require a higher dose (250 mg)

 Dosing Tips

- Dose requirements can escalate over time due to autoinduction. A drug holiday may restore effectiveness of lower dose
- In patients with shift work disorder, take 1 hour prior to beginning a shift

Overdose

- No reported deaths. Insomnia, restlessness, agitation, anxiety, tachycardia, nausea, and hypertension have been reported

Long-Term Use

- Although most initial trials were only a few months, appears safe. Periodically re-evaluate need for use

Habit Forming

- Class IV medication, but rarely abused in clinical practice

How to Stop

- Withdrawal is not problematic, unlike traditional stimulants. Symptoms of sleepiness may recur

Pharmacokinetics

- Metabolized by amide hydrolysis and CYP3A4/5 in the liver. T_{max} 2–4 hours. 60% protein bound. Elimination predominantly in urine and the half-life is 15 hours. Reaches steady state at 7 days. Although having similar half-life and T_{max} to modafinil, the average plasma concentration of armodafinil is higher than that of modafinil

 Drug Interactions

- It weakly induces CYP1A2 and 3A and inhibits CYP2C19. Dose reduction may be required for CYP2C19 substrate (e.g., phenytoin, diazepam, propranolol, omeprazole, TCAs)
- Strong CYP3A4 inhibitor (e.g., protease inhibitors, macrolides, azole antifungals, nefazodone) can increase armodafinil concentration
- Strong CYP3A4 inducer (e.g., carbamazepine, phenytoin, phenobarbital, rifampin, glucocorticoid, St. John's wort) can decrease armodafinil concentration
- Armodafinil can affect warfarin effectiveness, requiring closer monitoring of PTINR
- May interact with MAOIs

Other warnings/ precautions

- May adversely affect mood. Can cause activation of psychosis or mania

Do Not Use

- Known hypersensitivity to the drug, severe hypertension or cardiac arrhythmias

SPECIAL POPULATIONS

Renal Impairment

- No known effect. May require lower dose

Hepatic Impairment

- Reduce dose in patients with severe impairment

Cardiac Impairment

- Do not use in patients with ischemic ECG changes, chest pain, left ventricular hypertrophy, or recent myocardial infarction

Elderly

- No known effects

Children and Adolescents
- Not studied in children

 Pregnancy
- Category C. Generally not used in pregnancy

Breast Feeding
- Unknown if excreted in breast milk. Do not use

THE ART OF NEUROPHARMACOLOGY

Potential Advantages
- Less risk of addiction, withdrawal symptoms, and abuse compared to other stimulants. Longer duration of action than modafinil

Potential Disadvantages
- May be less effective than other stimulants. Drug interactions

Primary Target Symptoms
- Sleepiness, fatigue, concentration difficulties

 Pearls
- The Epworth sleepiness scale is a reliable way to measure daytime sleepiness and response to treatment. It is a self-administered 8-item questionnaire with scores of 0–24. A score of 10 or greater indicates excessive daytime sleepiness. A reduction of 4 or more points on the Epworth is considered a good response to treatment
- Narcolepsy is characterized by excessive daytime sleepiness, uncontrollable sleep, and observed cataplexy. Hypnagogic or hypnopompic hallucinations or sleep paralysis suggest the diagnosis. In sleep studies, a sleep latency of 8 minutes or less and quick onset of REM sleep confirm the diagnosis. The maintenance of wakefulness test can monitor response to treatment or be used to document safety in patients in which wakefulness is important for public safety (e.g., pilots). An increase of 1–2 minutes in maintenance of wakefulness is considered a good response to treatment
- Does not appear to affect sleep architecture
- Technically not a psychostimulant and has minimal abuse potential
- May be useful for treating fatigue in a variety of disorders (e.g., MS, HIV, sarcoidosis, fibromyalgia, depression, cancer, post-stroke)
- It may have positive augmentation effect when coupled with standard treatments of bipolar depression. It may reduce manic behaviors

 Suggested Reading

Darwish M, Kirby M, Hellriegel ET, Robertson P Jr. Armodafinil and modafinil have substantially different pharmacokinetic profiles despite having the same terminal half-lives: analysis of data from three randomized, single-dose, pharmacokinetic studies. *Clin Drug Investig.* 2009;29(9):613–23.

Lankford DA. Armodafinil: a new treatment for excessive sleepiness. *Expert Opin Investig Drugs.* 2008;17(4):565–73.

Nishino S, Okuro M. Armodafinil for excessive daytime sleepiness. *Drugs Today (Barc).* 2008;44(6):395–414.

Parmentier R, Anaclet C, Guhennec C, Brousseau E, Bricout D, Giboulot T, Bozyczko-Coyne D, Spiegel K, Ohtsu H, Williams M, Lin JS. The brain H3-receptor as a novel therapeutic target for vigilance and sleep-wake disorders. *Biochem Pharmacol.* 2007;73(8):1157–71.

Sienaert P, Lambrichts L, Dols A, De Fruyt J. Evidence-based treatment strategies for treatment-resistant bipolar depression: a systematic review. *Bipolar Disord.* 2012;15(1):61–9.

ASPIRIN (ACETYLSALICYLIC ACID)

Brands

- Bayer Aspirin, Ecotrin, Halfprin, Heartline, Empirin, Alka-Seltzer, Asprimox, Magnaprin, Bufferin, Ascriptin, Aspergum, ZORprin

Generic?

- Yes

Class

- Antiplatelet agent, NSAID

Commonly Prescribed for

(FDA approved in bold)

- **To reduce risk of recent myocardial infarction (MI), transient ischemic attack (TIA), ischemic stroke (IS) due to fibrin platelet emboli (aortic arch atheroma, intracranial artery severe stenosis, bioprosthetic heart valve, carotid/ vertebral arterial dissection)**
- **Angina (unstable or stable)**
- **Revascularization procedures: coronary artery bypass graft (CABG), angioplasty, and carotid endarterectomy**
- **Analgesic/antipyretic**
- **Rheumatoid disease: spondyloarthropathies, rheumatoid arthritis, osteoarthritis, pleurisy associated with systemic lupus erythematosus**
- Reducing risk of stroke in high-risk populations, such as non-valvular atrial fibrillation, when anticoagulants are contraindicated
- Toxemia of pregnancy
- Kawasaki disease
- Polycythemia vera

How the Drug Works

- By irreversibly acetylating cyclo-oxygenase-1 (COX-1), aspirin inhibits synthesis of thromboxane A_2, a prostaglandin derivative that is a potent vasoconstrictor and inducer of platelet aggregation
- Irreversibly inhibits platelet aggregation even at low doses
- At larger doses, it interferes with COX-1 and COX-2 in arterial walls, affecting prostaglandin production. It counteracts

fever by reducing prostaglandin E_2 within the hypothalamus, and dilation of peripheral blood vessels, allowing dissipation of excess heat

How Long Until It Works

- A single dose of aspirin inhibits platelet aggregation for the life of the platelet (7–10 days). In pain, effective within 1–2 hours

If It Works

- Continue to use for prevention of MI, IS, or TIA, and for pain

If It Doesn't Work

- Only reduces risk of MI or IS. Warfarin is superior for cardiogenic stroke. Control all IS risk factors such as smoking, hyperlipidemia, and hypertension. For acute events, admit patients for treatment and diagnostic testing. Consider screening for aspirin resistance

Best Augmenting Combos for Partial Response or Treatment-Resistance

- Recent stroke/TIA due to severe ($\geq$ 70%) stenosis of major intracranial artery: clopidogrel and aspirin for 90 days
- Minor stroke or TIA: clopidogrel and aspirin for 90 days
- Stroke/TIA and atrial fibrillation but unable to take oral anticoagulants: aspirin and clopidogrel might be reasonable
- Rheumatic mitral valve under adequate vitamin K antagonist (VKA) but still stroke/ TIA: VKA and aspirin might be considered
- Mechanical mitral/aortic valve with history of stroke/TIA: VKA and aspirin is recommended
- Unstable angina, coronary artery stenting, MI with left ventricular thrombus: VKA/dual antiplatelet therapy
- Pain: in acute migraine, add caffeine and/or acetaminophen, antiemetics, or triptans

Tests

- None required

How the Drug Causes AEs

- Antiplatelet effects increase bleeding risk

Notable AEs

- Stomach pain, heartburn, nausea and vomiting

 Life-Threatening or Dangerous AEs

- GI, intracranial, or intraocular bleeding. Risk increases with higher doses

Weight Gain

- Unusual

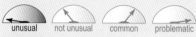

Sedation

- Unusual

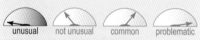

What to Do About AEs

- For significant GI or intracranial bleeding stop drug

Best Augmenting Agents to Reduce AEs

- Proton pump inhibitors reduce risk of GI bleeding

DOSING AND USE

Usual Dosage Range

- MI, TIA, or IS prevention: 50–1300 mg/day
- Pain: 325–1000 mg per dose

Dosage Forms

- Chewable tablets: 81 mg
- Tablets: 325 mg, 500 mg
- Gum tablets: 227.5 mg
- Enteric-coated: 81 mg, 165 mg, 325 mg, 500 mg, 650 mg
- Extended- or controlled-release: 650 mg, 800 mg
- Suppositories: 120 mg, 200 mg, 300 mg, 600 mg

How to Dose

- For stroke prevention, stable angina: 50–325 mg once daily
- Carotid endarterectomy: 80 mg once daily to 625 mg twice daily
- Acute myocardial infarction: 160–325 mg once daily

- For pain: 324–1000 mg every 4–6 hours up to a maximum of 4000 mg/day. With extended release, take 650–1300 mg every 8 hours as needed, maximum 3900 mg/day

 Dosing Tips

- Taking with food decreases absorption and reduces GI AEs

Overdose

- Early salicylism (> 200 mcg/mL): respiratory alkalosis, resulting in hyperpnea and tachypnea. Nausea and vomiting, hypokalemia, dizziness, tinnitus, dehydration, hyperthermia, thrombocytopenia, and easy bruising
- Late salicylism (> 400 mcg/mL): coma, pulmonary edema, respiratory failure, renal failure, hypoglycemia. Mixed respiratory alkalosis and metabolic acidosis may occur. Treat with emesis or gastric lavage and monitor salicylate levels and electrolytes. In severe cases, hemodialysis is effective

Long-Term Use

- Cautious for potential toxicity

Habit Forming

- No

How to Stop

- No need to taper

Pharmacokinetics

- Aspirin half-life is 20 minutes. > 99% protein binding. Hepatic metabolism and renal excretion

 Drug Interactions

- Alcohol increases risk of GI ulceration and may prolong bleeding time
- Urinary acidifiers (ascorbic acid, methionine) decrease secretion and increase drug effect
- Antacids and urinary alkalinizers may decrease drug effect
- Carbonic anhydrase inhibitors may increase risk of salicylate intoxication, and aspirin may displace acetazolamide from protein binding sites, leading to toxicity
- Activated charcoal decreases aspirin absorption and effect

- Corticosteroids may increase clearance and decrease serum levels
- Use with heparin or oral anticoagulants has an additive effect and can increase bleeding risks
- Aspirin may cause unexpected hypotension after treatment with nitroglycerin
- Aspirin use with NSAIDs may decrease NSAID serum levels and increases risk of GI AEs
- May displace valproic acid from binding sites and increase pharmacological effects
- May blunt effectiveness of β-blockers and ACE inhibitors
- May decrease effect of loop diuretics and spironolactone
- Increases drug levels of methotrexate
- Reduces the uricosuric effects of probenecid and sulfinpyrazone
- Large doses (> 2 g/day) may produce hypoglycemia when used with insulin or sulfonylureas in diabetics

 Other Warnings/ Precautions

- The use of aspirin or other salicylates in children or teens with influenza or chickenpox may be associated with Reye's syndrome. Symptoms include vomiting and lethargy that may progress to delirium or coma
- Tinnitus and dizziness are symptoms of aspirin toxicity
- Aspirin intolerance is not rare, especially in asthmatics (4–19%). Symptoms include bronchospasm, angioedema, severe rhinitis, or shock. It is possible to desensitize patients in a hospital setting, but they will need to maintain daily aspirin to avoid recurrence

Do Not Use

- Known hypersensitivity to salicylates, acute asthma or hay fever, severe anemia or blood coagulation defects, children or teenagers with chickenpox or flu symptoms

Renal Impairment

- Use with caution in chronic renal insufficiency. May temporarily worsen renal function or cause interstitial nephritis

Hepatic Impairment

- Use with caution in patients with significant disease including those with hypoprothrombinemia or vitamin K deficiency. High doses can cause hepatotoxicity

Cardiac Impairment

- No known effects

Elderly

- Use > 325 mg/day in high-risk groups (> 75 years old, corticosteroid, antiplatelet, anticoagulants) increases risk of GI bleeding or ulcer. Gastroprotective agent suggested

 Children and Adolescents

- Not recommended for prevention of IS or TIA in children younger than age 12. Dehydrated febrile children are prone to salicylate intoxication

 Pregnancy

- Category D. Crosses the placenta and is associated with anemia, ante- or post-partum hemorrhage, prolonged gestation and labor, and constriction of ductus arteriosus. Do not use, especially in third trimester

Breast Feeding

- Excreted in breast milk in low concentrations. Risk to infants and their platelet function is unknown

Potential Advantages

- Effective and inexpensive medication for prevention of both IS and other vascular diseases, such as MI

Potential Disadvantages

- May be less effective in some patients for ischemic stroke prevention. Risk of GI bleeding/ulcer, aspirin resistance. Drug interaction

Primary Target Symptoms

- Prevention of the neurological complications that result from ischemic stroke
- Headache or other pain

Pearls

- Aspirin monotherapy or the combination of aspirin and extended-release dipyridamole is the first-line drug for secondary prevention of non-cardioembolic IS or TIA. Clopidogrel monotherapy is a reasonable option, especially when allergic to aspirin or have stroke while taking aspirin
- May be less effective than clopidogrel for patients with peripheral vascular disease
- The combination of aspirin and clopidogrel might be considered for initiation within 24 hours of a minor IS or TIA and for continuation for 21 days. Long-term use increases the risk of hemorrhage
- For patients with small lacunar infarcts, there is no evidence for using combination therapy with clopidogrel
- In surgical procedure with moderate to high cardiovascular event risk (e.g., CABG), continue aspirin. In surgical procedure with minor cardiovascular event risk, stop aspirin 7–10 days before surgery. Simple dental procedure or cataract surgery is fine
- Standard coagulation tests do not accurately reflect the effect of aspirin. Bleeding times are often unreliable. Multiple assays are now available to measure the effect of a given aspirin on platelet function. These include standard platelet aggregometry and tests measuring the effect on COX-1 by measuring thromboxane metabolites
- Increasing aspirin dose may overcome resistance, but patients may develop aspirin resistance over time on a stable dose
- At this point, there are no guidelines to suggest when to screen for aspirin resistance. It is unclear if aspirin failures should simply increase their dose, change to another agent, or take another agent in combination with aspirin
- Retrospective studies suggest clopidogrel is more effective than aspirin in persons suffering stroke while on aspirin. However, for lacunar stroke at least, there is no evidence that clopidrogel is superior
- Antiplatelets may be as effective as anticoagulants for prevention of recurrent arterial dissection and secondary stroke
- In pain/migraine, combination products containing caffeine and/or acetaminophen may be more effective. Adding antiemetics such as metaclopramide is useful in migraine
- For bioprosthetic mitral/aortic valve with history of stroke/TIA and beyond 3–6 months from valve replacement, long-term therapy of aspirin is recommended in preference to anticoagulation
- A recent study found association of long-term aspirin use with reduced subarachnoid hemorrhage (SAH) risk compared with control. The clinical value of aspirin in SAH has yet to be confirmed

Suggested Reading

Bhatt DL, Fox KA, Hacke W, Berger PB, Black HR, Boden WE, et al; CHARISMA Investigators. Clopidogrel and aspirin versus aspirin alone for the prevention of atherothrombotic events. *N Engl J Med.* 2006;354(16):1706–17.

Diener HC, Lampl C, Reimnitz P, Voelker M. Aspirin in the treatment of acute migraine attacks. *Expert Rev Neurother.* 2006;6 (4):563–73.

García-Rodríguez LA, Gaist D, Morton J, Cookson C, González-Pérez A. Antithrombotic drugs and risk of hemorrhagic stroke in the general population. *Neurology.* 2013;81 (6):566–74.

Goldstein J, Silberstein SD, Saper JR, Ryan RE Jr, Lipton RB. Acetaminophen, aspirin, and caffeine in combination versus ibuprofen for acute migraine: results from a multicenter, double-blind, randomized, parallel-group, single-dose, placebo-controlled study. *Headache.* 2006; 46(3):444–53.

Kernan WN, Ovbiagele B, Black HR, Bravata DM, Chimowitz MI, Ezekowitz MD, et al. Guidelines for the prevention of stroke in patients with stroke and transient ischemic attack: a guideline for healthcare professionals from the American Heart Association/American Stroke Association. *Stroke.* 2014;45(7): 2160–236.

Lenz T, Wilson A. Clinical pharmacokinetics of antiplatelet agents used in the secondary prevention of stroke. *Clin Pharmacokinet.* 2003;42(10):909–20.

Serebruany VL, Malinin AI, Sane DC, Jilma B, Takserman A, Atar D, et al. Magnitude and time course of platelet inhibition with Aggrenox and Aspirin in patients after ischemic stroke: the AGgrenox versus Aspirin Therapy Evaluation (AGATE) trial. *Eur J Pharmacol.* 2004;499(3):315–24.

AZATHIOPRINE

THERAPEUTICS

Brands
- Imuran, Azasan, Azamun, Imurel

Generic?
- Yes

Class
- Immunosuppressant

Commonly Prescribed for
(FDA approved in bold)
- **Prophylaxis of organ rejection in patients with allogenic renal transplants**
- **Reducing signs and symptoms of rheumatoid arthritis**
- Myasthenia gravis (MG) (monotherapy or adjunctive)
- Lambert-Eaton myasthenia syndrome
- Inflammatory myopathies: polymyositis (PM) and dermatomyositis (DM)
- Multiple sclerosis (MS)
- Neuromyelitis optica
- Crohn's disease, ulcerative colitis
- Lupus nephritis

How the Drug Works
- Azathioprine, a derivative of 6-mercaptopurine, inhibits the synthesis of purine. This interferes with DNA and RNA synthesis as well as repair and replication of T and B leukocytes
- The mechanism of action in autoimmune diseases is unclear, but it appears to suppress cellular cytotoxicity and blunt hypersensitivity reactions

How Long Until It Works
- At least 3 months. Full effect may occur after 1–2 years

If It Works
- MG: improves strength and muscle fatigue. Often used as an adjunctive to corticosteroids or acute treatment such as immune globulin or plasma exchange. Taper corticosteroids if clinical symptoms improve
- PM/DM: may allow improvement in strength and discontinuation or reduced dose of corticosteroids. (Corticosteroids are usually tapered first.) Taper slowly over 6 months if clinical remission occurs
- MS: may reduce relapses and new lesions on MRI

If It Doesn't Work
- MG: effectiveness may not occur until 1 year. For patients with severe disability, consider more rapid-acting treatments, such as IV immune globulin
- DM/PM: question the diagnosis (inclusion-body myositis, hypothyroidism, muscular dystrophy), rule out corticosteroid-induced myopathy, and evaluate for undiagnosed malignancy (especially in DM). Change to methotrexate
- MS: if clearly not helpful, change to another agent

Best Augmenting Combos for Partial Response or Treatment-Resistance
- MG: usually combined with corticosteroids or other treatments in MG. Most patients also use symptomatic medication, such as pyridostigmine
- DM/PM: usually used in combination with corticosteroids as a sparing agent
- MS: occasionally combined with other treatments for the treatment of MS

Tests
- Obtain CBC weekly the first month, then twice monthly the second and third months, then monthly unless dose changes
- Before starting treatment, screen for thiopurine methyltransferase deficiency. Heterozygous patients often need a lower dose and closer monitoring. Homozygous patients are at risk for severe bone marrow toxicity

ADVERSE EFFECTS (AEs)

How the Drug Causes AEs
- Blocking purine synthesis and hindering DNA and RNA synthesis

Notable AEs
- Anorexia, nausea, or vomiting
- Skin rash, alopecia, arthralgias
- Idiosyncratic reaction (fever, myalgia, malaise) in about 10%: usually but not always within days of first dose

Life-Threatening or Dangerous AEs

- Bone marrow suppression: severe leukopenia, macrocytic anemia, thrombocytopenia, or pancytopenia. Dose-dependence can occur at any time during treatment
- Pancreatitis, liver toxicity
- Serious infection

Weight Gain

- Unusual

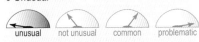

Sedation

- Not unusual

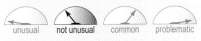

What to Do About AEs

- Reducing dose or temporary withdrawal allows reversal of bone marrow toxicity. Check serum amylase for symptoms of pancreatitis and discontinue if elevated

Best Augmenting Agents to Reduce AEs

- H_2-blockers may relieve GI symptoms

DOSING AND USE

Usual Dosage Range

- MG: 2–3 mg/kg daily
- DM/PM: 50–200 mg/day
- MS: 2–3 mg/kg daily

Dosage Forms

- Tablets: 25, 50, 75, 100 mg
- Injection: 100 mg/vial

How to Dose

- Start at 50 mg daily. Increase every 2–4 weeks to maintenance dose of 2–3 mg/kg/day

 ### Dosing Tips

- For patients with significant GI AEs, divide doses

Overdose

- Nausea and vomiting, diarrhea, leukopenia, and liver function abnormalities have been reported. Very large doses can cause severe bleeding, infection, or death

Long-Term Use

- Safe with appropriate monitoring

Habit Forming

- No

How to Stop

- In patients with clinical remission, taper by about 25 mg every 4 weeks and monitor for recurrence

Pharmacokinetics

- Azathioprine is cleaved to mercaptopurine. Drug is cleared by oxidation by xanthine oxidase and by thiol methylation by thiopurine methyltransferase. Peak levels of drug and metabolites in 1–2 hours and half-life 5 hours

 ### Drug Interactions

- Concurrent use with ACE inhibitors may induce severe leukopenia
- Allopurinol (a purine analog) may increase effects
- Methotrexate increases plasma levels of metabolite
- May decrease action of anticoagulants, such as warfarin
- Decreases cyclosporine levels
- May reverse actions of neuromuscular blockers

 ### Other Warnings/ Precautions

- May increase risk of malignancy

Do Not Use

- Known hypersensitivity, previous treatment with alkylating agents such as cyclophosphamide (due to risk of neoplasia)

SPECIAL POPULATIONS

Renal Impairment

- Unclear to what extent renal disease predicts effectiveness or toxicity. Consider reducing dose

Hepatic Impairment
- Hepatotoxicity is an uncommon AE. Use with caution and monitor closely

Cardiac Impairment
- No known effects

Elderly
- No known effects

 ## Children and Adolescents
- Effectiveness and safety unknown

 ## Pregnancy
- Category D. Multiple fetal abnormalities have been reported. Generally not used except in renal transplant patients

Breast Feeding
- Do not breast feed while on drug

THE ART OF NEUROPHARMACOLOGY

Potential Advantages
- Generally well-tolerated first-line treatment in MG. Useful corticosteroid-sparing agent in PM/DM

Potential Disadvantages
- Very slow onset of action. Effectiveness in MG may be less than other drugs

Primary Target Symptoms
- Reduce symptoms and progression from diseases such as MG, PM, DM, or MS

 ## Pearls
- It remains the first choice for long-term immunosuppressive therapy of MG. Slow onset of action in MG limits effectiveness. It is usually started in combination with prednisone. Not proven effective in 1 year in small clinical trials, but did show significant effect in 2 and 3 years. The average patient was able to discontinue prednisone treatment in 3 years but may still require lifelong immunosuppression
- In patients with contraindications to corticosteroids and less severe disability, may be used as monotherapy
- In a nationwide study in Denmark, azathioprine use in non-thymoma MG is associated with a slight increase of overall cancer (e.g., non-melanoma skin cancer)
- In DM or PM, azathioprine is an effective corticosteroid-sparing agent. Generally a first-line treatment, especially in those with interstitial lung or liver disease
- Improvement in muscle strength is a better predictor of improvement in PM or DM than a decrease in creatine kinase
- Anti-Jo-1 antibodies are predictive of worsening response in PM and DM
- PM in general is less likely to respond to corticosteroids (about 50%) than DM (over 80%), but DM patients may have a more difficult time tapering corticosteroids
- Small clinical trials demonstrate decrease in number of new MRI lesions in relapsing-remitting MS at doses up to 3 mg/kg/day. Larger trials are needed to conclusively demonstrate effectiveness
- In open-label studies it is effective in preventing progressive disability in neuromyelitis optica
- Therapeutic effects may correlate with increasing mean corpuscular volume in CBC. Start to consider tapering corticosteroids after this increase
- Azathioprine effectiveness may be optimized by TPMT gene polymorphism
- Based on two Cochrane reviews, azathioprine does not induce remission in Crohn's disease but may be more effective than placebo for maintenance of remission in ulcerative colitis

Suggested Reading

Casetta I, Iuliano G, Filippini G. Azathioprine for multiple sclerosis. *J Neurol Neurosurg Psychiatry.* 2009;80(2):131–2.

Costanzi C, Matiello M, Lucchinetti CF, Weinshenker BG, Pittock SJ, et al. Azathioprine: tolerability, efficacy, and predictors of benefit in neuromyelitis optica. *Neurology.* 2011;77(7): 659–66.

Hart IK, Sathasivam S, Sharshar T. Immunosuppressive agents for myasthenia gravis. *Cochrane Database Syst Rev.* 2007;(4): CD0052244.

Havrdova E, Zivadinov R, Krasensky J, Dwyer MG, Novakova I, et al. Randomized study of interferon beta-1a, low-dose azathioprine, and low-dose corticosteroids in multiple sclerosis. *Mult Scler.* 2009;15(8):965–76.

Hengstman GJ, van den Hoogen FH, van Engelen BG. Treatment of the inflammatory myopathies: update and practical recommendations. *Expert Opin Pharmacother.* 2009;10(7):1183–90.

Massacesi L, Parigi A, Barilaro A, Repice AM, Pellicanò G, Konze A, Siracusa G, Taiuti R, Amaducci L. Efficacy of azathioprine on multiple sclerosis new brain lesions evaluated using magnetic resonance imaging. *Arch Neurol.* 2005;62(12): 1843–7.

Palace J, Newsom-Davis J, Lecky B. A randomized double-blind trial of prednisolone alone or with azathioprine in myasthenia gravis. Myasthenia Gravis Study Group. *Neurology.* 1998;50(6):1778–83.

THERAPEUTICS

Brands
- Lioresal, Kemstro, Gablofen

Generic?
- Yes

Class
- Muscle relaxant

Commonly Prescribed for
(FDA approved in bold)
- **Spasticity and pain related to disorders such as multiple sclerosis (MS) or spinal cord diseases**
- Trigeminal neuralgia
- Alcohol withdrawal
- Gastroesophageal reflux disease (GERD)
- Gilles de la Tourette syndrome (GTS)
- Tardive dyskinesias
- Chorea in Huntington's disease
- Acquired peduncular nystagmus

How the Drug Works
- Baclofen is a GABA$_B$ agonist. Through mechanisms in addition to GABA$_B$'s inhibitory effect, it depresses monosynaptic and polysynaptic reflex transmission at spinal level but not neuromuscular transmission. However, the exact mechanism of action is unknown. It also has CNS depressant properties

How Long Until It Works
- Pain: hours to weeks

If It Works
- Slowly titrate to most effective dose as tolerated. Many patients will need gradual titration to maintain response and limit sedation

If It Doesn't Work
- Make sure to increase to highest tolerated dose – as high as 200 mg/day. If ineffective, slowly taper and consider alternative treatments for pain. In general, baclofen is more effective for spasticity related to MS or spinal cord disease than for other causes of spasticity

Best Augmenting Combos for Partial Response or Treatment-Resistance
- For focal spasticity, i.e., post-stroke spasticity, botulinum toxin is often more effective and is better tolerated
- Use other centrally acting muscle relaxants with caution due to potential synergistic CNS depressant effect
- Baclofen is usually used in combination with neuroleptics for the treatment of tardive dyskinesias or chorea
- Trigeminal neuralgia often responds to AEDs. Pimozide is another option. For truly refractory patients, surgical interventions may be required

Tests
- None required

ADVERSE EFFECTS (AES)

How the Drug Causes AEs
- Most AEs are related to CNS depression

Notable AEs
- Drowsiness, dizziness, weakness, fatigue are most common. Nausea, constipation, hypotension, and confusion

Life-Threatening or Dangerous AEs
- Worsening of seizure control
- The most dangerous AEs occur with rapid baclofen withdrawal including high fever, confusion, hallucinations, rebound spasticity, muscle rigidity and, in severe cases, rhabdomyolysis, multi-system organ failure, and death

Weight Gain
- Unusual

   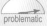

unusual not unusual common problematic

Sedation
- Problematic

unusual not unusual common problematic

What to Do About AEs

- Lower the dose and titrate more slowly

Best Augmenting Agents to Reduce AEs

- Most AEs cannot be reduced by an augmenting agent. MS-related fatigue can respond to CNS stimulants, such as modafinil, but in most cases it is easier to temporarily lower the baclofen dose until tolerance develops

DOSING AND USE

Usual Dosage Range

Spasticity
- Oral: 40–80 mg/day in divided doses
- Intrathecal: 300–800 mcg/day, rarely more than 1000 mcg/day

Dosage Forms

- Tablets: 10, 20 mg
- Orally disintegrating tablets: 10, 20 mg
- Intrathecal: Gablofen: 0.05, 0.5, 1, 2 mg/mL, Lioresal: 0.02, 0.5, 2 mg/mL, in prefilled syringe. For use with Medtronic Implantable Programmable Infusion Pumps

How to Dose

- Oral: start at 15 mg daily in 3 divided doses. Increase by 15 mg every 3 days as tolerated to 60 mg/day in 3 divided doses or until desired clinical effect. Patients may further benefit from increasing dose to 80 mg/day. Doses above 80 mg/day are usually not recommended but doses up to 200 mg/day have been used in patients that tolerate the medication well
- Intrathecal: patients must demonstrate a positive clinical response to treatment. A dose of 50 mcg is given on day 1 over greater than 1 minute. Observe 4–8 hours for a clinical response. If the response is inadequate, can repeat with dose of 75 mcg 24 hours later and again observe 4–8 hours for improvement. If no response, inject 100 mcg on day 3. Patients who do not respond to a dose of 100 mcg are not candidates for intrathecal treatment
- If the positive effect of the test dose lasts less than 8 hours, the starting dose should be doubled with the bolus dose given over 24 hours. If the response lasts over 8 hours, use the bolus dose as the original daily dose.

In patients with spasticity of spinal cord origin, increase the daily dose by 10–30% after 24 hours and then every 24 hours until the desired clinical effect is achieved. In patients with spasticity related to cerebral origin and in children increase the dose more slowly – about 5–15% each increase per 24 hours until desired effect reached
- When to consider intrathecal baclofen: for treatment of spasticity related to a stable, irreversible neurological disease or trauma that disables the patient or causes severe pain. The patient must have failed at least 3–4 oral medications or experience intolerable side effects at effective doses. The patient or the caregiver must understand the risks and benefits of the pump and the required follow-up care

 Dosing Tips

- About 5% of patients will become refractory to increasing doses of intrathecal baclofen. In those patients, consider careful withdrawal and treatment with other antispasticity agents for 2–4 weeks, then restart at the initial continuous infusion dose

Overdose

- Vomiting, hypotonia, drowsiness, coma, respiratory depression, and seizures. In an alert patient induce emesis and lavage. In obtunded patients, intubation is often required

Long-Term Use

- Safe for long-term use. Effectiveness may decrease over time and tolerance to clinical effects occurs in about 5%

Habit Forming

- No

How to Stop

- To avoid withdrawal symptoms, taper slowly over a week or more depending on the dose and time on drug
- Abrupt withdrawal of intrathecal baclofen (pump, battery failure, catheter clog, etc.) can mimic neuroleptic malignant syndrome

Pharmacokinetics

- Orally: rapidly absorbed (C_{max} 2–4 hours) with excretion half-life 3–4 hours. Intrathecal: bolus lasts 4–8 hours, with initial onset 0.5–1 hour after bolus. Continuous infusion lasts 6–8 hours. The peak action is 4 hours after a bolus and 24–48 hours after starting continuous infusion. Excreted 70% unchanged in urine

Drug Interactions

- Use with other CNS depressants will exacerbate sedation. No hepatic metabolism, therefore no major drug interactions to consider

Other Warnings/ Precautions

- Decreased spasticity can be problematic for some patients who require tone to maintain upright posture, balance, and ambulate
- May cause an increase in ovarian cysts
- May worsen symptoms of psychiatric disorders, such as schizophrenia or confusional states
- May worsen control of epilepsy
- Use with caution in patients with history of stroke and porphyria. Not recommended for patients with Parkinson's disease or rheumatoid disorder

Do Not Use

- Known hypersensitivity. Never start intrathecal baclofen in patients with an active infection

SPECIAL POPULATIONS

Renal Impairment

- Since baclofen is renally excreted, lower the dose with significant renal dysfunction

Hepatic Impairment

- No known effects

Cardiac Impairment

- No known effects

Elderly

- Titrate carefully but no contraindications. Increased risk of injury

Children and Adolescents

- Children over age 12 have similar dose requirements to adults. Children under 12 usually have a lower dose requirement for intrathecal baclofen – on average 274 mcg/day. For small children, start with a test dose of 25 mcg

Pregnancy

- Category C. Use only if benefits of medication outweigh risks

Breast Feeding

- Oral baclofen is excreted in breast milk. Do not use

THE ART OF NEUROPHARMACOLOGY

Potential Advantages

- First-line treatment for spasticity in MS and spinal cord injury patients. Effect is maintained with extended use

Potential Disadvantages

- Poor effectiveness and tolerability in patients with spasticity unrelated to MS or spinal cord injuries. Severe withdrawal AEs. Sedation often limits use

Primary Target Symptoms

- Spasticity, pain

Pearls

- Effective and important adjunctive medication for MS and spinal-cord injury spasticity and pain. With slow titration, baclofen is usually well tolerated. Recommended by National Institute for Health and Care Excellence (NICE) as first-line drug for the treatment of spasticity in MS
- Baclofen is generally NOT effective for spasticity related to Parkinson's disease, stroke, and traumatic brain injury, although it occasionally is used in severe cases. In general these patients are much more susceptible to AEs

- Early use of intrathecal baclofen implant in acquired brain injury patients may reduce spasticity and spasm frequency. However, FDA suggests waiting at least 1 year after injury before considering Gablofen therapy
- Intrathecal baclofen should be administered in centers that commonly treat MS and spinal cord diseases
- Intrathecal (not oral) baclofen may reduce spasticity but not associated pain, which is commonly managed by gabapentin or pregabalin. For patients on intrathecal baclofen with rapidly escalating dose requirements or new-onset depression, fever, or confusion, consider the possibility of a shunt catheter malfunction
- Some spasticity can be helpful for patients with MS or spinal cord injuries to support circulatory function, prevent deep vein thrombosis, and optimize activities of daily living
- A second-line treatment for trigeminal neuralgia, usually at doses of 60 mg/day or less. Level C evidence for trigeminal neuralgia
- Baclofen has been used off-label for many other conditions such as chorea, migraine, and neuropathic pain. These studies have been mostly negative
- May reduce belching and regurgitation in GERD
- May be useful for treatment of alcohol dependence. The effect is greater with 20 mg 3 times daily than 10 mg 3 times daily

Suggested Reading

Addolorato G, Leggio L, Ferrulli A, Cardone S, Bedogni G, Caputo F, et al. Dose-response effect of baclofen in reducing daily alcohol intake in alcohol dependence: secondary analysis of a randomized, double-blind, placebo-controlled trial. *Alcohol Alcohol.* 2011;46(3):312–17.

Attal N, Cruccu G, Baron R, Haanpää M, Hansson P, Jensen TS, et al. EFNS guidelines on the pharmacological treatment of neuropathic pain: 2010 revision. *Eur J Neurol.* 2010;17(9):1113–88.

Coffey RJ, Edgar TS, Francisco GE, Graziani V, Meythaler JM, Ridgely PM, et al. Abrupt withdrawal from intrathecal baclofen: recognition and management of a potentially life-threatening syndrome. *Arch Phys Med Rehabil.* 2002;83(6):735–41.

Cossentino MJ, Mann K, Armbruster SP, Lake JM, Maydonovitch C, Wong RKH. Randomised clinical trial: the effect of baclofen in patients with gastro-oesophageal reflux – a randomised prospective study. *Aliment Pharmacol Ther.* 2012;35(9):1036–44.

Metz L. Multiple sclerosis: symptomatic therapies. *Semin Neurol.* 1998;18(3):389–95.

Nair KPS, Marsden J. The management of spasticity in adults. *BMJ.* 2014;349:g4737.

Nielsen JF, Hansen HJ, Sunde N, Christensen JJ. Evidence of tolerance to baclofen in treatment of severe spasticity with intrathecal baclofen. *Clin Neurol Neurosurg.* 2002;104(2):142–5.

Posteraro F, Calandriello B, Galli R, Logi F, Iardella L, Bordi L. Timing of intrathecal baclofen therapy in persons with acquired brain injury: Influence on outcome. *Brain Inj.* 2013;27(13-14):1671–5.

Teasell RW, Mehta S, Aubut J-AL, Foulon B, Wolfe DL, Hsieh JTC, et al. A systematic review of pharmacologic treatments of pain after spinal cord injury. *Arch Phys Med Rehabil.* 2010;91(5):816–31.

Vender JR, Hughes M, Hughes BD, Hester S, Holsenback S, Rosson B. Intrathecal baclofen therapy and multiple sclerosis: outcomes and patient satisfaction. *Neurosurg Focus.* 2006;21(2):e6.

BENZTROPINE

THERAPEUTICS

Brands
- Cogentin

Generic?
- Yes

Class
- Antiparkinson agent, anticholinergic

Commonly Prescribed for
(FDA approved in bold)
- **Extrapyramidal disorders**
- **Parkinsonism**
- Acute dystonic reactions
- Idiopathic generalized dystonia
- Focal dystonias
- Dopa-responsive dystonia

How the Drug Works
- In Parkinson's disease (PD), there is a relative excess of cholinergic input. Benztropine is a synthetic anticholinergic with relatively greater CNS activity than most other anticholinergics. May also inhibit the reuptake and storage of dopamine at central dopamine receptors, prolonging dopamine action

How Long Until It Works
- PD/extrapyramidal disorders: minutes to hours

If It Works
- PD: do not abruptly discontinue or change doses of other PD treatments. Usually most effective in combination with other antiparkinsonian medications

If It Doesn't Work
- PD: generally benztropine is an adjunctive medication for common PD symptoms, such as tremor, rigidity, and drooling. Other cardinal PD symptoms, such as bradykinesia and gait difficulties, are most likely to improve with other PD treatments, such as levodopa, dopamine agonists, amantadine, or monoamine oxidase (MAO)-B inhibitors
- Acute dystonic reactions: diphenhydramine is another option, if not effective consider benzodiazepines. If possible, discontinue

the agent that precipitated the extrapyramidal AE

Best Augmenting Combos for Partial Response or Treatment-Resistance
- For bradykinesia or gait disturbances causing significant functional disturbance, levodopa is most effective. For idiopathic PD patients, especially younger patients with normal cognition and milder disability, dopamine agonists are a good first choice. Amantadine and MAO-B inhibitors may also be useful
- Depression is common in PD and may respond to low-dose SSRIs

Tests
- None

ADVERSE EFFECTS (AEs)

How the Drug Causes AEs
- Prevents the action of acetylcholine on muscarinic receptors

Notable AEs
- Dry mouth, tachycardia, palpitations, hypotension, disorientation, confusion, hallucinations, constipation, nausea/vomiting, dilation of colon, rash, blurred vision, diplopia, urinary retention, elevated temperature, decreased sweating, erectile dysfunction

Life-Threatening or Dangerous AEs
- May precipitate narrow-angle glaucoma. Risk of heat stroke, especially in elderly patients. Can cause tachycardia, cardiac arrhythmias, and hypotension in susceptible patients. May cause urinary retention in patients with prostate hypertrophy

Weight Gain
- Unusual

unusual   not unusual   common   problematic

Sedation
- Common

unusual   not unusual   **common**   problematic

What to Do About AEs

- Confusion, hallucinations: stop benztropine and any other anticholinergics
- Sedation: can take entire dose at night or lower dose
- Dry mouth: chewing gum or water can help
- Urinary retention: if drug cannot be discontinued, obtain urological evaluation

Best Augmenting Agents to Reduce AEs

- Most AEs cannot be reduced with the use of an augmenting agent

DOSING AND USE

Usual Dosage Range

- PD: 0.5–6 mg/day
- Extrapyramidal reactions: 2–8 mg/day

Dosage Forms

- Tablets: 0.5, 1, and 2 mg
- Injection: 1 mg/mL

How to Dose

- PD: use oral tablets. Start at 0.5 mg once daily and increase by 0.5 mg at 5–6 day intervals until reaching best tolerated and effective dose. Patients may take either once daily at night to improve sleep and allow for easier rising in the morning, or divide doses 2–4 times per day
- Drug-induced extrapyramidal disorders: 1–4 mg once or twice a day orally or parenterally. If the reaction occurs soon after the initiation of neuroleptic drugs (i.e., phenothiazines) they are likely to be transient. Attempt to withdraw benztropine after 1–2 weeks to determine if still needed. Disorders that develop after prolonged neuroleptic use may not respond to treatment
- Acute dystonic reactions: 1–2 mg injection (IV or IM) and tablets 1–2 mg twice per day prevent recurrence

 Dosing Tips

- Taking with meals can reduce AEs. IM and IV dosing are equally effective and fast acting

Overdose

- Complications may include circulatory collapse, cardiac arrest, respiratory depression or arrest, CNS depression or stimulation, psychosis, shock, coma, seizures, ataxia, combativeness, anhidrosis and hyperthermia, fever, dysphagia, decreased bowel sounds, and sluggish pupils. Induce emesis, use gastric lavage or activated charcoal. Oxygen or intubation may be needed for respiratory depression. Catheterize for urinary retention. Treat hyperthermia appropriately with cooling devices, local miotics for mydriasis/cycloplegia. Use physostigmine to reverse cardiac effects and use fluids and vasopressors if needed

Long-Term Use

- Safe for long-term use. Effectiveness may decrease over time (years) in PD, and AEs such as sedation and cognitive impairment can worsen

Habit Forming

- No

How to Stop

- No need to taper

Pharmacokinetics

- Half-life is 36 hours, but the greatest effect lasts about 6–8 hours. Mostly renal excretion. Bioavailability and metabolism not well understood

 Drug Interactions

- Use with amantadine may increase AEs
- Benztropine and all other anticholinergics may increase serum levels and effects of digoxin
- Can lower concentration of haloperidol and other phenothiazines, causing worsening of schizophrenia symptoms. Phenothiazines tend to increase anticholinergic AEs with concurrent use
- Can decrease gastric motility, resulting in increased gastric deactivation and hence reduced efficacy of levodopa

Other Warnings/ Precautions

- Use with caution in hot weather: may increase susceptibility to heat stroke
- Anticholinergics have additive effects when used with drugs of abuse such as cannabinoids, barbiturates, opioids, and alcohol

Do Not Use

- Patients with known hypersensitivity to the drug, glaucoma (especially angle-closure type), pyloric or duodenal obstruction, stenosing peptic ulcers, prostate hypertrophy or bladder neck obstructions, achalasia, or megacolon

SPECIAL POPULATIONS

Renal Impairment

- Use with caution but no known effects

Hepatic Impairment

- Use with caution but no known effects

Cardiac Impairment

- Use with caution in patients with known arrhythmias, especially tachycardia

Elderly

- Use with caution. More susceptible to AEs

Children and Adolescents

- Do not use in ages 3 or less. Generalized dystonias may respond to anticholinergic treatment and young patients usually tolerate the medication better than the elderly. Typical dose 0.05 mg/kg once or twice daily

Pregnancy

- Category C. Use only if benefit of medication outweighs risks

Breast Feeding

- Concentration in breast milk unknown. May inhibit lactation. Use only if benefits outweigh risk

THE ART OF NEUROPHARMACOLOGY

Potential Advantages

- Useful adjunctive agent for some PD patients, especially post-encephalitic. Long duration of action. First-line agent for extrapyramidal disorders related to neuroleptics, especially in acute setting

Potential Disadvantages

- Multiple dose-dependent AEs associated with antimuscarinic effects limit use. Not effective for most idiopathic PD patients. Patients with long-standing extrapyramidal disorders may not respond to treatment. Less established as treatment for generalized dystonias than trihexyphenidyl

Primary Target Symptoms

- Tremor, akinesia, rigidity, drooling

 Pearls

- Useful adjunct in younger PD patients with tremor, but trihexyphenidyl more commonly is used
- Useful in the treatment of post-encephalitic PD and for extrapyramidal reactions, other than tardive dyskinesias
- Sedation limits use, especially in older patients. Patients with mental impairment do poorly
- Post-encephalitic PD patients usually tolerate higher doses better than idiopathic PD patients
- Generalized dystonias are more likely to benefit from anticholinergic therapy than focal dystonias. Trihexyphenidyl is used more commonly than benztropine
- May be useful for treating secondary progressive multiple sclerosis by enhancing remyelination

Suggested Reading

Brocks DR. Anticholinergic drugs used in Parkinson's disease: an overlooked class of drugs from a pharmacokinetic perspective. *J Pharm Pharm Sci.* 1999;2(2):39–46.

Colosimo C, Gori MC, Inghilleri M. Post-encephalitic tremor and delayed-onset parkinsonism. *Parkinsonism Relat Disord.* 1999;5(3):123–4.

Costa J, Espírito-Santo C, Borges A, Ferreira JJ, Coelho M, Sampaio C. Botulinum toxin type A versus anticholinergics for cervical dystonia. *Cochrane Database Syst Rev.* 2005;1:CD004312.

Deshmukh VA, Tardif V, Lyssiotis CA, Green CC, Kerman B, Kim HJ, et al. A regenerative approach to the treatment of multiple sclerosis. *Nature.* 2013;502(7471):327–32.

Hai NT, Kim J, Park ES, Chi SC. Formulation and biopharmaceutical evaluation of transdermal patch containing benztropine. *Int J Pharm.* 2008;357(1–2):55–60.

BEVACIZUMAB

THERAPEUTICS

Brands
- Avastin

Generic?
- No

Class
- Antineoplastic agent

Commonly Prescribed for
(FDA approved in bold)
- **Monotherapy for glioblastoma following prior therapy**
- **Metastatic colorectal cancer**
- **Metastatic renal cell carcinoma**
- **Metastatic breast cancer**
- **Non-squamous non-small cell lung cancer**
- Schwannomatosis
- Ovarian cancer
- Age-related macular degeneration

How the Drug Works
- A recombinant humanized monoclonal immunoglobulin (IgG1) that binds to vascular endothelial growth factor (VEGF) and prevents the interaction of VEGF with its receptors (Flt-1 and KDR) on the surface of endothelial cells. It downregulates angiogenesis, improves vascular normalization, and enhances the efficacy of both radiotherapy and chemotherapy

How Long Until It Works
- Days to weeks. May rapidly reduce peritumoral edema, but the actual tumor shrinking effect may take months

If It Works
- Continue every 2 weeks

If It Doesn't Work
- Usually used for symptomatic glioblastomas in an advanced stage but other salvage therapies can be considered depending on the clinical situation

Best Augmenting Combos for Partial Response or Treatment-Resistance
- Generally given to ill and symptomatic patients. Usually given along with

dexamethasone, but bevacizumab may allow tapering of corticosteroids
- May be given along with temozolomide, although this is not standard practice
- Coadministration with irinotecan may increase survival

Tests
- Monitor blood pressure (may increase) during treatment
- Urinalysis for proteinuria
- CBC and hepatic function testing during treatment are required

ADVERSE EFFECTS (AEs)

How the Drug Causes AEs
- Many serious AEs (poor wound healing, severe GI complications) are directly related to inhibition of angiogenesis

Notable AEs
- Epistaxis, headache, hypertension, rhinitis, proteinuria, taste alteration, dry skin, rectal hemorrhage, lacrimation disorder, exfoliative dermatitis
- Less common: rash, diarrhea, thrombocytopenia, neutropenia

Life-Threatening or Dangerous AEs
- Wound healing delays or dehiscence, CSF leak, necrotizing fasciitis
- Hypertensive crisis
- Arterial or venous thromboembolic events
- Severe hemorrhage including retroperitoneal
- Febrile neutropenia, pancytopenia
- Congestive heart failure (rare)
- Hepatotoxicity (rare)
- Ovarian failure
- Gallbladder perforation

Weight Gain
- Unusual

unusual   not unusual   common   problematic

Sedation
- Not unusual

unusual   not unusual   common   problematic

What to Do About AEs

- For relatively benign AEs such as mild infusion reactions, continue treatment, especially if there is clinical benefit
- Avoid using immediately after surgery and stop 1 month before elective surgery
- Venous thromboembolic events can be treated with anticoagulation but arterial events usually require drug discontinuation

Best Augmenting Agents to Reduce AEs

- For infusion reactions, pretreat with acetaminophen and antihistamines. Pretreatment with IV glucocorticoids may also help. Hypertension is generally treatable with standard medications

DOSING AND USE

Usual Dosage Range

- 5–10 mg/kg every 2 weeks IV

Dosage Forms

- Injection: 25 mg/mL in 4 or 16 mL vials (100 or 400 mg)

How to Dose

- Glioblastoma: 10 mg/kg IV every 2 weeks. In glioblastoma usually given alone but for other non-brain cancers it is often combined with other agents
- Metastatic colorectal cancer: 5–10 mg/kg IV every 2 weeks, in combination with IV 5-fluorouracil-based chemotherapy
- Metastatic renal cell carcinoma: 10 mg/kg IV every 2 weeks in combination with interferon-α
- Non-squamous non-small cell lung cancer: 15 mg/kg IV every 3 weeks in combination with carboplatin and paclitaxel
- Age-related macular degeneration: 1.25–2.5 mg monthly

 Dosing Tips

- Deliver the initial dose over 90 minutes. If tolerated, then the infusion can be shortened to 60 and 30 minutes gradually
- Temporary suspension is recommended in patients with severe infusion reaction, severe hypertension, or moderate to severe proteinuria

Overdose

- Headaches are common with higher doses (20 mg/kg) but there are no reports of overdose

Long-Term Use

- May allow reduction in corticosteroid dosing. Multiple potential AEs require close monitoring. Average length of response is months, not years

Habit Forming

- No

How to Stop

- No need to taper, but monitor for recurrence of neurological disorder

Pharmacokinetics

- The estimated half-life of bevacizumab is approximately 20 days with a predicted time to reach steady state of 100 days

 Drug Interactions

- May lower paclitaxel levels when given in combination with carboplatin or paclitaxel
- May decrease irinotecan clearance
- Use with caution with any medication that can increase bleeding risk

 Other Warnings/ Precautions

- GI perforation: up to 2.4% of treated patients
- Increased risk of severe hemorrhage in avastin-treated patients

Do Not Use

- Do not initiate for 28 days following major surgery and until surgical wound is fully healed

SPECIAL POPULATIONS

Renal Impairment

- No known effects

Hepatic Impairment

- No known effects

Cardiac Impairment

- May rarely cause congestive heart failure, but this may be reversible

Elderly

- AEs such as cerebrovascular accidents, transient ischemic attacks, myocardial infarction, thrombocytopenia, neutropenia, headache, and fatigue are all more common in patients over age 65

Children and Adolescents

- Effectiveness and safety are unknown

Pregnancy

- Category C. Animal reproduction have shown an adverse effect on the fetus and there are no adequate and well-controlled studies in humans, but potential benefits may warrant use of the drug in pregnant women despite potential risks

Breast Feeding

- Discontinue until drug levels are not detectable

THE ART OF NEUROPHARMACOLOGY

Potential Advantages

- One of few available treatments and fairly rapid clinical effect for aggressive or recurrent glioblastoma

Potential Disadvantages

- High toxicity and unclear survival benefit

Primary Target Symptoms

- Tumor progression and edema, disability

Pearls

- Generally used as a salvage or rescue treatment for recurrence after initial therapy
- Use within the first postoperative month is problematic due to effects on wound healing
- In the phase II GLARIUS trial, 79.6% of patients treated with bevacizumab and irinotecan were free of progression at 6 months, compared with 41.3% of patients randomized to receive temozolomide. The median overall survival was 16.6 months for the former group, compared with 14.8 months for the latter group
- In a 2014 trial, there was no evidence of bevacizumab effectiveness for newly diagnosed glioblastoma or anaplastic astrocytoma. First-line use of bevacizumab did not improve overall survival in patients with newly diagnosed glioblastoma. Progression-free survival was prolonged but did not reach the prespecified improvement target
- T_1-hyperintense lesions with restrictive diffusion on MRI after bevacizumab treatment correspond to tumor calcifications and may predict favorable outcome
- Minor clinical fluctuations are common in those with glioblastoma, but rapid deterioration should raise concern for tumor bleeding, infection, or non-convulsive status epilepticus
- Synergy between bevacizumab and chemoradiotherapy is attractive but remains to be studied in efficacy and safety
- Bevacizumab has been reported to reduce tumor size in a patient with schwannomatosis associated with neurofibromatosis

Suggested Reading

Bähr O, Harter PN, Weise LM, You SJ, Mittelbronn M, Ronellenfitsch MW, et al. Sustained focal antitumor activity of bevacizumab in recurrent glioblastoma. *Neurology.* 2014;83(3):227–34.

Chamberlain MC. Bevacizumab for the treatment of recurrent glioblastoma. *Clin Med Insights Oncol.* 2011;5:117–29.

Friedman HS, Prados MD, Wen PY, Mikkelsen T, Schiff D, Abrey LE, et al. Bevacizumab alone and in combination with irinotecan in recurrent glioblastoma. *J Clin Oncol.* 2009;27(28):4733–40.

Gilbert MR, Dignam JJ, Armstrong TS, Wefel JS, Blumenthal DT, Vogelbaum MA, et al. A randomized trial of bevacizumab for newly diagnosed glioblastoma. *N Engl J Med.* 2014;370(8):699–708.

Gilbert MR, Wang M, Aldape KD, Stupp R, Hegi ME, Jaeckle KA, et al. Dose-dense temozolomide for newly diagnosed glioblastoma: a randomized phase III clinical trial. *J Clin Oncol.* 2013;31(32): 4085–91.

Omuro A, DeAngelis LM. Glioblastoma and other malignant gliomas: a clinical review. *JAMA.* 2013;310(17):1842–50.

Seystahl K, Wiestler B, Hundsberger T, Happold C, Wick W, Weller M, et al. Bevacizumab alone or in combination with irinotecan in recurrent WHO grade II and grade III gliomas. *Eur Neurol.* 2013;69(2):95–101.

BOTULINUM TOXIN TYPE A

THERAPEUTICS

Brands

- Onabotulinumtoxin A (Botox, Botox cosmetic), Abobotulinumtoxin A (Dysport), Incobotulinumtoxin A (Xeomin), Vistabel, Neuronox

Generic?

- No

Class

- Neurotoxin

Commonly Prescribed for

(FDA approved in bold)

- **Prophylaxis of chronic migraine**
- **Upper limb spasticity in adult patients**
- **Cervical dystonia (CD) in adult patients**
- **Overactive bladder (OAB) with an inadequate response to or if patients are intolerant of an anticholinergic medication**
- **Severe axillary hyperhidrosis**
- **Blepharospasm associated with dystonia in patients ≥ 12 years of age**
- **Strabismus in patients ≥ 12 years of age**
- **Glabellar lines**
- Focal dystonia
- Essential tremor
- Palmar hyperhidrosis
- Cosmetic use
- Hemifacial spasm
- Spasmodic torticollis
- Spasmodic dysphonia (laryngeal dystonia)
- Writer's cramp and other task-specific dystonias
- Spasticity associated with stroke
- Dynamic muscle contracture in cerebral palsy
- Acquired nystagmus
- Oscillopsia
- Sialorrhea (drooling)
- Temporomandicular joint dysfunction
- Diabetic neuropathic pain
- Myofascial pain
- Tics
- Achalasia (esophageal motility disorder)

How the Drug Works

- It blocks acceptor nerve terminals, entering the nerve terminals, and inhibiting the release of acetylcholine and other neurotrasmitters (e.g., glutamates, substance P, calcitonin gene-related peptide), and subsequently their downstream activation. The heavy chain (HC) binds to presynaptic gangliosides on the cell surface and promotes translocation of light chain (LC) into cytosolic endosomes. Once released into cytosol, LC (a zinc endopeptidase) cleaves SNAP-25 (synaptosomal-associated protein 25), a protein integral to the successful docking and release of neurotransmitters from vesicles situated within nerve endings. It may also affect membrane trafficking of other receptors and channel proteins

- It acts locally (due to limited diffusion from its large size), as well as distally possibly via axonal transports to central terminals, transcytosis to second-order neurons and glia, and even possible hematogenous spread

- It produces partial chemical denervation of the muscle and sweat gland, detrusor efferent activity, and facilitates pain. However, it has no role in acute antinociception peripherally

How Long Until It Works

- Migraine: time of onset of the therapeutic effect on migraine is observed from week 12 with meaningful reduction in headache at 56 weeks

- Dystonia: initial effect can be seen from days to less than 2 weeks, with maximal effect around 6 weeks

If It Works

- Continue the treatment but monitor for AEs

If It Doesn't Work

- Retreatment should be tailored to the degree and pattern of the dystonia/spasticity/spasm
- Concomitant use of systemic medication is often helpful

 ### Best Augmenting Combos for Partial Response or Treatment-Resistance

- For migraine: combination of preventive medications (e.g., topiramate, valproate, TCAs, SNRIs) is usually helpful
- Patients can develop neutralizing antibodies from prior exposure. Response to a test dose of 15 units in the frontalis muscle

indicates a physiological response. Antibody neutralization has not been reported with newer type-A formulations

Tests

• No available test

ADVERSE EFFECTS (AEs)

How the Drug Causes AEs

• Direct effect of the toxin on surrounding tissues

Notable AEs

• Injection site: pain, hemorrhage, infection, pruritus
• OAB: urinary tract infection, dysuria, urinary retention
• Migraine: neck pain, headache
• Spasticity: extremity pain
• CD: dysphagia, upper respiratory tract infection, neck pain, headache, cough, flu syndrome, back pain, rhinitis
• Axillary hyperhidrosis: injection site pain, hemorrhage, non-axillary sweating, pharyngitis, flu syndrome
• Blepharospasm/strabismus: ptosis, diplopia, dry or watery eyes, keratitis (from reduced blinking)
• Spasmodic dysphonia: hypophonia ("breathy" voice)
• Writer's cramp: hand weakness

 Life-Threatening or Dangerous AEs

• Spread of toxin effect; swallowing and breathing difficulties leading to death. Rarely patients may experience severe dysphagia requiring a feeding tube or leading to aspiration pneumonia
• Use with caution in patients with motor neuropathies or neuromuscular junctional disorders. These patients may be at greater risk for systemic weakness or respiratory problems
• Hypersensitivity to botulinum toxin or the components in the formulation

Weight Gain

• Unusual

unusual　　not unusual　　common　　problematic

Sedation

• Unusual

unusual　　not unusual　　common　　problematic

What to Do About AEs

• Reduce dose or hold the treatment for longer period. Most AEs will decrease with time (weeks)

Best Augmenting Agents to Reduce AEs

• None

DOSING AND USE

Usual Dosage Range

• CD: Botox mean dose 236u (usually 150–300u). Per muscle: sternocleidomastoid 12.5–70u, trapezius 25–100u, levator scapulae 25–60u, splenius 20–100u, scalenus 15–50u. Dysport: typical dose 250–1000u
• Blepharospasm: 1.25–5u at each site (15–100u total)
• Oromandibular dystonia: masseter 10–75u, temporalis 5–50u, medial and lateral pterygoids 5–40u each
• Spasmodic dysphonia: 2.5–5u
• Sialorrhea: 7.5–40u
• Limb dystonia: intrinsic hand muscles 2.5–12.5u, arm 5–45u, intrinsic foot muscles 35–85u, leg muscles 50–200u
• Primary axillary hyperhidrosis: 50u per axilla
• Headache: 50–200u
• Upper limb spasticity: 75–360u

Dosage Forms

• Injection, lyophilized powder: Botox (900 kDa; 50, 100, 200 u per vial), Dysport (500–900 kDa; 300, 500 u per vial), Xeomin (150 kDa; 50, 100 u per vial)

How to Dose

• Blepharospasm: initial 1.25–2.5 u IM. Increase every 3 months. Maximum 5 u per site
• CD: 200–300 u IM divided among the affected muscle. Maximum 50 u per site. Limit 100 u to sternocleidomastoid muscle

- Chronic migraine: 155 units IM at 31 sites. Repeat every 12 weeks
- OAB: 100 units IM into the detrusor. Requires infection prophylaxis
- Axillary hyperhidrosis: 50 units intradermally
- Oromandibular dystonia: masseter 10–75 units, temporalis 5–50 units, medial and lateral pterygoids 5–40 units each
- Spasmodic dysphonia: 2.5–5 units
- Sialorrhea: 7.5–40 units

 Dosing Tips

- Do not exceed the recommended dosage and frequency of administration
- Physicians should be familiar with the anatomy of the injection site and the specific disorders
- Reconstitute with 0.9% sodium chloride. Rotate gently to mix with the saline. Administer within 4 hours
- Dilute with 1, 2, 4, or 8 mL depending on the type of injections to be performed. Dilute more when injecting smaller muscles (such as ocular muscles) that require fewer units
- When injecting for blepharospasm, avoid the levator palpebrae superioris to reduce incidence of ptosis

Overdose

- Symptoms of overdose are likely not to be present immediately following injection. Cautious on pharyngeal, laryngeal, or respiratory muscle weakness, which causes dysphagia and breathing difficulties. Antidote is available from the Centers for Disease Control (CDC)

Long-Term Use

- Safe for long-term use

Habit Forming

- No

How to Stop

- No risk in abrupt discontinuation

Pharmacokinetics

- No systemic kinetic profile. However, the half-life of onabotulinumtoxinA is more than 4 months. Half-life varies among other serotypes

 Drug Interactions

- Concomitant use of aminoglycosides may enhance neuromuscular blocking action
- Concomitant use of anticholinergic agents may potentiate systemic anticholinergic effects
- Concomitant use of agents interfering with neuromuscular transmission may enhance neuromuscular blocking action and prolong respiratory depression

 Other Warnings/Precautions

- Corneal exposure and ulceration due to reduced blinking
- Retrobulbar hemorrhage
- Autonomic dysreflexia
- Immunogenicity
- Contains albumin, a blood derivative that can theoretically carry risk of viral infection or Creutzfeldt-Jacob disease
- Potential exacerbation in patients with preexisting peripheral motor neuropathic disorder and neuromuscular junction disorder

Do Not Use

- Hypersensitivity to the formulation of botulinum toxin A
- Infection at the proposed injection sites
- OAB with acute urinary tract infection

SPECIAL POPULATIONS

Renal Impairment

- No adjustment needed

Hepatic Impairment

- No adjustment needed

Cardiac Impairment

- Reports of arrhythmia and infarction

Elderly

- Starting at low dose

 Children and Adolescents

- Safety has not been evaluated in patients less than 12 years of age. Studied in children 12 and older for strabismus and blepharospasm, 16 and older for CD, and 18 and over for hyperhidrosis. Used for treatment of sialorrhea in cerebral palsy

 Pregnancy

• Category C. Use only if potential benefit outweighs risk to the fetus

Breast Feeding

• Not recommended

THE ART OF NEUROPHARMACOLOGY

Potential Advantages

• Effective local treatment for focal dystonia/blepharospasm/spasticity. Reduces headache frequency and severity in chronic migraineurs

Potential Disadvantages

• Potential spread of toxin

Primary Target Symptoms

• Headache frequency and severity
• Abnormal muscle dystonia or spasticity
• Sweating or drooling

 Pearls

• Botulinum toxin type A and type B are equally effective in focal dystonias. Generalized dystonias can be treated with anticholinergic therapy, especially in younger, cognitively normal patients
• Tolerance may occur if given more frequently than every 3 months. Very rarely, patient may develop neutralizing antibody-induced therapy failure
• For migraine, Botox doses between 150 u and 195 u are efficacious (headache days, crystal clear days) with limited side effects. It usually takes around 2–3 cycles of treatment to reach full effectiveness. It was

more effective than steroid but not better than topiramate, valproate, or amitriptyline in reducing chronic migraine frequency. However, patient compliance is better for onabotulinumtoxin due to fewer AEs
• Migraines with imploding and ocular headaches respond better than exploding ones. Not effective for episodic migraine or chronic tension-type headache
• Consider as an alternative for patients with focal "nummular" (coin-shaped) headache and trigeminal neuralgia
• May be useful in treating trigeminal neuralgia, SUNCT (short-lasting unilateral neuralgiform headache attacks with conjunctival injection and tearing), SUNA (short-lasting unilateral neuralgiform headache attacks with cranial autonomic symptoms), or hemicranias continua. However, strong evidence is lacking
• Botox to Xeomin conversion factor 1:1. Botox to Dysport conversion factor roughly 1:3. Type A to type B conversion factor roughly 1:40–66.6
• Anterocollis (forward neck flexion) is often associated with neuroleptic exposure and parkinsonism and is the most difficult CD to treat. Injections of sternocleidomastoid and anterior scalene muscles are standard but fluoroscopic injections of deep cervical flexors may reduce clinical failures
• In oromandibular dystonia, botulinum toxin appears more effective in jaw-closing dystonias than jaw-opening or mixed dystonias
• Meige syndrome is a combination of dystonias, including blepharospasm plus oromandibular dystonia. Symptoms may also include tongue protrusion, light sensitivity, muddled speech, contraction of the platysma muscle, and laryngeal dystonia. In addition to the usual sites for blepharospasm and oromandibular dystonia, consider injections of zygomaticus (usually 2.5–7.5 u) and risorius (2.5–10 u)
• May be useful for Gilles de la Tourette syndrome and essential tremor

Suggested Reading

Albanese A, Asmus F, Bhatia KP, Elia AE, Elibol B, Filippini G, et al. EFNS guidelines on diagnosis and treatment of primary dystonias. *Eur J Neurol.* 2011;18(1):5–18.

Batla A, Stamelou M, Bhatia KP. Treatment of focal dystonia. *Curr Treat Options Neurol.* 2012;14(3):213–29.

Delgado MR, Hirtz D, Aisen M, Ashwal S, Fehlings DL, McLaughlin J, et al. Practice parameter: pharmacologic treatment of spasticity in children and adolescents with cerebral palsy (an evidence-based review): report of the Quality Standards Subcommittee of the American Academy of Neurology and the Practice Committee of the Child Neurology Society. *Neurology.* 2010;74(4):336–43.

Hu Y, Guan X, Fan L, Li M, Liao Y, Nie Z, et al. Therapeutic efficacy and safety of botulinum toxin type A in trigeminal neuralgia: a systematic review. *J Headache Pain.* 2013;14(1):72.

Jackson JL, Kuriyama A, Hayashino Y. Botulinum toxin A for prophylactic treatment of migraine and tension headaches in adults: a meta-analysis. *JAMA.* 2012;307(16): 1736–45.

Ramachandran R, Yaksh TL. Therapeutic use of botulinum toxin in migraine: mechanisms of action. *Br J Pharmacol.* 2014;171(18): 4177–92.

Ramirez-Castaneda J, Jankovic J, Comella C, Dashtipour K, Fernandez HH, Mari Z. Diffusion, spread, and migration of botulinum toxin. *Mov Disord.* 2013;28(13):1775–83.

Zesiewicz TA, Elble RJ, Louis ED, Gronseth GS, Ondo WG, Dewey RB, et al. Evidence-based guideline update: treatment of essential tremor: report of the Quality Standards subcommittee of the American Academy of Neurology. *Neurology.* 2011;77(19): 1752–5.

BOTULINUM TOXIN TYPE B

THERAPEUTICS

Brands
• Rimabotulinumtoxin B (Myobloc, Neurobloc)

Generic?
• No

 Class
• Neurotoxin

Commonly Prescribed for
(FDA approved in bold)
• **Cervical dystonia (CD)**
• Glabellar lines
• Axillary hyperhidrosis
• Strabismus and blepharospasm associated with dystonia
• Hemifacial spasm
• Spasmodic torticollis
• Spasmodic dysphonia (laryngeal dystonia)
• Writer's cramp and other task-specific dystonias
• Spasticity associated with stroke
• Dynamic muscle contracture in cerebral palsy
• Sialorrhea (drooling)
• Headache
• Myofascial pain

 How the Drug Works
• Blocks neuromuscular transmission by cleaving the vesicle-associated membrane protein (VAMP; synaptobrevin), which inhibits the vesicular release of acetylcholine from nerve terminals
• In CD and other dystonias, produces partial denervation of muscle and localized reduction in muscle activity. In hyperhidrosis, produces chemical denervation of sweat glands
• Also appears to inhibit release of neurotransmitters involved in pain transmission (including glutamate, calcitonin gene-related peptide, and substance P) and may enter CNS via retrograde axonal transport

How Long Until It Works
• Usually 1–3 days with peak effect beginning at 2 weeks

If It Works
• Continue to use as long as effective, but monitor for clinical effects

If It Doesn't Work
• Increase dose or change injection technique. Some pain disorders may respond better to oral medications

 Best Augmenting Combos for Partial Response or Treatment-Resistance
• Increase dose or number of injections or change site of location

Tests
• None

ADVERSE EFFECTS (AEs)

How the Drug Causes AEs
• Most AEs are related to muscle weakness adjacent to the site of injection. Serious systemic AEs are rare, but injectors should use the lowest dose and be familiar with injection technique to minimize AEs

Notable AEs
• Injection site pain and hemorrhage, dry mouth, infection, fever, headache, pruritus, and myalgia. Most AEs depend on site of injection
• CD: dysphagia, neck weakness, upper respiratory infection
• Spasmodic dysphonia: hypophonia ("breathy" voice)

 Life-Threatening or Dangerous AEs
• Rarely patients may experience severe dysphagia requiring a feeding tube or leading to aspiration pneumonia
• Use with caution in patients with motor neuropathies or neuromuscular junctional disorders. These patients may be at greater risk for systemic weakness or respiratory problems

Weight Gain
- Unusual

unusual   not unusual   common   problematic

Sedation
- Unusual

unusual   not unusual   common   problematic

What to Do About AEs
- Most AEs will decrease with time (weeks)

Best Augmenting Agents to Reduce AEs
- Most AEs cannot be reduced with an augmenting agent

DOSING AND USE

Usual Dosage Range
- CD: total dose 5000–10,000 units (u)
- Hemifacial spasm: total dose 200–800 u
- Spasmodic dysphonia: 50–250 u
- Sialorrhea: 1000 u each side, up to 2500 bilaterally

Dosage Forms
- Lyophilized powder, 700 kDa. 2500, 5000, 10000 u per vial

How to Dose
- Administer every 3 months using the lowest effective dose
- CD: start at a low dose and adjust as needed. Limiting the dose injected into the sternocleidomastoid muscles to 2000 u or less may decrease incidence of dysphagia
- Spasmodic dysphonia: for more common adductor type inject 50–100 u into each side of the thyroarytenoid muscles, for abductor type inject the posterior cricoarytenoid
- Sialorrhea: inject 500–10000 u into each parotid gland and 250 u into each submandibular gland. The mandibular glands may also be injected

 Dosing Tips
- Physicians should be familiar with the anatomy of the injection site and the specific disorders

- Inject using a needle or hollow electrode
- EMG recording helps to indentify muscle involved in complex dystonias
- May dilute with saline but administer within 4 hours as product does not contain a preservative

Overdose
- Signs and symptoms of overdose may be delayed for several weeks. If accidental overdose occurs, monitor for signs of systemic weakness or paralysis

Long-Term Use
- Safe for long-term use

Habit Forming
- No

How to Stop
- No need to taper

Pharmacokinetics
- Does not reach peripheral blood after injection with recommended doses

 Drug Interactions
- Use with caution in patients taking medications, such as aminoglycosides or curare-like compounds, that can interfere with neuromuscular transmission

 Other Warning/Precautions
- Contains albumin, a blood derivative that can theoretically carry risk of viral infection or Creutzfeldt-Jacob disease

Do Not Use
- Hypersensitivity to the drug or any of its components; infection at the proposed injection sites

SPECIAL POPULATIONS

Renal Impairment
- No known effects

Hepatic Impairment
- No known effects

Cardiac Impairment
- No known effects

Elderly
- No known effects

Children and Adolescents
- Safety and effectiveness unknown

Pregnancy
- Category C. Use only if benefit of medication outweighs risks

Breast Feeding
- Concentration in breast milk unknown. Use only if benefits outweigh risk

THE ART OF NEUROPHARMACOLOGY

Potential Advantages
- Effective in CD and most likely other pain disorders, with very few AEs or drug interactions. Compared to type A may have faster onset of action

Potential Disadvantages
- Cost and need for frequent injections to maintain effect. Dose requirement increases with muscle size. Effect may wear off sooner than with type A formulations

Primary Target Symptoms
- Dystonia, spasticity, pain, drooling, or sweating (depending on indication)

 Pearls
- Botulinum toxin type A and type B are equally effective in focal dystonias. Generalized dystonias can be treated with anticholinergic therapy, especially in younger, cognitively normal patients
- It often takes a series of injections to determine the optimal dose for a given patient
- Botulinum toxin type B has not been extensively studied for the treatment of headache, neuropathic pain, or blepharospasm
- Some studies indicate that type B starts working earlier and produces a quicker recovery than type A, but that the duration of effect might be less. This could be due to the inability to convert doses, making it difficult to compare different formulations
- Type B may disperse from injection sites to a greater extent than type A toxin; this could also be due to conversion error between two formulations
- Type B seems to have more affinity for the autonomic system than type A toxin
- To date, there does not appear to be antibody production against type B toxin
- Type A to type B conversion factor roughly 1:40–66.6

Suggested Reading

Albanese A, Asmus F, Bhatia KP, Elia AE, Elibol B, Filippini G, et al. EFNS guidelines on diagnosis and treatment of primary dystonias. *Eur J Neurol.* 2011;18(1):5–18.

Batla A, Stamelou M, Bhatia KP. Treatment of focal dystonia. *Curr Treat Options Neurol.* 2012;14(3):213–29.

Delgado MR, Hirtz D, Aisen M, Ashwal S, Fehlings DL, McLaughlin J, et al. Practice parameter: pharmacologic treatment of spasticity in children and adolescents with cerebral palsy (an evidence-based review): report of the Quality Standards Subcommittee of the American Academy of Neurology and the Practice Committee of the Child Neurology Society. *Neurology.* 2010;74(4): 336–43.

Ramirez-Castaneda J, Jankovic J, Comella C, Dashtipour K, Fernandez HH, Mari Z. Diffusion, spread, and migration of botulinum toxin. *Mov Disord.* 2013;28(13):1775–83.

BROMOCRIPTINE

THERAPEUTICS

Brands
- Parlodel, Serocryptin, Cycloset

Generic?
- Yes

Class
- Antiparkinson agent, ergot

Commonly Prescribed for
(FDA approved in bold)
- **Parkinson's disease (PD)**
- **Acromegaly**
- **Hyperprolactinemia**
- **Adjunct therapy for type 2 diabetes mellitus**

How the Drug Works
- Dopamine agonist, with high affinity for the D_2 receptor (less potent than pergolide or cabergoline). This action is the reason for effectiveness. Also has weak α agonist and $5-HT_{1A/1D}$ agonist activity. In the treatment of hormone-secreting pituitary adenomas, bromocriptine works as a dopamine agonist, which inhibits prolactin-secreting cells in the anterior pituitary, reducing tumor size
- Bromocriptine alters neurotransmitter levels within hypothalamic circadian centers and affects glucose and lipid metabolism

How Long Until It Works
- PD: weeks

If It Works
- PD: may require dose adjustments over time or augmentation with other agents. Most PD patients will eventually require carbidopa-levodopa to manage their symptoms

If It Doesn't Work
- PD: bradykinesia, gait, and tremor should improve. Non-motor symptoms including autonomic symptoms such as postural hypotension, depression, and bladder dysfunction do not improve. If the patient has significantly impaired functioning, add or replace with levodopa

Best Augmenting Combos for Partial Response or Treatment-Resistance
- For suboptimal effectiveness, add carbidopa-levodopa with or without a catechol-O-methyltransferase (COMT) inhibitor. Monoamine oxidase (MAO)-B inhibitor may also be beneficial
- For younger patients with bothersome tremor: anticholinergics may help
- For severe motor fluctuations and/or dyskinesias with good "on" time, functional neurosurgery (deep brain stimulation) is an option
- Depression is common in PD and may respond to low-dose SSRIs
- Cognitive impairment/dementia is common in mid- to late-stage PD and may improve with acetylcholinesterase inhibitors
- For patients with late-stage PD experiencing hallucinations or delusions, withdraw bromocriptine and consider oral atypical neuroleptics (quetiapine, olanzapine, clozapine). Acute psychosis is a medical emergency that may require hospitalization and low-dose haloperidol for stabilization

Tests
- None required

ADVERSE EFFECTS (AEs)

How the Drug Causes AEs
- Direct effect on dopamine receptors

Notable AEs
- Nausea/vomiting, constipation, orthostatic hypotension/syncope, confusion, dyskinesias, hallucinations, nervousness, drowsiness, and anorexia
- Signs of ergotism such as digital vasospasm, tingling in the fingertips, Raynaud phenomenon, cold feet, and muscle cramps are uncommon, especially at lower doses

Life-Threatening or Dangerous AEs
- May cause somnolence or sudden-onset sleep, often without warning

- Rare pulmonary or retroperitoneal fibrosis, pleural or pericardial effusions
- High doses are associated with confusion, mental disturbances and hallucinations
- Rare but significant increases in blood pressure can occur, often delayed until a week after initiating therapy. Seizures or strokes have occurred rarely, often preceded by severe progressive headaches or visual disturbances. Less commonly myocardial infarction has occurred

Weight Gain

- Unusual

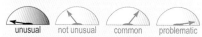

Sedation

- Common

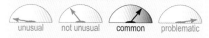

What to Do About AEs

- Nausea can be problematic when starting – titrate slowly
- Hallucinations or delusions may require stopping the medication
- Warn patients about the risk of excessive sleepiness while driving

Best Augmenting Agents to Reduce AEs

- Amantadine may help suppress dyskinesias
- Orthostatic hypotension: adjust dose or stop antihypertensives, add dietary salt, and consider fludrocortisone or midodrine
- Urinary incontinence: reducing PM fluids, voiding schedules, oxybutynin, desmopressin nasal spray, hyoscyamine sulfate, urological evaluation

DOSING AND USE

Usual Dosage Range

- PD: 5–40 mg daily, divided into 2 daily doses
- Hyperprolactinemia: 2.5–15 mg daily
- Acromegaly: 20–60 mg daily

Dosage Forms

- Tablets: 2.5 and 5 mg
- Cycloset: 0.8 mg

How to Dose

- Start at 1.25 or 2.5 mg at bedtime to increase tolerance, then dose twice daily. Increase the daily dose by 1.25 or 2.5 mg every 1–2 weeks

 Dosing Tips

- Slow titration will minimize nausea and dizziness

Overdose

- Symptoms may include nausea/vomiting, constipation, diaphoresis, dizziness, severe hypotension, lethargy, malaise, and hallucinations. Treatment of hypotension with vasopressors may be required in severe cases

Long-Term Use

- Retroperitoneal fibrosis has been reported with patients using for more than 2 years at high doses (30 mg or more). Effectiveness may decrease over time in PD

Habit Forming

- No

How to Stop

- Discontinue over a period of 1 week. PD symptoms may worsen, but serious AEs from discontinuation are rare. In patients using for pituitary disorders, tumor regrowth can occur

Pharmacokinetics

- Metabolized by CYP3A4. About 28% of drug is absorbed. Elimination half-life 2–8 hours. Highly protein bound

 Drug Interactions

- Increases the effect of levodopa
- Erythromycin increases levels
- Dopamine antagonists, such as phenothiazines and metoclopramide, diminish effectiveness
- Use with caution in patients on antihypertensive medications due to orthostatic hypotension
- Sympathomimetics such as isometheptene, phenylpropanolamine can increase AEs and case reports of ventricular tachycardia and cardiac dysfunction exist

- CYP3A4 inhibitors (protease inhibitors, macrolides, azoles) and inducers (carbamazepine, phenytoin, phenobarbital, rifampin, corticosteroid, pioglitazone) can alter bromocriptine's serum concentration

 Other Warnings/ Precautions

- During the first days of treatment, hypotensive reactions may occasionally occur and result in reduced alertness; particular care should be exercised when driving a vehicle or operating machinery

Do Not Use

- Known hypersensitivity to the drug or other ergots. Uncontrolled hypertension. Patients with eclampia, preeclampsia or pregnancy-induced hypertension, or post-partum patients with coronary artery disease or other severe cardiovascular condition

SPECIAL POPULATIONS

Renal Impairment

- No known effects

Hepatic Impairment

- No known effects

Cardiac Impairment

- Infrequently causes cardiac arrhythmias, rarely ventricular tachycardia. Use with caution

Elderly

- No known effects

 Children and Adolescents

- Use in PD is not studied in children (PD is rare) but does appear effective for the treatment of prolactin-secreting tumors in ages 16 and up. Has been used in children as young as 11

 Pregnancy

- Category B. Safety has not been established. For PD, use only if benefits of medication outweigh risks. In patients with prolactin-secreting adenomas, do a pregnancy test

every 4 weeks as long as no menses occur. If pregnancy is established, discontinue bromocriptine and monitor closely for signs of tumor regrowth

Breast Feeding

- Inhibits prolactin secretion. Do not use

THE ART OF NEUROPHARMACOLOGY

Potential Advantages

- In PD, may delay need for levodopa and decreases risk of motor dyskinesias. Less likely to cause sleep disturbances than non-ergot agonists

Potential Disadvantages

- Generally less effective than levodopa and more AEs such as hallucinations, somnolence, and orthostatic hypotension. Risk of serious complications (retroperitoneal fibrosis) with long-term use

Primary Target Symptoms

- PD: motor dysfunction including bradykinesia, hand coordination, gait and rest tremor

 Pearls

- More serious AEs than some of the newer dopamine agonists, which limits use
- For patients with mildly symptomatic disease, dopamine agonists are also appropriate for initial therapy, but for patients with significant disability, use levodopa early. Patients with poor response to levodopa will not benefit from bromocriptine
- Bromocriptine has minimal effect on the secretion of pituitary hormones other than prolactin and growth hormone. About 75% of patients with galactorrhea respond to therapy, usually within 12 weeks. Menses are usually reinitiated prior to complete cessation of galactorrhea, on average in 6–8 weeks
- Carbegoline is more favorable than bromocriptine in the treatment of hyperprolactinemia on prolactin normalization and with fewer adverse effects
- No evidence suggests its role in the treatment of tardive syndrome

Suggested Reading

Bhidayasiri R, Fahn S, Weiner WJ, Gronseth GS, Sullivan KL, Zesiewicz TA; American Academy of Neurology. Evidence-based guideline: treatment of tardive syndromes: report of the Guideline Development Subcommittee of the American Academy of Neurology. *Neurology* 2013;81:463–9.

Brocks DR. Anticholinergic drugs used in Parkinson's disease: an overlooked class of drugs from a pharmacokinetic perspective. *J Pharm Pharm Sci.* 1999;2(2):39–46.

Costa J, Espírito-Santo C, Borges A, Ferreira JJ, Coelho M, Sampaio C. Botulinum toxin type A versus anticholinergics for cervical dystonia. *Cochrane Database Syst Rev.* 2005;1: CD004312.

Defronzo RA. Bromocriptine: a sympatholytic, d2-dopamine agonist for the treatment of type 2 diabetes. *Diabetes Care.* 2011;34(4): 789–94.

dos Santos Nunes V, Dib El R, Boguszewski CL, Nogueira CR. Cabergoline versus bromocriptine in the treatment of hyperprolactinemia: a systematic review of randomized controlled trials and meta-analysis. *Pituitary.* 2011; 14(3):259–65.

Mizuno Y, Yanagisawa N, Kuno S, Yamamoto M, Hasegawa K, Origasa H, Kowa H; Japanese Pramipexole Study Group. Randomized, double-blind study of pramipexole with placebo and bromocriptine in advanced Parkinson's disease. *Mov Disord.* 2003;18(10):1149–56.

van Hilten JJ, Ramaker CC, Stowe R, Ives NJ. Bromocriptine versus levodopa in early Parkinson's disease. *Cochrane Database Syst Rev.* 2007 Oct 17;4:CD002258.

BUPROPION

THERAPEUTICS

Brands
- Wellbutrin, Wellbutrin SR, Wellbutrin XL, Aplenzin, Forfivo XL, Zyban, Contrave

Generic?
- Yes

Class
- Atypical antidepressant

Commonly Prescribed for
(FDA approved in bold)
- **Major depressive disorder**
- **Seasonal affective disorder (Wellbutrin XL only)**
- **Smoking cessation (Zyban only)**
- **Weight loss (Contrave only)**
- Neuropathic pain
- Attention deficit hyperactivity disorder
- Hypoactive sexual desire disorder
- Methamphetamine withdrawal

How the Drug Works
- Both bupropion and its metabolite (hydroxybupropion; half as potent as bupropion) inhibit reuptake of norepinephrine and dopamine
- It also blocks nicotinic acetylcholine receptors
- It does not block reuptake of serotonin nor inhibit monoamine oxidase

How Long Until It Works
- It may take more than 1 month for full effect

If It Works
- Continue to use and monitor for AEs. May continue for 1 year following first depression episode or indefinitely if > 1 episode of depression

If It Doesn't Work
- Increase to highest tolerated dose. Change to another agent or add a second agent

Best Augmenting Combos for Partial Response or Treatment-Resistance
- Low-dose polytherapy with 2 or more drugs may be better tolerated and more effective than high-dose monotherapy

Tests
- Not available. Monitor blood pressure, seizures, suicidality, and unusual psychiatric behavior

ADVERSE EFFECTS (AEs)

How the Drug Causes AEs
- By increasing dopamine and norepinephrine concentrations at non-therapeutic responsive receptors throughout the body. Most AEs are dose- and time-dependent

Notable AEs
- ≥ 5%: agitation, dry mouth, constipation, headache, nausea, vomiting, dizziness, hyperhidrosis, tremor, insomnia, blurred vision, tachycardia, confusion, rash, hostility, cardiac arrhythmia, hypertension, auditory disturbance

Life-Threatening or Dangerous AEs
- Worsening of depression and suicidality
- Rare hepatitis
- Rare activation of mania or suicidal ideation
- Rare worsening of coexisting seizure disorders

Weight Gain
- Unusual

unusual   not unusual   common   problematic

Sedation
- Unusual

unusual   not unusual   common   problematic

What to Do About AEs

- For minor AEs, lower dose, titrate slower, or switch to another agent. For serious AEs, lower dose and consider stopping, taper to avoid withdrawal symptoms

Best Augmenting Agents to Reducing AEs

- Try magnesium for constipation

DOSING AND USE

Usual Dosage Range

- 75–450 mg/day

Dosage Forms

- Tablet (immediate-release): 75, 100 mg
- Tablet (extended release; 12 h [ER-12h]): 100, 150, 200 mg
- Tablet (extended release; 24 h [ER-24h]): 150, 300, 450 mg
- Tablet (extended release): 174, 348, 522 mg

How to Dose

MDD:
- Immediate release: initial 200 mg/day in 2 divided doses. Maintenance 300 mg/day in 3 divided doses. Maximum 450 mg/day in 3–4 divided doses
- ER-12h: initial 150 mg once daily. Maintenance 150 mg twice daily.
- ER-24h: initial 150 mg once daily. Maintenance 300 or 450 mg once daily

Seasonal affective disorder (Wellbutrin XL):
- Initial 150 mg/day. Maintenance 300 mg/day

Smoking cessation (Zyban):
- Initial 150 mg/day. Increase to 300 mg/day after 3 days. Typically use for 3–6 months

 Dosing Tips

- Higher doses are typically used for pain. Extended-release formulation allows for once-a-day dosing and may be better tolerated. Extended-release tablets should be swallowed whole

Overdose

- Signs and symptoms may include seizure, hallucination, altered mental status, arrhythmia, fever, muscle rigidity, hypotension, stupor, coma

Long-Term Use

- Safe for long-term use. Increases the risk of seizure and hepatitis

Habit Forming

- No

How to Stop

- Taper slowly to avoid withdrawal (taper to 150 mg/day for 2 weeks before discontinuation)

Pharmacokinetics

- Extensively metabolized via the CYP2B6 isoenzyme
- Wellbutrin: Bupropion C_{max} 2 hours. Hydroxybupropion C_{max} 3 hours
- Wellbutrin XL: Bupropion C_{max} 5 hours. Hydroxybupropion C_{max} 7 hours
- Wellbutrin SR: Bupropion C_{max} 3 hours. Hydroxybupropion C_{max} 6 hours
- Forfivo XL: Bupropion C_{max} 5 hours (fasted) or 12 hours (fed) O Hydroxybupropion C_{max} 10 hours (fasted) and 16 hours (fed)
- Half-life 20 hours. Eliminated via urine (87%) and feces (10%)

 Drug Interactions

- CYP2B6 inhibitors (orphenadrine, thiotepa, cyclophosphamide, ticlopidine, clopidogrel) reduce the hydroxybupropion concentration. Coadministration not recommended
- CYP2B6 inducers (rifampin, phenobarbital, ritonavir, efavirenz) reduce bupropion concentration. Patients may require increased dose but should not exceed the maximum recommended dose
- Bupropion/hydroxybupropion inhibits CYP2D6, affecting venlafaxine, nortriptyline, imipramine, paroxetine, fluoxetine, antipsychotics (haloperidol, risperidone), β-blocker (metoprolol), antiarrhythmics (propafenone), mexiletine, lidocaine, and chlorpromazine
- Drugs that lower seizure threshold: antipsychotics, other antidepressants, theophylline, and systemic corticosteroids

 Other Warnings/ Precautions

- Increased risk of seizure

- Patients should be observed closely for clinical worsening, suicidality, and changes in behavior in known or unknown bipolar disorder

Do Not Use

- Seizure disorder
- Current or prior diagnosis of bulimia or anorexia nervosa
- Undergoing abrupt discontinuation of alcohol or sedative
- Proven hypersensitivity to drug
- Concurrently with MAOI; allow at least 14 days after discontinuation of an MAOI
- Uncontrolled angle-closure glaucoma

SPECIAL POPULATIONS

Renal Impairment

- Use with caution. Decrease usual dose by 25–50%
- Not recommended for Forfivo XL

Hepatic Impairment

- Use with caution. Decrease usual dose by 50%
- In moderate to severe hepatic impairment, maximum dose is 75 mg/day (Wellbutrin), 100 mg/day (Wellbutrin SR), and 150 mg/2 days (Wellbutrin XL). Forfivo XL is not recommended

Cardiac Impairment

- Use with caution. Dose-dependent effect on blood pressure

Elderly

- Reduce dose and monitor renal and hepatic function

Children and Adolescents

- Safety and efficacy not established. Use with caution. Observe closely for clinical worsening, suicidality, and changes in behavior in known or unknown bipolar disorder. Parents should be informed and advised of the risks

Pregnancy

- Category C. Generally not recommended during pregnancy

Breast Feeding

- Some drug is found in breast milk and use while breast feeding is not recommended

THE ART OF NEUROPHARMACOLOGY

Potential Advantages

- Can promote weight loss. Lack of sexual side effects. Less sedation

Potential Disadvantages

- Risk of seizure, serotonin syndrome, and suicidality

Primary Target Symptoms

- Reduction in depression
- Reduce nicotine withdrawal syndrome

Pearls

- Compared with other SSRIs, it has less sexual dysfunction and weight gain side effect
- Bupropion prolongs REM sleep latency and increases REM density (a measure of the number of eye movements in the period) and activity during the first REM sleep period
- Bupropion SR improves neuropathic pain for at least 6 weeks
- Bupropion SR or XL can be a second-line agent for ADHD
- Bupropion/Naltrexone (Contrave) extended release is used as an adjunct therapy to behavioral modification (e.g., reduced-calorie diet and increased physical activity) for chronic weight management. Bupropion increases pro-opiomelanocortin (POMC) neuron firing within hypothalamus (arcuate nucleus), releasing α-melanocyte-stimulating hormone (mild anorectic) and β-endorphin (autoinhibitory effect via opioid receptors on POMC). Naltrexone prevents this autoinhibition on POMC thus promoting the weight loss effect. Weight loss of 5–9% in the first year but its effectiveness may wane in the second year. Combination of zonisamide and bupropion is currently under investigation for the treatment of obesity
- It may have positive effect on various aspects of sexual function (e.g., sexual arousal, orgasm completion, sexual satisfaction) in premenopausal women diagnosed with hypoactive sexual desire disorder

Suggested Reading

Carroll FI, Blough BE, Mascarella SW, Navarro HA, Lukas RJ, Damaj MI. Bupropion and bupropion analogs as treatments for CNS disorders. In Dwoskin LP, ed. *Emerging Targets & Therapeutics in the Treatment of Psychostimulant Abuse* Vol. 69 *(Advances in Pharmacology).* San Diego: Academic Press, 2014; pp. 177–216.

Kooij SJJ, Bejerot S, Blackwell A, Caci H, Casas-Brugué M, Carpentier PJ, et al. European consensus statement on diagnosis and treatment of adult ADHD: The European Network Adult ADHD. *BMC Psychiatry.* 2010;10:67.

Semenchuk MR, Sherman S, Davis B. Double-blind, randomized trial of bupropion SR for the treatment of neuropathic pain. *Neurology.* 2001;57(9):1583–8.

CARBAMAZEPINE

THERAPEUTICS

Brands

- Tegretol, Carbatrol, Tegretol XR, Equetro, Teril, Timonil, Carbagen, Arbil, Epimaz, Mazepine, Novo-Carbamaz

Generic?

- Yes

 Class

- Antiepileptic drug (AED)

Commonly Prescribed for

(FDA approved in bold)
- **Complex partial seizures with or without secondary generalization (adults and children, monotherapy and adjunctive)**
- **Generalized tonic-clonic seizures**
- **Mixed seizure patterns (except absence seizures, juvenile myoclonic epilepsy)**
- **Trigeminal neuralgia**
- **Bipolar I disorder (acute manic and mixed episodes)**
- Glossopharyngeal neuralgia
- Lennox-Gastaut syndrome
- Neuropathic pain
- Alcohol withdrawal
- Restless leg syndrome
- Psychosis/schizophrenia (adjunctive)

 How the Drug Works

- Blocks voltage-dependent sodium channels
- Modulates sodium and calcium (L type) channels and NMDA glutamate transmission

How Long Until It Works

- Seizures: 2 weeks or less
- Trigeminal neuralgia or neuropathic pain: hours to weeks
- Mania: weeks

If It Works

- Seizures: goal is the remission of seizures. Continue as long as effective and well tolerated. Consider tapering and slowly stopping after 2 years without seizures, depending on the type of epilepsy
- Trigeminal neuralgia: should dramatically reduce or eliminate attacks, pain may recur. Periodically attempt to reduce to lowest effective dose or discontinue

If It Doesn't Work

- Increase to highest tolerated dose. Subject to autoinduction, meaning that dose requirements can change over time
- Epilepsy: consider changing to another agent, adding a second agent, using a medical device, or a referral for epilepsy surgery evaluation. When adding a second agent, keep drug interactions in mind. Check level if compliance is in question
- Trigeminal neuralgia: try an alternative agent. For truly refractory patients referral to tertiary headache center, consider surgical or other procedures

 Best Augmenting Combos for Partial Response or Treatment-Resistance

- Epilepsy: drug interactions can complicate multi-drug therapy
- Pain: can combine with other AEDs (gabapentin or pregabalin) or TCAs

Tests

- Baseline CBC, liver, kidney, and thyroid tests
- Check CBC biweekly for 2 months then every 3 months
- Liver, kidney, and thyroid tests every 6–12 months
- Check sodium levels for symptoms of hyponatremia

ADVERSE EFFECTS (AEs)

How the Drug Causes AEs

- CNS AEs are probably caused by sodium channel blockade effects
- Mild anticholinergic side effects

Notable AEs

- Sedation, dizziness, ataxia, headache, nystagmus
- Nausea, vomiting, abdominal pain, constipation, pancreatitis, loss of sex drive
- Aching joints and leg cramps
- Elevated liver enzymes. Hyponatremia
- Benign leukopenia (transient; in up to 10%)

Life-Threatening or Dangerous AEs

- Rare blood dyscrasias: aplastic anemia, agranulocytosis (mean exposure 49 days to onset; mean duration 6 days)
- Dermatological reactions including toxic epidermal necrolysis and Stevens-Johnson syndrome (SJS; more common in patients with HLA-B*1502 or HLA-A*3101 alleles). Can aggravate rash of lupus
- Can reduce thyroid function
- Hyponatremia/SIADH (syndrome of inappropriate antidiuretic hormone secretion)
- May increase seizure frequency in patients with generalized seizure disorders

Weight Gain

- Not unusual

unusual   not unusual   common   problematic

Sedation

- Problematic

unusual   not unusual   common   problematic

- May limit use

What to Do About AEs

- Take with food, split dose, and take higher dose at night to improve tolerability
- Extended-release form may be better tolerated
- Rashes are common but usually not severe. Usually resolve with time or decreased dose. If severe stop drug. Do HLA typing prior to use in Asian patients
- Elevated liver enzymes usually resolve spontaneously

Best Augmenting Agents to Reduce AEs

- Topical corticosteroids or antihistamines for rash

DOSING AND USE

Usual Dosage Range

- Epilepsy: 800–1200 mg/day, twice daily. Maximum 1600 mg/day

- Trigeminal neuralgia: 400–800 mg/day. Maximum 1200 mg/day
- Bipolar disorder: 400–1600 mg/day

Dosage Forms

- Chewable tablets: 100 mg; tablets: 200 mg; oral solution: 100 mg/5 mL; extended-release tablets: 100, 200, or 400 mg; extended-release capsules 100, 200, or 300 mg

How to Dose

- Epilepsy: age > 12: start at 200 mg/day in 2 divided doses. Titrate by 200 mg/week, in 2 doses/day for extended release and 3–4 doses/day for other formulations, until optimal. Age < 12: start and titrate in half dose. Maximum 1000 mg/day. Age < 6: 10–20 mg/kg/day in 2 divided doses. Maximum 35 mg/kg/day
- Trigeminal neuralgia/pain: start at 200 mg/day and increase by 200 mg/week to goal dose
- Do not check levels in the first few weeks due to autoinduction
- Adjust dose as needed when using with AEDs or other drugs that affect levels

 Dosing Tips

- Take with food to avoid GI side effects
- Slow titration will help avoid blood dyscrasias and other AEs
- Carbamazepine induces its own metabolism (autoinduction), meaning the effect can decrease with time
- Oral suspension has higher peak levels than other formulations. Start at a lower dose and titrate more slowly

Overdose

- Coma, ataxia, nystagmus, cerebellar signs, dizziness. Less commonly urinary retention, chorea, or seizures. Intraventicular conduction delay. Manage with stomach lavage or hemodialysis

Long-Term Use

- Safe for long-term use. Monitor CBC, sodium, liver, kidney, and thyroid function

Habit Forming

- No

How to Stop
- Taper slowly
- Abrupt withdrawal can lead to seizures in patients with epilepsy

Pharmacokinetics
- Hepatic metabolism via CYP450 system, CYP3A4. Inducer of CYP3A4 metabolism
- Highly protein bound, renally excreted
- Bioavailability is 75–85%
- Peak levels at 4–8 hours, plasma half-life 18–55 hours initially, decreasing to 5–26 hours after autoinduction

 Drug Interactions
- Carbamazepine decreases levels of many AEDs (valproate, clonazepam, topiramate, zonisamide, tiagabine, and ethosuxamide) and also warfarin, doxycycline, acetaminophen, haloperidol, nortriptyline, nifedipine, trazadone, alprazolam, among many
- Carbamazepine increases levels of flunarizine, digitalis, lithium, furosemide, isoniazid, and MAOIs
- Variable effect on phenytoin and phenobarbital
- Level decreased by CYP3A4 inducers (carbamazepine, lamotrigine, phenytoin, primidone, phenobarbital, felbamate, and others)
- Level increased by CYP3A4 inhibitors (acetazolamide, caffeine, verapamil, fluozetine, desipramine and many others)
- Valproate and clonazepam have a variable effect on levels

 Other Warnings/Precautions
- CNS AEs increase when used with other CNS depressants
- Rare systemic disorders: dermatomyositis, diabetes insipidus
- Rare worsening of acute angle-closure glaucoma
- Long-term treatment may affect bone metabolism
- May cause alterations in sex hormone levels and impair effectiveness of oral contraceptives
- Decrease of sex drive or fertility
- May worsen absence or mixed absence epilepsy syndromes

- Asian patients have a greater risk of SJS
- Do not take with MAOI

Do Not Use
- Patients with a proven allergy to carbamazepine

Renal Impairment
- Highly protein bound, makes easier to use. Patients with severe renal insufficiency may need lower dose

Hepatic Impairment
- Use with caution in patients with moderate to severe disease and monitor for AEs with regular hepatic function panels. Stop if any worsening

Cardiac Impairment
- Can produce arrhythmias in patients with cardiac disease or conduction disease. Use with caution and obtain baseline ECG

Elderly
- May need lower dose. More likely to experience AEs except rash. Increased risk of aplastic anemia

 Children and Adolescents
- Ages 6–12: start at 200 mg/day in divided doses. Increase by 100 mg/day every 1–2 weeks to goal dose, usually less than 1000 mg/day
- Age < 6: start at 10–20 mg/kg/day in divided doses, increase by 5–10 mg/kg/day every week until goal dose, usually 35 mg/kg/day or less
- Children have less risk of rash

 Pregnancy
- Category D. Teratogenicity includes increased rate of neural tube defects with use in first trimester
- Drug does cross placenta
- Plasma levels and effectiveness may change during pregnancy – monitor serum levels

- Supplementation with 0.4 mg of folic acid before and during pregnancy is recommended
- Patients taking for headache, pain, or bipolar disorder should generally stop before considering pregnancy

Breast Feeding

- 10–30% of mother's blood drug level found in breast milk
- Generally recommendations are to discontinue drug or bottle feed
- Monitor infant for sedation, poor feeding, or irritability

THE ART OF NEUROPHARMACOLOGY

Potential Advantages

- Proven effectiveness as monotherapy for adult with partial seizures
- Effective for trigeminal neuralgia

Potential Disadvantages

- Ineffective for many primary generalized epilepsies
- Multiple interactions with other AEDs and other drugs, and potential AEs
- Need for blood monitoring. Oxcarbazepine is often better tolerated

Primary Target Symptoms

- Seizure frequency and severity
- Chronic neuropathic pain
- Mood stabilization

Pearls

- Effective for partial epilepsies but may worsen absence, atonic, or myoclonic seizures
- May worsen or improve generalized tonic-clonic seizure control
- Autoinduction means dose requirements can increase after initial titration
- First-line drug for trigeminal neuralgia, effective in about 70% of patients, often in hours or days. Benefit may not be sustained
- Second-line treatment for SUNCT (short-lasting unilateral neuralgiform headache with conjunctival injection and tearing)
- Little evidence for use in migraine
- Useful in mania and mixed bipolar states, not necessarily depression
- Provides better pain relief than placebo in chronic neuropathic pain conditions (trigeminal neuralgia, painful diabetic neuropathy, post-herpetic neuralgia, and central post-stroke pain)
- Based on a Cochrane review that compares immediate release to extended release, no conclusion on superiority regarding seizure frequency. A trend on extended release for fewer AEs

Suggested Reading

Glauser T, Ben-Menachem E, Bourgeois B, Cnaan A, Guerreiro C, Kälviäinen R, et al. Updated ILAE evidence review of antiepileptic drug efficacy and effectiveness as initial monotherapy for epileptic seizures and syndromes. *Epilepsia.* 2013;54(3):551–63.

Harden CL, Pennell PB, Koppel BS, Hovinga CA, Gidal B, Meador KJ, et al; American Academy of Neurology; American Epilepsy Society. Practice parameter update: management issues for women with epilepsy – focus on pregnancy (an evidence-based review): vitamin K, folic acid, blood levels, and breastfeeding: report of the Quality Standards Subcommittee and Therapeutics and Technology Assessment Subcommittee of the American Academy of Neurology and American Epilepsy Society. *Neurology.* 2009;73(2):142–9.

Powell G, Saunders M, Rigby A, Marson AG. Immediate-release versus controlled-release carbamazepine in the treatment of epilepsy. *Cochrane Database Syst Rev.* 2014;12:CD007124.

Tomson T, Battino D, Bonizzoni E, Craig J, Lindhout D, Sabers A, et al. Dose-dependent risk of malformations with antiepileptic drugs: an analysis of data from the EURAP epilepsy and pregnancy registry. *Lancet Neurol.* 2011;10(7):609–17.

Wiffen PJ, Derry S, Moore RA, McQuay HJ. Carbamazepine for acute and chronic pain in adults. *Cochrane Database Syst Rev.* 2011;1: CD005451.

CARISOPRODOL

THERAPEUTICS

Brands
- Soma, Sanoma, Carisoma, Rela

Generic?
- Yes

Class
- Muscle relaxant

Commonly Prescribed for
(FDA approved in bold)
- **Acute painful musculoskeletal conditions**
- Muscle spasm
- Insomnia

How the Drug Works
- Sedative. Both carisoprodol and its active metabolite (meprobamate) bind to $GABA_A$ and may block interneuronal activity, depressing transmission of polysynaptic neurons in the descending reticular formation (sedation) and spinal cord (decreasing pain)

How Long Until It Works
- Pain: as little as 30 minutes and typically lasts 2–6 hours

If It Works
- Titrate to most effective tolerated dose

If It Doesn't Work
- Increase dose. If ineffective, consider alternative medications

Best Augmenting Combos for Partial Response or Treatment-Resistance
- Analgesic pain management often used in combination
- Botulinum toxin is effective, especially as an adjunct for focal spasticity (e.g., post-stroke or head injury affecting the upper limbs)
- Use other centrally acting muscle relaxants with caution due to potential additive CNS depressant effect

Tests
- None required

ADVERSE EFFECTS (AEs)

How the Drug Causes AEs
- Most are related to sedative effects

Notable AEs
- Drowsiness, dizziness, vertigo, ataxia, depression, nausea/vomiting, tachycardia, postural hypotension, facial flushing

Life-Threatening or Dangerous AEs
- Hypersensitivity reactions rarely occur after the first dose. Symptoms include extreme weakness, ataxia, vision loss, dysarthria, and euphoria. Serious allergic reactions, such as erythema multiforme, eosinophilia, asthmatic episodes, fever, angioedema, and anaphylactoid shock have been reported

Weight Gain
- Unusual

unusual | not unusual | common | problematic

Sedation
- Common

unusual | not unusual | common | problematic

What to Do About AEs
- Reduce dosing frequency for mild AEs and discontinue for serious AEs

Best Augmenting Agents to Reduce AEs
- Most AEs cannot be reduced by an augmenting agent

DOSING AND USE

Usual Dosage Range
- 1 tablet 3–4 times daily

Dosage Forms
- Tablets: 250, 350 mg

How to Dose
- Give 1 tablet 3 times a day and at bedtime

Dosing Tips

- May start by dosing at night; 250 mg may be better tolerated

Overdose

- Can produce stupor, coma, shock, respiratory depression, and rarely death. Additive effects when using with other CNS depressants. Use respiratory assistance and pressors if needed. Dialysis or hemodialysis may be helpful in some cases

Long-Term Use

- Not well studied

Habit Forming

- Potentially yes. Often mixed with other recreational drugs

How to Stop

- Patients on low doses do not need to taper. Withdrawal symptoms can occur in patients on higher doses. These may include anxiety, tremor, insomnia, hallucinations, and confusion

Pharmacokinetics

- Hepatic metabolism via CYP2C19 into active metabolite meprobamate (anxiolytic). Excreted via renal and non-renal pathways. Half-life 2.5 hours

 Drug Interactions

- Use with CNS depressants or psychotropic drugs may be additive
- Strong CYP2C19 inhibitor (moclobemide, fluvoxamine, chloramphenicol, proton pump inhibitors, azoles) increases carisoprodol concentration
- CYP2C19 inducer (rifamipicin, carbamazepine, steroid) lowers carisoprodol concentration
- CYP2C19 polymorphism. 15–20% Asians, 3–5% Whites or Blacks are poor metabolizers

Do Not Use

- Hypersensitivity to the drug. Patients with acute intermittent porphyria. Use with caution in addiction-prone individuals

Renal Impairment

- Use with caution, as decreased drug clearance may increase toxicity

Hepatic Impairment

- Use with caution, as decreased drug metabolism may increase toxicity

Cardiac Impairment

- No known effects

Elderly

- May be more prone to AEs

 Children and Adolescents

- Not studied in children

 Pregnancy

- Category C. Use only if there is a clear need

Breast Feeding

- Drug is excreted in breast milk and can cause sedation. Do not use

Potential Advantages

- Quick onset of action

Potential Disadvantages

- Risk of abuse and dependence. Sedation and potential for overdose

Primary Target Symptoms

- Pain, muscle spasm

 Pearls

- Usage in clinical practice has decreased compared to other agents for muscle spasm due to risk of addiction, sedation, and risk of serious hypersensitivity reactions
- Misused by opioid-addicted patients to increase the effect of smaller opioid doses. It particularly affects codeine-derived semi-synthetics, such as codeine, oxycodone, and hydrocodone

Suggested Reading

Chou R, Peterson K, Helfand M. Comparative efficacy and safety of skeletal muscle relaxants for spasticity and musculoskeletal conditions: a systematic review. *J Pain Symptom Manage.* 2004;28(2):140–75.

Littrell RA, Hayes LR, Stillner V. Carisoprodol (Soma): a new and cautious perspective on an old agent. *South Med J.* 1993;86(7):753–6.

Reeves RR, Beddingfield JJ, Mack JE. Carisoprodol withdrawal syndrome. *Pharmacotherapy.* 2004;24(12): 1804–6.

THERAPEUTICS

THERAPEUTICS

Brands
- BiCNU, Gliadel (wafer)

Generic?
- Yes (as infusion)

Class
- Antineoplastic agent

Commonly Prescribed for
(FDA approved in bold)
- **Brain tumors (including glioblastoma, brainstem glioma, medulloblastoma, astrocytoma, ependymoma, and metastatic tumors)**
- **Multiple myeloma**
- **Hodgkin's disease**
- Colorectal carcinoma
- Melanoma

How the Drug Works
- A nitrosourea that alkylates DNA and RNA. Drug metabolites may be responsible for clinical effectiveness and toxicity

How Long Until It Works
- Used to prolong survival. Clinical benefits may be difficult to determine for weeks to months

If It Works
- Wafer is only used postoperatively
- Infusions may be continued every 6–8 weeks

If It Doesn't Work
- Discontinue treatment; consider alternative salvage chemotherapy such as bevacizumab or temozolomide, or corticosteroids such as dexamethasone depending on clinical situation

Best Augmenting Combos for Partial Response or Treatment-Resistance
- Most patients will receive co-treatment with radiotherapy
- For glioblastomas, carmustine is usually given after treatment with temozolomide has ceased to be effective

- Alkyl guanine transferase inhibitors such as O-6-benzylguanine may increase effectiveness by inhibiting DNA repair

Tests
- Obtain pulmonary function testing before using
- Monitor CBC (platelets and white blood cells especially) weekly
- Monitor liver function tests and renal function periodically or as symptoms arise

ADVERSE EFFECTS (AEs)

How the Drug Causes AEs
- Similar to other alkylating dugs, AEs are related to carmustine's effects on rapidly dividing cells

Notable AEs
- Most common: leukopenia, thrombocytopenia, nausea, vomiting, headache
- Less common: abdominal pain, vision changes, allergic reactions, anemia

Life-Threatening or Dangerous AEs
- Pulmonary fibrosis: may be delayed
- Azotemia and renal failure (relatively rare)
- Severe hepatic toxicity (rare)
- Wafer only: CSF leak, intracranial hypertension
- Leukemia or bone marrow dysplasias

Weight Gain
- Unusual

unusual | not unusual | common | problematic

Sedation
- Unusual

unusual | not unusual | common | problematic

What to Do About AEs
- Leukopenia peaks at 5–6 weeks and thrombocytopenia at 4 weeks. These are used for evaluating subsequent doses
- Many toxicities such as pulmonary fibrosis are dose related

Best Augmenting Agents to Reduce AEs
- Antiemetics for nausea/vomiting

DOSING AND USE

Usual Dosage Range
- 150–200 mg/m^2 over 1 or 2 days (injection)
- 7.7 mg wafer polifeprosan 20 polymer (wafer)

Dosage Forms
- Vials for injection contain 100 mg in 3 mL

How to Dose
- Administer over 1 day or 2 consecutive days. Check CBC at least weekly for 6 weeks. Do not repeat dosing for at least 6 weeks and when CBC have returned to normal. Use the nadir CBC to guide further dosing:
- If lowest leukocyte count > 3000 and platelets > 75 000 then give 100% of initial dose
- If either lowest leukocyte count is between 2000 and 2999 or platelets between 25 000 and 74 999 then give 70% of initial dose
- If lowest leukocyte count < 2000 or platelets < 25 000 then give 50% of initial dose
- Gliadel wafer: placed intraoperatively during initial craniotomy

 Dosing Tips
- Divide infusion dose over 2 days for sensitive patients
- Rapid infusion increases risk of flushing response and local skin reactions

Overdose
- No known effects

Long-Term Use
- Monitoring for pulmonary symptoms and CBC are essential

Habit Forming
- No

How to Stop
- No need to taper after use, but monitor clinical symptoms and neuroimaging to assess response

Pharmacokinetics
- Carmustine is rapidly metabolized with no intact drug detectable after 15 minutes. Over 60% is excreted in urine after 4 days and some as respiratory carbon dioxide. Very high lipid solubility and relative lack of ionization leads to effective BBB crossing

 Drug Interactions
- Cimetidine appears to increase toxicity

 Other Warnings/ Precautions
- Long-term use of nitrosoureas has been reported to be associated with the development of secondary malignancies
- Most such adverse reactions are reversible if detected early. The drug should be reduced in dosage or discontinued and appropriate corrective measures should be taken according to the clinical judgment of the physician

Do Not Use
- Hypersensitivity to drug

SPECIAL POPULATIONS

Renal Impairment
- Renal failure may occur and is dose related. Use with caution, especially in elderly patients

Hepatic Impairment
- Use with caution, monitor for hepatotoxicity

Cardiac Impairment
- Carmustine may cause hypotension or tachycardia

Elderly
- No known effects except more likely to experience renal insufficiency. Start with relatively lower doses

Children and Adolescents

- Safety and toxicity is not established
- Delayed pulmonary toxicity (up to 17 years after use) may occur and increases with higher cumulative infusion doses

 Pregnancy

- Category D. Associated with multiple malformations in animal testing. Do not use

Breast Feeding

- Unknown if present in breast milk. Breast feeding is generally not recommended

THE ART OF NEUROPHARMACOLOGY

Potential Advantages

- Available as focal treatment after initial craniotomy. FDA approved for the treatment of multiple types of brain cancers

Potential Disadvantages

- Unclear if toxicities outweigh survival benefit

Primary Target Symptoms

- Tumor progression, disability

 Pearls

- Salvage treatment as infusion, adjunctive treatment as wafer
- Usually given in recurrent tumors such as glioblastoma
- Carmustine wafer appears to improve survival but adverse events such as seizures, edema, and infection have limited its use
- Minor clinical fluctuations are common in those with aggressive brain tumors but rapid deterioration should raise concern for tumor bleeding, infection, or non-convulsive status epilepticus

 Suggested Reading

Friedman HS, Pluda J, Quinn JA, et al. Phase I trial of carmustine plus O6-benzylguanine for patients with recurrent or progressive malignant glioma. *Clin Oncol.* 2000;18(20): 3522–8.

Garside R, Pitt M, Anderson R, et al. The effectiveness and cost-effectiveness of carmustine implants and temozolomide for the treatment of newly diagnosed high-grade glioma: a systematic review and economic evaluation. *Health Technol Assess.* 2007;11(45): iii–iv, ix–221.

Omuro A, DeAngelis LM. Glioblastoma and other malignant gliomas: a clinical review. *JAMA.* 2013;310(17):1842–50.

Westphal M, Hilt DC, Bortey E, et al. A phase 3 trial of local chemotherapy with biodegradable carmustine (BCNU) wafers (Gliadel wafers) in patients with primary malignant glioma. *Neuro Oncol.* 2003;5(2):79–88.

CHLORPROMAZINE

THERAPEUTICS

Brands
- Thorazine, Largactil, Sonazine, Promapar

Generic?
- Yes

Class
- Antiemetic, antipsychotic

Commonly Prescribed for
(FDA approved in bold)
- **Antiemetic**
- **Intractable hiccups**
- **Psychosis, schizophrenia**
- **Manic depression in bipolar disorder**
- **Acute intermittent porphyria**
- **Adjunct treatment for tetanus**
- **Restlessness and apprehension before surgery**
- **Hyperactivity and behavioral problems (children)**
- Acute treatment for migraine

How the Drug Works
- It is an aliphatic phenothiazine derivative with high antagonistic effect for α_1-adrenergic, H_1, M_1, and $5\text{-}HT_2$ receptors, but low affinity for D_{1-4} receptors; hence it has high risk for sedation, weight gain, and orthostatic hypotension but lower risk for dyskinesia than haloperidol

How Long Until It Works
- Migraine: 1 hour (oral) or less than 30 minutes (IV)

If It Works
- Use at lowest required dose
- Monitor QTc interval

If It Doesn't Work
- Change to another agent

Best Augmenting Combos for Partial Response or Treatment-Resistance
- For migraine, can be used with dihydroergotamine or NSAIDs

Tests
- Obtain blood pressure and pulse before initial IV and monitor QTc with ECG

ADVERSE EFFECTS (AEs)

How the Drug Causes AEs
- Anticholinergic effects produce most AEs (sedation, blurred vision, dry mouth). Hypotension and dizziness are related to α-adrenergic blockade, and motor AEs are related to dopamine blocking effects

Notable AEs
- Dizziness, sedation, orthostatic hypotension, tachycardia, urinary retention, depression
- Akathisia, extrapyramidal symptoms, parkinsonism
- Long-term use: weight gain, glucose intolerance, sexual dysfunction, hyperprolactinemia

Life-Threatening or Dangerous AEs
- Tardive dyskinesias
- Neuroleptic malignant syndrome (rare)
- Jaundice
- Rare agranulocytosis (mean exposure of 45 days to onset; mean duration of 11 days)

Weight Gain
- Common (with chronic use)

unusual   not unusual   **common**   problematic

Sedation
- Problematic

unusual   not unusual   common   **problematic**

What to Do About AEs
- Lowering dose or changing to another antiemetic improves most AEs
- Rarely causes ECG changes. Use with caution in patients if QTc is above 450 (females) or 440 (males) and do not administer with QTc greater than 500
- If excessive sedation, use only as a rescue agent for intractable migraine in hospitalized

patients or when patients can lie down or sleep

Best Augmenting Agents to Reduce AEs

- Give fluids to avoid hypotension, tachycardia, and dizziness
- Give anticholinergics (diphenhydramine or benztropine) or benzodiazepines for extrapyramidal reactions
- Amantadine may improve motor AEs

DOSING AND USE

Usual Dosage Range

- Migraine: up to 200 mg/day IV, IM, or oral in divided doses

Dosage Forms

- Tablets: 10, 25, 50, 100, 200 mg
- Injection: 25 mg/mL
- Syrup: 10 mg/5mL
- Oral concentrate: 30, 100 mg/mL
- Suppository: 25, 100 mg

How to Dose

- Oral: give 10–25 mg and repeat as needed every 4–6 hours. Patients with previous exposure and few significant AEs may increase dose and use up to 200 mg/day in divided doses
- IV/IM: give 12.5–50 mg every 4–8 hours up to 200 mg/day

 Dosing Tips

- In hospitalized patients, start with lower dose to ensure drug is tolerated and increase as needed to effective dose
- Warn patients not to drive
- Check ECG daily while patients are treated and monitor blood pressure

Overdose

- CNS depression, hypotension, or extrapyramidal reactions are most common. Tachycardia, restlessness, convulsions, and respiratory depression may occur

Long-Term Use

- Safe for long-term use with appropriate monitoring. Tardive dyskinesias may be irreversible

Habit Forming

- No

How to Stop

- No need to taper

Pharmacokinetics

- Metabolized by CYP2D6. T_{max} 1–4 hours and half-life 8–33 hours. 90% protein bound

 Drug Interactions

- Use with CNS depressants (barbiturates, opiates, general anesthetics) potentiates CNS AEs
- Potent CYP2D6 inhibitors (e.g., fluoxetine, paroxetine, bupropion, quinidine) may increase chlorpromazine serum concentration
- Use with alcohol or diuretics may increase hypotension
- It is a CYP2D6 inhibitor that may increase the drug concentration of imipramine, amitriptyline, SSRIs, venlafaxine, other antipsychotics, β-blockers
- May decrease effectiveness of dopaminergic agents
- Reduces effectiveness of anticoagulants
- May increase phenytoin levels
- The combination of lithium and neuroleptics has been reported to produce an encephalopathy similar to neuroleptic malignant syndrome
- Greater risk for QTc prolongation, especially if concomitant use of ziprasidone, zuclopenthixol

 Other Warnings/Precautions

- Neuroleptic malignant syndrome is characterized by fever, rigidity, confusion, and autonomic instability, and is most common with IV typical neuroleptics such as chlorpromazine

Do Not Use

- Hypersensitivity to drug, CNS depression, or QTc greater than 500

Renal Impairment
• No known effects

Hepatic Impairment
• No known effects

Cardiac Impairment
• May worsen orthostatic hypotension. Risk of QTc prolongation and torsade de pointes

Elderly
• More sensitive to CNS AEs, use lower doses

 Children and Adolescents
• Appears safe in children over age 1, but mostly used for behavioral problems. Not a first-line agent in pediatric migraine

 Pregnancy
• Category C. Use only if benefit outweighs risks

Breast Feeding
• Some drug is found in breast milk and may cause sedation or movement problems in infants. Do not use for migraine

THE ART OF NEUROPHARMACOLOGY

Potential Advantages
• Effective drug for severe migraine. Sedation may be helpful for some patients and akathisia may be less common than with other antiemetics

Potential Disadvantages
• Significant AEs, including extrapyramidal reactions, sedation, and hypotension. Children and elderly patients may tolerate poorly. Risk of torsade de pointes

Primary Target Symptoms
• Headache, nausea

 Pearls
• Effective in refractory migraine and status migrainosus. Often combined with dihydroergotamine, given about 30 minutes after chlorpromazine
• Pretreat or combine with diphenhydramine, 25–50 mg, to reduce rate of akathisia and dystonic reactions
• Generally used as a "rescue" treatment in severe migraine when first-line medications (triptans, dihydroergotamine, NSAIDs) have failed
• May be more effective in preventing migraine recurrence than IV lidocaine or dihydroergotamine

 ### Suggested Reading

Evans RW, Young WB. Droperidol and other neuroleptics/antiemetics for the management of migraine. *Headache*. 2003; 43(7):811–13.

Leucht S, Wahlbeck K, Hamann J, Kissling W. New generation antipsychotics versus low-potency conventional antipsychotics: a systematic review and meta-analysis. *Lancet* 2003;361:1581–9.

Marmura MJ. Use of dopamine antagonists in treatment of migraine. *Curr Treat Options Neurol*. 2012;14(1):27–35.

CITALOPRAM

Brands
- Celexa

Generic?
- Yes

Class
- Selective serotonin reuptake inhibitor (SSRI)

Commonly Prescribed for
(FDA approved in bold)
- **Major depressive disorder (adolescent and adult)**
- Generalized anxiety disorder
- Obsessive-compulsive disorder (OCD)
- Post-traumatic stress disorder
- Cataplexy

How the Drug Works
- Both citalopram (50:50 S-,R-enantiomer) and escitalopram (S-enantiomer of citalopram) block serotonin reuptake pumps, increasing serotonin levels within hours, but antidepressant effect takes weeks. Escitalopram (Ki = 1.1 nM) is 100-fold more potent than the R-enantiomer in inhibiting SERT
- No affinity for NET, serotonergic, adrenergic, muscarinic, H_1, dopamine, opiate, GABA receptors, and Ca^{2+}, Na^+, K^+, Cl^- channels

How Long Until It Works
- May start to see improvement in 1–2 weeks, but usually it takes longer period for full effect

If It Works
- Continue to use and monitor for AEs

If It Doesn't Work
- Increase to highest tolerated dose. Consider adding a second agent or changing to another one

Best Augmenting Combos for Partial Response or Treatment-Resistance
- For some patients, low-dose polytherapy with 2 or more drugs may be better

tolerated and more effective than high-dose monotherapy

Tests
- Check ECG for QTc prolongation at baseline and when increasing dose, especially in those with a personal or family history of QTc prolongation, cardiac arrhythmia, heart failure, or recent myocardial infarction

How the Drug Causes AEs
- By increasing serotonin on non-therapeutic responsive receptors throughout the body. Most AEs are dose- and time-dependent

Notable AEs
- Incidence $\geq$ 5%: insomnia, nausea, fatigue, somnolence, hyperhidrosis, decreased libido, ejaculation delay, and anorgasmia

Life-Threatening or Dangerous AEs
- QTc prolongation, torsade de pointes, and rarely death
- Serotonin syndrome
- Rare activation of mania or suicidal ideation, especially during the initial few months
- Angle-closure glaucoma
- Rare worsening of existing seizure disorders
- Rare hyponatremia and abnormal bleeding

Weight Gain
- Not unusual

unusual · not unusual · common · problematic

Sedation
- Not unusual

unusual · not unusual · common · problematic

What to Do About AEs
- For minor AEs, lower dose, titrate more slowly, or switch to another agent. For serious AEs, lower dose and consider stopping, taper to avoid withdrawal symptoms

Best Augmenting Agents to Reduce AEs

- Cyproheptadine can be used for serotonin syndrome by blocking 5-HT receptors and SERT
- Sexual dysfunction (anorgasmia, impotence) may be reversed by agents with α_2-adrenergic antagonist activity (e.g., buspirone, amantadine, bupropion, mirtazapine, ginkgo biloba, etc.)

DOSING AND USE

Usual Dosage Range

- Citalopram: 20–80 mg/day

Dosage Forms

- Tablet (40 mg), oral solution (2 mg/mL)

How to Dose

- Initial 20 mg/day. Titrate 20 mg weekly. Maximum 40 mg/day (MDD), 60 mg/day (binge eating), 80 mg/day (OCD)

 Dosing Tips

- Start at a low dose and titrate up every week as tolerated. Not affected by food

Overdose

- Often in combination with other drugs. Symptoms include convulsions, coma, dizziness, hypotension, insomnia, nausea, vomiting, sinus tachycardia, somnolence, and ECG changes (including QTc prolongation and very rare cases of torsade de pointes)
- Establish and maintain an airway. Gastric lavage with activated charcoal should be considered. Cardiac and vital sign monitoring is recommended, along with general symptomatic and supportive care. Due to the large volume of distribution of citalopram/escitalopram, forced diuresis, dialysis, hemoperfusion, and exchange transfusion are unlikely to be of benefit. There are no specific antidotes

Long-Term Use

- Safe for long-term use

Habit Forming

- No

How to Stop

- Taper slowly (no more than 50% reduction every 3–4 days until discontinuation) to avoid withdrawal symptoms (agitation, anxiety, confusion, dry mouth, dysphoria, etc.)

Pharmacokinetics

- Metabolized by CYP3A4, CYP2C19, and CYP2D6 (lesser extent). 20% eliminated by kidney. Bioavailability 80%. Half-life 20–40 hours. 56% protein bound

 Drug Interactions

- Serotonin syndrome may occur with concomitant use of MAOIs or serotonergic drugs
- Concomitant use of CYP450 inhibitors typically does not significantly affect the pharmacokinetics of citalopram due to the involvement of multiple enzyme systems
- Citalopram has mild but clinically insignificant inhibitory effect on CYP2D6
- Abnormal bleeding: use caution in concomitant use with NSAIDs, aspirin, warfarin, or other drugs that affect coagulation

 Other Warnings/ Precautions

- May increase risk of seizure

Do Not Use

- Concurrently with MAOI; allow at least 14 days between discontinuation of an MAOI and initiation of citalopram, or at least 7–14 days between discontinuation of citalopram and initiation of an MAOI
- Concurrent use of serotonin precursors (e.g., tryptophan)
- In patients with uncontrolled narrow angle-closure glaucoma
- In patients treated with linezolid or methylene blue IV

SPECIAL POPULATIONS

Renal Impairment
- Use with caution in patients with severe impairment. No dosage adjustment for patients with mild or moderate renal impairment

Hepatic Impairment
- 10 mg/day for patient with hepatic function impairment

Cardiac Impairment
- Do not use in patients with cardiac structural lesions (e.g., myocardial infarction, severe heart failure), hypokalemia, hypomagnesemia, and history of QTc prolongation

Elderly
- 10 mg/day for most elderly

Children and Adolescents
- Safety and effectiveness not established in pediatric MDD patients < 18 years old

Pregnancy
- Category C. Neonates exposed to SNRIs or SSRIs late in the third trimester have developed complications necessitating extended hospitalizations, respiratory support, and tube feeding. Respiratory distress, cyanosis, apnea, seizures, temperature instability, feeding difficulty, vomiting, hypoglycemia, hypotonia, hyperreflexia, tremor, jitteriness, irritability, and constant crying consistent with a toxic effect of the drug or drug discontinuation syndrome have been reported

Breast Feeding
- Some drug is found in breast milk and use while breast feeding is not recommended

THE ART OF NEUROPHARMACOLOGY

Potential Advantages
- The most potent SSRI

Potential Disadvantages
- Requires gradual titration. Sexual dysfunction potential

Primary Target Symptoms
- Depression and anxiety

 Pearls
- Based on pooled and meta-analysis studies on depression, escitalopram demonstrates superior efficacy compared with citalopram and other SSRIs. Escitalopram shows similar efficacy to SNRI but the number of trials in these comparisons is limited
- Based on a Cochrane review, citalopram was more efficacious than paroxetine and reboxetine and more acceptable than TCAs, reboxetine, and venlafaxine; however, it seemed to be less efficacious than escitalopram
- In an animal study to investigate the normalization of sucrose solution consumption in stressed rats, escitalopram takes 1 week, citalopram takes 2 weeks, and TCAs and MAOIs take 3–5 weeks
- Limited evidence supporting citalopram/ escitalopram as preventives for migraine or tension-type headache
- No strong evidence supporting citalopram as treatment for fibromyalgia. However, it may help depressive symptoms in patients with fibromyalgia
- Limited evidence for its use in treating diabetic neuropathy
- May reduce binge eating and improve abstinence rates but does not lead to weight loss
- Overall improves sleep quality in depressed patients (as most SSRIs). All SSRIs are associated with similar sleep architecture changes such as REM amount reduction, REM latency increase, slow wave sleep increase especially stages 1 and 2, and sleep fragmentation
- Overall decreases sleep quality in OCD patients
- May be effective for cataplexy but not narcolepsy

Suggested Reading

Ali MK, Lam RW. Comparative efficacy of escitalopram in the treatment of major depressive disorder. *Neuropsychiatr Dis Treat.* 2011;7:39–49.

Arnold LM. Duloxetine and other antidepressants in the treatment of patients with fibromyalgia. *Pain Med.* 2007;8 Suppl 2:S63–74.

Brownley KA, Berkman ND, Sedway JA, Lohr KN, Bulik CM. Binge eating disorder treatment: a systematic review of randomized controlled trials. *Int J Eat Disord.* 2007;40(4):337–48.

Cipriani A, Purgato M, Furukawa TA, Trespidi C, Imperadore G, Signoretti A, et al. Citalopram versus other anti-depressive agents for depression. *Cochrane Database Syst Rev.* 2012;7:CD006534.

Drago A. SSRIs impact on sleep architecture: guidelines for clinician use. *Clin Neuropsychiatry.* 2008;5:115–31.

Dworkin RH, O'Connor AB, Backonja M, Farrar JT, Finnerup NB, Jensen TS, et al. Pharmacologic management of neuropathic pain: evidence-based recommendations. *Pain.* 2007;132(3):237–51.

Smitherman TA, Walters AB, Maizels M, Penzien DB. The use of antidepressants for headache prophylaxis. *CNS Neurosci Ther.* 2010;17(5): 462–9.

CLOBAZAM

THERAPEUTICS

Brands
• Onfi, Frisium (EU)

Generic?
• No

Class
• Benzodiazepine, antiepileptic drug (AED)

Commonly Prescribed for
(FDA approved in bold)
• **Adjunctive treatment of seizures associated with Lennox-Gastaut syndrome (LGS) in patients 2 years of age or older**
• Adjunctive therapy for refractory focal seizure, general tonic-clonic seizure, Dravet syndrome, benign epilepsy with centrotemporal spikes, Panayiotopoulos syndrome, catamenial seizure, cluster seizure
• Acute or chronic anxiety

How the Drug Works
• Potentiation of GABAergic neurotransmission resulting from binding to the GABA$_A$ receptor

How Long Until It Works
• T$_{max}$ = 0.5–4 hours. May take days to weeks

If It Works
• May consider tapering after seizure free for 2 years, depending on the seizure type

If It Doesn't Work
• Consider changing to another agent, adding a second agent, using a medical device, or a referral for epilepsy surgery evaluation. When adding a second agent, keep drug interactions in mind

Best Augmenting Combos for Partial Response or Treatment-Resistance
• Consider a tertiary care or switch to other agents

Tests
• Not required

ADVERSE EFFECTS (AEs)

How the Drug Causes AEs
• CNS inhibitory effect from actions on benzodiazepine receptors

Notable AEs
• Constipation, somnolence, pyrexia, lethargy, drooling, and withdrawal symptoms

Life-Threatening or Dangerous AEs
• Stevens-Johnson syndrome (SJS), toxic epidermal necrolysis (TEN)

Weight Gain
• Not unusual

unusual   not unusual   common   problematic

Sedation
• Not unusual

unusual   not unusual   common   problematic

What to Do About AEs
• If SJS or TEN, hospitalization is required
• Discontinue or switch to another agent

Best Augmenting Agents to Reduce AEs
• Most AEs cannot be reduced by an augmenting agent

DOSING AND USE
• 20–40 mg/day twice daily

Dosage Forms
• Tablet: 10 and 20 mg
• Oral suspension: 2.5 mg/mL in 120 mL bottles

How to Dose
• ≤ 30 kg: starting dose 5 mg; starting 7th day 10 mg; starting 14th day 20 mg
• 30 kg: starting dose 10 mg; starting 7th day 20 mg; starting 14th day 40 mg

Dosing Tips

- Dosage adjustment based on clinical presentation, age, body weight, renal/hepatic conditions, presence of CYP2C19/CYP3A4 inducers/inhibitors
- Crushing or use with food does not affect absorption

Overdose

- Management: gastric lavage, activated charcoal, IV fluid, control airway, supportive measures
- Flumazenil can lead to withdrawal symptoms, which is not recommended in patients with epilepsy

Long-Term Use

- Less sedation and tolerance than typical benzodiazepine over time

Habit Forming

- Can be abused, with dependence and withdrawal symptoms

How to Stop

- Gradually. 5–10 mg/day weekly

Pharmacokinetics

- Half-life 2–3 days. Metabolized extensively in liver. CYP3A4 converts clobazam to N-desmethylclobazam (the major active metabolite), which is then metabolized by CYP2C19; 11% is excreted in feces and 82% in urine

 Drug Interactions

- Clobazam is a weak CYP3A4 inducer, which may affect some hormonal contraceptives
- CYP2C19 inhibitor (e.g., fluconazole, omeprazole) increases exposure to N-desmethylclobazam up to 5-fold
- Concomitant use of other CNS depressants may increase the risk of sedation
- Alcohol increases clobazam blood level by 50%

 Other Warnings/Precautions

- May develop dependence, tolerance after long-term use
- Acute withdrawal increases risk of seizure

Do Not Use

- Hypersensitivity to the drug, significant renal or hepatic impairment

Renal Impairment

- No significant concentration change with mild or moderate renal impairment. Not known in end-stage kidney disease

Hepatic Impairment

- Titrate slowly for mild or moderate hepatic impairment. Not known in severe impairment
- CYP2C19 poor metabolizer: titrate slowly

Cardiac Impairment

- No known effects

Elderly

- Titrate slowly

 Children and Adolescents

- Not for < 2 years old. Half dose for patients with body weight < 30 kg

 Pregnancy

- Category C. Neonatal flaccidity, respiratory and feeding difficulties, hypothermia, and withdrawal symptoms have been reported in infants born to mothers who received benzodiazepines, including clobazam, late in pregnancy

Breast Feeding

- Clobazam is excreted in human milk

THE ART OF NEUROPHARMACOLOGY

Potential Advantages

- High response rates in refractory epilepsy, relatively less sedation than other benzodiazepines

Potential Disadvantages

- Sedation and tolerance. Not a first-line AED

Primary Target Symptoms

• Seizure frequency and severity

Pearls

• Can be valuable for quick add-on to bridge AED transitions.

• Useful short-term treatment for catamenial seizures
• For children with newly diagnosed or untreated partial-onset seizure (Level of Evidence D)
• Compared with other benzodiazepines, clobazam has longer half-life and less sedative side effect

Suggested Reading

Glauser T, Ben-Menachem E, Bourgeois B, Cnaan A, Guerreiro C, Kälviäinen R, et al. Updated ILAE evidence review of antiepileptic drug efficacy and effectiveness as initial monotherapy for epileptic seizures and syndromes. *Epilepsia.* 2013; 54(3):551–63.

Sirven JI, Noe K, Hoerth M, Drazkowski J. Antiepileptic drugs 2012: recent advances and trends. *Mayo Clin Proc.* 2012;87(9):879–89.

CLONAZEPAM

THERAPEUTICS

Brands
- Klonopin, Rivotril

Generic?
- Yes

Class
- Benzodiazepine, antiepileptic drug (AED)

Commonly Prescribed for
(FDA approved in bold)
- **Seizure disorders. Used as monotherapy or adjunctive for the treatment of Lennox-Gastaut syndrome, akinetic, myoclonic, or absence seizures**
- **Panic disorder, with or without agoraphobia**
- Periodic leg movements disorder (PLMD)
- Restless legs syndrome (RLS)
- Tic disorders
- Parkinsonian (hypokinetic) dysarthria
- Tardive dyskinesia
- Muscle relaxation
- Insomnia
- Burning mouth syndrome
- Generalized anxiety disorder
- Schizophrenia (adjunctive)
- Acute mania in bipolar disorder

How the Drug Works
- Benzodiazepines bind to and potentiate the effect of GABA$_A$ receptors, which are ligand-gated chloride channels activated by GABA. It boosts chloride conductance across cell membranes, hyperpolarizes the membrane potential, and increases the threshold potential. There are at least 2 benzodiazepine receptors, 1 of which is associated with sleep mechanisms, the other with memory, sensory, and cognitive functions. Benzodiazepines act at spinal cord, brainstem, cerebellum, limbic, and cortical areas
- In petit mal seizures clonazepam suppresses spike and wave discharges, and in motor seizures decreases the frequency, amplitude, duration, and spread of discharge

How Long Until It Works
- There is often an immediate effect in treatment of epilepsy, PLMD, RLS, insomnia, and panic disorders, but usually weeks are required for optimal dose adjustments and maximal therapeutic benefit

If It Works
- Seizures: goal is the remission of seizures. Continue as long as effective and well tolerated. Consider tapering and slowly stopping after 2 years seizure-free, depending on the type of epilepsy
- PLMD, RLS, tic disorders: continue to adjust dose to find the lowest dose that produces relief of symptoms with fewest AEs
- Anxiety: often used only on a short-term basis. Consider adding an SSRI or SNRI for long-term treatment

If It Doesn't Work
- Epilepsy: consider changing to another agent, adding a second agent, using a medical device, or a referral for epilepsy surgery evaluation. When adding a second agent, keep drug interactions in mind
- PLMD, RLS: change to or use in combination with a dopamine agonist or an AED such as gabapentin or carbamazepine. Rule out iron deficiency; if obese, weight loss may be helpful

Best Augmenting Combos for Partial Response or Treatment-Resistance
- Epilepsy: often used in combination with other AEDs for optimal control but sedation can increase
- PLMD, RLS: dopamaine agonists or gabapentin
- Anxiety: SSRI or SNRIs. In most cases it is best to avoid combining with other benzodiazepines
- Insomnia: may be combined with low-dose TCAs (amitriptyline), or tetracyclics (trazodone, mirtazapine)

Tests
- None required

ADVERSE EFFECTS (AEs)

How the Drug Causes AEs

- Actions on benzodiazepine receptors including augmentation of inhibitory neurotransmitter effects

Notable AEs

- Most common: sedation, fatigue, depression, weakness, ataxia, nystagmus, confusion, and psychomotor retardation
- Less common: bradycardia, anorexia, hypotonia, and anterograde amnesia

 Life-Threatening or Dangerous AEs

- CNS depression and decreased respiratory drive, especially in combination with opiates, barbiturates, or alcohol
- Rare blood dyscrasias or liver function abnormalities

Weight Gain

- Unusual

unusual   not unusual   common   problematic

Sedation

- Not unusual

   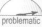
unusual   not unusual   common   problematic

What to Do About AEs

- May decrease or remit in time as tolerance develops
- Lower the total dose and take more at bedtime
- For severe, life-threatening AEs, administer flumazenil to reverse effects. Be cautious on any withdrawal seizure development

Best Augmenting Agents to Reduce AEs

- Most AEs cannot be reduced by adding an augmenting agent

DOSING AND USE

Usual Dosage Range

- Epilepsy: up to 20 mg/day in adults in divided dose

- PLMD, RLS: 0.5–2 mg/night
- Panic/anxiety disorders: usually best dose in panic disorder is 1 mg/day in divided doses. Maximum is generally 4 mg/day

Dosage Forms

- Tablets: 0.5, 1, and 2 mg
- Orally disintegrating (wafer): 0.125, 0.25, 0.5, 1, and 2 mg

How to Dose

- Epilepsy: start at 0.5 mg twice or three times daily. Increase dose in increments of 0.5 mg to 1 mg every 3 days until seizures are adequately controlled or AEs develop. Use the largest dose at bedtime. Tolerance to drug occasionally requires increasing dose to a maximum of 20 mg/day in divided doses 2–3 times daily
- RLS: start at 0.5 mg at bedtime. Increase by 0.5 mg every few nights until symptoms improve to maximum of 2 mg at night
- Panic disorder: start at 0.25 mg twice daily and increase to either 0.5 mg twice daily or 1 mg at night in 3 days

 Dosing Tips

- Dose in epilepsy often requires adjustment over time due to tolerance. Tolerance and dependence are less common in doses used to treat RLS or anxiety
- Assess need to continue treatment in all disorders
- Use disintegrating tablets for patients with swallowing difficulties

Overdose

- Confusion, drowsiness, decreased reflexes, incoordination, and lethargy are common. Ataxia, hypotension, coma, and death are rare. Coma, respiratory or circulatory depression are rare when used alone. Use with other CNS depressants such as alcohol, narcotics, or barbituates places patients at greater risk. Induce vomiting and use supportive measures along with gastric lavage or ipecac and in severe cases forced diuresis. Flumazenil reverses effect of clonazepam but provokes seizures in patients with epilepsy

Long-Term Use

- Safe for long-term use with appropriate monitoring

Habit Forming

- Schedule 4 drug with risk of tolerance and dependence. Dependence is most common with use after 6 weeks or more. Patients with a history of drug or alcohol abuse have an increased risk of dependency

How to Stop

- Taper slowly, as abrupt withdrawal can cause seizures, even in patients without epilepsy. The seizures often occur over a week after stopping drug due to long half-life
- Taper by 0.25 mg/day every 3 days to reduce risk of withdrawal symptoms. Once at a lower dose (1.5 mg/day or less) decrease speed of taper to as little as 0.125 mg/week or less. Slow tapers are especially recommended for patients on clonazepam for many months or years
- Monitor for re-emergence of disease symptoms (seizures, RLS, or anxiety)

Pharmacokinetics

- Peak plasma level at 1–2 hours but long elimination half-life compared to other benzodiazepines (18–50 hours). 97% protein bound and bioavailability over 80%. Mostly metabolized by CYP3A4 isoenzyme

 Drug Interactions

- Alcohol and CNS depressants (barbiturates, narcotics) increase CNS AEs
- CYP3A4 inhibitors such as nefazodone, fluoxetine, fluvoxamine, ketoconazole, clarithromycin, and many antivirals decrease clearance of drug but dose adjustment is rarely needed
- Antacids may alter the rate of absorption
- May increase serum concentrations of digoxin and phenytoin, leading to toxicity

 Other Warnings/ Precautions

- May increase salivation. Use with caution in patients with chronic respiratory disease
- May cause drowsiness and impair ability to drive or perform tasks that require alertness

Do Not Use

- Patients with a proven allergy to clonazepam or any benzodiazepine.

Significant liver disease or narrow angle-closure glaucoma

Renal Impairment

- Metabolites are renally excreted. Reduce dose

Hepatic Impairment

- Do not use in patients with significant disease

Cardiac Impairment

- No known effects

Elderly

- May clear drug more slowly and have lower dose requirement. Due to slower drug clearance, elderly patients may better tolerate benzodiazepines with a shorter half-life, such as diazepam

 Children and Adolescents

- In infants and children under 10 or under 30 kg body weight, initial dose should be between 0.01 and 0.03 mg/kg/day in 2 or 3 divided doses and maximal dose no more than 0.05 mg/kg/day. Increase dose by 0.25 or 0.5 mg every 3 days to a maximum maintenance dose of 0.1–0.2 mg/kg/day
- Not studied for use in anxiety/panic disorders

 Pregnancy

- Risk category D. Drug crosses placenta and accumulates in fetal circulation. May increase risk of fetal malformations. Use during labor can cause "floppy infant" syndrome with hypotonia, lethargy, and sucking difficulties
- In epilepsy, use with caution due to risk of seizures in pregnancy or change to another agent. Do not use for treatment of anxiety or RLS

Breast Feeding

- Can be found in breast milk
- Generally recommendations are to discontinue drug or bottle feed
- Monitor infant for sedation, poor feeding, or irritability

THE ART OF NEUROPHARMACOLOGY

Potential Advantages

- Rapid onset of action in epilepsy, RLS, and anxiety disorders, with longer duration of action compared to other benzodiazepines. Useful in even intractable seizure disorders and can be used in children. Most commonly used medication for PLMD

Potential Disadvantages

- Not a first-line agent in most patients with epilepsy. Development of tolerance and CNS depression can be problematic. Potential for abuse. Not as effective as diazepam or lorazepam for seizure emergencies (status epilepticus)

Primary Target Symptoms

- Seizure frequency and severity
- Pain in PLMD, RLS
- Anxiety or panic attacks

 Pearls

- The most commonly used benzodiazepine for the treatment of epilepsy
- As initial therapy: adult or children with partial-onset seizure (Level D)
- The use of clonazepam with divalproate may exacerbate absence seizures
- In patients with multiple types of seizures, may increase the incidence or precipitate generalized tonic-clonic (grand mal) seizures
- As an adjunctive therapy for PLMD/RLS that also improves sleep quality. Treat RLS patients with ropinirole and pramipexole as first line
- In most patients with anxiety, used as an adjunctive medication with an SSRI or SNRI. Longer half-life makes it easier to taper and may have less abuse potential than other benzodiazepines
- Clonazepam probably improves tardive dyskinesia and ginkgo biloba probably improves tardive syndrome (both Level B)

 Suggested Reading

Aurora RN, Kristo DA, Bista SR, Rowley JA, Zak RS, Casey KR, et al. The treatment of restless legs syndrome and periodic limb movement disorder in adults – an update for 2012: practice parameters with an evidence-based systematic review and meta-analyses: an American Academy of Sleep Medicine Clinical Practice Guideline. *Sleep.* 2012;35(8):1039–62.

Bhidayasiri R, Fahn S, Weiner WJ, Gronseth GS, Sullivan KL, Zesiewicz TA, et al. Evidence-based guideline: treatment of tardive syndromes: report of the Guideline Development Subcommittee of the American Academy of Neurology. *Neurology.* 2013;81(5): 463–9.

Biary N, Pimental PA, Langenberg PW. A double-blind trial of clonazepam in the treatment of parkinsonian dysarthria. *Neurology.* 1988;38(2):255–8.

DeVane CL, Ware MR, Lydiard RB. Pharmacokinetics, pharmacodynamics, and treatment issues of benzodiazepines: alprazolam, adinazolam, and clonazepam. *Psychopharmacol Bull* 1991;27:463–73.

Glauser T, Ben-Menachem E, Bourgeois B, Cnaan A, Guerreiro C, Kälviäinen R, et al. Updated ILAE evidence review of antiepileptic drug efficacy and effectiveness as initial monotherapy for epileptic seizures and syndromes. *Epilepsia.* 2013;54(3):551–63.

Isojärvi JI, Tokola RA. Benzodiazepines in the treatment of epilepsy in people with intellectual disability. *J Intellect Disabil Res.* 1998;42 Suppl 1:80–92.

Zakrzewska JM, Forssell H, Glenny AM. Interventions for the treatment of burning mouth syndrome. *Cochrane Database Syst Rev.* 2005;1:CD002779.

CLONIDINE

THERAPEUTICS

Brands
- Catapres, Dixarit, Clorpres, Duraclon (injection only), Kapvay, Jenloga

Generic?
- Yes

Class
- α_2-adrenergic agonist

Commonly Prescribed for
(FDA approved in bold)
- **Hypertension (immediate release only)**
- **Attention deficit hyperactivity disorder (ADHD) (extended release only)**
- **Severe pain in cancer patients**
- Postanesthetic shivering
- Withdrawal (alcohol, opiate, methadone)
- Gilles de la Tourette syndrome (GTS), tics
- Smoking cessation
- Growth delay
- Ulcerative colitis
- Menopausal symptoms such as hot flushes
- Neuropathic pain
- Ascites
- Hyperhidrosis
- Anesthesia premedication
- Restless legs syndrome (RLS)

How the Drug Works
- α_2 agonist with similar potency at 2A/2B/2C receptors. These adrenergic receptors are distributed throughout the CNS, with α_{2A} and α_{2C} being more in the CNS and α_{2B} more in the periphery (e.g., heart, lung, kidney, liver). Stimulating these presynaptic receptors (α_{2A}, α_{2C}) inhibits norepinephrine release, decreases sympathetic tone, and reduces blood pressure and heart rate. Sedation and analgesia is mediated by centrally located α_{2A}-receptors, while peripheral α_{2B}-receptors mediate vascular constriction. May also reduce plasma renin activity and catecholamine excretion. Additional antihypertensive effect may come from imidazoline I_1 receptor agonism

How Long Until It Works
- Hypertension, withdrawal: less than 2 hours
- GTS: weeks to months
- RLS: days

If It Works
- In neurological conditions such as tics, continue to assess effect of the medication and whether it is still needed

If It Doesn't Work
- GTS/tics: neuroleptics are often effective, but their use should be reserved for patients with significant social isolation or embarrassment
- RLS: generally used as an adjunctive agent. Dopamine agonists are more effective

Best Augmenting Combos for Partial Response or Treatment-Resistance
- In hypertension, combine with treatments less likely to affect heart rate or cause orthostasis (ACE inhibitors, diuretics)
- Tics and GTS symptoms may change over time. Many patients improve with age. Behavioral and psychological therapies are useful, and education and reassurance are all that is needed in mild cases
- Identify and treat comorbid conditions such as ADHD or obsessive-compulsive disorder

Tests
- Monitor blood pressure and pulse at office visits

ADVERSE EFFECTS (AEs)

How the Drug Causes AEs
- Related to α_2 agonist effect – hypotension and sedation

Notable AEs
- Dry mouth, hypotension/syncope, weakness, fatigue, sedation, dizziness, impotence, vivid dreams/nightmares, rash or pruritus, nausea, and depression

Life-Threatening or Dangerous AEs
- Bradycardia, AV block, and prolongation of QTc interval may occur with higher doses. Rapid withdrawal can cause rebound hypertension

Weight Gain
- Unusual

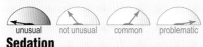

Sedation
- Common

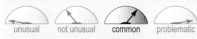

What to Do About AEs
- Lower the dose and take the highest dose in the evening. Many AEs are reduced with time

Best Augmenting Agents to Reduce AEs
- Most AEs cannot be reduced by an augmenting agent

DOSING AND USE

Usual Dosage Range
- 0.1–0.8 mg/day in 2 divided doses

Dosage Forms
- Tablets: 0.1, 0.2, 0.3 mg
- Tablets, extended release: 0.1, 0.2 mg
- Transdermal extended-release patches: 0.1/24 h, 0.2/24 h, 0.3/24 h
- Injection: 1 mg/10 mL, 5 mg/10 mL,
- 0.09 mg/mL suspension is equivalent to 0.1 mg/mL immediate release

How to Dose
- Hypertension: start 0.05 or 0.1 mg twice daily, and increase by 0.1 mg/day weekly with tablets or start with 0.1 mg patch and increase by 0.1 mg/week as tolerated
- GTS/tics: start at 0.05 twice daily and increase weekly by 0.05 or 0.1 mg/day as tolerated with tablets. Can take a larger dose in evening if sedation is problematic. The patch is rarely used in neurological disorders: if used titrate more slowly
- Shivering: 0.3mg/kg single IV dose
- Cancer pain: 30–40 mcg/h epidural infusion
- Withdrawal symptoms: 0.1–0.3 mg 3–4 times per day

 Dosing Tips
- Take the final dose before bedtime

- Rebound hypertension usually occurs 2–4 days after discontinuation

Overdose
- Hypertension may occur first, followed by severe hypotension, bradycardia, respiratory depression, hypothermia, drowsiness, decreased reflexes, weakness, or coma. Consider gastric lavage or activated charcoal for large ingestions

Long-Term Use
- Safe, but tolerance to antihypertensive effects is common

Habit Forming
- There are reports of abuse in opioid-dependent patients

How to Stop
- Taper slowly to avoid rebound tachycardia and hypertension. Other withdrawal symptoms may include nervousness, tremor, agitation, and headache

Pharmacokinetics
- Half-life is 12 hours in most, but sometimes longer. The peak effect is at 2–4 hours. Bioavailability is 75–95%, with about half of the drug metabolized into inactive metabolites and the other half excreted unchanged in urine

 Drug Interactions
- Clonidine may reduce effectiveness of levodopa
- Prazosin and TCAs may block the antihypertensive effects of clonidine
- Use with β-blockers, digitalis, or verapamil can have a synergistic effect, possibly causing AV block
- Use with other CNS depressants increases sedation

 Other Warnings/Precautions
- Do not discontinue therapy perioperatively and monitor blood pressure closely
- Therapeutic blood levels do not occur until about 2–3 days of starting transdermal patch
- In animal studies, corneal lesions (with concurrent amitriptyline) and retinal degeneration occurred

Do Not Use

• Known hypersensitivity to the drug

Renal Impairment

• Clearance is reduced in patients with severe renal insufficiency. Consider reducing dose

Hepatic Impairment

• No known effects

Cardiac Impairment

• Avoid using in patients with known coronary artery disease, conduction disturbances, recent myocardial infarction, or cerebrovascular events. Concurrent β-blocker or digitalis use may exacerbate AEs

Elderly

• No known effects

 Children and Adolescents

• Children may be more sensitive to CNS AEs than adults. Doses for GTS and tics are similar to adults but titrate more slowly. Consider giving the entire oral dose at night

 Pregnancy

• Category C. Use only if there is a clear need

Breast Feeding

• Excreted in breast milk. Do not use

Potential Advantages

• Fewer AEs than neuroleptics in the treatment of GTS and tic disorders. Useful agent for multiple neurological conditions, including ADHD

Potential Disadvantages

• Less effective than neuroleptics for GTS or tics. Hypotension, sedation, and rebound hypertension may limit use

Primary Target Symptoms

• Tics, attention deficit, hyperactivity, pain, sweating, and hot flushes

 Pearls

• The first clinical decision in the treatment of GTS or tics is to decide if pharmacological treatment is indicated. If the patient is not severely disabled, then reassure the patient and family that symptoms may improve and the prognosis is good. For patients with significant disability, clonidine is a good initial choice due to lack of long-term AEs, especially in patients with coexisting ADHD
• Guanfacine is a similar α_2-adrenergic agonist occasionally used for GTS or tics. It is not as well studied as clonidine
• In patients with severe ADHD, stimulants are generally more effective
• Useful in anxiety disorders and opioid withdrawal due to blocking of autonomic symptoms, such as sweating or palpitations
• Chemically similar to another α_2-adrenergic agonist, tizanidine, but much more effective for lowering blood pressure. Because the treatment of spasticity related to spinal cord injury often requires high doses, clonidine is not used in these patients
• May be synergistic with intrathecal local anesthetics for surgery but is associated with intraoperative hypotension
• Perioperative systemic clonidine decreases postoperative opioid consumption, pain intensity, and nausea
• It does not seem to prevent migraine occurrence
• 0.1% topical clonidine may help neuropathic pain
• As diagnostic test, it can be used for growth hormone stimulation test and suppression test for pheochromocytoma
• Apraclonidine (α_2 and weak α_1 agonist) can be used for diagnosis of Horner syndrome. Its weak α_1 agonist activity activates the denervated (hypersensitive) pupillary dilator muscle, causing reversal of anisocoria of the affected Horner eye

Suggested Reading

Blaudszun G, Lysakowski C, Elia N, Tramèr MR. Effect of perioperative systemic A2 agonists on postoperative morphine consumption and pain intensity: systematic review and meta-analysis of randomized controlled trials. *Anesthesiology* 2012;116: 1312–22.

Chen K, Lu Z, Xin YC, Cai Y, Chen Y, Pan SM. Alpha-2 agonists for long-term sedation during mechanical ventilation in critically ill patients. *Cochrane Database Syst Rev* 2015;1: CD010269.

Elia N, Culebras X, Mazza C, Schiffer E, Tramèr MR. Clonidine as an adjuvant to intrathecal local anesthetics for surgery: systematic review of randomized trials. *Reg Anesth Pain Med* 2008;33:159–67.

Kurlan RM. Treatment of Tourette syndrome. *Neurotherapeutics* 2014;11:161–5.

Peppin JF, Albrecht PJ, Argoff C, Gustorff B, Pappagallo M, Rice FL, et al. Skin matters: a review of topical treatments for chronic pain. Part two: treatments and applications. *Pain Ther* 2015;4:33–50.

Roessner V, Plessen KJ, Rothenberger A, Ludolph AG, Rizzo R, Skov L, et al. European clinical guidelines for Tourette syndrome and other tic disorders. Part II: pharmacological treatment. *Eur Child Adolesc Psychiatry* 2011;20:173–96.

CLOPIDOGREL

THERAPEUTICS

Brands
- Plavix, clopidogrel bisulfate

Generic?
- Yes

Class
- Antiplatelet agent

Commonly Prescribed for
(FDA approved in bold)
- **Acute coronary syndrome/non-ST-segment elevation myocardial infarction (ACS/NSTEMI): decrease the rate of a combined endpoint of cardiovascular death, myocardial infarction (MI), or stroke**
- **ST-segment elevation myocardial infarction (STEMI): reduce the rate of death from any cause and the rate of a combined endpoint of death, reinfarction, or stroke. The benefit for patients who undergo primary percutaneous intervention is unknown**
- **Recent MI, recent stroke, or established peripheral arterial disease: reduce the combined endpoint of new ischemic stroke, new MI, and other vascular death**
- Pain in peripheral artery disease
- Prevention of clots following angioplasty with stenting

How the Drug Works
- Inhibitor of platelet aggregation. Clopidogrel, once metabolized by CYP2C19, irreversibly binds to the platelet $P2Y_{12}$ class of adenosine diphosphate (ADP) receptor and inhibits the activation of the GPIIb/IIIa complex

How Long Until It Works
- Inhibition of platelet aggregation begins as soon as 2 hours after a single oral dose of clopidogrel. Platelets are affected for their lifespan (7–10 days)

If It Works
- Continue to use for MI or stroke prevention

If It Doesn't Work
- Check CYP2C19 dysfunctional genotype (2% White, 4% Black, 14% Chinese). Avoid concomitant use of proton pump inhibitor (e.g., omeprazole). Warfarin is superior for atrial fibrillation embolic stroke. Control all stroke risk factors such as smoking, hyperlipidemia, and hypertension. For acute events, admit patients for treatment and diagnostic testing

Best Augmenting Combos for Partial Response or Treatment-Resistance
- Based on CHANCE study, combination of clopidogrel and aspirin is superior to aspirin alone in reducing the risk of a secondary stroke in the first 90 days and does not increase the risk of hemorrhage

Tests
- None required

ADVERSE EFFECTS (AEs)

How the Drug Causes AEs
- Antiplatelet effect increases bleeding risk

Notable AEs
- Bleeding, thrombotic thrombocytopenic purpura

Life-Threatening or Dangerous AEs
- GI hemorrhage (2%), intracranial hemorrhage (0.1–0.4%), or intraocular bleeding leading to vision loss

Weight Gain
- Unusual

unusual   not unusual   common   problematic

Sedation
- Unusual

unusual   not unusual   common   problematic

What to Do About AEs
- No antidote. Discontinue clopidogrel

Best Augmenting Agents to Reduce AEs
- Most AEs cannot be reduced by an augmenting agent

DOSING AND USE

Usual Dosage Range
• 75 mg daily

Dosage Forms
• Tablets: 75 mg

How to Dose
• Ischemic stroke prevention: 75 mg/day
• ACS/NSTEMI: 300 mg loading, 75 mg once daily
• STEMI: 75 mg once daily with aspirin 75–100 mg once daily
• After stenting: at least 6 months
• Stop clopidogrel 5 days before surgery or procedures. Restart 1–2 days after surgery

 Dosing Tips
• Food does not affect absorption

Overdose
• Unknown but platelet transfusion may restore clotting ability

Long-Term Use
• Safe for long-term use

Habit Forming
• No

How to Stop
• No need to taper

Pharmacokinetics
• Metabolized by esterase (85%, inactive derivative) or multiple CYP450 enzymes (15%, active derivative). Onset of action in 2 hours with half-life of 6 hours. Inhibitory steady state 3–7 days after daily use; duration of action 7–10 days

 Drug Interactions
• Increases GI bleeding or bleeding time when used with NSAIDS, other antiplatelets, or anticoagulants
• CYP2C19 inhibitors (e.g., omeprazole, esomeprazole, ketoconazole, fluoxetine, cimetidine) decrease clopidogrel antiplatelet activity

 Other Warnings/ Precautions
• Thrombotic thrombocytopenic purpura is a rare complication that can occur in as little as 2 weeks and is characterized by thrombocytopenia, hemolytic anemia, neurological dysfunction, renal dysfunction, and fever. Requires urgent plasmapheresis
• Neutropenia/agranulocytosis is a common AE (0.8%) of ticlopidine, a chemically similar drug to clopidogrel. The risk of myelotoxicity with clopidogrel is quite low

Do Not Use
• Known hypersensitivity to the drug or active pathological bleeding, such as a peptic ulcer or intracranial hemorrhage

SPECIAL POPULATIONS

Renal Impairment
• Reduced platelet inhibition in patients with CrCl ≤ 60 mL/min

Hepatic Impairment
• No dosage adjustment needed. But patients with severe disease have an increased risk of bleeding complications

Cardiac Impairment
• No known effects

Elderly
• No known effects

 Children and Adolescents
• No safety profile in children

 Pregnancy
• Category B but not fully studied. Only use in pregnancy if clearly needed

Breast Feeding
• Excreted in breast milk. Do not use

THE ART OF NEUROPHARMACOLOGY

Potential Advantages

- Avoids issue of aspirin resistance. Useful for prevention of both stroke and MI. May be especially useful in patients with coronary artery stenting or peripheral vascular disease

Potential Disadvantages

- Cost. Combination of clopidogrel and aspirin increases bleeding risk. Activated by CYP2C19, which has genotype variation and is affected by other drugs

Primary Target Symptoms

- Prevention of the neurological complications that result from ischemic stroke

 Pearls

- First-line drug for secondary prevention of ischemic stroke along with aspirin or extended-release dipyridamole plus aspirin
- From PROGRESS and PRoFESS studies, tighter blood pressure control and dual aspirin/clopidogrel do not prevent cognitive decline
- Recent stroke/transient ischemic attack (TIA) attributable to severe stenosis (> 70%) of major intracranial artery, clopidogrel + aspirin for 90 days followed by monotherapy might be reasonable (Class IIb, Level of Evidence B)
- Recent stroke/TIA attributable to > 50% stenosis of major intracranial artery, data on clopidogrel or aggrenox are insufficient (Class IIb, Level of Evidence C)
- Recent stroke/TIA with atrial fibrillation unable to take oral anticoagulants, aspirin (Class I, Level of Evidence A) or clopidogrel + aspirin (Class IIb, Level of Evidence B) might be reasonable
- Recent stroke/TIA with extracranial carotid or vertebral arterial dissection, either antiplatelet or anticoagulant therapy for at least 3–6 months is reasonable (Class IIa; Level of Evidence B)
- Minor stroke/TIA, initiate aspirin + clopidogrel within 24 hours and continue for 90 days (Class IIb, Level of Evidence B)
- Combination of oral anticoagulants and antiplatelet is not recommended for recent stroke/TIA but reasonable in acute coronary syndrome or stent placement (Class IIb, Level of Evidence C)
- In patients with coronary artery disease, stenting, or peripheral vascular disease, clopidogrel may be superior to aspirin for the secondary prevention of vascular disease
- Based on a meta-analysis, no significant effect in non-ST elevation ACS but increases the risk of major bleeding
- In the CAPRIE trial comparing aspirin 325 mg/day and clopidogrel 75 mg/day, there was a relative risk reduction with clopidogrel but no statistically significant difference between the two groups for stroke prevention. The risk reduction in the clopidogrel group was greatest in patients with peripheral artery disease
- The MATCH trial compared clopidogrel to clopidogrel plus aspirin 325 mg. The CHARISMA trial compared aspirin 75–162 mg to aspirin 75–162 mg plus clopidogrel. In both trials there was no significant difference in stroke prevention between the two groups, but bleeding complications were higher (1.3% absolute increase) in the combination groups
- Recent retrospective studies suggest clopidogrel is more effective than aspirin in persons suffering stroke while on aspirin. However for lacunar stroke at least, there is no evidence that clopidrogel is superior
- Aspirin + clopidogrel has greater overall bleeding risk but less intracranial bleeding risk than warfarin monotherapy
- If antacid therapy is required, H_2-blocker (other than cimetidine) or pantoprazole (weak CYP2C19 inhibitor) should be considered to avoid drug interaction
- More diarrhea and rash than aspirin. Fewer other GI symptoms and hemorrhage than aspirin
- Newer $P2Y_{12}$ antiplatelet agents (ticagrelor, prasugrel), compared to clopidogrel, may reduce the rate of death from vascular causes, MI, or stroke but increase rate of bleeding. For stroke prevention in patients with history of stroke, both agents have more intracranial bleeding
- Vorapaxar, a new class of antiplatelet via protease-activated receptor 1 antagonist, was introduced for MI and peripheral arterial disease. But it has greater risk of intracranial hemorrhage in patients with history of stroke or TIA

Suggested Reading

Bellemain-Appaix A, Kerneis M, O'Connor SA, Silvain J, Cucherat M, Beygui F, et al. Reappraisal of thienopyridine pretreatment in patients with non-ST elevation acute coronary syndrome: a systematic review and meta-analysis. *BMJ*. 2014;349:g6269.

Hansen ML, Sørensen R, Clausen MT, Fog-Petersen ML, Raunsø J, Gadsbøll N, et al. Risk of bleeding with single, dual, or triple therapy with warfarin, aspirin, and clopidogrel in patients with atrial fibrillation. *Arch Intern Med*. 2010;170(16):1433–41.

Kernan WN, Ovbiagele B, Black HR, Bravata DM, Chimowitz MI, Ezekowitz MD, et al. Guidelines for the prevention of stroke in patients with stroke and transient ischemic attack: a guideline for healthcare professionals from the American Heart Association/American Stroke Association. *Stroke*. 2014;45(7):2160–236.

Levine GN, Bates ER, Blankenship JC, Bailey SR, Bittl JA, Cercek B, et al. 2011 ACCF/AHA/SCAI Guideline for Percutaneous Coronary Intervention. A report of the American College of Cardiology Foundation/American Heart Association Task Force on Practice Guidelines and the Society for Cardiovascular Angiography and Interventions. *J Am Coll Cardiol*. 2011;58 (24):e44–122.

Sacco RL, Diener HC, Yusuf S, Cotton D, Ounpuu S, Lawton WA, et al; PRoFESS Study Group. Aspirin and extended-release dipyridamole versus clopidogrel for recurrent stroke. *N Engl J Med*. 2008;359(12):1238–51.

Wang Y, Wang Y, Zhao X, Liu L, Wang D, Wang C, et al. Clopidogrel with aspirin in acute minor stroke or transient ischemic attack. *N Engl J Med*. 2013;369(1):11–19.

CLOZAPINE

THERAPEUTICS

Brands
- Clozaril, Clopine, Fazaclo ODT, Versacloz, Denzapine, Zaponex, Leponex

Generic?
- Yes

 Class
- Antipsychotic

Commonly Prescribed for
(FDA approved in bold)
- **Treatment-resistant schizophrenia**
- **Reducing suicidal behavior in patients with schizophrenia or schizoaffective disorder**
- Dyskinesia
- Psychosis in patients with Parkinson's disease (PD) or dementia with Lewy bodies (DLB)
- Bipolar disorder (treatment resistant)
- Severe psychosis
- Post-traumatic stress disorder

 How the Drug Works
- It is a dibenzodiazepine derivative of high affinity for 5-HT$_2$, $\alpha_{1/2}$, M$_{1-5}$, and H$_1$ receptors and moderate affinity for D$_{2/4}$ receptors. The effect is likely from antagonizing D$_2$ receptors (for positive symptoms) and 5-HT$_{2A}$ receptors (for negative symptoms)

How Long Until It Works
- Psychosis: may be effective in days, more commonly takes weeks or months to determine best dose and achieve best clinical effect

If It Works
- Continue to use at lowest required dose with appropriate monitoring. Patients with PD and DLB may improve more than patients with schizophrenia

If It Doesn't Work
- Increase dose
- In psychosis related to PD or DLB, eliminate or reduce dose of offending medications, such as dopamine agonists or amantadine

 Best Augmenting Combos for Partial Response or Treatment-Resistance
- PD and DLB: cholinesterase inhibitors may reduce psychotic symptoms
- In dementia, SSRIs may improve behavioral symptoms

Tests
- Obligatory. Prior to starting treatment, obtain CBC, including white count and absolute neutrophil count. Repeat weekly for 6 weeks, then every other week as long as patient is on medication and for 4 weeks after stopping. Also monitor blood sugar periodically

ADVERSE EFFECTS (AEs)

How the Drug Causes AEs
- Motor AEs: blocking of D$_2$ receptors
- Sedation, weight gain: blocking of H$_1$ receptors
- Hypotension: blocking of $\alpha_{1/2}$-adrenergic receptors
- Dry mouth, constipation: blocking of muscarinic receptors (anticholinergic)

Notable AEs
- Most common: CNS (sedation, dizziness/vertigo, headache, tremor); cardiovascular (tachycardia, orthostatic hypotension, syncope); autonomic (hypersalivation, sweating, dry mouth, visual disturbance, urinary retention); GI reaction (GI hypomotility, constipation, nausea); and fever

 Life-Threatening or Dangerous AEs
- Tardive dyskinesia
- Neuroleptic malignant syndrome
- Metabolic syndrome (hyperglycemia, diabetic ketoacidosis, dyslipidemia)
- Seizures
- Myocarditis
- Agranulocytosis (mean exposure of 56 days to onset; mean duration of 12 days)

Weight Gain
- Problematic

unusual   not unusual   common   problematic

Sedation

- Problematic

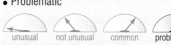

What to Do About AEs

- Take at bedtime and use low dose whenever possible
- Stop drug for absolute neutrophil count below 1000/mm^3
- Stop drug for eosinophil count over 4000/mm^3 and do not restart until under 3000/mm^3

Best Augmenting Agents to Reduce AEs

- Most AEs cannot be reduced with an augmenting agent

DOSING AND USE

Usual Dosage Range

- Bipolar disorder/schizophrenia: 300–450 mg/day
- Psychosis in PD/DLB: 25–100 mg/day

Dosage Forms

- Tablets: 12.5, 25, 50, 100 mg
- Oral disintegrating tablets: 12.5, 25, 50, 100, 150, 200 mg

How to Dose

- Start at 12.5 mg twice a day for acute psychosis or mania. Increase by 25–50 mg every 1–2 days until effective dose is reached
- For psychosis with PD or DLB, consider giving all the medication at night. Start at 6.25–12.5 mg at night. Increase by 6.25–12.5 mg every 1–2 days until symptoms improve. Most patients respond to a dose of 50 mg/day or less

 Dosing Tips

- Prescriptions are given 1 week at a time (due to risk of aganulocytosis) for 6 months, then every 2 weeks
- Disintegrating tablets may be useful in PD and DLB

Overdose

- Sedation, respiratory depression, excessive salivation, seizures, arrhythmias, and death have been reported

Long-Term Use

- Safe for long-term use with appropriate monitoring

Habit Forming

- No

How to Stop

- Taper over 1–2 weeks to avoid rebound psychosis and cholinergic rebound (diarrhea, headache)

Pharmacokinetics

- Hepatic metabolism via CYP1A2 (main), 3A4, and 2D6. Half-life 8–12 hours, peak effect at 2.5 hours

 Drug Interactions

- Use with CNS depressants (barbiturates, opiates, general anesthetics) potentiates CNS AEs
- Potent CYP1A2 (fluoroquinolones, fluvoxamine, verapamil), 3A4 (protease inhibitors, clarithromycin, ketoconazole, nefazodone), and 2D6 (fluoxetine, paroxetine, bupropion) inhibitors may increase levels
- Caffeine may increase levels
- Concomitant use of strong CYP3A4 inducer (e.g., carbamazepine, phenytoin, phenobarbital, rifampin, corticosteroid, St. John's wort) not recommended
- Valproic acid and cigarettes (CYP2C19 inducer) may lower levels
- May enhance effects of antihypertensives

 Other Warnings/ Precautions

- Use with caution in patients with enlarged prostate or glaucoma
- Possible association with cardiomyopathy

Do Not Use

- Proven hypersensitivity to drug, CNS depression, myeloproliferative disorders, or granulocytopenia

SPECIAL POPULATIONS

Renal Impairment

- No dose adjustment needed

Hepatic Impairment
• Use with caution. May need to lower dose

Cardiac Impairment
• May worsen orthostatic hypotension. Moderate risk of QTc prolongation with rare reports of torsade de pointes. Use with caution

Elderly
• At risk for CNS AEs and anticholinergic toxicity. Start with lower doses

Children and Adolescents
• Efficacy and safety unknown

Pregnancy
• Category B. PD and DLB are uncommon in women of childbearing age. Use only if benefit outweighs risks

Breast Feeding
• Probably excreted in breast milk based on animal studies. Use while breast feeding is generally not recommended

---

THE ART OF NEUROPHARMACOLOGY

Potential Advantages
• Most effective drug for refractory psychosis associated with PD or DLB. Effective at relatively low doses, with very low risk of drug-induced parkinsonism or tardive dyskinesias. Minimal prolactin elevation

Potential Disadvantages
• Safety and need for frequent monitoring. Sedation and weight gain

Primary Target Symptoms
• Psychosis

Pearls
• Very effective, but dangerous, antipsychotic. Reduces suicide in schizophrenia
• Efficacious in reducing dyskinesia in PD. It may be useful for treating tardive dyskinesia caused by other neuroleptics. Clonazepam, ginkgo biloba, tetrabenazine, and reserpine probably are more effective in treating tardive dyskinesia
• Clozapine was formerly the first-line agent for psychosis with PD, but now often a second-line agent due to risk of agranulocytosis. Quetiapine is now the most commonly used drug, although it remains investigational. Other atypical neuroleptics may also be effective but often cause motor AEs
• Was previously believed useful in treating psychosis in patients with Alzheimer's dementia, but subsequently shown to worsen cognitive function with significant AEs
• May be used for REM sleep behavior disorder
• Based on a recent Cochrane review, clozapine was associated with more sedation and hypersalivation than olanzapine, quetiapine, and risperidone and with more seizures than olanzapine and risperidone. There was a higher incidence of white blood cell decrease in clozapine groups than olanzapine groups and more weight gain than in risperidone groups. On the other hand clozapine produced fewer movement disorders than risperidone and less prolactin increase than olanzapine, quetiapine

Suggested Reading

Asenjo Lobos C, Komossa K, Rummel-Kluge C, Hunger H, Schmid F, Schwarz S, et al. Clozapine versus other atypical antipsychotics for schizophrenia. *Cochrane Database Syst Rev.* 2010;11:CD006633.

Aurora RN, Zak RS, Maganti RK, Auerbach SH, Casey KR, Chowdhuri S, et al. Best practice guide for the treatment of REM sleep behavior disorder (RBD). *J Clin Sleep Med.* 2010;6(1): 85–95.

Bhidayasiri R, Fahn S, Weiner WJ, Gronseth GS, Sullivan KL, Zesiewicz TA, et al. Evidence-based guideline: treatment of tardive syndromes: report of the Guideline Development Subcommittee of the American Academy of Neurology. *Neurology.* 2013;81(5):463–9.

Fox SH, Katzenschlager R, Lim S-Y, Ravina B, Seppi K, Coelho M, et al. The Movement Disorder Society Evidence-Based Medicine Review Update: Treatments for the motor symptoms of Parkinson's disease. *Mov Disord.* 2011;26 Suppl 3:S2–41.

Lauterbach EC. The neuropsychiatry of Parkinson's disease. *Minerva Med.* 2005;96(3):155–73.

Lieberman JA. Maximizing clozapine therapy: managing side effects. *J Clin Psychiatry* 1998;59 (Suppl 3): 38–43.

Poewe W. When a Parkinson's disease patient starts to hallucinate. *Pract Neurol.* 2008;8(4): 238–41.

Zahodne LB, Fernandez HH. Pathophysiology and treatment of psychosis in Parkinson's disease: a review. *Drugs Aging.* 2008;25(8): 665–82.

CORTICOTROPIN

THERAPEUTICS

Brands
- Acthar, H.P. Acthar Gel, Cosyntropin, Cortrosyn, Tetracosactide

Generic?
- Yes

Class
- Corticosteroid

Commonly Prescribed for
(FDA approved in bold)
- **Treatment of infantile spasms in infants and children under 2 years of age**
- **Treatment of exacerbations of multiple sclerosis (MS) in adults**
- **Disorders and diseases: adrenal, pituitary, rheumatic, collagen, dermatological, allergic states, ophthalmic, respiratory, and edematous state**
- **Diagnostic testing of adrenal function**

How the Drug Works
- Similar to endogenous adrenocorticotropic hormone (ACTH), it stimulates the adrenal cortex to secrete cortisol, corticosterone, aldosterone, and a number of weakly androgenic substances. Prolonged large-dose administration can induce hyperplasia and hypertrophy of the adrenal cortex and continuous high output of cortisol, corticosterone, and weak androgens. Glucocorticoids have anti-inflammatory effects, modify immune responses to stimuli, and have numerous metabolic effects. The extra-adrenal effects include increased melanotropic activity, increased growth hormone secretion, and an adipokinetic effect

How Long Until It Works
- Infantile spasm: 7–12 days
- MS: days
- Diagnostic testing: 30–60 minutes

If It Works
- Complete a course of treatment. May repeat if necessary. Monitor for long-term corticosteroid-related adverse effects

If It Doesn't Work
- Infantile spasm: consider switch to vigabatrin or other AEDs. If with underlying tuberous sclerosis, may consider surgical evaluation or everolimus
- MS: if no improvement, confirm the diagnosis of relapsing-remitting MS. Start long-term disease-modifying therapy

 ### Best Augmenting Combos for Partial Response or Treatment-Resistance
- MS: use disease-modifying treatments to reduce relapses that require corticosteroids

Tests
- Monitor blood pressure, blood glucose, body weight, and electrolytes with long-term therapy

ADVERSE EFFECTS (AEs)

How the Drug Causes AEs
- Most AEs are due to immunosuppression, metabolic, or endocrine effects

Notable AEs
- General: fluid retention, potassium loss, glucose intolerance, hypertension, behavioral and mood change, increased appetite and weight gain
- Specific reactions in children < 2: increased risk of infection, cushingoid symptoms, cardiac hypertrophy, stomach upset, diarrhea, weight gain, hypertension, irritability, acne, rash

 ### Life-Threatening or Dangerous AEs
- Osteopenic fracture. Fractures, aseptic necrosis of femoral or humoral heads
- Posterior subcapsular cataract, glaucoma
- Adrenal insufficiency
- Hypokalemia may cause cardiac arrhythmias
- Diabetic ketoacidosis, hyperosmolar coma
- May mask symptoms of infection and prevent ability of patient to prevent dissemination. May activate latent amebiasis or tuberculosis. May prolong coma in cerebral malaria
- Hypersensitivity

Weight Gain

- Problematic

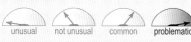

Sedation

- Unusual

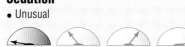

What to Do About AEs

- Avoid food with high sodium content. Potassium supplementation
- Control and monitor blood sugar
- Antibiotics, antivirals, or antifungals if severe infection
- H$_2$-blocker or proton pump inhibitor for gastric ulcer prevention
- Slow tapering

Best Augmenting Agents to Reduce AEs

- With prolonged treatment, use daily calcium and vitamin D supplements and bisphosphonates to prevent osteoporosis and fractures, and H$_2$-blocker or proton pump inhibitors to prevent peptic ulcers

DOSING AND USE

Usual Dosage Range

- Infantile spasm (Acthar gel): 150 units per unit body surface area (m^2), divided into twice daily IM
- MS (Acthar gel): 80–120 units
- ACTH stimulation test (Cortrosyn): 0.25–0.75 mg ($\geq$ 2 years old), 0.125 mg (< 2 years old) IV/IM

Dosage Forms

- Acthar gel: 5 mL multi-dose vial containing 80 USP units per mL. It is derived from porcine pituitary
- Cortrosyn: 0.25 mg (lyophilized powder; identical to 25 units) and 10 mg of mannitol to be constituted with 1 mL of 0.9% sodium chloride injection. It is a synthetic peptide containing the first 24 amino acids of natural ACTH

How to Dose

- Infantile spasm: Acthar gel IM 150 U/m^2 divided dose daily over 2 weeks then slowly

taper: 30, 15, 10 U/m^2 in the morning every 3 days, and 10 U/m^2 every other morning for 6 days. Body surface area: square root [weight (kg) $\times$ height (cm)/3600]
- MS: Acthar gel IM 80–120 units for 2–3 weeks followed by a taper

 Dosing Tips

- In patients improving on long-term treatment, consider converting to every-other-day dosing to reduce AEs
- Acthar should be warmed to room temperature before injection. Rotate site each time to avoid muscular injury from repeated injections

Overdose

- Rare and not fully studied. In corticosteroid, acute overdose can produce psychosis, hypertension, arrhythmia, Na/K imbalance, fluid retention

Long-Term Use

- Associated with side effects related to excess mineralocorticoids or corticosteroids. Usually not recommended for long-term use unless clinically necessary

Habit Forming

- No

How to Stop

- For long-term user with altered hypothalamus-pituitary-adrenal axis, taper slowly

Pharmacokinetics

- Half-life 15 minutes following IV administration. Half-life following IM administration has not been studied

 Drug Interactions

- May accentuate the electrolyte loss associated with diuretic therapy
- It induces the synthesis of corticosteroid, which is a weak CYP450 isoenzyme inducer

 Other Warnings/ Precautions

- Do not administer live or attenuated vaccines to patients on immunosuppressive doses

- Neutralizing antibodies with chronic administration may lead to a loss of endogenous corticotropin activity
- Symptoms of diabetes and myasthenia gravis may be worsened during the treatment

Do Not Use

- Cortrosyn is contraindicated for previous hypersensitivity to drug
- Acthar is contraindicated for use in scleroderma, osteoporosis, systemic fungal infections, ocular herpes simplex, recent surgery, history of or the presence of a peptic ulcer, congestive heart failure, uncontrolled hypertension, sensitivity to proteins of porcine origin, children under 2 with suspected congenital infections, administration of live or live attenuated vaccines under immunosuppressive state, primary adrenocortical insufficiency, adrenocortical hyperfunction, or IV administration

SPECIAL POPULATIONS

Renal Impairment

- Patients are more likely to develop edema with corticosteroids. Use with caution

Hepatic Impairment

- May have enhanced effect in those with liver cirrhosis

Cardiac Impairment

- May cause hypertension

Elderly

- Consider lower doses due to lower plasma volumes and decreased muscle mass. Monitor blood pressure, glucose, and electrolytes at least every 6 months

 Children and Adolescents

- Adverse reactions seen in infants and children under 2 years of age treated for infantile spasms are similar to those seen in older patients. Long-term use may have negative effects on growth and physical development in children

 Pregnancy

- Category C. It has embrocidal effect. No adequate and well-controlled studies in pregnancy. It should be used only if the potential benefit justifies the potential risk to the fetus

Breast Feeding

- It is not known whether this drug is excreted in human milk. Avoid breast feeding with high-dose, long-term treatment

THE ART OF NEUROPHARMACOLOGY

Potential Advantages

- Can be effective for infantile spasm

Potential Disadvantages

- Cost for repository gel

Primary Target Symptoms

- Depending on disorder: Treating and preventing neurological complications in MS, infantile spasm, and other disorders treatable with corticosteroid

 Pearls

- AAN guideline: low-dose corticotropin (20–30 units) should be considered for treatment of infantile spasms. Corticotropin or vigabatrin may be useful for short-term treatment of infantile spasms, with corticotropin considered preferentially over vigabatrin. Hormonal therapy (corticotropin or prednisolone) may be considered for use in preference to vigabatrin in infants with cryptogenic infantile spasms, to possibly improve developmental outcome. A shorter lag time to treatment of infantile spasms with either hormonal therapy or vigabatrin possibly improves long-term developmental outcomes
- Infantile spasm may remit, but relapse is not uncommon. No data guiding repeated usage
- Vigabatrin should be considered drug of choice for infantile spasms patients with tuberous sclerosis. The risk of visual changes is minor compared to poor outcomes of untreated infantile spasms

- H.P. Acthar Gel is almost 29 times more expensive than Cortrosyn in the US
- No evidence that corticotropin is superior to other corticosteroid for the treatment of MS relapses

- Synthetic ACTH (Cosyntropin) is quicker onset for ACTH test and less immunogenic than corticotropin

Suggested Reading

Gettig J, Cummings JP, Matuszewski K. H.P. Acthar Gel and Cosyntropin review: clinical and financial implications. *P&T.* 2009;34:250–7.

Go CY, Mackay MT, Weiss SK, Stephens D, Adams-Webber T, Ashwal S, Snead OC; Child Neurology Society; American Academy of Neurology. Evidence-based guideline update: medical treatment of infantile spasms. Report of the Guideline Development Subcommittee of the American Academy of Neurology and the Practice Committee of the Child Neurology Society. *Neurology.* 2012;78:1974–80.

CYCLOBENZAPRINE

THERAPEUTICS

Brands
- Flexeril, Fexmid, Amrix, Apo-Cyclobenzaprine

Generic?
- Yes

Class
- Muscle relaxant

Commonly Prescribed for
(FDA approved in bold)
- **Muscle spasm**
- Neck pain/lower back pain
- Myofascial pain
- Fibromyalgia

How the Drug Works
- A tricyclic compound structurally similar to amitriptyline. It blocks serotonin and norepinephrine reuptake pumps and has anticholinergic effects. Acts on locus coeruleus and via gamma fibers to inhibit the alpha motor neurons in the ventral horn of the spinal cord, hence decreased muscle tone. Reduces tonic somatic motor activity

How Long Until It Works
- Pain: May work within hours but maximal effect occurs in 4–14 days

If It Works
- Titrate to most effective tolerated dose

If It Doesn't Work
- Increase to highest tolerated dose. If ineffective, consider alternative medications or other modalities

Best Augmenting Combos for Partial Response or Treatment-Resistance
- Use other centrally acting muscle relaxants with caution due to potential additive CNS depressant effect
- Combine with non-pharmacological treatments such as exercise/physical therapy, massage, heat/ice, or acupuncture

Tests
- Consider checking ECG for QTc prolongation at baseline and when increasing dose

ADVERSE EFFECTS (AEs)

How the Drug Causes AEs
- Anticholinergic and antihistaminic properties are causes of most common AEs

Notable AEs
- Dry mouth, dizziness, fatigue, constipation, weakness, sweating, and nausea are most common. Somnolence is more common with the intermediate-acting form

Life-Threatening or Dangerous AEs
- Orthostatic hypotension, tachycardia, QTc prolongation, and rarely death
- Increased intraocular pressure
- Paralytic ileus, hyperthermia
- Rare activation of mania or suicidal ideation
- Rare worsening of existing seizure disorders
- Serotonin syndrome

Weight Gain
- Not unusual

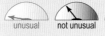

| unusual | not unusual | common | problematic |

Sedation
- Common

| unusual | not unusual | common | problematic |

What to Do About AEs
- For somnolence or fatigue, change to once-daily formulation or decrease dose. For any serious AEs, discontinue

Best Augmenting Agents to Reduce AEs
- Most AEs cannot be reduced by use of augmenting agent

DOSING AND USE

Usual Dosage Range
- 15–30 mg/day

Dosage Forms

- Tablets: 5, 7.5, 10 mg
- Extended-release capsules: 15, 30 mg

How to Dose

- Start at 5 mg 3 times a day and increase as tolerated (for best effect) to 7.5 or 10 mg 3 times a day. The extended-release capsule should be taken 4–6 hours before bedtime

Dosing Tips

- Take the largest dose in the evening to avoid somnolence with the immediate-release form. The extended-release capsule peaks at about 6–8 hours. Taking the extended-release form just before bedtime can lead to excess fatigue before awakening. Peak concentrations are greater when taking with food

Overdose

- Cardiac arrhythmias and ECG changes; death can occur. CNS depression and tachycardia are most common. Convulsions or severe hypotension are less common. Least commonly, agitation, ataxia, tremor, vomiting, or coma can occur. Patients should be hospitalized. Sodium bicarbonate can treat arrhythmias and hypotension. Treat shock with vasopressors, oxygen, or corticosteroids

Long-Term Use

- Not studied but probably safe

Habit Forming

- No

How to Stop

- Not usually tapered but may cause withdrawal symptoms similar to those of TCA (insomnia, nausea, headache) withdrawal

Pharmacokinetics

- Metabolized by CYP3A4, CYP1A2, and to a lesser extent CYP2D6. It is excreted as glucuronides via the kidney. 93% protein bound. Half-life 18 hours. All forms take 3–4 days to reach steady state and at usual doses exhibit linear pharmacokinetics

Drug Interactions

- Strong CYP3A4 inhibitors (protease inhibitors, macrolides, azoles, nefazodone) and strong CYP1A2 inhibitors (fluoroquinolones, fluvoxamine, verapamil) may decrease cyclobenzaprine concentration
- Strong CYP3A4 inducers (carbamazepine, phenytoin, phenobarbital, rifampin, corticosteroid) may reduce cyclobenzaprine concentration
- Use with anticholinergics can increase AEs (i.e., risk of ileus)
- May enhance effects of CNS depressants
- Use with MAOI, such as rasagiline or selegiline, can cause hypertensive crisis, seizures, or death
- May alter effects of antihypertensive medications, such as guanethidine (blocking effect)
- Use with tramadol may increase seizure risk

Other Warnings/Precautions

- Because of its atropine-like action cyclobenzaprine should be used with caution in patients with a history of urinary retention, angle-closure glaucoma, increased intraocular pressure, and in patients taking anticholinergic medication

Do Not Use

- Proven hypersensitivity to drug or other TCAs
- Contraindicated with MAOIs
- In acute recovery after myocardial infarction or uncompensated heart failure
- In conjunction with antiarrhythmics that prolong QTc interval

SPECIAL POPULATIONS

Renal Impairment

- Use with caution. May need to lower dose

Hepatic Impairment

- Increased plasma concentrations with moderate to severe liver dysfunction. Use with caution at low doses if at all

Cardiac Impairment
- Do not use in patients with recent myocardial infarction, severe heart failure, a history of QTc prolongation, or orthostatic hypotension

Elderly
- Plasma levels are higher and may be at greater risk of AEs. Use with caution, especially over age 65. Increased risk of injury

Children and Adolescents
- Not studied in children under age 15

Pregnancy
- Category B. Use only if there is a clear need

Breast Feeding
- Unknown if excreted in breast milk. Do not use

THE ART OF NEUROPHARMACOLOGY

Potential Advantages
- Effective antispasmodic with effectiveness in acute muscle spasm and pain. Low risk of addiction/dependence compared to carbisodol. Available as once-daily dose

Potential Disadvantages
- Sedation can be problematic, especially with immediate-acting form. Not effective for spasticity due to CNS disorders (e.g., multiple sclerosis [MS], spinal cord injury)

Primary Target Symptoms
- Muscle spasm, pain

Pearls
- Similar to TCA class in structure, pharmacology, and AEs. In long-standing pain disorders such as migraine, chronic neck pain, or fibromyalgia, consider using TCAs for long-term treatment
- Do not use for spasticity related to CNS disorders, including MS, spinal cord injury, and cerebral palsy. Baclofen or tizanidine are more effective agents for these conditions
- Usually used as a short-term adjunctive agent (2–6 weeks) for acute muscle spasm and pain. No longer-term studies have been done, but due to similarities with TCAs, probably safe to use for months or years

Suggested Reading

Carette S, Bell MJ, Reynolds WJ, Haraoui B, McCain GA, Bykerk VP, Edworthy SM, Baron M, Koehler BE, Fam AG, et al. Comparison of amitriptyline, cyclobenzaprine, and placebo in the treatment of fibromyalgia. A randomized, double-blind clinical trial. *Arthritis Rheum.* 1994;37(1):32–40.

Chou R, Peterson K, Helfand M. Comparative efficacy and safety of skeletal muscle relaxants for spasticity and musculoskeletal conditions: a systematic review. *J Pain Symptom Manage.* 2004;28(2):140–75.

See S, Ginzburg R. Choosing a skeletal muscle relaxant. *Am Fam Physician.* 2008;78(3):365–70.

Tofferi JK, Jackson JL, O'Malley PG. Treatment of fibromyalgia with cyclobenzaprine: a meta-analysis. *Arthritis Rheum.* 2004;51(1):9–13.

Toth PP, Urtis J. Commonly used muscle relaxant therapies for acute low back pain: a review of carisoprodol, cyclobenzaprine hydrochloride, and metaxalone. *Clin Ther.* 2004;26(9):1355–67. Review

CYCLOPHOSPHAMIDE

Brands
- Revimmune, Cytoxan, Neosar, Endoxan, Procytox

Generic?
- Yes

Class
- Immunosuppressant

Commonly Prescribed for
(FDA approved in bold)
- **Treatment of malignancies, including lymphomas (lymphocytic, mixed-cell type, histiocytic, Burkitt's, and Hodgkin's disease), disseminated neuroblastoma, ovarian adenocarcinoma, and breast**
- Other malignancies: bronchogenic, small cell lung, endometrial, prostate, testicular, and sarcomas
- **Mycosis fungoides**
- **"Minimal change" nephrotic syndrome in children**
- Myasthenia gravis (MG)
- Multiple sclerosis (MS) (relapsing-remitting)
- Neuromyelitis optica
- Polymyositis and dermatomyositis
- Multifocal motor neuropathy
- Vasculitis including Wegener's granulomatosis, polyarteritis nodosa
- Rheumatoid arthritis
- Systemic lupus erythematosus
- Bone marrow transplantation

How the Drug Works
- An alkylating agent and non-specific cell-cycle inhibitor with metabolites that interfere with the growth of rapidly proliferating normal and malignant cells, most likely by cross-linking of tumor cell DNA

How Long Until It Works
- Within a week, but effect on neurological diseases may take months

If It Works
- MG: may allow improvement in symptoms or reduction in dose or discontinuation of corticosteroids or other agents

- MS: may reduce relapses and new lesions on MRI
- Other disorders: improves symptoms (weakness, sensory changes) and clinical marker of the disease

If It Doesn't Work
- Usually used as a disease modifying agent in refractory cases when first-line agents have failed

Best Augmenting Combos for Partial Response or Treatment-Resistance
- Often used in combination with other agents depending on the disease in question, such as corticosteroids for vasculitis or MG and plasma exchange for multifocal motor neuropathy

Tests
- Obtain CBC regularly during treatment to determine WBC and platelet counts. Examine urine for red cells (hemorrhagic cystitis)

How the Drug Causes AEs
- Immunosupression, lymphopenia, and risk of secondary neoplasia

Notable AEs
- Nausea and vomiting, anorexia, abdominal pain, diarrhea, darkening of the skin/nails, alopecia, delay in wound healing, and lethargy. Hemorrhagic cystitis is common but preventable with the detoxifying agent mesna. May cause sterility (usually temporary) in women (amenorrhea is common) and men (decreased sperm count and increased gonadotropin levels)

Life-Threatening or Dangerous AEs
- Leukopenia occurs in all patients and is dose related, less commonly thrombocytopenia and anemia. Recovery from leukopenia begins 7–10 days after cessation of therapy
- Severe congestive heart failure due to hemorrhagic myocarditis or myocardial necrosis

- Increases risk of new malignancy, usually several years after treatment – bladder, myeloproliferative, or lymphoproliferative are most common
- Interstitial pulmonary fibrosis

Weight Gain

- Unusual

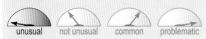

Sedation

- Unusual

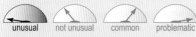

What to Do About AEs

- Treat infections appropriately and reduce dose if possible

Best Augmenting Agents to Reduce AEs

- Hydration or mesna should be used to prevent hemorrhagic cystitis

DOSING AND USE

Usual Dosage Range

- Oral: 1–5 mg/kg/day adjusted based on WBC
- IV: 1–3 g/m² not to exceed 85 mg/kg

Dosage Forms

- Tablets 25, 50 mg
- Capsule: 25, 50 mg
- Injection, powder: 100, 200, 500, 1000, 2000 mg/vial

How to Dose

- Oral: start at 2–3 mg/kg/day and adjust to maintain a WBC between 2500 and 4000/mm³ and lymphocyte count below 1000/mm³. For more significant leukopenia or other AEs, patients may skip doses
- IV: many different regimens exist. 40–50 mg/kg over 2–5 days every 3–4 weeks, 10–15 mg/kg every 7–10 days, or 3–5 mg/kg twice weekly are examples. In neurological disorders, a typical regimen is 1–3 g/m², given over an 8-day period on days 1, 2, 4, 6, and 8, equally divided. The 4th and 5th doses are given only if the WBC is greater than 3500/mm³. Obtain a CBC

before each dose. Alternatively give a total dose of 1 g/m² every 4–5 weeks

 Dosing Tips

- Optimal availability with oral formulation when taken without food. With IV administration, give adequate hydration and treat nausea if necessary

Overdose

- Unknown

Long-Term Use

- Usually used on a short-term basis for refractory disorders

Habit Forming

- No

How to Stop

- No need to taper but monitor for recurrence of neurological disorder

Pharmacokinetics

- Peak action of metabolites at 2–3 hours and half-life 3–12 hours. Hepatic metabolism to active metabolites and renal excretion

 Drug Interactions

- Allopurinol and thiazide diuretics increase its myelosuppressive effects, potentially increasing AEs
- Phenobarbital and chloramphenicol may decrease effectiveness
- Can increase anticoagulant effect, cardiotoxicity from doxorubicin, and neuromuscular blockade of succinylcholine
- May decrease digoxin serum levels and antimicrobial effects of fluoroquinolones

 Other Warnings/ Precautions

- Anaphylactic reactions have been reported
- Possible cross-sensitivity with other alkylating agents has been reported

Do Not Use

- Known hypersensitivity to the drug or severely depressed bone marrow function. Urinary outflow obstruction

Renal Impairment
• No known effects

Hepatic Impairment
• No known effects

Cardiac Impairment
• Can cause cardiac toxicity, especially at high doses. Use with caution

Elderly
• No known effects. Use with caution

Children and Adolescents
• Effectiveness and safety are unknown. Rarely used due to long-term AEs

Pregnancy
• Category D. Use contraception during treatment to avoid pregnancy

Breast Feeding
• Do not breast feed while on drug

Potential Advantages
• Useful for many refractory autoimmune neurological disorders when usual first-line disease-modifying agents fail

Potential Disadvantages
• Multiple AEs complicate use

Primary Target Symptoms
• Preventive treatment of complications from diseases, such as MG or MS

Pearls
• Appears to be effective in MG. Patients experienced increased strength and decreased prednisone doses at 12 months in one study. Treatment consisted of pulse doses 500 mg/m^2 monthly for 6 months

• In one study, a one-time treatment with cyclophosphamide (1–12 g based on level of leukopenia over 1–2 weeks) in relapsing MS resulted in decreased relapse rates. Now rarely used for MS due to emerging new therapies and AEs

• Used in combination with corticosteroids for refractory cases of systemic or CNS vasculitis, such as polyarteritis nodosa. Treatment consists of IV cyclophosphamide until remission (usually at least 6 and up to 12 pulses) and then patients are transitioned to maintenance therapy (azathioprine or methotrexate). Cyclophosphamide is used in most cases of systemic Wegener's granulomatosis, either orally or IV. Pulse doses are given every 3–4 weeks at a dose of 0.5–0.7 g/m^2

• In polymyositis and dermatomyositis, usually used in cases refractory to corticosteroids and azathioprine. Assess treatment success by following muscle strength and creatine kinase levels

• In multifocal motor neuropathy, IV cyclophosphamide is used for 6 months in cases refractory to IV immune globulin and often combined with plasma exchange. Follow clinical improvement and reduction of anti-GM1 antibodies

• Useful in fulminant cases of CNS vasculitis refractory to standard treatment

Suggested Reading

Gladstone DE, Brannagan TH 3rd, Schwartzman RJ, Prestrud AA, Brodsky I. High dose cyclophosphamide for severe refractory myasthenia gravis. *J Neurol Neurosurg Psychiatry.* 2004;75(5):789–91.

Gonzalez-Duarte A, Higuera-Calleja J, Flores F, Davila-Maldonado L, Cantú-Brito C. Cyclophosphamide treatment for unrelenting CNS vasculitis secondary to tuberculous meningitis. *Neurology.* 2012;78(16):1277–8.

Hart IK, Sathasivam S, Sharshar T. Immunosuppressive agents for myasthenia gravis. *Cochrane Database Syst Rev.* 2007;4: CD005224

Hengstman GJ, van den Hoogen FH, van Engelen BG. Treatment of the inflammatory myopathies: update and practical recommendations. *Expert Opin Pharmacother.* 2009;10(7):1183–90.

Neuhaus O, Kieseier BC, Hartung HP. Immunosuppressive agents in multiple sclerosis. *Neurotherapeutics.* 2007;4(4):654–60.

Schwartzman RJ, Simpkins N, Alexander GM, Reichenberger E, Ward K, Lindenberg N, Topolsky D, Crilley P. High-dose cyclophosphamide in the treatment of multiple sclerosis. *CNS Neurosci Ther.* 2009;15(2):118–27.

CYCLOSPORINE (CICLOSPORIN)

Brands
- Gengraf, Neoral, Sandimmune, Cicloral

Generic?
- Yes

Class
- Immunosuppressant

Commonly Prescribed for
(FDA approved in bold)
- **Prophylaxis of organ rejection in patients with allogenic kidney, liver, and heart transplants**
- **Rheumatoid arthritis**
- **Psoriasis**
- Myasthenia gravis (MG)
- Neuromyelitis optica
- Acute disseminated encephalomyelitis
- Leukemia refractory to routine treatment
- Aplastic anemia
- Ulcerative colitis

How the Drug Works
- It binds to cyclophilin thus inhibiting the phosphatase activity of calcineurin, with a resultant decrease in activation of nuclear factor of activated T-lymphocytes (NFATs). It also blocks the activation of JNK and p38 signaling pathways. Overall, it inhibits lymphokine (e.g., interleukin 2) production and release, and reduces T-lymphocyte (especially T-helper cell) activation

How Long Until It Works
- Most patients with MG improve 1–2 months after starting treatment, but maximum improvement takes 6 or more months

If It Works
- Decrease dose of corticosteroids. Gradually reduce to the minimum dose needed to maintain clinical improvement

If It Doesn't Work
- Consider alternative disease-modifying therapy or thymectomy

Best Augmenting Combos for Partial Response or Treatment-Resistance
- Often used with corticosteroids (prednisone), especially in the initial stages of treatment

Tests
- Obtain baseline CBC, magnesium, potassium, uric acid, lipids, blood urea nitrogen, and creatinine. Measure trough levels 1 month after starting to determine dosing. Measure creatinine every 2–4 weeks for the first few months, then monthly, and then every 2–3 months when stable or when new medications are added. Measure CBC, uric acid, potassium, and lipids every 2 weeks for the first 3 months, then monthly. Monitor blood pressure frequently (at least monthly)

How the Drug Causes AEs
- Uncertain

Notable AEs
- Hypertension, hirsutism, cramps, diarrhea, infection, hypomagnesemia
- Tremor, convulsions, paresthesias

Life-Threatening or Dangerous AEs
- Renal failure. Elevations of blood urea nitrogen and creatinine are common and are dose related. Nephrotoxicity occurs in over 20% of patients
- Thrombocytopenia and microangiopathic hemolytic anemia
- Hyperkalemia
- Hepatotoxicity, usually in first month of therapy

Weight Gain
- Unusual

unusual | not unusual | common | problematic

Sedation
- Not unusual

unusual | not unusual | common | problematic

What to Do About AEs

- Renal function generally improves with dose reductions. Creatinine should be below 150% of baseline. Reduce dose by 25–50% for laboratory abnormalities

Best Augmenting Agents to Reduce AEs

- Most AEs cannot be reduced

DOSING AND USE

Usual Dosage Range

- MG: 200–600 mg/day in 2 divided doses

Dosage Forms

- Capsules: 25, 50, 100 mg
- Oral solution: 100 mg/mL
- Injection: 50 mg/mL

How to Dose

- Start at dose of 4–6 mg/kg/day in 2 doses per day about 12 hours apart
- Adjust dose for a trough level of 75–150 ng/mL every month

 Dosing Tips

- Take at about the same times daily, with or without food

Overdose

- There is minimal experience with overdose. Forced emesis is of value up to 2 hours after ingestion

Long-term Use

- Safe for long-term use

Habit Forming

- No

How to Stop

- Taper slowly, as MG symptoms may worsen

Pharmacokinetics

- Incompletely absorbed from GI tract. Most drugs are metabolized in the liver by the CYP450 3A4 enzyme. Peak effect is 3.5 hours for Sandimmune formulation and 1.5–2 hours for Neoral and Gengraf. Half-life is 19 hours for Sandimmune and 8.4 hours for Neoral and Gengraf

 Drug Interactions

- Concomitant NSAID use can worsen hypertension and renal disease
- Avoid medications, such as orlistat, that decrease absorption
- CYP3A4 inhibitors reduce metabolism and can increase levels and toxicity. Drugs that increase levels include verapamil, diltiazem, ketoconazole, fluconazole, azithromycin, erythromycin, allopurinol, oral contraceptives, colchicine, and amiodarone
- Corticosteroids, fluoroquinolones (ciprofloxacin), metaclopramide, bromocriptine, and β-blockers can also increase levels
- HIV protease inhibitors likely also increase levels
- SSRIs that are CYP3A4 inhibitors, such as fluvoxamine or fluoxetine, may increase levels and toxicity
- CYP3A4 inducers, such as phenytoin, phenobarbital, carbamazepine, rifampin, and St. John's wort, may decrease levels
- Use with potassium-sparing drugs, including ACE inhibitors and angiotensin II receptor antagonists, can cause hyperkalemia
- May cause myopathy or rhabdomyolysis with HMG-CoA reductase inhibitors
- Decreases concentrations of methotrexate and sirolimus
- Grapefruit juice can increase concentrations and should be avoided

 Other Warnings/ Precautions

- Patients with malabsorption may have difficulty reaching therapeutic levels
- Vaccines may be less effective and patients should not be given live vaccines due to risks of illness

Do Not Use

- Hypersensitivity to drug or components, uncontrolled hypertension, new-onset renal failure, or malignancy

SPECIAL POPULATIONS

Renal Impairment

- Renal function commonly worsens on drug. Monitor function closely

Hepatic Impairment

- Liver transplant patients are more likely to develop encephalopathy. Use with caution

Cardiac Impairment

- May cause new-onset or worsen existing hypertension

Elderly

- More prone to development of systolic hypertension and renal failure. Use with caution

 Children and Adolescents

- Poorly studied but no unusual AEs have been observed in children as young as 6 months

 Pregnancy

- Category C. Embryotoxic and fetotoxic in animals. Complications such as prematurity, low birth weight, preeclampsia or eclampsia, and fetal losses are common in the pregnancies of women on cyclosporine. Do not use for treatment of MG during pregnancy

Breast Feeding

- Excreted in breast milk. Discontinue the drug or bottle feed

THE ART OF NEUROPHARMACOLOGY

Potential Advantages

- Fairly effective disease-modifying agent in MG. May be effective as second-line treatment for many refractory immune-mediated neurological disorders

Potential Disadvantages

- Multiple AEs and need for frequent monitoring by physicians familiar with immunosuppressive therapy

Primary Target Symptoms

- To improve weakness, visual problems, respiratory symptoms associated with MG

 Pearls

- In small clinical trials, improved strength and lowered antireceptor antibody titers, allowing lowering of corticosteroid doses in MG
- Relatively fast onset of action compared to other corticosteroid-sparing agents
- Prevents opening of mitochondrial permeability pore, which inhibits the release of cytochrome c, a stimulator of apoptosis. This may be protective and could prevent complications of head injury and neurodegenerative diseases
- Intrathecal cyclosporine prolongs survival of late-stage ALS (amyotrophic lateral sclerosis) mice
- May be effective, in combination with corticosteroids, for the treatment of neuromyelitis optica
- Cyclosporine ophthalmic emulsion is used for ocular inflammation associated with keratoconjunctivitis sicca

CYCLOSPORINE (continued)

Suggested Reading

Appel SH, Stewart SS, Appel V, Harati Y, Mietlowski W, Weiss W, et al. A double-blind study of the effectiveness of cyclosporine in amyotrophic lateral sclerosis. *Arch Neurol.* 1988;45(4): 381–6.

Ciafaloni E, Nikhar NK, Massey JM, Sanders DB. Retrospective analysis of the use of cyclosporine in myasthenia gravis. *Neurology.* 2000;55(3):448–50.

Hart IK, Sathasivam S, Sharshar T. Immunosuppressive agents for myasthenia gravis. *Cochrane Database Syst Rev.* 2007;4: CD005224.

Hatton J, Rosbolt B, Empey P, Kryscio R, Young B. Dosing and safety of cyclosporine in patients with severe brain injury. *J Neurosurg.* 2008;109(4):699–707.

Kageyama T, Komori M, Miyamoto K, Ozaki A, Suenaga T, Takahashi R, et al. Combination of cyclosporine A with corticosteroids is effective for the treatment of neuromyelitis optica. *J Neurol.* 2013;260(2):627–34.

Lavrnic D, Vujic A, Rakocevic-Stojanovic V, Stevic Z, Basta I, Pavlovic S, et al. Cyclosporine in the treatment of myasthenia gravis. *Acta Neurol Scand.* 2005;111(4):247–52.

CYPROHEPTADINE

THERAPEUTICS

Brands
- Periactin, Cypromar, Periavit, Pyrohep

Generic?
- Yes

Class
- Antihistamine

Commonly Prescribed for
(FDA approved in bold)
- **Hypersensitivity reactions**
- Migraine prophylaxis (children and adults)
- Tension-type headache prophylaxis
- Nightmares/post-traumatic stress disorder
- Serotonin syndrome

How the Drug Works
- As an antagonist, it has high affinity for histamine (H_1), muscarine (M_{1-5}), serotonin ($5-HT_{1A/2A/2B/2C}$, serotonin transporter), and dopamine (D_3) receptors and perhaps for calcium channel receptors. The relative importance of each action in headache prophylaxis is unclear. Prevention of cortical spreading depression may be one mechanism of action for all migraine preventatives

How Long Until It Works
- Migraines may decrease in as little as 2 weeks, but can take up to 2 months to see full effect

If It Works
- Migraine: goal is a 50% or greater decrease in migraine frequency or severity. Consider tapering or stopping if headaches remit for more than 6 months or if considering pregnancy

If It Doesn't Work
- Increase to highest tolerated dose
- Migraine: address other issues, such as medication overuse, other coexisting medical disorders, such as anxiety, and consider changing to another agent or adding a second agent

Best Augmenting Combos for Partial Response or Treatment-Resistance
- Migraine: for some patients with migraine, low-dose polytherapy with 2 or more drugs may be better tolerated and more effective than high-dose monotherapy. May use in combination with AEDs, antidepressants, natural products, and non-medication treatments, such as biofeedback, to improve headache control

Tests
- Monitor weight during treatment

ADVERSE EFFECTS (AEs)

How the Drug Causes AEs
- Most are related to antihistamine and anticholinergic activity

Notable AEs
- Sedation, dizziness, dry mouth, postural hypotension, photosensitivity, and weight gain

Life-Threatening or Dangerous AEs
- Bradycardia, ECG changes, including QTc prolongation
- Hypersensitivity reactions

Weight Gain
- Problematic

unusual   not unusual   common   **problematic**

Sedation
- Common

unusual   not unusual   **common**   problematic

What to Do About AEs
- Lower dose or switch to another agent. For serious AEs, do not use

Best Augmenting Agents to Reduce AEs
- No treatment for most AEs other than lowering dose or stopping drug

DOSING AND USE

Usual Dosage Range
- 8–32 mg/day

Dosage Forms
- Tablets: 4 mg
- Syrup: 2 mg/5mL

How to Dose
- Migraine/tension-type headache: initial dose is usually 2 mg at night. Increase by 2 mg every 3–7 days in 3 divided doses until beneficial or AEs develop

 Dosing Tips
- Take the largest dose at night to minimize drowsiness

Overdose
- CNS depression is most common, but hypotension, cardiac collapse or ECG changes, and respiratory depression may occur. Anticholinergic effects include fixed pupils, flushing, and hyperthermia. Convulsions indicate poor prognosis. Protect against aspiration, correct electrolyte disturbances and acidosis, and give activated charcoal with a cathartic. Give diazepam for convulsions and consider physostigmine for central anticholinergic effects

Long-Term Use
- Safe for long-term use

Habit Forming
- No

How to Stop
- No need to taper, but migraine often returns after stopping

Pharmacokinetics
- Peak levels at 1–2 hours, duration 4–6 hours. Hepatic metabolism (glucuronide conjugation, N-demethylation, etc.) with renal excretion of metabolites and some unchanged drug

 Drug Interactions
- MAOIs, ketoconazole, and erythromycin may increase plasma levels and toxicity

- Cyproheptadine may lower effectiveness of SSRIs due to serotonin antagonism
- May diminish expected pituitary-adrenal response to metyrapone
- Excess sedation with other CNS depressants (alcohol, barbiturates) can occur

 Other Warnings/ Precautions
- Avoid in patients with respiratory disease such as sleep apnea or chronic obstructive pulmonary disease

Do Not Use
- Hypersensitivity to drug, angle-closure glaucoma, bladder neck obstruction, patients using MAOIs, symptomatic prostatic hypertrophy

SPECIAL POPULATIONS

Renal Impairment
- No known effects

Hepatic Impairment
- May reduce metabolism. Titrate more slowly

Cardiac Impairment
- Rarely causes arrhythmias and ECG changes. Use with caution

Elderly
- More likely to experience AEs, especially anticholinergic. Avoid using for headache prophylaxis

 Children and Adolescents
- Drug is used most often for pediatric headache disorders, but may decrease alertness or produce paradoxical excitation

 Pregnancy
- Category B. Use only if potential benefit outweighs risk to the fetus

Breast Feeding
- Unknown if excreted in breast milk. Patient should not breast feed while on drug

THE ART OF NEUROPHARMACOLOGY

Potential Advantages

- Commonly used pediatric migraine preventive, especially for younger children

Potential Disadvantages

- No large studies that demonstrate effectiveness and many AEs that limit use

Primary Target Symptoms

- Headache frequency and severity

Pearls

- In one study, superior to placebo but inferior to methysergide
- Antiserotonin effects are most likely responsible for effectiveness, but can cause depression despite previously successful treatment when used with SSRIs
- 4–8 mg every 6 hours may be used for treating serotonin syndrome. Antagonism of 5-HT receptors suggests usefulness in the treatment of serotonin syndrome and MAOI toxicity
- In one study, 4 mg/day was as effective as propranolol 80 mg/day in migraine prophylaxis
- May be useful for post-traumatic nightmare

Suggested Reading

Holland S, Silberstein SD, Freitag F, Dodick DW, Argoff C, Ashman E; Quality Standards Subcommittee of the American Academy of Neurology and the American Headache Society. Evidence-based guideline update: NSAIDs and other complementary treatments for episodic migraine prevention in adults: report of the Quality Standards Subcommittee of the American Academy of Neurology and the American Headache Society. *Neurology*. 2012;78:1346–53.

Iqbal MM, Basil MJ, Kaplan J, Iqbal MT. Overview of serotonin syndrome. *Ann Clin Psychiatry*. 2012;24:310–18.

Lewis DW, Yonker M, Winner P, Sowell M. The treatment of pediatric migraine. *Pediatr Ann*. 2005;34(6):448–60.

Meythaler JM, Roper JF, Brunner RC. Cyproheptadine for intrathecal baclofen withdrawal. *Arch Phys Med Rehabil*. 2003; 84(5):638–42.

DABIGATRAN ETEXILATE

THERAPEUTICS

Brands
- Pradaxa

Generic?
- No

Class
- Anticoagulant

Commonly Prescribed for
(FDA approved in bold)
- **Prevention of stroke and systemic embolism in adult patients with non-valvular atrial fibrillation (NVAF)**
- Primary prevention of venous thromboembolic (VTE) events in adult patients who have undergone elective total hip or knee arthroplasty
- Prevention of stroke and systemic embolism in patients with left ventricular thrombosis

How the Drug Works
- Dabigatran etexilate is a prodrug that is rapidly converted to its active compound, dabigatran, by non-specific esterase in the plasma and liver. Dabigatran is a reversible inhibitor for factor IIa (thrombin, free and clot-bound), thereby reducing the conversion of fibrinogen into fibrin and thrombus formation. Thrombin-induced platelet aggregation is also inhibited

How Long Until It Works
- Peak concentration in 1–2 hours

If It Works
- Monitor for signs of bleeding. Assess renal function periodically as clinically indicated

If It Doesn't Work
- Correct the underlying disorder. Use a higher dose or switch to different anticoagulant

Best Augmenting Combos for Partial Response or Treatment-Resistance
- Based on RE-LY study, concomitant antiplatelet therapy has little effect on the relative advantages of dabigatran in comparison with warfarin on AF management

Tests
- A prolonged aPTT ($> 1\times$ control) is consistent with the presence of dabigatran, but the degree of prolongation does not correlate well with plasma concentrations. aPTT > 2 upper limit (after 12–24 hours) or thrombin time > 65 seconds may indicate greater bleeding risks. The Hemoclot thrombin clotting time is more accurate but not available in the US. aPTT $< 1\times$ control is at low risk of bleeding events

ADVERSE EFFECTS (AEs)

How the Drug Causes AEs
- Reduced coagulation due to inhibited thrombin

Notable AEs
- Bleeding and GI events (e.g., diarrhea, dyspepsia, abdominal pain, hemorrhage)
- Compared with warfarin, dabigatran has lower rates of intracranial bleeding and life-threatening bleeding, but higher GI bleeding

Life-Threatening or Dangerous AEs
- Life-threatening bleed (1.5%), intracranial hemorrhage (0.3%), major GI bleed (1.6%), anaphylactic shock ($< 0.1\%$)

Weight Gain
- Unusual (0.45%)

unusual   not unusual   common   problematic

Sedation
- Unusual (0.01%)

unusual   not unusual   common   problematic

What to Do About AEs
- Discontinue treatment, supportive care, hemodialysis

Best Augmenting Agents to Reduce AEs

- Antiplatelet agent, fibrinolytic agent, other anticoagulants, long-term NSAID, amiodarone, and ketoconazole

DOSING AND USE

Usual Dosage Range

- 150 mg twice daily

Dosage Forms

- Capsule

How to Dose

- NVAF: 150 mg twice daily
- Acute VTE: 150 mg twice daily for 6 months
- Post-total knee arthroplasty VTE prophylaxis: 150 mg or 220 mg once daily for 6 months
- Renal impairment: reduce to half dose if CrCl 15–50 mL/min
- Converting from warfarin: discontinue warfarin and start dabigatran when INR is below 2
- Surgical procedure: discontinue 1–2 days. Consider longer times if major surgery

 Dosing Tips

- Capsule should be swallowed whole; not to be broken, chewed, or emptied. Not affected by food

Overdose

- May lead to hemorrhagic complications. Can use hemodialysis. Investigational antidote (aripazine, idarucizumab)

Long-Term Use

- Safe for long-term use

Habit Forming

- No

Pharmacokinetics

- Hydrolyzed to acyl glucuronides then excreted in urine (80%) or feces (20%). Half-life 14–17 hours. Bioavailability 3–7%

 Drug Interactions

- Anticoagulants such as heparin, vitamin K antagonists increase bleeding risk

- Antiplatelet agents such as aspirin, dipyridamole, clopidogrel, and abciximab may increase bleeding risk
- Long-term NSAIDs may increase risk of GI bleed
- P-glycoprotein inhibitor (amiodarone, dronedarone, ketoconazole, quinidine, and verapamil) increases drug concentration
- P-glycoprotein inducer (rifampin and St. John's wort) lowers drug concentration

 Other Warnings/ Precautions

- Procedure with minor bleeding risk: stop 1 day before procedure and start 12–24 hours after procedure. If CrCl < 50 mL/min stop 2 days before, and consider stopping earlier if < 30 mL/min
- Procedure with major bleeding risk: stop 2 days before procedure and start 2–3 days after procedure. If CrCl < 50 mL/min stop 4 days before, and consider stopping 5 days beforehand if < 30 mL/min

Do Not Use

- History of mechanical heart valve replacement
- Hypersensitivity to the drug
- Evidence of major bleeding (e.g., intracranial, intra-abdominal, retroperitoneal, intra-articular, etc.)
- Serious trauma
- Prior to major surgery
- Patients with renal failure

SPECIAL POPULATIONS

Renal Impairment

- CrCl 15–50 mL/min: 75 mg twice daily
- CrCl < 15 mL/min: no recommendation available. Use with extreme caution

Hepatic Impairment

- Contraindicated in severe hepatic impairment. May be safer than warfarin in mild to moderate hepatic impairment

Cardiac Impairment

- Should not be used in patients with AF and mechanical heart valves due to increased risk of stroke or myocardial infarction (MI). (Level of Evidence B)

• During AF ablation, periprocedural dabigatran use increases the risk of bleeding or thromboembolic complications compared with uninterrupted warfarin therapy

Elderly

• Patients over 75 are more likely to have bleeding complications

 Children and Adolescents

• Not studied in children

 Pregnancy

• Category C. Use if potential benefit outweighs risks. Increased risk of uterine hemorrhage during labor in rat studies

Breast Feeding

• Unknown if present in breast milk, use with caution

THE ART OF NEUROPHARMACOLOGY

Potential Advantages

• Proven treatment for stroke and systemic embolism prevention in adults with AF. Less risk for intracranial hemorrhage and life-threatening bleeding than conventional anticoagulants. Not affected by CYP450 enzymes

Potential Disadvantages

• Increased risk of bleeding. Lack of antidote or monitoring lab test. Increased incidence of GI adverse reactions (35% vs. 24% on warfarin; risk ratio 1.41). Case reports of life-threatening GI bleeding. During AF ablation, periprocedural dabigatran use increases the risk of bleeding or thromboembolic complications compared with uninterrupted warfarin therapy

Primary Target Symptoms

• Reduce recurrent attacks of cerebral embolism caused by cardiogenic thrombi due to AF

 Pearls

• According to the American Heart Association (AHA) guideline, warfarin therapy (Class I; Level of Evidence A), apixaban (Class I; Level of Evidence A), and dabigatran (Class I; Level of Evidence B) are all indicated for the prevention of recurrent stroke in patients with NVAF, whether paroxysmal or permanent. Dabigatran, rivaroxaban, or apixaban for 3 months may be considered as an alternative to warfarin therapy for prevention of recurrent stroke or transient ischemic attack in patients with acute MI complicated by left ventricular thrombus (Class IIb; Level of Evidence C)

• May be useful for heparin-induced thrombocytopenia

• For cerebral venous thrombosis, despite a lack of evidence, it is often recommended to use warfarin for 3–12 months. Longer duration is reserved for those with severe coagulopathies or recurrent VTE. For newer anticoagulants, although no evidence available, their lower intracranial bleeding rate might offer them a potential role for cerebral venous thrombosis

• Based on RE-LY study, the rate of intracranial hemorrhage per year was 0.76% (warfarin INR 2–3), 0.31% (dabigatran 150 mg twice daily), and 0.23% (dabigatran 110 mg twice daily)

• No clear benefit in stroke prevention in patients with valve replacement or non-cardiogenic stroke

• AF patients with chronic kidney disease are at greater risk for major bleeding with dabigatran compared to warfarin

Suggested Reading

Dans AL, Connolly SJ, Wallentin L, Yang S, Nakamya J, Brueckmann M, et al. Concomitant use of antiplatelet therapy with dabigatran or warfarin in the Randomized Evaluation of Long-Term Anticoagulation Therapy (RE-LY) Trial. *Circulation*. 2013;127(5):634–40.

Gonsalves WI, Pruthi RK, Patnaik MM. The new oral anticoagulants in clinical practice. *Mayo Clin Proc*. 2013;88(5):495–511.

Hart RG, Diener H-C, Yang S, Connolly SJ, Wallentin L, Reilly PA, et al. Intracranial hemorrhage in atrial fibrillation patients during anticoagulation with warfarin or dabigatran: the RE-LY trial. *Stroke*. 2012;43(6):1511–17.

January CT, Wann LS, Alpert JS, Calkins H, Cleveland JC, Cigarroa JE, et al. 2014 AHA/ACC/HRS guideline for the management of patients with atrial fibrillation: a report of the American College of Cardiology/American Heart Association Task Force on practice guidelines and the Heart Rhythm Society. *Circulation*. 2014;130(23):e199–267. Erratum in *Circulation*. 2014;130(23):e272–4.

DALFAMPRIDINE

THERAPEUTICS

Brands
- Ampyra, Fampyra, 4-aminopyridine

Generic?
- No

Class
- Potassium channel blocker

Commonly Prescribed for
(FDA approved in bold)
- **To improve walking in patients with multiple sclerosis (MS)**
- Spinal cord injury

How the Drug Works
- It is a broad-spectrum potassium channel antagonist that improves walking strength and speed in MS patients. Neurological improvement is probably associated with potassium channel inhibition that prolongs action potential and improves conduction in demyelinated axons. It may exert immunomodulatory effect on viable neurons through potassium channel blockade on microglia, macrophages, and lymphocytes that influence the autoimmune process in MS

How Long Until It Works
- Hours to days

If It Works
- Continue treatment. Monitor kidney function and any seizure activity

If It Doesn't Work
- Treat underlying MS with disease-modifying agents and symptomatic treatments

Best Augmenting Combos for Partial Response or Treatment-Resistance
- There is no other drug approved for improving walking in patients with MS. Does not affect MS progression

Tests
- Check kidney function before starting and periodically afterwards

ADVERSE EFFECTS (AEs)

How the Drug Causes AEs
- Potassium channel blockade

Notable AEs
- Asthenia, balance disorder, dizziness, headache, insomnia, nausea, urinary tract infection

Life-Threatening or Dangerous AEs
- Seizure (10 and 15 mg twice daily: 0.4% and 1.7% seizure incidence in clinical trial)
- Hypersensitivity reactions

Weight Gain
- Unusual

| unusual | not unusual | common | problematic |

Sedation
- Unusual

| unusual | not unusual | common | problematic |

What to Do About AEs
- Lower the dose or discontinue. Examine kidney function

Best Augmenting Agents to Reduce AEs
- Most AEs cannot be reduced

DOSING AND USE

Usual Dosage Range
- 10 mg, every 12 hours

Dosage Forms
- Tablet, extended release: 10 mg

How to Dose
- 10 mg twice daily, 12 hours apart
- CrCl 51–80 mL/min: standard dose may result in plasma level similar to 15 mg twice daily with a potential risk of seizure

Dosing Tips
- Do not chew or cut tablet

- Do not take double or take an extra dose if a dose is missed

Overdose

- May develop seizure, confusion, diaphoresis, and amnesia. Short-term memory difficulty may continue for longer period

Long-Term Use

- Safe for long-term use with appropriate monitoring

Habit Forming

- No

How to Stop

- No need to taper

Pharmacokinetics

- Plasma protein binding 1–3%. Bioavailability 96%. 90% eliminated as unchanged via kidneys. Some metabolized by CYP2E1. Half-life is 5–6 hours

 Drug Interactions

- It does not affect CYP isoenzymes or P-glycoprotein transporter

 Other Warnings/ Precautions

- Consider alerting patients to the risk of seizures

Do Not Use

- History of seizures. CrCl < 50 mL/min. Hypersensitivity to dalfampridine or 4-aminopyridine

Renal Impairment

- Contraindicated in moderate or severe renal impairment

Hepatic Impairment

- Not studied. Hepatic impairment is not expected to significantly affect its pharmacokinetics

Cardiac Impairment

- No known effects. It does not prolong QTc interval

Elderly

- Use with caution, may be more prone to AEs

 Children and Adolescents

- Safety and effectiveness in patients younger than 18 years old have not been established

 Pregnancy

- Category C. Use of dalfampridine in animals during pregnancy resulted in decreased offspring viability and growth

Breast Feeding

- It is not known whether dalfampridine is excreted in milk

Potential Advantages

- Effective for improving walking strength and speed in MS

Potential Disadvantages

- Potential risk for seizure

Primary Target Symptoms

- Walking speed and strength in MS

 Pearls

- Dalfampridine extended release 10 mg twice daily improved walking ability in patients with MS in 2 phase III trials
- The overall improvement from baseline in walking speed (13.4% vs. 5.8%) and timed walk responder rates (37.3% vs. 8.9%) was significantly ($p < 0.001$) higher in dalfampridine extended release 10 mg twice daily recipients (n = 394) than in placebo recipients (n = 237)
- Target patients with mild to moderate gait dysfunction. Patients with minimal gait impairment and wheelchair-bound patients with severe disability may not be candidates for this drug
- It may improve the subjective global impression and spasticity in patients with spinal cord injury

Suggested Reading

Blight AR. Treatment of walking impairment in multiple sclerosis with dalfampridine. *Ther Adv Neurol Disord.* 2011;4(2):99–109.

Chwieduk CM, Keating GM. Dalfampridine extended release: in multiple sclerosis. *CNS Drugs.* 2010;24 (10):883–91.

Sedehizadeh S, Keogh M, Maddison P. The use of aminopyridines in neurological disorders. *Clin Neuropharmacol.* 2012;35:191–200.

DANTROLENE

THERAPEUTICS

Brands
- Dantrium, Dantamacrin, Dantrolen, Revonto, Ryanodex

Generic?
- Yes

 ### Class
- Muscle relaxant

Commonly Prescribed for
(FDA approved in bold)
- **Chronic spasticity**
- **Malignant hyperthermia (MT)**
- Exercise-induced muscle pain
- Heat stroke
- Neuroleptic malignant syndrome

 ### How the Drug Works
- Dantrolene produces relaxation by directly interfering with the release of calcium from the sarcoplasmic reticulum, and weakening muscle contraction. It blocks RYR_1 receptors, which show prolonged open state during malignant hyperthermia

How Long Until It Works
- MT: immediate
- Pain: hours to days

If It Works
- Discontinue use once MT symptoms remit. For chronic spasticity, continue to use with standard precautions

If It Doesn't Work
- For spasticity, increase to highest tolerated dose. If ineffective, stop after 45 days and consider alternative treatments. In MT cases, stop all anesthetics

Best Augmenting Combos for Partial Response or Treatment-Resistance
- For focal spasticity, i.e., post-stroke spasticity, botulinum toxin is often more effective and is better tolerated
- Use other centrally acting muscle relaxants with caution due to potential synergistic CNS depressant effect

- 100% oxygen, cold gastric lavage, cooling blankets, and cold IV fluids may be useful in MT

Tests
- Obtain baseline liver function studies then do periodically

ADVERSE EFFECTS (AEs)

How the Drug Causes AEs
- Some are related to CNS depression, others hepatic disease

Notable AEs
- Fatigue, diarrhea, drowsiness, weakness, respiratory failure, rash, labile blood pressure, confusion/depression, abdominal cramps, crystalluria, chills, and fever. Thrombophlebitis (highly irritating to peripheral veins) and extravasation tissue necrosis

 ### Life-Threatening or Dangerous AEs
- Hepatotoxicity is not rare even after only short-term use, especially in patients that are females, over 35, taking multiple medications, or taking dose greater than 800 mg
- Less common: heart failure, pulmonary edema, and hematological abnormalities have been reported

Weight Gain
- Unusual

unusual | not unusual | common | problematic

Sedation
- Problematic

unusual | not unusual | common | problematic

What to Do About AEs
- If symptoms of hepatotoxicity develop (clinically or based on elevated hepatic enzymes), discontinue drug. For sedation, lower the dose and titrate more slowly. Do not let patient drive or perform hazardous tasks

Best Augmenting Agents to Reduce AEs

- Most AEs cannot be reduced by an augmenting agent

DOSING AND USE

Usual Dosage Range

- Spasticity: 75–300 mg/day in divided doses
- MT: 1–10 mg/kg/day

Dosage Forms

- Capsules: 25, 50, and 100 mg
- Infusion: 20 mg/vial (with 3 g mannitol)

How to Dose

- Oral: start at 25 mg daily. Increase dose every 7 days and change to 3 times daily, dosing as follows: 25 mg, 50 mg, and 100 mg. Wait at least 7 days between dose increases to assess response. If increasing a dose does not produce added benefit, then decrease to the previous lower dose. For MT, give 4–8 mg/kg in 3–4 divided doses for 1–2 days before surgery. If needed following a crisis, give for 1–3 days to prevent recurrence
- Injection: preoperatively give 2.5 mg/kg about 1¼ hours before anticipated anesthesia. For recognized MT, give minimum of 1 mg/kg (usually 2) as an IV bolus until symptoms improve or a maximum of 10 mg/kg

 Dosing Tips

- For chronic spasticity with reversible symptoms, slow oral titration until improvement occurs
- For MT, oral dantrolene can be used preoperatively but with prompt use of IV dantrolene when indicated

Overdose

- Weakness, lethargy, coma, vomiting, diarrhea

Long-Term Use

- Safety with long-term use not established

Habit Forming

- No

How to Stop

- No need to taper

Pharmacokinetics

- Hepatic metabolism. Half-life of 8–9 hours on average, with peak levels at 4–5 hours
- Some drug is protein bound. Excreted in feces and urine as active drug and metabolites

 Drug Interactions

- Use with other CNS depressants can worsen sedation
- Hepatotoxicity more common in women on oral estrogens
- Use with verapamil can cause hyperkalemia or myocardial depression
- Use with vecuronium may potentiate neuromuscular block
- Warfarin and clofibrate lower plasma protein binding of drug
- May affect concentrations of CYP3A4 medications

 Other Warnings/ Precautions

- At high doses carcinogenic in animals, although not proven in humans
- Patients who rely on spasticity to sustain upright posture and balance in walking should not use

Do Not Use

- Hypersensitivity to the drug or active hepatic disease

SPECIAL POPULATIONS

Renal Impairment

- No known effects

Hepatic Impairment

- Do not use

Cardiac Impairment

- May worsen existing heart failure, change blood pressure, or produce tachycardia. Use with caution

Elderly

- Very susceptible to AEs, including hepatotoxicity. Titrate carefully and use with extreme caution

Children and Adolescents

- Children over age 5 may use, but potential for carcinogenesis with long-term use. Titrate as follows: 0.5 mg/kg once daily for 7 days, then 0.5 mg/kg 3 times daily for 7 days, then 1 mg/kg 3 times daily for 7 days, then 2 mg/kg 3 times daily

 Pregnancy

- Category C. Use only if benefits of medication outweigh risks

Breast Feeding

- Do not use

THE ART OF NEUROPHARMACOLOGY

Potential Advantages

- Most effective medication in the treatment of MT

Potential Disadvantages

- Multiple serious AEs, including hepatic toxicity and sedation, along with lack of long-term data make it a second-line agent for the treatment of chronic spasticity

Primary Target Symptoms

- Spasticity, pain, fever

 Pearls

- The introduction of dantrolene reduced mortality of MT from about 70% to 10%
- Drug works best for MT if given early in the setting of illness
- The dose and usage of dantrolene for treatment of neuroleptic malignant syndrome (1 mg/kg, up to 10 mg/kg) is similar to that of acute MT, but is of unproven effectiveness
- It may be useful for treating ventricular fibrillation

 Suggested Reading

Dressler D, Benecke R. Diagnosis and management of acute movement disorders. *J Neurol.* 2005;252(11):1299–306.

Krause T, Gerbershagen MU, Fiege M, Weisshorn R, Wappler F. Dantrolene – a review of its pharmacology, therapeutic use and new developments. *Anaesthesia.* 2004;59(4): 364–73.

Perry PJ, Wilborn CA. Serotonin syndrome vs neuroleptic malignant syndrome: a contrast of causes, diagnoses, and management. *Ann Clin Psychiatry.* 2012;24(2):155–62.

Roden DM, Knollmann BC. Dantrolene: from better bacon to a treatment for ventricular fibrillation. *Circulation.* 2014;129(8): 834–6.

Saulino M, Jacobs BW. The pharmacological management of spasticity. *J Neurosci Nurs.* 2006;38(6):456–9.

Velamoor VR, Swamy GN, Parmar RS, Williamson P, Caroff SN. Management of suspected neuroleptic malignant syndrome. *Can J Psychiatry.* 1995;40(9): 545–50.

Verrotti A, Greco R, Spalice A, Chiarelli F, Iannetti P. Pharmacotherapy of spasticity in children with cerebral palsy. *Pediatr Neurol.* 2006;34(1):1–6.

DESVENLAFAXINE

THERAPEUTICS

Brands
- Khedezla, Pristiq

Generic?
- Yes

Class
- Serotonin and norepinephrine reuptake inhibitor (SNRI)

Commonly Prescribed for
(FDA approved in bold)
- **Major depressive disorder**
- Generalized anxiety disorder
- Panic disorder
- Social phobia
- Migraine or tension-type headache prophylaxis
- Diabetic neuropathy
- Other painful peripheral neuropathies
- Cancer pain (neuropathic)
- Depression secondary to stroke
- Stress urinary incontinence
- Fibromyalgia
- Binge-eating disorder
- Post-traumatic stress disorder
- ADHD
- Perimenopausal/menopausal hot flushes
- Cataplexy

How the Drug Works
- Both venlafaxine and its active metabolite (desvenlafaxine) are potent inhibitors of serotonin and norepinephrine reuptake transporters (SERT, NET), increasing serotonin and norepinephrine levels within hours, but antidepressant effects take weeks. Effect is more likely related to adaptive changes in serotonin and norepinephrine receptor systems over time
- Weakly blocks dopamine reuptake pump (dopamine transporter)
- Interacts with μ-opioid receptors and α_2-adrenergic receptor

How Long Until It Works
- Migraines: effective in as little as 2 weeks, but can take up to 10 weeks on a stable dose to see full effect

- Tension-type headache prophylaxis: effective in 4–8 weeks
- Neuropathic pain: usually some effect within 4 weeks
- Diabetic neuropathy: may have significant improvement with high doses within 6 weeks
- Depression: 2 weeks but up to 2 months for full effect

If It Works
- Migraine/tension-type headache: goal is a 50% or greater reduction in headache frequency or severity. Consider tapering or stopping if headaches remit for more than 6 months or if considering pregnancy
- Neuropathic pain: the goal is to reduce pain intensity and symptoms, but usually does not produce remission. Continue to use and monitor for AE
- Diabetic neuropathy: the goal is to reduce pain intensity and reduce use of analgesics, but usually does not produce remission. Continue to use and maintain strict glycemic control and diabetic management
- Depression: continue to use and monitor for AEs. May continue for 1 year following first depression episode or indefinitely if > 1 episode of depression

If It Doesn't Work
- Increase to highest tolerated dose
- Migraine and tension-type headache: address other issues, such as medication overuse, and other coexisting medical disorders, such as anxiety, and consider changing to another agent or adding a second agent
- Neuropathic pain: either change to another agent or add a second agent

Best Augmenting Combos for Partial Response or Treatment-Resistance
- Headache: for some patients, low-dose polytherapy with 2 or more drugs may be better tolerated and more effective than high-dose monotherapy. May use in combination with AEDs, antihypertensives, natural products, and non-medication treatments, such as biofeedback, to improve headache control
- Neuropathic pain: TCAs, AEDs (gabapentin, pregabalin, carbamazepine, lamotrigine), SNRIs (duloxetine, venlafaxine, milnacipran,

mirtazapine, bupropion), capsaicin, and mexiletine are agents used for neuropathic pain. Opioids (morphine, tramadol) may be appropriate for long-term use in some cases but require careful monitoring

Tests

- Check blood pressure at baseline and when increasing dose
- Monitor sodium, intraocular pressure, suicidality, and unusual changes in behavior

ADVERSE EFFECTS (AEs)

How the Drug Causes AEs

- By increasing serotonin and norepinephrine on non-therapeutic responsive receptors throughout the body. Most AEs are dose- and time-dependent

Notable AEs

- Constipation, dry mouth, sweating, blurry vision, mydriasis, anorexia, nausea, weight loss or gain, hypertension, headache, asthenia, dizziness, tremor, dream disorder, insomnia, somnolence, abnormal ejaculation, impotence, orgasm disorder, sweating, itching, sedation, nervousness, restlessness, cholesterol/triglyceride elevation

 Life-Threatening or Dangerous AEs

- Serotonin syndrome
- Rare hepatitis
- Rare activation of mania or suicidal ideation
- Rare worsening of coexisting seizure disorders

Weight Gain

- Not unusual

unusual   not unusual   common   problematic

Sedation

- Not unusual

unusual   not unusual   common   problematic

- May cause insomnia in some patients

What to Do About AEs

- For minor AEs, lower dose, titrate more slowly, or switch to another agent. For serious AEs, lower dose and consider stopping, taper to avoid withdrawal symptoms

Best Augmenting Agents to Reduce AEs

- Try magnesium for constipation
- Cyproheptadine can be used for serotonin syndrome by blocking 5-HT receptors and SERT
- Sexual dysfunction (anorgasmia, impotence) may be reversed by agents with α_2-adrenergic antagonist activity (e.g., buspirone, amantadine, bupropion, mirtazapine, ginkgo biloba, etc.)

DOSING AND USE

Usual Dosage Range

- 37.5–375 mg/day

Dosage Forms

- Tablet (extended release): 50, 100 mg

How to Dose

- 50 mg daily. 50 mg every other day if CrCl < 30 mL/min

 Dosing Tips

- Higher doses are typically used for pain. Extended-release formulation allows for once-a-day dosing and may be better tolerated. It should be swallowed whole and not be crushed or chewed

Overdose

- Signs and symptoms may include cardiac arrhythmias, usually tachycardia, ECG changes (prolonged QTc interval or bundle branch block), sedation, seizures, bowel perforation, serotonin syndrome, fever, rhabdomyolysis, hyponatremia, blood pressure abnormalities, extrapyramidal effects, headache, nervousness, tremor; death can occur

Long-Term Use

- Safe for long-term use with monitoring of blood pressure and suicidality

Habit Forming

- No

How to Stop

- Taper slowly (no more than 50% reduction every 3–4 days until discontinuation) to avoid withdrawal symptoms (agitation, anxiety, confusion, dry mouth, dysphoria, etc.). Pain often worsens shortly after decreasing dose

Pharmacokinetics

- Desvenlafaxine is metabolized by conjugation (major) and CYP3A4 (minor); CYP2D6 is not involved. Half-life 11 hours. < 30% protein bound. 45% excreted unchanged in urine

 Drug Interactions

- Reduce dose in the presence of CYP3A4 inhibitors (clarithromycin, ketoconazole, itraconazole)
- Increase dose in the presence of strong CYP3A4 inducer (phenytoin, rifampin, carbamazepine, dexamethasone, barbiturates, St. John's wort)
- The release of serotonin by platelets is important for maintaining hemostasis. Combined use of SSRIs or SNRIs (such as venlafaxine) and NSAIDs, and/or drugs that have anticoagulant effects has been associated with an increased risk of bleeding
- May decrease effects of antihypertensive medications, such as metoprolol
- May decrease clearance and increase effect of antipsychotics (haloperidol, clozapine)
- May increase the risk of seizure or serotonin syndrome with tramadol
- May cause serotonin syndrome when used within 14 days of MAOIs
- May increase risk of cardiotoxicity and arrhythmia when used with TCAs

 Other Warnings/ Precautions

- May increase risk of seizure
- Patients should be observed closely for clinical worsening, suicidality, and changes in behavior in known or unknown bipolar disorder

Do Not Use

- Proven hypersensitivity to drug
- Concurrently with MAOI; allow at least 14 days between discontinuation of an MAOI and initiation of venlafaxine or at least 7–14 days between discontinuation of venlafaxine and initiation of an MAOI
- Concurrent use of serotonin precursors (e.g., tryptophan)
- In patients with uncontrolled narrow angle-closure glaucoma
- In patients treated with linezolid or methylene blue IV

SPECIAL POPULATIONS

Renal Impairment

- Use with caution. Decrease usual dose by 25–50%

Hepatic Impairment

- Use with caution. Decrease usual dose by 50%

Cardiac Impairment

- Use with caution. Dose-dependent effect on blood pressure. Venlafaxine may prolong QTc, particularly of elderly; insufficient data on desvenlafaxine

Elderly

- No adjustments necessary

 Children and Adolescents

- Safety and efficacy not established. Use with caution. Observe closely for clinical worsening, suicidality, and changes in behavior in known or unknown bipolar disorder. Parents should be informed and advised of the risks

 Pregnancy

- Category C. Generally not recommended for the treatment of headaches or neuropathic pain during pregnancy. Neonates exposed to venlafaxine or other SNRIs or SSRIs late in the third trimester have developed complications necessitating extended hospitalizations, respiratory support, and tube feeding. Respiratory distress, cyanosis, apnea, seizures, temperature instability, feeding difficulty, vomiting, hypoglycemia, hypotonia, hyperreflexia, tremor, jitteriness, irritability, and constant crying consistent with a toxic effect of the drug or drug discontinuation syndrome have been reported

Breast Feeding

- Some drug is found in breast milk and use while breast feeding is not recommended

 THE ART OF NEUROPHARMACOLOGY

Potential Advantages

- Very effective in the treatment of multiple pain disorders. Effective for treatment of comorbid depression and anxiety in chronic pain. Less sedation than tertiary amine TCAs (i.e., amitriptyline)

Potential Disadvantages

- May cause or worsen hypertension. Usually higher doses are needed for pain disorders than for depression

Primary Target Symptoms

- Reduction in headache frequency, duration, and/or intensity
- Reduction in neuropathic pain
- Reduction in depression, anxiety

 Pearls

- Desvenlafaxine functions as SNRI at higher doses (> 100 mg/day). This may explain why higher doses are needed in pain disorders than in depression and anxiety
- Although there is no study on desvenlafaxine for headache and neuropathic pain, desvenlafaxine in theory acts similarly to venlafaxine, especially at higher doses
- Combination use of SNRI and triptans usually will not lead to serotonin syndrome, which requires activation of 5-HT$_{2A}$ receptors and a possible limited role of 5-HT$_{1A}$. However, triptans are agonists at the 5-HT$_{1B/1D/1F}$ receptor subtypes, with weak affinity for 5-HT$_{1A}$ receptors and no activity at the 5-HT$_2$ receptors. Thus, given the seriousness of serotonin syndrome, caution is certainly warranted and clinicians should be vigilant to serotonin toxicity symptoms and signs to insure prompt treatment

Suggested Reading

Aran A, Einen M, Lin L, Plazzi G, Nishino S, Mignot E. Clinical and therapeutic aspects of childhood narcolepsy-cataplexy: a retrospective study of 51 children. *Sleep*. 2010;33(11): 1457–64.

Evans RW, Tepper SJ, Shapiro RE, Sun-Edelstein C, Tietjen GE. The FDA alert on serotonin syndrome with use of triptans combined with selective serotonin reuptake inhibitors or selective serotonin-norepinephrine reuptake inhibitors: American Headache Society position paper. *Headache*. 2010;50(6): 1089–99.

Ozyalcin SN, Talu GK, Kiziltan E, Yucel B, Ertas M, Disci R. The efficacy and safety of venlafaxine in the prophylaxis of migraine. *Headache*. 2005;45(2):144–52.

Saarto T, Wiffen PJ. Antidepressants for neuropathic pain: a Cochrane review. *J Neurol Neurosurg Psychiatry*. 2010;81(12):1372–3.

Wellington K, Perry CM. Venlafaxine extended-release: a review of its use in the management of major depression. *CNS Drugs*. 2001;15(8): 643–69.

Zissis NP, Harmoussi S, Vlaikidis N, Mitsikostas D, Thomaidis T, Georgiadis G, Karageorgiou K. A randomized, double-blind, placebo-controlled study of venlafaxine XR in out-patients with tension-type headache. *Cephalalgia*. 2007; 27(4):315–24.

DEXAMETHASONE

THERAPEUTICS

Brands
- Decadron, Decadron-LA, Dexone

Generic?
- Yes

 Class
- Corticosteroid

Commonly Prescribed for
(FDA approved in bold)
- **Nervous system: acute exacerbation of multiple sclerosis; cerebral edema associated with primary or metastatic brain tumor, craniotomy, or head injury**
- **Dermatological diseases: pemphigus, bullous dermatitis herpetiformis, Stevens-Johnson syndrome, exfoliative erythroderma, mycosis fungoides, severe psoriasis, severe seborrheic dermatitis**
- **Endocrine disorders: primary or secondary adrenocortical insufficiency, congenital adrenal hyperplasia, non-suppurative thyroiditis, hypercalcemia associated with cancer**
- **Hematological disorders: idiopathic thrombocytopenic purpura in adult, autoimmune hemolytic anemia, pure red cell aplasia, congenital hypoplastic anemia**
- **GI diseases: to tide over a critical period of ulcerative colitis or regional enteritis**
- **Neoplastic diseases: palliative management of leukemias and lymphomas**
- **Respiratory diseases: symptomatic sarcoidosis, Loeffler syndrome not manageable by other means, berylliosis, fulminating or disseminating pulmonary tuberculosis, aspiration pneumonitis, idiopathic eosinophilic pneumonias**
- **Renal diseases: to induce remission of proteinuria in the nephrotic syndrome, without uremia, of the idiopathic type or due to lupus erythematosus**
- **Rheumatic disorders: adjunctive therapy for short-term treatment in psoriatic arthritis, rheumatoid arthritis, acute rheumatic carditis, ankylosing spondylitis, acute bursitis, acute synovitis of osteoarthritis, epicondylitis, dermatomyositis, polymyositis, systemic lupus erythematosus, temporal arteritis**

- **Severe allergic state: allergic rhinitis, bronchial asthma, contact dermatitis, atopic dermatitis, serum sickness, drug hypersensitivity reactions**
- **Diagnostic testing: adrenocortical hyperfunction**
- Migraine headache
- Cluster headache
- Acute demyelinating encephalomyelitis (ADEM)
- Acute brain injury
- CNS lymphoma
- Infantile hemangioma
- Prevention or acute treatment of altitude sickness
- Chemotherapy-induced nausea and vomiting

 How the Drug Works
- Glucocorticoids have anti-inflammatory effects, modify immune responses to stimuli, and have numerous metabolic effects. They cross cell membranes and bind with glucocorticoid receptors, then bind to DNA glucocorticoid response elements that in turn modify the protein synthesis required for inflammation. Dexamethasone is more potent than prednisolone and cortisone for suppression of inflammation but has minimal mineralocorticoid effect

How Long Until It Works
- Peritumoral edema, migraine, cluster: hours to days

If It Works
- Migraine: usually used for intractable headache or status migrainosus for short periods of time. After resolution, revert to safer preventive and abortive therapy
- Cluster: start preventive therapy and prednisone at the beginning of a cycle
- Peritumoral edema: use to alleviate symptoms. Lower dose if able based on symptoms, response to treatment, and disease progression

If It Doesn't Work
- Migraine: start preventive therapy. IV neuroleptics or dihydroergotamine may be needed to treat status migrainosus
- Cluster: start preventive therapy

- Peritumoral edema: discussions with family on prognosis and treatment goals are important. Increasing doses may improve symptoms but increase AEs

 Best Augmenting Combos for Partial Response or Treatment-Resistance

- Migraine/cluster: antiemetics and migraine-specific agents may be used with corticosteroids for acute attacks
- Peritumoral edema: used in combination with measures to treat underlying tumor such as surgery, radiation, or chemotherapy

Tests

- Monitor blood pressure, glucose, and electrolytes with long-term therapy

ADVERSE EFFECTS (AEs)

How the Drug Causes AEs

- Most AEs are due to immunosuppression, metabolic or endocrine effects

Notable AEs

- Convulsion, vertigo, paresthesias, aggravation of psychiatric conditions, insomnia
- Amenorrhea, cushingoid state, increased sweating, increased insulin requirement in diabetics, hyperglycemia
- Pancreatitis, abdominal distension, esophagitis, bowel perforation, weight gain
- Cataracts, glaucoma
- Impaired wound healing, petechiae, erythema, hirsutism, Cushing's syndrome
- Sodium and fluid retention, hypokalemia, metabolic acidosis
- Muscle weakness, myopathy, muscle mass loss, tendon rupture, osteoporosis
- Thrombophlebitis, hypertension
- Infection, excessive stomach acid secretion, increased hunger

 Life-Threatening or Dangerous AEs

- Fractures, aseptic necrosis of femoral or humoral heads
- Hypokalemia may cause cardiac arrhythmias

- Diabetic ketoacidosis, hyperosmolar coma
- May mask symptoms of infection and prevent ability of patient to prevent dissemination. May activate latent amebiasis or tuberculosis. May prolong coma in cerebral malaria
- Adrenal suppression with long-term use
- Psychosis with clouded sensorium, severe depression, personality changes, or insomnia, usually within 15–30 days after starting treatment. Female sex and higher doses are risk factors

Weight Gain

- Problematic

unusual   not unusual   common   problematic

Sedation

- Unusual

unusual   not unusual   common   problematic

What to Do About AEs

- For diseases such as migraine or cluster, avoid using for prolonged periods of time (i.e., weeks) and stop for most significant AEs
- In diseases requiring long-term treatment, consider using corticosteroid-sparing agents – often starting these treatments with prednisone to reduce the dose requirement and possibly allow discontinuation as clinical symptoms improve
- Weight-bearing exercises are recommended to promote bone protection and minimize muscle wasting
- Weight gain: avoid other medications that may exacerbate, dietary modification
- Hypertension: discontinue drug if possible

Best Augmenting Agents to Reduce AEs

- With prolonged treatment, use daily calcium and vitamin D supplements and bisphosphonates to prevent osteoporosis and fractures, and H_2-blocker or proton pump inhibitors to prevent peptic ulcers

DOSING AND USE

Usual Dosage Range
- 1–20 mg daily. (The range of doses varies dramatically depending on the disease being treated)

Dosage Forms
- Tablet: 0.25, 0.5, 0.75, 1, 1.5, 2, 4, 6 mg
- Oral concentrate: 1 mg/mL (30% alcohol)
- Oral elixir: 0.5 mg/5mL
- Injection: 4, 10 mg/mL in 1, 5, 10, 30 mL vials, 1 mL syringe

How to Dose
- Migraine: no standard regimen. Usually used for less than 1 week for status migrainosus at doses of 4–12 mg daily with rapid taper
- Cluster: often used for 2–3 weeks at a time. Doses of 4–12 mg/day appear effective. Start with a higher dose and taper over 1–3 weeks
- Peritumoral edema: initial doses range from 12 to 16 mg/day in divided doses. Usually tapered if possible

Dosing Tips
- Give with food to avoid GI upset

Overdose
- Large doses often produce cushingoid changes, including moonface, central obesity, hirsutism, acne, hypertension, osteoporosis, sexual dysfunction, diabetes, hyperlipidemia, peptic ulcer, and electrolyte and fluid imbalance

Long-Term Use
- Not usually used for long periods of time in migraine or cluster. Weigh AEs against clinical benefit and patient/family wishes in cases of peritumoral edema

Habit Forming
- No

How to Stop
- Taper rapidly for exacerbation of acute disorder, such as migraine
- Taper slowly over days to weeks and monitor for recurrence of symptoms in cases of peritumoral edema

- Acute adrenal insufficiency can occur with too rapid withdrawal. Symptoms include nausea, anorexia, hypoglycemia, dizziness, orthostatic hypotension, fever, and myalgias. Return of normal adrenal and pituitary function may take up to 9 months

Pharmacokinetics
- T_{max} 1–4 hours. 70% protein bound. Metabolized by CYP3A4 with elimination half-life 36–54 hours

 Drug Interactions
- Do not give live vaccines during therapy with high doses
- Strong CYP3A4 inhibitor (e.g., protease inhibitors, macrolides, azole antifungals, nefazodone) can increase dexamethasone concentration
- Strong CYP3A4 inducer (e.g., carbamazepine, phenytoin, phenobarbital, rifampin, glucocorticoid, St. John's wort) can decrease dexamethasone concentration
- Dexamethasone at doses used clinically increases CYP3A4 activity with extensive intersubject variability. It may lower the concentration of CYP3A4 substrates
- It suppresses estrogen action at the pituitary level
- May cause severe hypokalemia with potassium-depleting diuretics, increasing the risk of digitalis toxicity
- Reduces salicylate levels and effectiveness
- May inhibit growth-promoting effect of somatrem
- May decrease levels of isoniazid
- May alter activity of warfarin or theophylline

 Other Warnings/ Precautions
- May suppress reactions to skin tests
- Although occasionally used for chronic active hepatitis, may actually be harmful for hepatitis B carrier

Do Not Use
- Hypersensitivity to drug, systemic fungal infection, administration of live virus vaccine

Renal Impairment

- Patients are more likely to develop edema with corticosteroids. Use with caution

Hepatic Impairment

- No known effects

Cardiac Impairment

- Associated with left ventricular free wall rupture after recent myocardial infarction. Use with caution

Elderly

- Consider lower doses due to lower plasma volumes and decreased muscle mass. Monitor blood pressure, glucose, and electrolytes at least every 6 months

 Children and Adolescents

- Appears safe. Frequently used in asthma, Duchenne's muscular dystrophy, but may cause growth problems with long-term use

 Pregnancy

- Category C. Relatively lower placental transport compared to other corticosteroids. May cause hypoadrenalism in infants

Breast Feeding

- Appears in breast milk and may suppress growth. Avoid breast feeding with high-dose, long-term treatment

THE ART OF NEUROPHARMACOLOGY

Potential Advantages

- Effective treatment for acute migraine and cluster headache. Relatively fast-acting treatment for peritumoral edema

Potential Disadvantages

- Effectiveness varies depending on the disorder. Numerous AEs, especially with long-term use

Primary Target Symptoms

- Depending on disorder: treating and preventing neurological complications in patients with peritumoral edema. Reducing pain in headache disorders. Anti-inflammation

 Pearls

- In migraine studies, primary benefit appears to be prevention of headache recurrence. When effective in migraine, patients usually improve within 24 hours
- In cluster headache, effective as a short-term treatment usually early in a cycle
- The majority of patients experience recurrence after completing the taper, so preventive therapy should be started when initiating treatment
- Shorter corticosteroid courses, to reduce AEs, may be appropriate in cluster headache depending on disease severity and frequency of cycles: for patients with frequent cycles (more than 1/year) consider a taper of 10 days or less. Do not give as a daily medication for either migraine or cluster headache
- Cardiac arrhythmias are most common with rapid IV administration of methylprednisolone (1 g in 10 minutes) rather than with oral dexamethasone therapy
- Dexamethasone is preferred to prednisone for the treatment of cerebral edema related to primary or metastatic brain tumors or head trauma
- Oral dexamethasone is comparable to IV given high bioavailability
- Despite its frequent use, there is little evidence that dexamethasone or corticosteroids in general improve long-term outcomes after acute brain injury
- May be effective in CNS lymphoma due to induction of apoptosis and decrease in tumor size. The use of corticosteroids, however, may affect the ability to confirm the diagnosis
- Prednisone 5 mg is equal to hydrocortisone 20 mg, cortisone 25 mg, dexamethasone 0.75 mg, and methylprednisolone 4 mg
- Steroid taper is needed if used > 3 weeks, presence of cushingoid feature and no response to adrenocorticotropic hormone (ACTH) stimulation testing

Suggested Reading

Becker WJ. Cluster headache: conventional pharmacological management. *Headache.* 2013;53(7):1191–6.

Dearden NM, Gibson JS, McDowall DG, Gibson RM, Cameron MM. Effect of high-dose dexamethasone on outcome from severe head injury. *J Neurosurg.* 1986;64(1): 81–8.

Huang Y, Cai X, Song X, Tang H, Huang Y, et al. Steroids for preventing recurrence of acute severe migraine headaches: a meta-analysis. *Eur J Neurol.* 2013;20(8):1184–90.

Kostaras X, Cusano F, Kline GA, Roa W, Easaw J. Use of dexamethasone in patients with high-grade glioma: a clinical practice guideline. *Curr Oncol.* 2014;21(3):e493–503.

DEXTROMETHORPHAN HYDROBROMIDE AND QUINIDINE SULFATE

Brands
- Nuedexta

Generic?
- No

Class
- NMDA receptor antagonist

Commonly Prescribed for
(FDA approved in bold)
- **Treatment of pseudobulbar affect (PBA) in patients with underlying amyotrophic lateral sclerosis (ALS) or multiple sclerosis (MS)**
- PBA in Alzheimer's disease or other dementia
- Agitation in Alzheimer's disease
- Depression

How the Drug Works
- Dextromethorphan is a serotonin transporter/norepinephrine transporter inhibitor, σ_1 receptor agonist, non-competitive NMDA receptor antagonist, and $\alpha_3\beta_4$- and $\alpha_4\beta_2$-nicotinic receptor antagonist. Quinidine is a specific CYP2D6 inhibitor that reduces its conversion to active metabolite dextrorphan and increases 20-fold the systemic bioavailability of dextromethorphan. The exact mechanism of action is unclear. It is possible many neurotransmitters, such as serotonin, GABA, norepinephrine, glutamate, and dopamine, participate in emotional expression involved in PBA

How Long Until It Works
- Typically less than a month

If It Works
- Continue use and monitor AEs

If It Doesn't Work
- May try increasing the dose of dextromethorphan. Evaluate the treatment efficacy for underlying disorders

Best Augmenting Combos for Partial Response or Treatment-Resistance
- There is no other drug approved for use in treating PBA

Tests
- Monitor potential QTc prolongation

How the Drug Causes AEs
- Quinidine may cause cardiac AEs

Notable AEs
- Headache, dizziness, cough, vomiting, asthenia, urinary tract infection, flatulence, diarrhea

Life-Threatening or Dangerous AEs
- Thrombocytopenia or other hypersensitivity reactions
- Leukopenia
- Hepatitis
- QTc prolongation
- Serotonin syndrome with concomitant SSRI use
- Worsening of myasthenia gravis

Weight Gain
- Unusual

unusual · not unusual · common · problematic

Sedation
- Unusual

unusual · not unusual · common · problematic

What to Do About AEs
- Discontinue if severe AEs occur

Best Augmenting Agents to Reduce AEs
- Most AEs are not treatable with medications

DOSING AND USE

Usual Dosage Range
• 1 capsule every 12 hours

Dosage Forms
• Capsule: dextromethorphan 20 mg, quinidine 10 mg

How to Dose
• Start once daily for 7 days then once every 12 hours

 Dosing Tips
• May take with or without food

Overdose
• Quinidine overdose has been associated with ventricular arrhythmia and hypotension
• Dextromethorphan overdose includes nausea, vomiting, stupor, coma, psychosis

Long-Term Use
• Generally safe for long-term use

Habit Forming
• Dextromethorphan abuse has been reported in adolescents

How to Stop
• No need to taper

Pharmacokinetics
• Dextromethorphan is rapidly metabolized by CYP3A4 and CYP2D6 to dextrorphan, which is rapidly glucuronidated and renally excreted. It is 60–70% protein bound. Half-life 3–6 hours. In the presence of quinidine, the half-life is 19 hours
• Quinidine is metabolized by CYP3A4 with 20% excreted unchanged in urine. It is 80–90% protein bound. Half-life 6–8 hours

 Drug Interactions
• Quinidine inhibits CYP2D6 that increases drug concentration (TCAs, SSRIs, opioids, antipsychotics, β-blocker, etc.)
• Quinidine inhibits P-glycoprotein transporter that increases drug

concentration (digoxin, antineoplastics, immunosuppressants)
• Strong CYP2D6 inhibitors (e.g., fluoxetine, paroxetine, bupropion, ritonavir) can increase dextromethorphan concentration
• Strong CYP3A4 inhibitors (e.g., protease inhibitors, macrolides, azole antifungals, nefazodone) can increase quinidine and dextromethorphan concentrations
• Approximately 7–8% of individuals of White descent, 3–6% of Black African descent, 2–3% of Arab descent, and 1–2% of Asian descent generally lack the capacity to metabolize CYP2D6 substrates and are classified as poor metabolizers
• Approximately 1–10% of individuals of White descent, 5–30% of Black African descent, 12–40% of Arab descent, and 1% of Asian descent exhibit increased metabolic activity for CYP2D6 substrates and are classified as ultra-rapid metabolizers

 Other Warnings/ Precautions
• Take precautions to reduce falls
• Monitor for worsening in myasthenia gravis and other possible anticholinergic side effects

Do Not Use
• Concomitant use with quinidine, quinine, or mefloquine
• Patients with a history of quinidine, quinine or mefloquine-induced thrombocytopenia, hepatitis, or other hypersensitivity reactions
• Patients with known hypersensitivity to dextromethorphan
• Use with an MAOI or within 14 days of stopping an MAOI. Allow 14 days after stopping Nuedexta before starting an MAOI
• Prolonged QTc interval, congenital long QT syndrome, history suggestive of torsade de pointes, or heart failure
• Complete AV block without implanted pacemaker, or patients at high risk of complete AV block
• Concomitant use with drugs that both prolong QTc interval and are metabolized by CYP2D6 (e.g., thioridazine or pimozide)

Renal Impairment
• Dose adjustment not required

Hepatic Impairment
• Dose adjustment not required

Cardiac Impairment
• Increase in QTc interval. Monitor ECG in patients with left ventricular dysfunction or hypertrophy

Elderly
• No known effects but limited experience in those over 65

 Children and Adolescents
• The safety and effectiveness of Nuedexta in pediatric patients below the age of 18 have not been established

 Pregnancy
• Category C. In oral studies conducted in rats and rabbits, a combination of dextromethorphan/quinidine demonstrated developmental toxicity, including teratogenicity (rabbits) and embryolethality, when given to pregnant animals

Breast Feeding
• It is not known whether dextromethorphan or quinidine is excreted in human milk

THE ART OF NEUROPHARMACOLOGY

Potential Advantages
• Effective for controlling PBA

Potential Disadvantages
• Drug interaction on CYP2D6. Risk of QTc prolongation

Primary Target Symptoms
• Involuntary emotional crying and laughing

 Pearls
• PBA was previously treated off-label by TCAs or SSRIs but their efficacy was not established. Nuedexta was coincidentally discovered in an ALS trial where patients reported it helped in controlling involuntary emotional outbursts, such as crying and laughing. The actual effect ranged from 7% to 95% in patients with MS
• In animal studies, Nuedexta exerts antidepressant-like effects that occur at least in part through a σ_1 receptor-dependent mechanism. σ_1 receptor is a non-opioid receptor residing specifically at the endoplasmic reticulum (ER)–mitochondrion interface called the MAM (mitochondrion-associated ER membrane). It serves as an inter-organelle signaling modulator locally at the MAM and remotely at the plasmalemma/plasma membrane. It is expressed particularly in limbic and motor regions and plays a role in emotional functions
• The effects are enhanced by quinidine, which suggests the drug of action is dextromethorphan but not dextrorphan, which has different receptor binding profiles. The dose of quinidine is at an amount 10–20 times lower than that used to treat arrhythmia
• Initial study suggests possible efficacy in treating agitation in people with Alzheimer's dementia. This could be an alternative to neuroleptics

Suggested Reading

Brooks BR, Thisted RA, Appel SH, Bradley WG, Olney RK, Berg JE, et al. Treatment of pseudobulbar affect in ALS with dextromethorphan/quinidine. *Neurology.* 2004;63(8):1364–70.

Miller A, Panitch H. Therapeutic use of dextromethorphan: key learnings from treatment of pseudobulbar affect. *J Neurol Sci.* 2007; 259(1–2):67–73.

Nguyen L, Robson MJ, Healy JR, Scandinaro AL, Matsumoto RR. Involvement of sigma-1 receptors in the antidepressant-like effects of dextromethorphan. *PLoS One.* 2014;9(2):e89985.

Rosen H. Dextromethorphan/quinidine sulfate for pseudobulbar affect. *Drugs Today (Barc).* 2008;44(9):661–8.

Schoenfeld S, Tariot P, Peskind E, Cummings J, Lyketsos C, Nguyen U, et al. Treatment of agitation in people with Alzheimer's dementia: Rationale for the clinical investigation of AVP-923 (dextromethorphan/quinidine). *Alzheimers Dement.* 2013;9(4):P757.

Su T-P, Hayashi T, Maurice T, Buch S, Ruoho AE. The sigma-1 receptor chaperone as an inter-organelle signaling modulator. *Trends Pharmacol Sci.* 2010;31(12):557–66.

DIAZEPAM

THERAPEUTICS

Brands
- Valium, Diastat, Diastat AcuDial, Diazepam Intensol, Dialar, Diazemuls, Rimapam, Stesolid, Tensium, Valclair, Alupram, Solis, Atensine, Evacalm, Valrelease

Generic?
- Yes

Class
- Benzodiazepine, antiepileptic drug (AED)

Commonly Prescribed for
(FDA approved in bold)
- **Seizure disorders. Adjunctively and to control bouts of increased seizure activity**
- **Anxiety disorders**
- **Acute alcohol withdrawal**
- **Muscle relaxant**
- **Preoperative medication**
- Status epilepticus
- Tetanus
- Insomnia
- Agitation
- Stiff person syndrome
- Spasticity due to upper motor neuron disorders
- Irritable bowel syndrome
- Panic attacks
- Nausea and vomiting (from chemotherapy)
- Emergency treatment of preeclampsia
- Dystonia
- Vertigo
- Opioid or other drug withdrawal
- Acute mania in bipolar disorder

 How the Drug Works
- Benzodiazepines bind to and potentiate the effect of GABA$_A$ receptors, which are ligand-gated chloride channels activated by GABA. It boosts chloride conductance across the cell membrane, hyperpolarizes the membrane potential, and increases the threshold potential. Specific GABA receptor subunits have been associated with diazepam's function (e.g., α_1: sedation, anterograde amnesia; α_2: anxiolytic effect; $\alpha_{1,2,3}$: AED effect). Benzodiazepines act at spinal cord, brainstem, cerebellum, and limbic and cortical areas

How Long Until It Works
- Works quickly (minutes to hours depending on formulation) in the treatment of seizures, acute anxiety, drug withdrawal, and muscle relaxation. In patients with chronic disorders such as spasticity, dystonia, or generalized anxiety it may take weeks to determine optimal dose for maximal therapeutic benefit

If It Works
- Seizures: rectal diazepam is used intermittently as an adjunctive for patients with known epilepsy with increased seizure frequency. IV diazepam is used for status epilepticus in conjunction with IV maintenance AEDs. In patients with epilepsy who benefit from oral diazepam as an adjunctive medication, consider tapering the medication after 2 years without seizures, depending on the type of epilepsy
- Spasticity: used as an adjunct medication. The cause of spasticity usually determines the duration of use. For acute muscle spasm, change to as needed use 1–3 weeks after onset
- Anxiety: generally used on a short-term basis. Consider adding an SSRI, SNRI, or buspirone for long-term treatment

If It Doesn't Work
- Epilepsy: for acute treatment only. Status epilepticus is a medical emergency requiring immediate medical attention. After using diazepam, start maintenance AEDs such as phenytoin and evaluate for the cause of worsening seizures
- Spasticity: if not effective change to another agent
- Anxiety: consider a secondary cause, mania, or substance abuse. Change to another agent or add an augmenting agent

 Best Augmenting Combos for Partial Response or Treatment-Resistance
- Epilepsy: often used in combination with other AEDs for optimal control but sedation can increase
- Spasticity: tizanidine, baclofen, and other CNS depressants may be used
- Anxiety: SSRI, SNRIs, or TCAs are helpful for chronic anxiety. In most cases it is best

to avoid combining with other benzodiazepines
- Insomnia: may be combined with low-dose TCAs (amitriptyline), or tetracyclics (trazadone, mirtazapine)

Tests
- None required

ADVERSE EFFECTS (AEs)

How the Drug Causes AEs
- Actions on benzodiazepine receptors including augmentation of inhibitory neurotransmitter effects

Notable AEs
- Most common: sedation, fatigue, depression, weakness, ataxia, nystagmus, confusion, and psychomotor retardation
- Less common: bradycardia, anorexia, hypotonia, and anterograde amnesia

 Life-Threatening or Dangerous AEs
- CNS depression and decreased respiratory drive, especially in combination with opiates, barbiturates, or alcohol
- Rare blood dyscrasias or liver function abnormalities
- With injection there is a 1.7% risk of serious AEs, such as hypotension, respiratory and cardiac arrest

Weight Gain
- Unusual

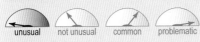
unusual　not unusual　common　problematic

Sedation
- Common

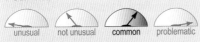
unusual　not unusual　**common**　problematic

What to Do About AEs
- May decrease or remit in time as tolerance develops
- Lower the total dose and take more at bedtime
- For severe, life-threatening AEs administer flumazenil to reverse effects

Best Augmenting Agents to Reduce AEs
- Most AEs cannot be reduced by adding an augmenting agent

DOSING AND USE

Usual Dosage Range
- Epilepsy: 2–10 mg 2–4 times daily
- Muscle spasm: 2–10 mg 3–4 times daily
- Panic/anxiety disorders: 2–10 mg 2–4 times daily

Dosage Forms
- Tablets: 2, 5, and 10 mg
- Capsule, extended release: 15 mg
- Oral solution: 5 mg/mL
- Rectal gel: 2.5, 10, and 20 mg (5 mg/mL)
- Injection: 5 mg/mL

How to Dose
- Epilepsy: used as adjunct in chronic epilepsy. Start at 2 mg 2–3 times daily and increase as tolerated to effective dose over days to weeks to maximum 10 mg 3–4 times daily
- Bouts of increased seizures in patients with epilepsy: dose based on age and weight. In patients 12 or older, give rectal diazepam 5 mg if 14–27 kg, 10 mg if 28–50 kg, 15 mg if 51–75 kg, and 20 mg to patients 76 kg or more
- Status epilepticus: 0.15–0.25 mg/kg in adults. Usually given 2–5 mg/min. IV or IM injection if no IV access available. After initial 5 or 10 mg, repeat every 10–15 minutes up to maximum of 30 mg in adults if seizures do not remit
- Spasticity: start at 2 mg at bedtime. Increase by 2–5 mg every few days as tolerated to most effective/best tolerated dose
- Panic disorder: start at 2 mg 2–3 times daily. Increase over 1–2 weeks as tolerated to most effective dose. Maximum 10 mg 4 times a day

 Dosing Tips
- Children usually require higher doses per unit body weight for acute seizure control
- Rectal administration or injections are useful for acute seizures including exacerbations in patients with chronic epilepsy

• Assess need to continue treatment in all disorders

Overdose

• Confusion, drowsiness, decreased reflexes, incoordination, and lethargy are common. Ataxia, hypotension, coma, and death are rare. Coma and respiratory or circulatory depression are rare when used alone. Use with other CNS depressants (such as alcohol, opioids, or barbiturates) places patients at greater risk for severe AEs. Induce vomiting and use supportive measures along with gastric lavage or ipecac and in severe cases forced diuresis
• Flumazenil, an antagonist, reverses effect of diazepam
• Physostigmine can reverse some AEs but either can provoke seizures in patients with epilepsy

Long-Term Use

• Safe for long-term use with appropriate monitoring

Habit Forming

• Schedule IV drug with risk of tolerance and dependence. Dependence is common after 6 weeks or more of use. Patients with a history of drug or alcohol abuse have an increased risk of dependency

How to Stop

• Taper slowly. Abrupt withdrawal can cause seizures, even in patients without epilepsy. Seizures can occur over a week after stopping drug
• Taper 1–2 mg/day every 3 days to reduce risk of withdrawal symptoms. Once at a lower dose, decrease speed of taper to as little as 1–2 mg/week or less. Slow tapers are especially recommended for patients on diazepam for many months or years
• Monitor for re-emergence of disease symptoms (seizures, muscle spasm, or anxiety)

Pharmacokinetics

• Peak plasma level at 0.5–2 hours and elimination half-life 20–80 hours. 98% protein bound. Mostly metabolized by CYP3A4 isoenzymes. Highly lipid soluble with good CNS penetration

 Drug Interactions

• Alcohol and other CNS depressants (barbiturates, opioids) increase CNS AEs
• Ranitidine may reduce GI absorption
• Inhibitors of hepatic metabolism (i.e., HIV antivirals, oral contraceptives, fluoxetine, isoniazid, ketoconazole, propranolol, valproic acid, metoprolol, grapefruit juice) can increase diazepam levels
• Antacids may alter the rate of absorption
• May increase serum concentrations of digoxin and phenytoin, leading to toxicity

 Other Warnings/ Precautions

• May cause drowsiness and impair ability to drive or perform tasks that require alertness
• Rare reports of death in patients with severe pulmonary impairment

Do Not Use

• Patients with a proven allergy to diazepam or any benzodiazepine. Significant liver disease or narrow angle-closure glaucoma

SPECIAL POPULATIONS

Renal Impairment

• Metabolites are renally excreted. Use with caution

Hepatic Impairment

• Do not use in patients with significant liver dysfunction

Cardiac Impairment

• No known effect

Elderly

• May clear drug more slowly and have lower dose requirement. Use lower doses than in younger adults

 Children and Adolescents

• For bouts of increased seizures in epilepsy, dose by age and weight.
• Age 2–5: 5 mg 6–11 kg, 10 mg 12–22 kg, 15 mg 23–33 kg, and 20 mg 34–44 kg

- Age 6–11: 5 mg 10–18 kg, 10 mg 19–37 kg, 15 mg 38–55 kg, and 20 mg 56 kg and up
- Status epilepticus: 0.1–1.0 mg/kg total dose at 2–5 mg/min
- Used in children as young as 6 months (oral) and neonates under 30 days of age (injection)
- Paradoxical excitement and rage may occur in psychiatric patients and hyperactive children

Pregnancy

- Category D. Drug crosses placenta and drug and its metabolites may accumulate. May increase risk of fetal malformations and infants can experience withdrawal. Use during labor can cause "floppy infant" syndrome with hypotonia, lethargy, and sucking difficulties
- Consider changing to another AED in patients that use as a daily preventative, but can be used for status epilepticus
- Do not use for treatment of anxiety

Breast Feeding

- Can be found in breast milk
- Generally recommendations are to discontinue drug or bottle feed
- Monitor infant for sedation, poor feeding, or irritability

THE ART OF NEUROPHARMACOLOGY

Potential Advantages

- Rapid onset of action in epilepsy, spasticity, and anxiety disorders. Useful in the emergency treatment of seizures and as an adjunctive medication in spasticity disorders

Potential Disadvantages

- Not a first-line maintenance agent in most patients with epilepsy. Development of tolerance and CNS depression often problematic. Significant potential for abuse

due to quick onset of action compared to clonazepam

Primary Target Symptoms

- Seizure frequency and severity
- Pain in spasticity disorders or dystonia
- Reduction in anxiety

Pearls

- Useful for treatment of acute seizures including status epilepticus, but patients typically require loading of a longer-lasting AED such as phenytoin
- In the treatment of status epilepticus aggressive treatment with simultaneous therapies may be more effective, but overtreatment may also lead to poor outcomes due to intubation. This is probably more of a consideration for patients with complex partial status epilepticus (as opposed to generalized tonic-clonic seizures)
- Nasal spray and autoinjector formulations are under development for the treatment of cluster seizures
- A first-line agent along with other benzodiazepines for stiff person syndrome symptoms, but not curative
- Effective for the short-term treatment of spasticity in children with cerebral palsy (Level of Evidence B). Tizanidine may be considered (Level of Evidence C)
- Lorazepam (0.1 mg/kg) IV or midazolam (0.2 mg/kg) IM is the first-line treatment for status epilepticus. Rectal diazepam is indicated in children for out-of-hospital treatment
- In cases of acute vertigo, benzodiazepines (diazepam, lorazepam, clonazepam) work to suppress vestibular function and improve symptoms. Treat every 4–6 hours with low dose (2 mg). May allow time for other treatments to work (i.e., vestibular therapy or preventive medication). Long-acting benzodiazepines are not helpful

Suggested Reading

Abbruzzese G. The medical management of spasticity. *Eur J Neurol.* 2002;9 Suppl 1:30–4; discussion 53–61.

Cesarani A, Alpini D, Monti B, Raponi G. The treatment of acute vertigo. *Neurol Sci.* 2004;25 Suppl 1:S26–30.

Delgado MR, Hirtz D, Aisen M, Ashwal S, Fehlings DL, et al. Practice parameter: pharmacologic treatment of spasticity in children and adolescents with cerebral palsy (an evidence-based review): report of the Quality Standards Subcommittee of the American Academy of Neurology and the Practice

Committee of the Child Neurology Society. *Neurology.* 2010;74(4):336–43.

Okoromah CN, Lesi FE. Diazepam for treating tetanus. *Cochrane Database Syst Rev.* 2004;1: CD003954.

Rey E, Tréluyer JM, Pons G. Pharmacokinetic optimization of benzodiazepine therapy for acute seizures. Focus on delivery routes. *Clin Pharmacokinet.* 1999;36(6):409–24.

Treiman DM. The role of benzodiazepines in the management of status epilepticus. *Neurology.* 1990;40(5 Suppl 2):32–42.

DICLOFENAC

THERAPEUTICS

Brands
- Cataflam, Cambia, Dyloject, Pennsaid, Solaraze, Voltaren, Zipsor, Zorvolex

Generic?
- Yes

Class
- Non-steroidal anti-inflammatory drug (NSAID)

Commonly Prescribed for
(FDA approved in bold)
- **Acute migraine attacks in adults (Cambia only)**
- **For relief of mild to moderate acute pain of osteoarthritis, rheumatoid arthritis, ankylosing spondylitis, gout, trauma, fractures, renal colic, surgery**
- **Primary dysmenorrhea**

How the Drug Works
- Like other NSAIDs, it binds competitively to cyclo-oxygenase (predominantly COX-1) thus inhibiting synthesis of proinflammatory thromboxane (TXA_2) and prostaglandins (PGE_2). The inhibition is serum concentration dependent
- Emerging evidence suggests it inhibits leukotriene synthesis, stimulates nitric oxide-cGMP antinociceptive pathway, increases plasma β-endorphin levels, and inhibits NMDA pathway. It may inhibit substrate P, NMDA receptor hyperalgesia, peroxisome proliferator activated receptor gamma (PPARgamma); block acid-sensing ion channels; and lower substance P and interleukin-6 production

How Long Until It Works
- Acute migraine: less than 2 hours
- Pain: within 30 minutes

If It Works
- Continue to use

If It Doesn't Work
- Migraine: add triptan, dihydroergotamine, antiemetic, or another NSAID

Best Augmenting Combos for Partial Response or Treatment-Resistance
- Migraine: combine with triptan or antiemetic

Tests
- Monitor blood pressure

ADVERSE EFFECTS (AEs)

How the Drug Causes AEs
- COX-1 is required for maintaining production of prostanoids, including prostacyclin (PGI_2) for GI mucosal protection and platelet aggregation inhibition

Notable AEs
- Dyspepsia, dizziness, nausea, diarrhea most common
- Inhibition of platelet aggregation is usually mild
- Elevation in hepatic transaminases (usually borderline)

Life-Threatening or Dangerous AEs
- Fatal cardiovascular thrombotic events (myocardial infarction, stroke)
- GI ulceration, perforation, and bleeding
- New-onset or worsening of hypertension
- Renal papillary necrosis or other renal injury
- Anaphylactoid reactions in patients with the aspirin triad (nasal polyps, asthma, aspirin intolerance)
- Stevens-Johnson syndrome, toxic epidermal necrolysis

Weight Gain
- Unusual

unusual | not unusual | common | problematic

Sedation
- Not unusual

unusual | not unusual | common | problematic

What to Do About AEs
- For significant GI or intracranial bleeding, stop the drug. Some AEs respond to lowering dose

Best Augmenting Agents to Reduce AEs

• Proton pump inhibitors may reduce risk of GI ulcers

DOSING AND USE

Usual Dosage Range

• Acute pain: 25–75 mg

Dosage Forms

• Submicron particle-filled capsules (Zorvolex): 18, 35 mg
• Liquid-filled capsule (Zipsor): 25 mg
• Extend-release tablet: 100 mg
• Tablet: 50, 75 mg
• Injection (Dyloject): 37.5 mg/mL
• Packet (Cambia): 50 mg

How to Dose

• Acute migraine: one packet (50 mg) in 1–2 ounces (30–60 mL) of water
• Acute pain: 37.5 mg/mL IV push (15 seconds) every 6 hours as needed. Maximum 150 mg/day
• Use the lowest effective dose for the shortest treatment duration

 Dosing Tips

• Taking with food decreases absorption and reduces GI AEs

Overdose

• GI distress, drowsiness, paresthesias, and numbness are most common. Severe overdose may cause hypertension, metabolic acidosis, hepatic or renal failure, and cardiac arrest. Consider multiple doses of activated charcoal or hemodialysis for severe cases

Long-Term Use

• Can increase the risk of AEs

Habit Forming

• No

How to Stop

• No need to taper

Pharmacokinetics

• T_{max} 15 minutes to 5 hours, depending on the formulation. It is metabolized in liver and eliminated through urine and bile. Half-life 2 hours. 100% bioavailability. 99% protein bound

 Drug Interactions

• Strong CYP inhibitor (e.g., ketoconazole) and inducer (e.g., rifampin) can alter diclofenac serum concentration
• Increased bleeding risk with alcohol, corticosteroid, aspirin, antiplatelets, and anticoagulants
• Cholestyramine may decrease absorption
• Cyclosporine and NSAIDs increase risk of nephrotoxicity
• It is a CYP1A2 inhibitor that increases concentration of antidepressants, antipsychotics, and others
• May increase drug levels and effects of digoxin, aminoglycosides, methotrexate, lithium, and phenytoin

 Other Warnings/ Precautions

• NSAIDs may cause an increased risk of serious cardiovascular thrombotic events, myocardial infarction, and stroke, which can be fatal. This risk may increase with duration of use. Patients with cardiovascular disease or risk factors for cardiovascular disease may be at greater risk
• NSAIDs cause an increased risk of serious GI adverse events including bleeding, ulceration, and perforation of the stomach or intestines, which can be fatal. These events can occur at any time during use and without warning symptoms. Elderly patients are at greater risk for serious GI events

Do Not Use

• Known hypersensitivity to diclofenac, its excipients, or other NSAIDs
• Preexisting asthma, urticaria, or allergic-type reactions after taking aspirin or other NSAIDs
• Use during the perioperative period in the setting of coronary artery bypass graft (CABG) surgery

Renal Impairment

- Use with caution in chronic renal insufficiency as may worsen renal function. Use low dose and monitor frequently

Hepatic Impairment

- Use with caution in patients with significant disease. May increase risk of GI bleeding and toxicity

Cardiac Impairment

- May cause fluid retention and decompensation in patients with cardiac failure. Higher risk of ischemic events. May cause hypertension or lower effectiveness of antihypertensives

Elderly

- More likely to experience GI bleeding or CNS AEs

 Children and Adolescents

- Safety in children 18 and under is not established

 Pregnancy

- Category C, except category D in third trimester. If used after 30th week, may cause premature closure of ductus arteriosus or prolonged labor. Use with caution

Breast Feeding

- Most NSAIDs are excreted in breast milk. Do not breast feed due to effects on infant cardiovascular system

Potential Advantages

- Simple effective pain medication. Useful as an alternative to triptans or in combination with other medications for migraine

Potential Disadvantages

- Cardiovascular risk, potential renal toxicity, GI bleeding

Primary Target Symptoms

- Pain and inflammation

 Pearls

- NSAIDs can be administered by different routes: pills, powder, injection (rapid onset), nasal spray (bypass GI tract for patients who are vomiting)
- For established migraine ($>$ 1 hour from onset), NSAIDs such as diclofenac may be more effective than oral triptans
- Less COX-1 inhibition than most other NSAIDs such as indomethacin or ketorolac
- One of the few NSAIDs with an indication for migraine
- Cambia T_{max} 15 minutes (tablet 1 hour), C_{max} 50% higher than diclofenac immediate-release tablet. Migraine 2-hour pain free: Cambia 25% vs. placebo 10%. The rapid kinetics is probably attributed to special combination of potassium salt and bicarbonate to enhance absorption
- Although NSAIDs do not cause vasoconstriction (unlike triptans or dihydroergotamine), they still increase the long-term risk of heart attack and stroke
- A 35 mg dose of diclofenac free acid is approximately equal to 37.6 mg of sodium diclofenac or 39.5 mg of potassium diclofenac

Suggested Reading

Diener HC, Montagna P, Gacs G, Lyczak P, Schumann G, Zoller B, et al. Efficacy and tolerability of diclofenac potassium sachets in migraine: a randomized, double-blind, cross-over study in comparison with diclofenac potassium tablets and placebo. *Cephalalgia*. 2006;26(5):537–47.

Gan TJ. Diclofenac: an update on its mechanism of action and safety profile. *Curr Med Res Opin*. 2010;26(7):1715–31.

Lipton RB, Grosberg B, Singer RP, Pearlman SH, Sorrentino JV, Quiring JN, et al. Efficacy and tolerability of a new powdered formulation of diclofenac potassium for oral solution for the acute treatment of migraine: Results from the International Migraine Pain Assessment Clinical Trial (IMPACT). *Cephalalgia*. 2010;30(11): 1336–45.

Rothrock JF. PRO-513 for acute migraine treatment. *Headache*. 2007;47(10):1459.

Tepper DE. Non-steroidal anti-inflammatories for the acute treatment of migraine. *Headache*. 2012;53(1):225–6.

Tepper DE. Nasal sprays for the treatment of migraine. *Headache*. 2013;53(3):577–8.

DIHYDROERGOTAMINE (DHE)

THERAPEUTICS

Brands
- Migranal, DHE-45, Dihydergot, Semprana

Generic?
- Yes

Class
- Ergot

Commonly Prescribed for
(FDA approved in bold)
- **Acute migraine treatment**
- **Acute cluster headache treatment**
- Status migrainosus

How the Drug Works
- Strong 5-HT$_{1B/1D}$ agonist (stronger than sumatriptan) with additional binding to $\alpha_{1,2}$-adrenergic, 5-HT$_{1A/2A/2B/2C}$, D$_2$ receptors
- In addition to vasoconstriction on meningeal vessels, its antinociceptive effect is likely due to blocking the transmission of pain signals at trigeminal nerve terminals (preventing the release of inflammatory neuropeptides) and synapses of second-order neurons in the trigeminal nucleus caudalis and third-order neurons in the thalamus. The site of pharmacological action, whether central or peripheral, remains to be studied

How Long Until It Works
- Migraine/cluster: within 1–2 hours

If It Works
- Continue to take as needed. Patients taking acute treatment more than 2 days/week are at risk for medication-overuse headache, especially if they have migraine

If It Doesn't Work
- Treat early in the attack (before severe pain)
- Address life style issues (e.g., stress, sleep hygiene), medication use issues (e.g., compliance, overuse), and other underlying medical conditions
- Change to higher dosage, another administration route, or combination of other medications (e.g., corticosteroid, antiemetics, NSAIDs). Add preventive medication when needed

Best Augmenting Combos for Partial Response or Treatment-Resistance
- Migraine: non-steroidal anti-inflammatory drugs (NSAIDs) or antiemetics are often used to augment response
- Cluster: oxygen (high-flow)
- Status migrainosus: combine with neuroleptics, ketorolac, diphenhydramine, IV valproate, IV magnesium, hydrate, and start preventative treatment

Tests
- Monitor blood pressure – especially after IV administration

ADVERSE EFFECTS (AEs)

How the Drug Causes AEs
- Actions on serotonin receptors cause vasoconstriction, nausea

Notable AEs
- Nausea, dizziness, sedation, dysphoria, chest or throat tightness, diarrhea, abdominal cramping
- Muscle pains, coldness, pallor, and cyanosis of digits
- Hypertension, flushing
- Altered taste, rhinitis (nasal spray), injection site reaction (IM)

Life-Threatening or Dangerous AEs
- Ergotism, cardiac (acute myocardial infarction, arrhythmia) or cerebrovascular events (hemorrhagic or ischemic stroke) are all rare

Weight Gain
- Unusual

unusual not unusual common problematic

Sedation
- Not unusual

unusual not unusual common problematic

What to Do About AEs
• Lower dose for nausea, stop for serious AEs

Best Augmenting Agents to Reduce AEs
• Pretreat before using (especially IV) with antiemetics

DOSING AND USE

Usual Dosage Range
• IV/IM: up to 3mg/day
• Nasal spray: up to 2 kits (4mg each)/day

Dosage Forms
• Nasal spray: 4mg/mL (0.5mg/spray)
• Injection: 1mg/mL

How to Dose
• IV: give 0.1–1mg 3–4 times daily as needed, usually for status migrainosus. Start with a test dose of 0.5mg in adults. Reduce dose for significant nausea (more than 10 minutes) after dose. If tolerated and pain not relieved, increase to 1mg dose. Give a maximum 3mg/day. Give up to 21mg for status migrainosus over 7 days
• IM: give 0.5–1mg as needed, up to 3mg/day
• Nasal spray: give 1 spray (0.5mg) in each nostril, repeat in 10–15 minutes up to twice a day
• Pretreatment with antiemetics is recommended for IV administration, but may not be necessary with IM or nasal spray. Pretreat with antiemetics (metoclopramide, droperidol, prochlorperazine; not aprepitant) 30 minutes before DHE
• In patients with risk factors for coronary artery disease, consult cardiologist. May give the first dose in a medical setting

 Dosing Tips
• IV push: slowly over 3 or more minutes to avoid nausea

Overdose
• Ergotamine poisoning may cause abdominal pain, nausea, vomiting, paresthesias, edema, muscle pain, cold hands and feet, and hypertension or hypotension. Confusion, depression, convulsions, and gangrene may occur. Unclear if DHE poses similar risks

Long-Term Use
• Appears safe, but monitor blood pressure and vascular risk factors with extended use

Habit Forming
• No

How to Stop
• No need to taper

Pharmacokinetics
• Bioavailability 100% (IV), 40% (intranasal), < 1% (oral). T_{max} 1–2 minutes (IV), 30 minutes (IM), 30–60 minutes (intranasal), 45 minutes (SC). Hepatic metabolism, mostly excreted in bile. Due to strong binding to the receptors, the effect of DHE is longer than its serum concentration

 Drug Interactions
• Use with caution with other vasoconstrictive agents, such as other ergot alkaloids or triptans
• Administration with potent CYP3A4 inhibitors (e.g., protease inhibitors, macrolide antibiotics, azole antifungals, nefazodone) and moderate CYP3A4 inhibitors (e.g., aprepitant, verapamil, grapefruit juice) can increase its serum concentration and the risk of vasospasm
• Nicotine may predispose to vasoconstriction
• May decrease effectiveness of nitrates

 Other Warnings/ Precautions
• For patients with risk factors predicative of coronary artery disease, it is strongly recommended that administration of the first dose of DHE take place in the setting of a physician's office or similar medically staffed and equipped facility unless the patient has previously received DHE

Do Not Use
• Uncontrolled hypertension, coronary artery vasospasm (Prinzmetal's angina), pregnancy, breast feeding, coronary arterial disease, or hypersensitivity to ergots

Renal Impairment

- Risks unknown. May be prone to hypertension and cardiac AEs

Hepatic Impairment

- Safety and effect of significant disease on drug metabolism unknown. Avoid in patients with severe disease

Cardiac Impairment

- Do not use in patients with hypertension or coronary artery disease

Elderly

- No known effects, but ensure safety before use (normal blood pressure, no coronary artery disease)

Children and Adolescents

- Not studied in children but likely safe

Pregnancy

- Category X. Associated with developmental toxicity and has oxytocic properties

Breast Feeding

- Likely excreted in breast milk. Do not breast feed after using

Potential Advantages

- Effective in status migrainosus, with low risk for medication overuse and fewer AEs than ergotamine. Effective in preventing migraine recurrence

Potential Disadvantages

- Compared to triptans: not available as oral form, as effective as sumatriptan injection in episodic migraine and acute cluster headache but more AEs

Primary Target Symptoms

- Headache pain, nausea, photo- and phonophobia

Pearls

- Effective for acute migraine even in those with refractory headache
- An ergotamine derivative with better safety profile than other ergots: less arterial constriction, less 5-HT$_{2B}$-induced fibrosis, less nausea and emesis, less oxytocic, and less likely to produce ergotism and gangrene
- Injections are more efficacious than nasal spray for acute migraine treatment
- Safety with other potentially vasoconstrictive drugs (e.g., triptans) is unknown. In general do not use within 24 hours of triptans
- Compared with sumatriptan, DHE may be less effective for acute headache with slower onset of action but lower rates of headache recurrence. Prolonged binding of 5-HT receptors may lead to sustained pain relief. Sometimes, it can be used for triptan non-responders. It is possibly effective in migraine with or without allodynia
- May be useful in the setting of status migrainosus and acute medication overuse. Medication overuse from opioids, barbiturates, or triptans can lead to treatment refractoriness
- An aerosol formulation of DHE (Semprana) that provides drug delivery using a pressurized, metered-dose Tempo inhaler for absorption through lung alveoli is currently awaiting approval

Suggested Reading

Ashkenazi A, Schwedt T. Cluster headache – acute and prophylactic therapy. *Headache.* 2011;51(2):272–86.

Dahlöf C, Maassen Van Den Brink A. Dihydroergotamine, ergotamine, methysergide and sumatriptan – basic science in relation to migraine treatment. *Headache.* 2012;52(4): 707–14.

Pringsheim T, Howse D. In-patient treatment of chronic daily headache using dihydroergotamine: a long-term follow-up study. *Can J Neurol Sci.* 1998;25(2): 146–50.

Raskin NH. Repetitive intravenous dihydroergotamine as therapy for intractable migraine. *Neurology.* 1986; 36(7):995–7.

Saper JR, Silberstein SD. Pharmacology of dihydroergotamine and evidence for efficacy and safety in migraine. *Headache.* 2006;46 Suppl 4: S171–81.

Silberstein SD, Kori SH. Dihydroergotamine: a review of formulation approaches for the acute treatment of migraine. *CNS Drugs.* 2013;27(5): 385–94.

Winner P, Ricalde O, Le Force B, Saper J, Margul B. A double-blind study of subcutaneous dihydroergotamine vs subcutaneous sumatriptan in the treatment of acute migraine. *Arch Neurol.* 1996;53(2):180–4.

DIMETHYL FUMARATE

THERAPEUTICS

Brands
- Tecfidera

Generic?
- No

 ### Class
- Immunomodulator

Commonly Prescribed for
(FDA approved in bold)
- **Patients with relapsing forms of multiple sclerosis (MS)**
- Psoriasis

 ### How the Drug Works
- The mechanism of action is unclear. The active metabolite, monomethyl fumarate (MMF), can suppress nuclear factor kappa B (NF-κB)-dependent transcription, regulate astrocyte histone deacetylase expression, activate Nrf2 pathway, reduce transendothelial migration of activated leukocytes, and induce detoxification enzymes in astrocytes and microglial cells. All of these play certain roles in anti-inflammation and antioxidation

How Long Until It Works
- It may take several months for the effect to be visible

If It Works
- Continue the drug. Monitor any AEs

If It Doesn't Work
- Switch to other disease-modifying agents

 ### Best Augmenting Combos for Partial Response or Treatment-Resistance
- For acute relapse, corticosteroid has the fastest response

Tests
- Obtain a CBC when initiating treatment, then every 6–12 months

ADVERSE EFFECTS (AEs)

How the Drug Causes AEs
- Serious AEs are related partially to anti-inflammation

Notable AEs
- Flushing (40%), abdominal pain, diarrhea, nausea
- Mildly elevated hepatic transaminases

 ### Life-Threatening or Dangerous AEs
- Anaphylaxis and angioedema
- Progressive multifocal leukoencephalopathy (PML) (one case report)
- Lymphopenia

Weight Gain
- Unusual

unusual · not unusual · common · problematic

Sedation
- Unusual

unusual · not unusual · common · problematic

What to Do About AEs
- Stop the drug if severe AEs develop

Best Augmenting Agents to Reduce AEs
- Flushing may improve by dosing after a meal, especially with fatty foods. Aspirin may improve flushing reaction. AEs generally lower when taken after a meal, especially high-fat meals

DOSING AND USE

Usual Dosage Range
- 240 mg twice daily

Dosage Forms
- Capsule, extended release: 120, 240 mg

How to Dose
- Start at 120 mg twice daily for 7 days
- Maintain at 240 mg twice daily after 7 days

Dosing Tips
- Capsule should be swallowed whole

Overdose
- Not well established

Long-Term Use
- Safe for long-term use with appropriate monitoring

Habit Forming
- No

How to Stop
- No need to taper but monitor for MS relapse

Pharmacokinetics
- Rapidly hydrolyzed by esterases to MMF in guts, tissues, and blood. T_{max} 2–2.5 hours. Plasma protein binding 27–54%. Eliminated mainly by CO_2 exhalation (60%), kidney (16%), and feces (1%). Half-life 1 hour

 Drug Interactions
- None well documented

 Other Warnings/ Precautions
- A transient increase in mean eosinophil counts may occur during the initial treatment period

Do Not Use
- Known hypersensitivity to the drug or its excipients

Renal Impairment
- No known effect

Hepatic Impairment
- Slight increase in hepatic transaminases primarily during the first 6 months

Cardiac Impairment
- No known effect

Elderly
- Not studied

 Children and Adolescents
- Safety and effectiveness have not been established

 Pregnancy
- Category C. In animals, adverse effects on offspring survival, growth, sexual maturation, and neurobehavioral function were observed

Breast Feeding
- It is not known whether this drug is excreted in human milk

Potential Advantages
- Effective in reducing MS relapse

Potential Disadvantages
- Risk of PML and lymphopenia. Frequent flushing and GI AEs

Primary Target Symptoms
- Neurological dysfunctions associated with MS

Pearls
- It was originally used as a biocide in furniture that later caused allergic contact dermatitis. It is currently banned in consumer products
- In clinical trials, 3–4% subjects discontinued the medication due to intolerable flushing and GI AEs
- DEFINE study (phase III): at 2 years, 240 mg twice or thrice daily has similar effect in reducing relapse and progression of disability/MRI as placebo
- CONFIRM study (phase III): at 2 years, dimethyl fumarate is superior to glatiramer in lower annualized relapse rate and MRI progression. Both drugs are not effective in reducing disability progression
- Relatively rapid onset of effect with improvements noted at week 12 in clinical trials
- The reported case of PML occurred in a patient with a very low lymphocyte count after 4 years of therapy

Suggested Reading

Fox RJ, Miller DH, Phillips JT, Hutchinson M, Havrdova E, Kita M, et al. Placebo-controlled phase 3 study of oral BG-12 or glatiramer in multiple sclerosis. *N Engl J Med.* 2012;367(12):1087–97.

Gold R, Kappos L, Arnold DL, Bar-Or A, Giovannoni G, Selmaj K, et al. Placebo-controlled phase 3 study of oral BG-12 for relapsing multiple sclerosis. *N Engl J Med.* 2012;367(12):1098–107.

Kappos L, Giovannoni G, Gold R, Phillips JT, Arnold DL, et al. Time course of clinical and neuroradiological effects of delayed-release dimethyl fumarate in multiple sclerosis. *Eur J Neurol.* 2015;22(4): 664–71.

DIPYRIDAMOLE AND ASPIRIN

Brands
- Aggrenox

Generic?
- Yes

Class
- Antiplatelet agent

Commonly Prescribed for
(FDA approved in bold)
- **To reduce risk of recurrent transient ischemic attack (TIA) or ischemic stroke (IS) due to thrombosis**
- **Adjunctive prophylaxis of thromboembolism after cardiac valve replacement (adjunctive with warfarin: use dipyridamole only)**

How the Drug Works
- Aspirin: by acetylating cyclo-oxygenase-1 (COX-1), aspirin irreversibly inhibits thromboxane synthetase, reducing synthesis of thromboxane A_2, a prostaglandin derivative that is a potent vasoconstrictor and inducer of platelet aggregation
- Dipyridamole: inhibits (1) thromboxane synthetase, (2) the cellular reuptake of adenosine into platelets, endothelial cells, and erythrocytes, and adenosine deaminase, which both increase extracellular adenosine levels leading to stimulation of platelet adenylate cyclase and inhibition of platelet aggregation, and (3) phosphodiesterase, augmenting the effect of endothelium-derived relaxing factor (nitric oxide)

How Long Until It Works
- 1–2 hours. Inhibits platelet aggregation for the life of the platelet (7–10 days)

If It Works
- Continue to use

If It Doesn't Work
- Only reduces risk of myocardial infarction (MI) or stroke. Warfarin is superior for

cardiogenic stroke. Control all stroke risk factors such as smoking, hyperlipidemia, and hypertension. For acute events, admit patients for treatment and diagnostic testing

 ## Best Augmenting Combos for Partial Response or Treatment-Resistance
- Combinations with other antiplatelet agents are not recommended

Tests
- None required

How the Drug Causes AEs
- Antiplatelet effects increase bleeding risk. Effects on nitric oxide may produce headache

Notable AEs
- Headache, abdominal pain, dyspepsia, nausea/vomiting, diarrhea, arthralgia, hypotension, epistaxis

 ## Life-Threatening or Dangerous AEs
- GI, intracranial, or intraocular bleeding. Rare hepatic failure

Weight Gain
- Unusual

unusual — not unusual — common — problematic

Sedation
- Unusual

unusual — not unusual — common — problematic

What to Do About AEs
- For significant GI or intracranial bleeding, stop drug. For intolerable headaches, switch to 1 capsule at bedtime and low-dose aspirin in the morning for 1 week (headaches usually resolve in 1 week or less)

Best Augmenting Agents to Reduce AEs

- Proton pump inhibitors reduce risk of GI bleeding

DOSING AND USE

Usual Dosage Range

- 200 mg extended-release dipyridamole/25 mg aspirin twice daily

Dosage Forms

- Capsules: 200 mg extended-release dipyridamole/25 mg aspirin

How to Dose

- 1 capsule twice daily

Dosing Tips

- Swallow whole capsule with or without food

Overdose

- Aspirin: respiratory alkalosis resulting in tachypnea, nausea, hypokalemia, tinnitus, thrombocytopenia, and easy bruising early. Can lead to pulmonary edema, respiratory failure, renal failure, and coma
- Dipyridamole: flushing, sweating, restlessness, dizziness, and a feeling of weakness can occur. Less commonly tachycardia and hypotension

Long-Term Use

- Safe for long-term use

Habit Forming

- No

How to Stop

- No need to taper

Pharmacokinetics

- Aspirin: half-life is about 20 minutes. > 99% protein binding. Hepatic metabolism and renal excretion
- Dipyridamole: peak levels at 2 hours. Hepatic metabolism into a glucuronide metabolite that is mostly excreted via bile into feces. Plasma half-life 13.6 hours

Drug Interactions

Aspirin:

- Alcohol increases risk of GI ulceration and may prolong bleeding time
- Urinary acidifiers (ascorbic acid, methionine) decrease secretion and increase drug effect
- Antacids and urinary alkalinizers may decrease drug effect
- Carbonic anhydrase inhibitors may increase risk of salicylate intoxication, and aspirin may displace acetazolamide from protein binding sites, leading to toxicity
- Activated charcoal decreases aspirin absorption and effect
- Corticosteroids may increase clearance and decrease serum levels
- Use with heparin or oral anticoagulants has an additive effect and can increase bleeding risks
- Aspirin may cause unexpected hypotension after treatment with nitroglycerin
- Use with NSAIDs may decrease NSAID serum levels and increases risk of GI AEs
- May displace valproic acid from binding sites and increase pharmacological effects
- May displace warfarin from binding sites and prolong PT
- May blunt effectiveness of β-blockers and ACE inhibitors
- May decrease effect of loop diuretics and spironolactone
- Increases drug levels of methotrexate
- Reduces the uricosuric effects of probenecid and sulfinpyrazone

Dipyridamole:

- Increases plasma levels and cardiac effects of adenosine
- May decrease effect of cholinesterase inhibitors, such as pyridostigmine, which may worsen symptoms of myasthenia gravis

Other Warnings/ Precautions

- The use of aspirin or other salicylates in children or teens with influenza or chickenpox may be associated with Reye's syndrome. Symptoms include vomiting and lethargy that may progress to delirium or coma

- Aspirin intolerance is not rare, especially in asthmatics. Symptoms include bronchospasm, angioedema, severe rhinitis, or shock

Do Not Use

- Known hypersensitivity to salicylates, NSAIDs, or dipyridamole, acute asthma or hay fever, severe anemia or blood coagulation defects, children or teenagers with chickenpox or flu symptoms

SPECIAL POPULATIONS

Renal Impairment

- Not studied. Use with caution with significant disease. May temporarily worsen renal function

Hepatic Impairment

- Not studied. Use with caution in patients with significant disease, including those with hypoprothrombinemia or vitamin K deficiency. Hepatotoxicity may occur

Cardiac Impairment

- Use with caution in patients with severe coronary artery disease, including recent MI or angina. The vasodilatory effect of dipyridamole can aggravate chest pain. May exacerbate hypotension if present. Aspirin content in Aggrenox may not provide adequate treatment for MI or angina

Elderly

- No known effects

Children and Adolescents

- Not studied in children younger than age 12. Do not use in setting of chickenpox or flu symptoms

Pregnancy

- Category B (dipyridamole)/D (aspirin). Crosses the placenta and is associated with anemia, ante- or post-partum hemorrhage, prolonged gestation and labor, and constriction of ductus arteriosus. Do not use, especially in third trimester

Breast Feeding

- Both products excreted in breast milk in low concentrations. Risk to infants is unknown

THE ART OF NEUROPHARMACOLOGY

Potential Advantages

- Effective medication for secondary stroke prevention

Potential Disadvantages

- Low aspirin doses may not provide adequate prophylaxis against cardiac disease. Cost

Primary Target Symptoms

- Prevention of the neurological complications that result from IS

 Pearls

- First-line drug for secondary prevention of stroke along with clopidogrel and aspirin
- Compared to clopidogrel, may be less effective in patients with peripheral vascular disease
- Stop 1 week before any surgical procedure, given its effect on platelet function
- Headache is a common AE that may raise concerns in the setting of recent IS. When starting drug, inform patients that headache is common in the first week of treatment
- This dipyridamole and aspirin combination is more effective than 25 mg aspirin twice daily, but it is unclear if it is more effective than higher aspirin doses
- Recent stroke/TIA attributable to > 50% stenosis of major intracranial artery, data on clopidogrel or Aggrenox are insufficient (Class IIb, Level of Evidence C)
- ESPS-2: compared with aspirin alone, Aggrenox reduced the stroke risk by 23%. More headache and GI symptoms
- PRoFESS: early discontinuation due to adverse effect more common in Aggrenox than clopidogrel (16.4% vs. 10.6%). Stroke recurrence in Aggrenox similar to clopidogrel (9.0% vs. 8.8%)
- Given the results of PRoFESS trial, has become less popular than clopidogrel, which does not cause headaches and can be taken once daily

Suggested Reading

Diener HC, Sacco RL, Yusuf S, Cotton D, Ounpuu S, Lawton WA, et al; Prevention Regimen for Effectively Avoiding Second Strokes (PRoFESS) study group. Effects of aspirin plus extended-release dipyridamole versus clopidogrel and telmisartan on disability and cognitive function after recurrent stroke in patients with ischaemic stroke in the Prevention Regimen for Effectively Avoiding Second Strokes (PRoFESS) trial: a double-blind, active and placebo-controlled study. *Lancet Neurol.* 2008;7(10):875–84.

Kernan WN, Ovbiagele B, Black HR, Bravata DM, Chimowitz MI, Ezekowitz MD, et al. Guidelines for the prevention of stroke in patients with stroke and transient ischemic attack: a guideline for healthcare professionals from the American Heart Association/American Stroke Association. *Stroke.* 2014;45(7):2160–236.

Lenz T, Wilson A. Clinical pharmacokinetics of antiplatelet agents used in the secondary prevention of stroke. *Clin Pharmacokinet.* 2003;42(10):909–20.

Redman AR, Ryan GJ. Aggrenox((R)) versus other pharmacotherapy in preventing recurrent stroke. *Expert Opin Pharmacother.* 2004;5(1):117–23.

Serebruany VL, Malinin AI, Sane DC, Jilma B, Takserman A, Atar D, et al. Magnitude and time course of platelet inhibition with Aggrenox and Aspirin in patients after ischemic stroke: the AGgrenox versus Aspirin Therapy Evaluation (AGATE) trial. *Eur J Pharmacol.* 2004;499(3):315–24.

Usman MH, Notaro LA, Nagarakanti R, Brahin E, Dessain S, Gracely E, et al. Combination antiplatelet therapy for secondary stroke prevention: enhanced efficacy or double trouble? *Am J Cardiol.* 2009;103(8):1107–12.

DONEPEZIL

THERAPEUTICS

Brands
- Aricept, Aricept Evess, Aricept ODT, Memorit

Generic?
- Yes

 Class
- Cholinesterase inhibitor

Commonly Prescribed for
(FDA approved in bold)
- **Alzheimer's dementia (AD) (mild, moderate, or severe)**
- Vascular dementia
- Mild cognitive impairment
- Dementia with Lewy bodies (DLB)
- HIV dementia
- Autism
- Attention deficit hyperactivity disorder

 How the Drug Works
- Increases the concentration of acetylcholine through reversible, non-competitive inhibition of acetylcholinesterase, which increases availability of acetylcholine. A deficiency of cholinergic function is felt to be important in producing the signs and symptoms of AD. May interfere with amyloid deposition
- Although symptoms of AD can improve, donepezil does not prevent disease progression

How Long Until It Works
- Typically 2–6 weeks at a given dose, but effect is best observed over a period of months

If It Works
- Continue to use but symptoms of dementia usually continue to worsen

If It Doesn't Work
- Consider adjusting dose
- Change to another cholinesterase inhibitor or NMDA antagonist (memantine)
- Non-pharmacological measures are the basis of dementia treatment. Maintain regular schedules and routines. Avoid prolonged travel, unnecessary medical procedures or emergency room visits, crowds, and large social gatherings
- Limit drugs with sedative properties such as opioids, hypnotics, AEDs, and TCAs
- Treat other disorders that can worsen symptoms, such as hyperglycemia or urinary difficulties

 Best Augmenting Combos for Partial Response or Treatment-Resistance
- Addition of the NMDA receptor antagonist memantine may be beneficial. In one study donepezil plus memantine reduced the rate of progression compared to that in those taking donepezil alone
- Treat depression or apathy with SSRIs but be cautious for increased risk of AEs (e.g., QTc prolongation, injurious falls). Avoid TCAs in demented patients due to risk of confusion. In dementia patients with severe depression, electroconvulsive therapy can be an option
- For significant confusion and agitation avoid neuroleptics (especially in DLB) because of the risk of neuroleptic malignant syndrome. Atypical antipsychotics (e.g., risperidone, clozapine, aripiprazole) or SSRIs can be used instead

Tests
- None required

ADVERSE EFFECTS (AEs)

How the Drug Causes AEs
- Acetylcholinesterase inhibition in the CNS and PNS

Notable AEs
- GI AEs (nausea, diarrhea, anorexia and weight loss) are most common
- Fatigue, depression, dizziness, muscle cramps, and sleep disturbances
- Bladder outflow obstruction

 Life-Threatening or Dangerous AEs
- Rarely bradycardia or heart block causing syncope
- Generalized convulsions

- Increases gastric acid secretions, which can predispose to GI bleeding
- Exaggerates succinylcholine-type muscle relaxation during anesthesia

Weight Gain

- Unusual

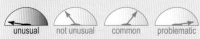

unusual   not unusual   common   problematic

Sedation

- Unusual

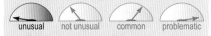

unusual   not unusual   common   problematic

What to Do About AEs

- In patients with dementia, determining if AEs are related to medication or another medical condition can be difficult. For CNS side effects, discontinuation of non-essential centrally acting medications may help. If a bothersome AE is clearly drug-related then lower the dose (especially for GI AEs) or discontinue donepezil

Best Augmenting Agents to Reduce AEs

- Most AEs do not respond to adding other medications

DOSING AND USE

Usual Dosage Range

- 5–10mg at night

Dosage Forms

- Tablets: 5, 10, 23mg
- Orally disintegrating: 5, 10mg
- Oral solution: 1mg/mL

How to Dose

- Start at 5mg in the evening. Increase to 10mg in 4–6 weeks if needed. If AEs occur, titrate more slowly
- If under 10mg daily for 3 months, can be switched to 23mg daily

 Dosing Tips

- Slow titration can reduce AEs. Food does not affect absorption

Overdose

- Symptoms of cholinergic crisis can occur: nausea/vomiting, hypotension, diaphoresis, convulsions, bradycardia/collapse. May cause muscle weakness and respiratory failure. Atropine with an initial dose of 1–2mg IV is a potential antidote

Long-Term Use

- Safe for long-term use. Effectiveness may decrease over time as the dementing illness progresses

Habit Forming

- No

How to Stop

- Abrupt discontinuation can produce rapid worsening of dementia symptoms, memory and behavioral disturbances. Taper slowly

Pharmacokinetics

- Metabolized by CYP2D6 and 3A4. Elimination half-life is 70 hours but peak effect at 3–4 hours. About 17% of drug is excreted unchanged in urine. Linear pharmacokinetics. Bioavailability 100%. Protein binding 96%

 Drug Interactions

- Increases the effect of anesthetics such as succinylcholine. Stop before surgery
- Anticholinergics interfere with effect of drug
- Other cholinesterase inhibitors, cholinergic agonists (bethanechol) and neuromuscular blockers (such as succinylcholine) may cause a synergistic effect
- CYP3A4 and 2D6 inhibitors (ketoconazole, quinidine) increase donepezil concentrations and inducers (carbamazepine, phenobarbital, phenytoin, rifampin, dexamethasone) reduce concentrations
- Bradycardia may occur when used with β-blockers
- A weak CYP1A2/2D6 inhibitor

 Other Warnings/ Precautions

- Weight loss is more common under 23mg (4.7%) than 10mg (2.5%) once daily

Do Not Use

- Hypersensitivity to the drug or piperidine derivatives (including meperidine and fentanyl)

Renal Impairment

- No known effects

Hepatic Impairment

- Patients with severe disease have 20% reduced clearance. This may not be clinically significant

Cardiac Impairment

- Significant heart block, bradycardia, and syncope are rare but have been reported

Elderly

- No known effects

Children and Adolescents

- Not studied. AD does not occur in children. May be useful for ADHD as adjunctive treatment

Pregnancy

- Category C. Use only if benefits of medication outweigh risks

Breast Feeding

- Unknown if excreted in breast milk. Do not use

Potential Advantages

- Proven effectiveness for AD, even with severe dementia. Low risk of the hepatotoxicity seen with other acetylcholinesterase inhibitors (tacrine), and lower GI AEs (nausea, anorexia) than rivastigmine. Once-daily dosing

Potential Disadvantages

- Cost and lack of effectiveness. Sleep disturbances such as insomnia are more common than with other AD treatments. Does not prevent progression of AD or other dementia

Primary Target Symptoms

- Confusion, agitation, memory, performing activities of daily living

 Pearls

- Cholinesterase inhibitors are efficacious for mild to moderate AD. Donepezil has greater cost-effectiveness than rivastigmine and galantamine. In most clinical trials, medication treatments for AD patients had a similar rate of benefit
- In patients with moderate or severe AD, continued treatment with donepezil and memantine was associated with cognitive benefits. Combination may have short-term additional benefit. Combining with other cholinesterase inhibitors is not recommended
- May be useful for behavioral problems in AD (delusion, anxiety, and apathy for example) as well as memory disturbance
- Shown to be effective for the cognitive and behavioral symptoms (agitation, apathy, hallucinations) of DLB
- When changing from one cholinesterase inhibitor to another, avoid a washout period which could precipitate clinical deterioration
- May delay the need for nursing home placement
- May help treat dementia in Down's syndrome, which has similar pathology to AD
- Most open-label studies of donepezil for ADHD did not demonstrate benefit, and AEs were common. For treatment of Tourette's in children with coexisting ADHD, donepezil appears to reduce tics, but AEs are problematic
- A recent study showed that it does not improve memory in multiple sclerosis

Suggested Reading

Bentué-Ferrer D, Tribut O, Polard E, Allain H. Clinically significant drug interactions with cholinesterase inhibitors: a guide for neurologists. *CNS Drugs.* 2003;17(13):947–63.

Birks J. Cholinesterase inhibitors for Alzheimer's disease. *Cochrane Database Syst Rev.* 2006;1: CD005593.

Bond M, Rogers G, Peters J, Anderson R, Hoyle M, Miners A, et al. The effectiveness and cost-effectiveness of donepezil, galantamine, rivastigmine and memantine for the treatment of Alzheimer's disease (review of Technology Appraisal No. 111): a systematic review and economic model. *Health Technol Assess.* 2012;16(21):1–470.

Downey D. Pharmacologic management of Alzheimer disease. *J Neurosci Nurs.* 2008;40(1): 55–9.

Howard R, McShane R, Lindesay J, Ritchie C, Baldwin A, Barber R, et al. Donepezil and memantine for moderate-to-severe Alzheimer's disease. *N Engl J Med.* 2012;366(10):893–903.

Krupp LB, Christodoulou C, Melville P, Scherl WF, Pai LY, Muenz LR, et al. Multicenter randomized clinical trial of donepezil for memory impairment in multiple sclerosis. *Neurology.* 2011;76(17):1500–7.

Porsteinsson AP, Grossberg GT, Mintzer J, Olin JT; Memantine MEM-MD-12 Study Group. Memantine treatment in patients with mild to moderate Alzheimer's disease already receiving a cholinesterase inhibitor: a randomized, double-blind, placebo-controlled trial. *Curr Alzheimer Res.* 2008;5(1):83–9.

Schmitt FA, van Dyck CH, Wichems CH, Olin JT; for the Memantine MEM-MD-02 Study Group. Cognitive response to memantine in moderate to severe Alzheimer disease patients already receiving donepezil: an exploratory reanalysis. *Alzheimer Dis Assoc Disord.* 2006;20(4): 255–62.

Stahl SM. The new cholinesterase inhibitors for Alzheimer's disease, Part 1: their similarities are different. *J Clin Psychiatry.* 2000;61(10): 710–11.

DROPERIDOL

THERAPEUTICS

Brands
- Inapsine

Generic?
- Yes

Class
- Antiemetic

Commonly Prescribed for
(FDA approved in bold)
- **Antiemetic for nausea and vomiting related to surgical and diagnostic procedures**
- Migraine (acute)
- Chemotherapy-induced nausea and vomiting

How the Drug Works
- Antidopaminergic, with mild α_1 adrenergic blockade and sedative effects

How Long Until It Works
- Migraine, nausea in less than 10 minutes

If It Works
- Use at lowest required dose
- Monitor QTc interval, potassium and magnesium level

If It Doesn't Work
- Change to another agent

Best Augmenting Combos for Partial Response or Treatment-Resistance
- For migraine, can be used with dihydroergotamine or NSAIDs

Tests
- Obtain ECG to monitor QTc

ADVERSE EFFECTS (AEs)

How the Drug Causes AEs
- Hypotension and dizziness are related to α-blockade, and abnormal movement AEs are related to dopamine blocking effects

Notable AEs
- Drowsiness, hypotension, tachycardia, chills
- Dystonia, akathisia, restlessness, anxiety, state of mental detachment
- Less common: elevated blood pressure, apnea, muscular rigidity

Life-Threatening or Dangerous AEs
- QTc prolongation and torsade de pointes have been reported, especially with higher doses

Weight Gain
- Unusual

unusual   not unusual   common   problematic

Sedation
- Common

unusual   not unusual   common   problematic

What to Do About AEs
- Lowering dose or changing to another antiemetic improves most AEs
- Use with caution in patients if QTc is above 450 (females) or 440 (males). Lower dose or change to another agent. Do not administer droperidol for QTc greater than 500
- For patients on daily IV therapy, continue to monitor with daily ECG, especially as dose increases

Best Augmenting Agents to Reduce AEs
- Give fluids to avoid hypotension and dizziness
- Give anticholinergics (diphenhydramine or benztropine) for extrapyramidal reactions

DOSING AND USE

Usual Dosage Range
- 0.625–2.5 mg every 6–8 hours

Dosage Forms
- Injection: 2.5 mg/mL

How to Dose
- After ensuring no QTc prolongation, give 0.625–2.5 mg as a single dose every 6–8 hours IV or as IM injection

 Dosing Tips
- In hospitalized patients, start with lower dose to ensure no QTc prolongation occurs and drug well tolerated and increase as needed to effective dose
- Check ECG daily while receiving treatment

Overdose
- Sedation, hypotension, extrapyramidal reactions, and arrhythmias, including QTc prolongation

Long-Term Use
- Safe for long-term use with appropriate monitoring

Habit Forming
- No

How to Stop
- No need to taper

Pharmacokinetics
- Onset of action in 3–10 minutes and peak levels at 30 minutes. Half-life 2.2 hours. Hepatic metabolism and excreted mostly as metabolites in urine and feces

 Drug Interactions
- Use with CNS depressants (barbiturates, opiates, general anesthetics) potentiates CNS AEs
- Epinephrine may worsen hypotension due to α_1-adrenergic blockade by droperidol
- Use with some forms of conduction anesthesia (spinal anesthesia, epidural anesthetics) can cause hypotension or peripheral vasodilation due to sympathetic blockade
- Fentanyl and droperidol may induce hypertension due to alterations in sympathetic pathway

 Other Warnings/ Precautions
Risk factors for QTc prolongation include:
- Significant bradycardia (less than 50 bpm)

- Cardiac disease
- Treatment with class I and III antiarrhythmics
- Treatment with MAOIs
- Treatment with medications known to prolong QTc intervals
- Electrolyte imbalance (hypokalemia, hypomagnesemia), as seen with some diuretics

Do Not Use
- Hypersensitivity to drug, QTc prolongation, including long QT syndrome

Renal Impairment
- Unknown effects. Use with caution

Hepatic Impairment
- Use with caution. May need to lower dose

Cardiac Impairment
- May worsen orthostatic hypotension. Avoid using in patients with arrhythmia

Elderly
- May be more sensitive to CNS AEs

 Children and Adolescents
- Appears safe in children over age 2. Reduce dose to 1 or 1.5 mg in young children

 Pregnancy
- Category C. Use only if benefit outweighs risks

Breast Feeding
- Unknown if found in breast milk. Use while breast feeding is generally not recommended

Potential Advantages
- Highly effective drug in the treatment of refractory migraine

Potential Disadvantages

- Need to monitor QTc interval. Extrapyramidal reactions

Primary Target Symptoms

- Headache, nausea

 Pearls

- Effective in refractory migraine and status migrainosus. Often combined with dihydroergotamine, given about 30 minutes after droperidol

- Droperidol is similar to prochlorperazine in pain reduction and incidence of akathisia
- Combine with diphenydramine, 25–50 mg, to reduce rate of akathisia and dystonic reactions
- Cases of torsade de pointes reported, all at dose of 5 mg IV or greater. Black-box warning due to risk of QTc prolongation and death, but with appropriate ECG monitoring and doses under 10 mg/day, this is extremely rare. Patients with QTc above 500 are at greatest risk

 Suggested Reading

Evans RW, Young WB. Droperidol and other neuroleptics/antiemetics for the management of migraine. *Headache*. 2003;43(7):811–13.

Kelley NE, Tepper DE. Rescue therapy for acute migraine, part 2: neuroleptics, antihistamines, and others. *Headache*. 2012; 52(2):292–306.

Nuttall GA, Eckerman KM, Jacob KA, Pawlaski EM, Wigersma SK, Marienau ME, Oliver WC, Narr BJ, Ackerman MJ. Does low-dose droperidol administration increase the risk of drug-induced QT prolongation and torsade de pointes in the general surgical population? *Anesthesiology*. 2007;107(4):531–6.

Silberstein SD, Young WB, Mendizabal JE, Rothrock JF, Alam AS. Acute migraine treatment with droperidol: a randomized, double-blind, placebo-controlled trial. *Neurology*. 2003; 60(2):315–21.

Wang SJ, Silberstein SD, Young WB. Droperidol treatment of status migrainosus and refractory migraine. *Headache*. 1997;37(6):377–82.

DROXIDOPA

THERAPEUTICS

Brands
- Northera

Generic?
- No

Class
- Catecholamine analog

Commonly Prescribed for
(FDA approved in bold)
- **Treatment of symptomatic neurogenic orthostatic hypotension (orthostatic dizziness, lightheadedness, syncope) in adult patients caused by primary autonomic failure (Parkinson's disease [PD], multiple system atrophy, pure autonomic failure, familial amyloid polyneuropathy), dopamine β-hydroxylase deficiency, and non-diabetic autonomic neuropathy**
- Freezing of gait in PD
- Postural tachycardia syndrome (POTS)
- Prevention of orthostasis in hemodialysis patients
- Fibromyalgia
- Attention deficit hyperactivity disorder
- Chronic fatigue

How the Drug Works
- It is a synthetic catecholamino acid analog that is directly metabolized by dopa-decarboxylase to increase the concentrations of norepinephrine and epinephrine throughout the body. It also crosses the BBB and exerts its pharmacological effects within the CNS. Peripherally, it increases blood pressure by inducing peripheral arterial and venous vasoconstriction. It induces small and transient rises in plasma norepinephrine
- The contribution of other actions of droxidopa to its pharmacological effect is not well understood

How Long Until It Works
- Few days

If It Works
- May continue for a longer time, although no available study on treatment more than 2 weeks so far

If It Doesn't Work
- Correct any treatable underlying disorders
- Volume expansion: high-salt diet, increased fluid intake, fluorohydrocortisone
- Vasoconstriction: desmopressin (vasopressin analog), midodrine (α_1 agonist)

Best Augmenting Combos for Partial Response or Treatment-Resistance
- Orthostasis: volume expansion and vasoconstriction
- POTS: volume expansion and vasoconstriction, exercise, cognitive behavioral therapy, propranolol, SNRIs, pyrostigmine
- Fibromyalgia: TCAs, SNRI, aerobic exercise, cognitive behavioral therapy

Tests
- None

ADVERSE EFFECTS (AEs)

How the Drug Causes AEs
- Elevated norepinephrine concentration

Notable AEs
- Headache, dizziness, nausea, supine hypertension, fatigue

Life-Threatening or Dangerous AEs
- Allergic reaction
- Neuroleptic malignant syndrome mimics (hyperpyrexia and confusion)
- May exacerbate existing ischemic heart disease, arrhythmias, and congestive heart failure

Weight Gain
- Unusual

unusual not unusual common problematic

Sedation
- Unusual

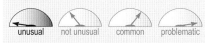

unusual | not unusual | common | problematic

What to Do About AEs
- Reduce or discontinue droxidopa

Best Augmenting Agents to Reduce AEs
- Most AEs cannot be reduced with the use of an augmenting agent

DOSING AND USE

Usual Dosage Range
- 100–600 mg 3 times a day

Dosage Forms
- Capsule: 100, 200, 300 mg

How to Dose
- Initial: 100 mg 3 times during the day
- Titration: 100 mg 3 times daily
- Maximum: 600 mg 3 times daily

 Dosing Tips
- Avoid supine hypertension during sleep: elevate head of the bed and last dose 3 hours prior to sleep
- Swallow whole, with or without food

Overdose
- There was only one incidence. A patient ingested 7700 mg droxidopa and developed a hypertensive crisis, which was resolved promptly with treatment. No antidote at the moment

Long-Term Use
- Not fully studied

Habit Forming
- No

How to Stop
- Taper in a few days

Pharmacokinetics
- T_{max} = 1–4 hours but plasma norepinephrine does not correlate well with dose. Droxidopa is metabolized by catechol-O-methyltransferase, dopa decarboxylase and others (not P450 system), and is eliminated in urine. It has a mean half-life of 2.5 hours

 Drug Interactions
- Risk of supine hypertension increases upon use of agents that increase blood pressure (norepinephrine, ephedrine, midodrine, triptans)
- Dopa-decarboxylase inhibitors (e.g, carbidopa, α-methyldopa, benserazide) can increase droxidopa serum concentration
- In clinical trials, dopamine agonists, amantadine derivatives, and monoamine oxidase (MAO)-B inhibitors did not appear to affect its clearance, and no dose adjustments were required. Also in clinical trials, although carbidopa and catechol-O-methyltransferase (COMT) inhibitors can affect droxidopa's clearance, no significant dose adjustment was required

 Other Warning/ Precautions
- Monitor supine blood pressure prior to and during treatment and more frequently when increasing doses

Do Not Use
- Known hypersensitivity to the drug

SPECIAL POPULATIONS

Renal Impairment
- Do not recommended if GFR < 30 mL/min

Hepatic Impairment
- Use with caution but no known effects

Cardiac Impairment
- May exacerbate existing ischemic heart disease, arrhythmias, and congestive heart failure

Elderly
- Use with caution. More susceptible to AEs

 Children and Adolescents
- Not fully studied

Pregnancy

- Category C. Use only if benefit of medication outweighs risks

Breast Feeding

- Concentration in breast milk unknown. Exposure of infant may lead to reduced weight gain and reduced survival

THE ART OF NEUROPHARMACOLOGY

Potential Advantages

- Treatment of orthostatic hypotension. No CYP450 interaction

Potential Disadvantages

- Long-term effect unknown. Supine hypertension

Primary Target Symptoms

- Orthostasis

Pearls

- Unlike midodrine, which improves standing systolic blood pressure but not symptoms, droxidopa improves both subjective and objective manifestation of neurogenic orthostatic hypotension for 2 weeks. Long-term effect remains to be studied
- Due to its involvement in central norepinephrine system, it is currently under investigation for managing cognitive impairment in PD, anxiety/depression in PD, pain, fibromyalgia, migraine, ADHD, seizure, and others
- In a case report, an individual with complete dopamine β-hydroxylase deficiency (severe orthostatic hypotension, inability to stand for more than 2 minutes without losing consciousness) may improve with droxidopa treatment (up to 1200 mg/day during 6-month training) to such an extent that patient successfully completed a marathon run
- Combination of COMT inhibitor (entacapone) and droxidopa may improve freezing of gait in PD (typically unresponsive to subthalamic nucleus deep brain stimulation [STN-DBS])
- Based on a rat study, it may be useful to improve renal perfusion in cirrhotic patients
- Atomoxetine, which inhibits presynaptic norepinephrine transporter, also can be used for treating POTS or freezing/cognitive performance in PD

Suggested Reading

Coll M, Rodriguez S, Raurell I, Ezkurdia N, Brull A, Augustin S, et al. Droxidopa, an oral norepinephrine precursor, improves hemodynamic and renal alterations of portal hypertensive rats. *Hepatology.* 2012;56(5):1849–60.

Fukada K, Endo T, Yokoe M, Hamasaki T, Hazama T, Sakoda S. L-threo-3,4-dihydroxyphenylserine (L-DOPS) co-administered with entacapone improves freezing of gait in Parkinson's disease. *Med Hypotheses.* 2013;80(2):209–12.

Garland EM, Raj SR, Demartinis N, Robertson D. Case report: Marathon runner with severe autonomic failure. *Lancet.* 2005;366 Suppl 1:S13.

Kaufmann H, Freeman R, Biaggioni I, Low P, Pedder S, Hewitt LA, et al. Droxidopa for neurogenic orthostatic hypotension: a randomized, placebo-controlled, phase 3 trial. *Neurology.* 2014;83(4): 328–35.

DULOXETINE

THERAPEUTICS

Brands
- Cymbalta, Xeristar, Yentreve, Ariclaim

Generic?
- Yes

Class
- Serotonin and norepinephrine reuptake inhibitor (SNRI)

Commonly Prescribed for
(FDA approved in bold)
- **Major depressive disorder**
- **Diabetic peripheral neuropathic pain**
- **Generalized anxiety disorder (GAD)**
- **Fibromyalgia**
- **Chronic musculoskeletal pain**
- Stress urinary incontinence
- Migraine or tension-type headache prophylaxis
- Other painful peripheral neuropathies
- Depression secondary to stroke
- Binge-eating disorder
- Post-traumatic stress disorder
- Attention deficit hyperactivity disorder
- Perimenopausal/menopausal hot flushes
- Cataplexy

How the Drug Works
- It blocks serotonin and norepinephrine reuptake transporters (SERT, NET), increasing serotonin and norepinephrine levels within hours, but antidepressant effects take weeks. Effect is more likely related to adaptive changes in serotonin and norepinephrine receptor systems over time
- Weakly blocks dopamine reuptake pump (dopamine transporter)
- Interacts with opioid receptors and α_2-adrenergic receptor
- Inhibition of serotonin and norepinephrine reuptake in Onuf's nucleus in the sacral spinal cord may increase urethral closure pressure
- Duloxetine has 100-fold or higher affinity for human and rat SERT and at least 300-fold higher affinity for NET in vitro compared to venlafaxine

How Long Until It Works
- Migraines: effective in as little as 2 weeks, but can take up to 10 weeks on a stable dose to see full effect
- Tension-type headache prophylaxis: effective in 4–8 weeks
- Neuropathic pain: usually some effect within 4 weeks
- Diabetic neuropathy: may have significant improvement with high doses within 6 weeks
- Depression: 2 weeks but up to 2 months for full effect

If It Works
- Migraine/tension-type headache: goal is a 50% or greater reduction in headache frequency or severity. Consider tapering or stopping if headaches remit for more than 6 months or if considering pregnancy
- Neuropathic pain: the goal is to reduce pain intensity and symptoms, but usually does not produce remission. Continue to use and monitor for AE
- Diabetic neuropathy: the goal is to reduce pain intensity and reduce use of analgesics, but usually does not produce remission. Continue to use and maintain strict glycemic control and diabetic management
- Depression: continue to use and monitor for AEs. May continue for 1 year following first depression episode or indefinitely if > 1 episode of depression

If It Doesn't Work
- Increase to highest tolerated dose
- Migraine and tension-type headache: address other issues, such as medication overuse, other coexisting medical disorders, such as anxiety, and consider changing to another agent or adding a second agent
- Neuropathic pain: either change to another agent or add a second agent

Best Augmenting Combos for Partial Response or Treatment-Resistance
- Fibromyalgia: SNRI such as milnacipran and/or AEDs, such as gabapentin, pregabalin, are agents that may be useful in managing fibromyalgia. May also use in combination with natural products and non-medication treatments, such as biofeedback or physical therapy, to improve pain control

- Headache: for some patients, low-dose polytherapy with 2 or more drugs may be better tolerated and more effective than high-dose monotherapy. May use in combination with AEDs, antihypertensives, natural products, and non-medication treatments, such as biofeedback, to improve headache control
- Neuropathic pain: TCAs, AEDs (gabapentin, pregabalin, carbamazepine, lamotrigine), SNRIs (duloxetine, venlafaxine, milnacipran, mirtazapine, bupropion), capsaicin, and mexiletine are agents used for neuropathic pain. Opioids (morphine, tramadol) may be appropriate for long-term use in some cases but require careful monitoring

Tests

- Check blood pressure and cholesterol at baseline and when increasing dose
- Monitor sodium, intraocular pressure, suicidality, unusual change in behavior

---

ADVERSE EFFECTS (AEs)

How the Drug Causes AEs

- By increasing serotonin and norepinephrine on non-therapeutic responsive receptors throughout the body. Most AEs are dose- and time-dependent, especially with concomitant medications (antihypertensives, CYP1A2 inhibitors, serotonergic drugs)

Notable AEs

- > 5%: constipation, nausea, dry mouth, sweating, somnolence, anorexia
- Others: blurry vision, mydriasis, weight loss or gain, hypertension, orthostatic hypotension, syncope, headache, asthenia, dizziness, tremor, dream disorder, insomnia, abnormal ejaculation, impotence, orgasm disorder, itching, nervousness, restlessness, cholesterol/triglyceride elevation, hyponatremia, increased HbA_{1c}, urinary hesitancy

Life-Threatening or Dangerous AEs

- Serotonin syndrome
- Rare hepatitis or hepatic failure
- Rare activation of mania or suicidal ideation

- Rare worsening of coexisting seizure disorders
- Stevens-Johnson syndrome

Weight Gain

- Not unusual

unusual   not unusual   common   problematic

Sedation

- Not unusual

unusual   not unusual   common   problematic

- May cause insomnia in some patients

What to Do About AEs

- For minor AEs, lower dose, titrate more slowly, or switch to another agent. For serious AEs, lower dose and consider stopping, taper to avoid withdrawal symptoms

Best Augmenting Agents to Reduce AEs

- Try magnesium for constipation
- Cyproheptadine can be used for serotonin syndrome by blocking 5-HT receptors and SERT
- Sexual dysfunction (anorgasmia, impotence) may be reversed by agents with α_2-adrenergic antagonist activity (e.g., buspirone, amantadine, bupropion, mirtazapine, ginkgo biloba, etc.)

DOSING AND USE

Usual Dosage Range

- 30–120 mg/day

Dosage Forms

- Delayed-release capsule: 20, 30, 60 mg. Coating dissolves under high pH

How to Dose

- Initial: 30 mg/day. Increment 30 mg weekly as tolerated
- Maintenance: 60 mg/day. Maximum 120 mg. Dose over 60 mg may not provide additional benefit except in headache prevention

Dosing Tips
- Swallowed whole, with or without food. Capsule should not be opened

Overdose
- Somnolence, coma, serotonin syndrome, seizures, syncope, tachycardia, hypotension, hypertension, vomiting. Standard support treatment. Caution on mixed drug use

Long-Term Use
- Safe for long-term use with monitoring of blood pressure. A significantly higher percentage of duloxetine-treated patients versus placebo discontinued due to AE

Habit Forming
- No

How to Stop
- Taper slowly to avoid withdrawal symptoms. Pain often worsens shortly after decreasing dose

Pharmacokinetics
- Metabolized via CYP2D6 and CYP1A2. 70% metabolites in urine and 20% in feces. Half-life 12 hours. > 90% protein bound

 Drug Interactions
- Concomitant heavy alcohol intake may be associated with severe liver injury
- Duloxetine is a substrate of CYP2D6 and CYP1A2. May need to reduce dose in the presence of CYP2D6 inhibitors (paroxetine, fluoxetine, bupropion, duloxetine, sertraline, citalopram, methadone, ranitidine, cimetidine, amiodarone), or CYP1A2 inhibitors (ciprofloxacin, quinolones, amiodarone, cimetidine, fluvoxamine), especially in patients with hypertension, hepatic impairment, and in elderly
- Duloxetine is a moderate CYP2D6 inhibitor, which may increase serum concentration of carvedilol, propranolol, amitriptyline, haloperidol, chlorpromazine, metoclopramide, mexiletine, tamoxifen, amphetamine
- The release of serotonin by platelets is important for maintaining hemostasis. Combined use of SSRIs or SNRIs (such as venlafaxine) and NSAIDs, and/or drugs that have anticoagulant effects has been associated with an increased risk of bleeding

 Other Warnings/ Precautions
- Slow gastric emptying may increase the risk of duloxetine hydrolysis to 1-naphthol, which is toxic to GI membrane
- May increase risk of seizure
- Patients should be observed closely for clinical worsening, suicidality, and changes in behavior in known or unknown bipolar disorder

Do Not Use
- Proven hypersensitivity to drug
- Concurrently with MAOI; allow at least 14 days between discontinuation of an MAOI and initiation of duloxetine or at least 7–14 days between discontinuation of duloxetine and initiation of an MAOI
- Concurrent use of serotonin precursors (e.g., tryptophan)
- In patients with uncontrolled narrow angle-closure glaucoma
- In patients treated with linezolid or methylene blue IV

SPECIAL POPULATIONS

Renal Impairment
- Avoid use in patients with severe renal impairment, GFR < 30 mL/min

Hepatic Impairment
- Avoid use in patients with chronic liver disease or cirrhosis

Cardiac Impairment
- Use with caution. Dose-dependent effect on blood pressure
- No effect on QTc

Elderly
- No adjustments necessary

 Children and Adolescents
- Use of duloxetine in a child or adolescent must balance the potential risks with the

clinical need. Safety and efficacy not established. Efficacy demonstrated in 7–17-year-old GAD patients but not in MDD patients

• Use with caution. Observe closely for clinical worsening, suicidality, and changes in behavior in known or unknown bipolar disorder. Parents should be informed and advised of the risks

 Pregnancy

• Category C. Generally not recommended for the treatment of headaches or neuropathic pain during pregnancy. Neonates exposed to SNRIs or SSRIs late in the third trimester have developed complications necessitating extended hospitalizations, respiratory support, and tube feeding. Respiratory distress, cyanosis, apnea, seizures, temperature instability, feeding difficulty, vomiting, hypoglycemia, hypotonia, hyperreflexia, tremor, jitteriness, irritability, and constant crying consistent with a toxic effect of the drug or drug discontinuation syndrome have been reported

Breast Feeding

• Some drug is found in breast milk and use while breast feeding is not recommended

THE ART OF NEUROPHARMACOLOGY

Potential Advantages

• Very effective in the treatment of multiple pain disorders. Effective for treatment of comorbid depression and anxiety in chronic pain. Less sedation than tertiary amine TCAs (i.e., amitriptyline). Less hypertension than other venlafaxine. No effect on QTc

Potential Disadvantages

• May cause or worsen hypertension. Potential hepatotoxicity. Drug interactions

Primary Target Symptoms

• Reduction in headache frequency, duration, and/or intensity
• Reduction in musculoskeletal pain, neuropathic pain, and fibromyalgia
• Reduction in depression and anxiety

 Pearls

• High-dose (90–120 mg/day) duloxetine may be effective in treating non-depressed migraineurs
• For fibromyalgia syndrome, it remains uncertain whether amitriptyline, duloxetine, or milnacipran is superior. Number needed to treat is 6 for 50% pain relief in fibromyalgia and painful diabetic neuropathy
• It becomes SNRI at dose > 60 mg/day. However, duloxetine 60 mg/day may be as effective as 120 mg/day in treating severe depression symptoms in hospitalized patients
• In one study for treating diabetic neuropathic pain, monotherapy (duloxetine 120 mg/day or pregabalin 600 mg/day) was as effective as polytherapy (duloxetine 60 mg/day plus 300 mg/day)
• In patients with diabetic neuropathic pain unresponsive to gabapentin, switching to duloxetine instead of pregabalin may be a better alternative
• For treating chemotherapy-induced neuropathic pain and multiple sclerosis-related neuropathic pain, if tolerated to 60 mg/day or higher
• Combining antipsychotics (e.g., quetiapine, ziprasidone) with duloxetine may increase the risk of urinary retention

Suggested Reading

Brecht S, Desaiah D, Marechal ES, Santini AM, Podhorna J, Guelfi JD. Efficacy and safety of duloxetine 60 mg and 120 mg daily in patients hospitalized for severe depression. *J Clin Psychiatry*. 2010;72(08):1086–94.

Hauser W, Petzke F, Uceyler N, Sommer C. Comparative efficacy and acceptability of amitriptyline, duloxetine and milnacipran in fibromyalgia syndrome: a systematic review with meta-analysis. *Rheumatology*. 2011; 50(3):532–43.

Smith EML, Pang H, Cirrincione C, Fleishman S, Paskett ED, Ahles T, et al. Effect of duloxetine on pain, function, and quality of life among patients with chemotherapy-induced painful peripheral neuropathy: a randomized clinical trial. *JAMA*. 2013;309(13):1359–67.

Tanenberg RJ, Clemow DB, Giaconia JM, Risser RC. Duloxetine compared with pregabalin for diabetic peripheral neuropathic pain management in patients with suboptimal pain response to gabapentin and treated with or without antidepressants: a post hoc analysis. *Pain Pract*. 2013;14(7):640–8.

Tesfaye S, Wilhelm S, Lledo A, Schacht A, Tölle T, Bouhassira D, et al. Duloxetine and pregabalin: high-dose monotherapy or their combination? The "COMBO-DN study"–a multinational, randomized, double-blind, parallel-group study in patients with diabetic peripheral neuropathic pain. *Pain*. 2013; 154(12):2616–25.

Vollmer TL, Robinson MJ, Risser RC, Malcolm SK. A randomized, double-blind, placebo-controlled trial of duloxetine for the treatment of pain in patients with multiple sclerosis. *Pain Pract*. 2013;14(8):732–44.

Young WB, Bradley KC, Anjum MW, Gebeline-Myers C. Duloxetine prophylaxis for episodic migraine in persons without depression: a prospective study. *Headache*. 2013;53(9):1430–7.

THERAPEUTICS

Brands
- Savaysa

Generic?
- No

Class
- Anticoagulant

Commonly Prescribed for
(FDA approved in bold)
- **To reduce the risk of stroke and systemic embolism in patients with non-valvular atrial fibrillation (NVAF)**
- **Treatment of deep vein thrombosis (DVT) and pulmonary embolism (PE) following 5–10 days of initial therapy with a parenteral anticoagulant**
- Prevention of DVT and PE
- Treatment of cerebral venous thrombosis

How the Drug Works
- Edoxaban is a selective inhibitor of the enzyme factor Xa (Stuart-Prower factor), which is the first member of the final common pathway of coagulation. It does not require antithrombin III for antithrombotic activity. It inhibits free factor Xa, and prothrombinase activity and inhibits thrombin-induced platelet aggregation. Inhibition of factor Xa in the coagulation cascade reduces thrombin generation and reduces thrombus formation

How Long Until It Works
- Peak effect in 1–2 hours

If It Works
- Monitor for signs of bleeding. Assess renal function periodically as clinically indicated

If It Doesn't Work
- Correct the underlying disorder. Use a higher dose or switch to different anticoagulant

 Best Augmenting Combos for Partial Response or Treatment-Resistance
- Combining with antiplatelet agent may not always improve efficacy but definitely increases bleeding risk

Tests
- The degree of anticoagulation does not need to be assessed; PT, aPTT highly variable
- Assess renal function (CrCl) regularly

ADVERSE EFFECTS (AEs)

How the Drug Causes AEs
- Reduced coagulation due to inhibited thrombin formation

Notable AEs
- Bleeding, nausea/vomiting, constipation, abnormal liver function test, rash

 Life-Threatening or Dangerous AEs
- From clinical trials, the yearly incidence of major bleeding is 3.1%, intracranial hemorrhage is 0.5%, GI bleeding 1.8%, and fatal bleeding (mostly intracranial hemorrhage) is 0.2%. Non-major bleeding 9.4%

Weight Gain
- Unusual

unusual   not unusual   common   problematic

Sedation
- Unusual

unusual   not unusual   common   problematic

What to Do About AEs
- Discontinue treatment, supportive care. Activated charcoal may reduce absorption
- Not effective: vitamin K, protamine sulfate, tranexamic acid, and hemodialysis

Best Augmenting Agents to Reduce AEs
- In most cases discontinuation and changing to another medication is

more practical than trying to reduce AEs with another medication

DOSING AND USE

Usual Dosage Range
- 60 mg once daily

Dosage Forms
- Tablet: 15, 30, 60 mg

How to Dose
Treatment of NVAF:
- 60 mg once daily: CrCl 50–95 mL/min
- 30 mg once daily: CrCl 15–50 mL/min
Treatment of DVT and PE:
- 60 mg once daily
- 30 mg once daily: CrCl 15–50 mL/min, body weight ≤ 60 kg, or under P-glycoprotein (P-gp) inhibitors

 Dosing Tips
- Can be taken with or without food

Overdose
- A specific reversal agent for edoxaban is not available. May lead to hemorrhagic complications

Long-Term Use
- Increased risk of bleeding

Habit Forming
- No

Pharmacokinetics
- T_{max} 1–2 hours. Bioavailability 62%. Plasma protein binding 55%. Steady state within 3 days. Minimal metabolism via hydrolysis, conjugation, and oxidation. Eliminated as unchanged drug in urine. Half-life 10–14 hours

 Drug Interactions
- It does not inhibit major P450 enzymes nor P-gp transporter
- P-gp inhibitors (e.g., ketoconazole, quinidine, verapamil, erythromycin, cyclosporine, amiodarone, captopril) increase edoxaban concentration. However,

no dose reduction is needed for treating NVAF
- P-gp inducer (e.g., carbamazepine, phenytoin, rifampin) can lower edoxaban concentration. Do not use concomitantly
- Coadministration of NSAIDs, anticoagulants, antiplatelets, and thrombolytics may increase the risk of bleeding

 Other Warnings/ Precautions
- Reduced efficacy and increased risk of stroke in NVAF patients with CrCl > 95 mL/min
- Premature discontinuation of edoxaban increases the risk of ischemic events
- Spinal/epidural hematoma following spinal puncture
- Procedure with minor bleeding risk: stop 1–2 days before procedure and start 12–24 hours after procedure
- Procedure with major bleeding risk: stop 2–4 days before procedure and start 2–3 days after procedure

Do Not Use
- Active pathological bleeding
- Mechanical heart valves or moderate to severe mitral stenosis

SPECIAL POPULATIONS

Renal Impairment
- In ENGAGE AF-TIMI 48 study, NVAF patients with CrCl > 95 mL/min had an increased rate of ischemic stroke with edoxaban 60 mg daily compared to patients treated with warfarin. Another anticoagulant should be used

Hepatic Impairment
- No adjustment needed in mild or moderate impairment. No information on severe impairment

Cardiac Impairment
- Safety information is lacking for use in patients with mechanical valve. Use is not recommended
- It does not prolong QTc interval

Elderly

- In clinical trials the efficacy and safety of SAVAYSA in elderly (65 years or older) and younger patients were similar

Children and Adolescents

- Safety and effectiveness in pediatric patients have not been established

Pregnancy

- Category C. There are no adequate and well-controlled studies in pregnant women. SAVAYSA should be used during pregnancy only if the potential benefit justifies the potential risk to the fetus

Breast Feeding

- It is not known if edoxaban is excreted in human milk

THE ART OF NEUROPHARMACOLOGY

Potential Advantages

- Proven treatment for stroke and systemic embolism prevention in adults with NVAF
- Better than aspirin, non-inferior to warfarin in reducing rate of stroke and systemic embolism from AF
- Has a lower risk than warfarin for hemorrhagic stroke and major bleeding, and marginally lower risk of death from any cause

Potential Disadvantages

- Increased risk of bleeding although less than warfarin. Lack of antidote or monitoring lab test. Not dialyzable

Primary Target Symptoms

- Reduce recurrent attacks of cerebral embolism caused by cardiogenic thrombi due to AF. Reduce venothromboembolism

Pearls

- In ENGAGE AF-TIMI 48 study, edoxaban (60 mg and 30 mg) was non-inferior to warfarin with respect to the prevention of stroke or systemic embolism and was associated with significantly lower rates of bleeding and death from cardiovascular causes
- In Hokusai-VTE study, edoxaban administered once daily after initial treatment with heparin was non-inferior to high-quality standard therapy and caused significantly less bleeding in a broad spectrum of patients with venous thromboembolism, including those with severe PE
- Prothrombin complex concentrate, activated prothrombin complex concentrate, and recombinant factor VIIa can potentially reverse edoxaban's effect
- No large head-to-head comparisons with other newer agents in clinical trials. However, indirect comparison analysis on four new oral anticoagulants showed edoxaban (60 mg) having similar efficacy to apixaban, rivaroxaban, and dabigatran (110 mg twice daily) but higher systemic embolism/stroke than dabigatran (150 mg twice daily). Edoxaban (60 mg) has similar bleeding risk to apixaban, dabigatran, but lower bleeding risk than rivaroxaban. Edoxaban (30 mg) is less effective with less bleeding risk
- For cerebral venous thrombosis, despite a lack of evidence, it is often recommended to use warfarin for 3–12 months. Longer duration is reserved for those with severe coagulopathies or recurrent VTE. For newer anticoagulants, although no evidence available, their lower intracranial bleeding rate might offer them a potential role for cerebral venous thrombosis

Suggested Reading

Fukuda T, Honda Y, Kamisato C, Morishima Y, Shibano T. Reversal of anticoagulant effects of edoxaban, an oral, direct factor Xa inhibitor, with haemostatic agents. *Thromb Haemost.* 2012;107(2):253–9.

Giugliano RP, Ruff CT, Braunwald E, Murphy SA, Wiviott SD, Halperin JL, et al. Edoxaban versus warfarin in patients with atrial fibrillation. *N Engl J Med.* 2013;369(22):2093–104.

Hokusai-VTE Investigators, Büller HR, Décousus H, Grosso MA, Mercuri M, Middeldorp S, et al. Edoxaban versus warfarin for the treatment of symptomatic venous thromboembolism. *N Engl J Med.* 2013;369(15):1406–15.

January CT, Wann LS, Alpert JS, Calkins H, Cleveland JC, Cigarroa JE, et al. 2014 AHA/ACC/HRS guideline for the management of patients with atrial fibrillation: a report of the American College of Cardiology/American Heart Association Task Force on practice guidelines and the Heart Rhythm Society. *Circulation.* 2014;130(23):e199–267. Erratum in *Circulation.* 2014;130(23):e272–4.

Skjøth F, Larsen TB, Rasmussen LH, Lip GYH. Efficacy and safety of edoxaban in comparison with dabigatran, rivaroxaban and apixaban for stroke prevention in atrial fibrillation. An indirect comparison analysis. *Thromb Haemost.* 2014;111(5):981–8.

EDROPHONIUM

THERAPEUTICS

Brands
- Enlon, Reversol, Tensilon, Enlon-Plus

Generic?
- Yes

Class
- Cholinesterase inhibitor

Commonly Prescribed for
(FDA approved in bold)
- **Myasthenia gravis (MG): diagnostic test**
- Curare antagonist (to reverse respiratory depression)

How the Drug Works
- Improves symptoms of MG by preventing the metabolism of acetylcholine by cholinesterase. This improves neuromuscular transmission in MG

How Long Until It Works
- Less than 1 minute

If It Works
- Usually assists with the differential diagnosis of MG. Pyridostigmine is used for long-term treatment

If It Doesn't Work
- If no effect with the 10 mg dose, question the diagnosis of MG

Best Augmenting Combos for Partial Response or Treatment-Resistance
- Not applicable

Tests
- None

ADVERSE EFFECTS (AEs)

How the Drug Causes AEs
- Pro-cholinergic properties of the drug

Notable AEs
- Diarrhea, abdominal cramps, nausea, increased salivation, miosis, increased bronchial secretions, worsening of bronchial asthma, fasciculations, muscle weakness, and diaphoresis

Life-Threatening or Dangerous AEs
- Bradycardia – possibly leading to hypotension – is most common

Weight Gain
- Unusual

unusual | not unusual | common | problematic

Sedation
- Unusual

unusual | not unusual | common | problematic

What to Do About AEs
- Give atropine to treat airway obstruction from bronchial secretions

Best Augmenting Agents to Reduce AEs
- Not applicable

DOSING AND USE

Usual Dosage Range
- MG: 10 mg in adults

Dosage Forms
- Injection: 10 mg/mL

How to Dose
- In adults, give 0.2 mL (2 mg) within 15–30 seconds. If no reaction occurs after 45 seconds, give the remaining 8 mg. Discontinue the test if any cholinergic reactions and monitor for any clinical changes
- Alternatively give 10 mg IM. In patients with hypersensitivity (cholinergic reaction), wait 30 minutes and give a lower dose (2 mg) to rule out a false-negative reaction

Dosing Tips
- Not applicable

Overdose
• Not applicable

Long-Term Use
• Not applicable

Habit Forming
• Not applicable

How to Stop
• Not applicable

Pharmacokinetics
• Onset of action < 1 minute IV and 2–10 minutes IM. Peak plasma levels < 7 minutes IV and 5–20 minutes IM. Eliminated through the kidneys and excreted in urine

 Drug Interactions
• Do not combine with other cholinesterase inhibitors
• May increase neuromuscular blocking effects of succinylcholine

 Other Warnings/ Precautions
• Anticholinesterase overdosage (cholinergic crisis) symptoms may mimic underdosage (myasthenic weakness)

Do Not Use
• Known hypersensitivity to the cholinesterase inhibitors. Mechanical intestinal or urinary obstruction

SPECIAL POPULATIONS

Renal Impairment
• Markedly increases half-life and plasma clearance

Hepatic Impairment
• No known effects

Cardiac Impairment
• Use with caution in patients with arrhythmias, hypotension, or bradycardia

Elderly
• May be more prone to cardiac events, such as bradycardia

 Children and Adolescents
• Safe for use. For children 34 kg or less, give 1 mg and if no response in 45 seconds give another 4 mg. For children over 34 kg give the adult dose (up to 10 mg)

 Pregnancy
• Category C. Use only if benefits of medication outweigh risks

Breast Feeding
• Unknown if excreted in breast milk. Do not use

THE ART OF NEUROPHARMACOLOGY

Potential Advantages
• Helpful in the diagnosis of MG. Rapid onset of action

Potential Disadvantages
• Not a long-term treatment. Need to give in a monitored setting due to risk of AEs

Primary Target Symptoms
• To improve weakness, visual problems, respiratory symptoms associated with MG

Pearls
• When using to diagnose MG, pick a specific testable symptom to measure before administration, such as muscle strength or extraocular eye movements
• Can differentiate between myasthenic and cholinergic crisis in established MG. Give 1–2 mg 1 hour after last dose of the agent used to treat MG (usually pyridostigmine). If muscle strength (ptosis, diplopia, dysphagia, respiration, limb strength) improves, then myasthenic crisis is confirmed. Decreased muscle strength, fasciculations, and severe pro-cholinergic AEs (lacrimation, diaphoresis, salivation, nausea) confirm cholinergic crisis. Cholinergic crisis is rare in patients with MG taking typically prescribed doses of anticholinesterase medication

Suggested Reading

Aquilonius SM, Hartvig P. Clinical pharmacokinetics of cholinesterase inhibitors. *Clin Pharmacokinet.* 1986;11(3):236–49.

Ing EB, Ing SY, Ing T, Ramocki JA. The complication rate of edrophonium testing for suspected myasthenia gravis. *Can J Ophthalmol.* 2000;35(3):141–4; discussion 145.

Scherer K, Bedlack RS, Simel DL. Does this patient have myasthenia gravis? *JAMA.* 2005;293(15):1906–14.

Brands
- Relpax, Relert

Generic?
- No

 Class
- Triptan

Commonly Prescribed for
(FDA approved in bold)
- **Acute treatment of migraine in adults**

 How the Drug Works
- Selective 5-HT$_{1B/1D/1F}$ receptor agonist. In addition to vasoconstriction of meningeal vessels, its antinociceptive effect is likely due to blocking the transmission of pain signals at trigeminal nerve terminals (preventing the release of inflammatory neuropeptides) and synapses of second-order neurons in trigeminal nucleus caudalis

How Long Until It Works
- 1 hour or less

If It Works
- Continue to take as needed. Patients taking acute treatment more than 2 days/week are at risk for medication-overuse headache, especially if they have migraine

If It Doesn't Work
- Treat early in the attack: triptans are less likely to work after the headache becomes moderate or severe, regardless of cutaneous allodynia, which is a marker of central sensitization
- Address life style issues (e.g., stress, sleep hygiene), medication use issues (e.g., compliance, overuse), and other underlying medical conditions
- Change to higher dosage, another triptan, another administration route, or combination of other medications. Add preventive medication when needed
- For patients with partial response or reoccurrence, other rescue medications include NSAIDs (e.g., ketorolac, naproxen), antiemetic (e.g., prochlorperazine, metoclopramide), neuroleptics (e.g., haloperidol, chlorpromazine), ergots, antihistamine, or corticosteroid

 Best Augmenting Combos for Partial Response or Treatment-Resistance
- NSAIDs or neuroleptics are often used to augment response

Tests
- None required

How the Drug Causes AEs
- Direct effect on serotonin receptors

Notable AEs
- Tingling, flushing, sensation of burning, vertigo, sensation of pressure, palpitations, heaviness, nausea

 Life-Threatening or Dangerous AEs
- Rare cardiac events including acute myocardial infarction, cardiac arrhythmias, and coronary artery vasospasm have been reported with eletriptan

Weight Gain
- Unusual

unusual / not unusual / common / problematic

Sedation
- Unusual

unusual / not unusual / common / problematic

What to Do About AEs
- In most cases, only reassurance is needed. Lower dose, change to another triptan, or use an alternative headache treatment

Best Augmenting Agents to Reduce AEs
- Treatment of nausea with antiemetics is acceptable. Other AEs decrease with time

DOSING AND USE

Usual Dosage Range
- 20–40 mg

Dosage Forms
- Tablets: 20 and 40 mg

How to Dose
- Tablets: most patients respond best at 40 mg oral dose. Give 1 pill at the onset of an attack and repeat in 2 hours for a partial response or if the headache returns. 80 mg also effective but associated with more AEs. Maximum 80 mg/day. Limit 10 days/month

 Dosing Tips
- Treat early in attack

Overdose
- May cause hypertension, cardiovascular symptoms. Other possible symptoms include seizure, tremor, extremity erythema, cyanosis, or ataxia. For patients with angina, perform ECG and monitor for ischemia for at least 20 hours

Long-Term Use
- Monitor for cardiac risk factors with continued use

Habit Forming
- No

How to Stop
- No need to taper. Patients who overuse triptans often experience withdrawal headaches lasting up to several days

Pharmacokinetics
- Half-life about 4–5 hours. T_{max} 60–90 minutes. Bioavailability is 50%. Metabolized by CYP3A4 enzyme. 85% protein binding

 Drug Interactions
- Concurrent propranolol use slightly increases peak concentrations
- CYP3A4 inhibitors may affect eletriptan's serum concentration

 Other Warnings/Precautions
- Not applicable

Do Not Use
- Within 24 hours of ergot-containing medications such as dihydroergotamine
- Patients with proven hypersensitivity to eletriptan, known cardiovascular disease, uncontrolled hypertension, or Prinzmetal's angina
- Eletriptan was not studied in patients with hemiplegic and basilar migraine
- May worsen symptoms in ischemic bowel disease
- Do not use within 72 hours of CYP3A4 inhibitors: ketoconazole, erythromycin, fluconazole, and verapamil

SPECIAL POPULATIONS

Renal Impairment
- No significant change in patients with severe renal impairment

Hepatic Impairment
- No dose adjustment needed for moderate or severe liver impairment. Not studied in severe impairment

Cardiac Impairment
- Do not use in patients with known cardiovascular or peripheral vascular disease

Elderly
- Decreased clearance. Increased blood pressure. May be at increased cardiovascular risk

 Children and Adolescents
- Safety and efficacy have not been established
- Triptan trials in children were negative, due to higher placebo response

 Pregnancy
- Category C. Use only if potential benefit outweighs risk to the fetus. Migraine often

improves in pregnancy, and other acute agents (opioids, neuroleptics, prednisone) have more proven safety

Breast Feeding

- Eletriptan is found in breast milk. Concentration in breast milk is lower than other triptans due to high protein binding. Use with caution

THE ART OF NEUROPHARMACOLOGY

Potential Advantages

- Effective and long-lasting, even compared to other oral triptans. May be drug of choice for patients with severe, long-lasting migraines. Less risk of abuse than opioids or barbiturate-containing treatments

Potential Disadvantages

- Cost, potential for medication-overuse headache. More AEs at 80 mg dose than other triptans

Primary Target Symptoms

- Headache pain, nausea, photo- and phonophobia

 Pearls

- Early treatment of migraine is most effective
- Best 24-hour pain-free response (33%, number needed to treat 5) among the triptans

- May not be effective when taking during aura, before headache begins
- In patients with "status migrainosus" (migraine lasting more than 72 hours) neuroleptics and dihydroergotamine are more effective
- Triptans were not originally studied for use in the treatment of basilar or hemiplegic migraine
- Patients taking triptans more than 10 days/ month are at increased risk of medication-overuse headache, which is less responsive to treatment
- May have more AEs than other triptans
- Chest and throat tightness are usually benign and may be related to esophageal spasm rather than cardiac ischemia. These symptoms occur more commonly in patients without cardiac risk factors
- Combination use of SNRI and triptans usually will not lead to serotonin syndrome, which requires activation of $5\text{-}HT_{2A}$ receptors and a possible limited role of $5\text{-}HT_{1A}$. However, triptans are agonists at the $5\text{-}HT_{1B/1D/1F}$ receptor subtypes, with weak affinity for $5\text{-}HT_{1A}$ receptors and no activity at the $5\text{-}HT_2$ receptors. Thus, given the seriousness of serotonin syndrome, caution is certainly warranted and clinicians should be vigilant for serotonin toxicity symptoms and signs to insure prompt treatment
- The site of pharmacological action, whether central or peripheral, remains to be studied. Although triptans generally do not penetrate BBB, it has been postulated that transient BBB breakdown may occur during a migraine attack

Suggested Reading

Dodick D, Lipton RB, Martin V, Papademetriou V, Rosamond W, MaassenVanDenBrink A, et al. Consensus statement: cardiovascular safety profile of triptans (5-HT1B/1D agonists) in the acute treatment of migraine. *Headache*. 2004; 44(5):414–25.

Evans RW, Tepper SJ, Shapiro RE, Sun-Edelstein C, Tietjen GE. The FDA alert on serotonin syndrome with use of triptans combined with selective serotonin reuptake inhibitors or selective serotonin-norepinephrine reuptake inhibitors: American Headache Society position paper. *Headache*. 2010;50(6):1089–99.

Ferrari MD, Roon KI, Lipton RB, Goadsby PJ. Oral triptans (serotonin 5-HT(1B/1D) agonists) in acute migraine treatment: a meta-analysis of 53 trials. *Lancet*. 2001;358(9294):1668–75.

Gladstone JP, Gawel M. Newer formulations of the triptans: advances in migraine management. *Drugs*. 2003;63(21):2285–305.

Goadsby PJ, Zanchin G, Geraud G, de Klippel N, Diaz-Insa S, Gobel H, et al. Early vs. non-early intervention in acute migraine – 'Act when Mild (AwM)'. A double-blind, placebo-controlled trial of almotriptan. *Cephalalgia*. 2008;28(4):383–91.

Goldstein JA, Massey KD, Kirby S, Gibson M, Hettiarachchi J, Rankin AJ, et al. Effect of high-dose intravenous eletriptan on coronary artery diameter. *Cephalalgia*. 2004;24(7):515–21.

ENTACAPONE

THERAPEUTICS

Brands
- Comtan, Stalevo

Generic?
- No

Class
- Antiparkinson agent

Commonly Prescribed for
(FDA approved in bold)
- **Parkinsonism, including Parkinson's disease (PD)**

How the Drug Works
- Highly selective peripherally acting inhibitor of catechol-*O*-methyltransferase (COMT), an important enzyme in dopamine metabolism. Use with carbidopa-levodopa enables more levodopa to enter the brain and prevents the end-of-dose wearing-off seen in PD. Entacapone has less activity on COMT in the brain, meaning the drug is not considered centrally active

How Long Until It Works
- PD: hours to weeks

If It Works
- PD: a majority (58%) of patients taking 800 mg or more per day of levodopa will lower levodopa dose, on average by 25% of the total after starting entacapone

If It Doesn't Work
- If end-of-dose wearing-off does not improve with entacapone and levodopa, decrease the dosing interval, add a dopamine agonist or monoamine oxidase B (MAO-B) inhibitor, or consider neurosurgical options. For sudden, unpredictable wearing-off, consider apomorphine

Best Augmenting Combos for Partial Response or Treatment-Resistance
- Entacapone is used only as an adjunctive medication in PD with levodopa
- For dyskinesias, lower dose of levodopa or add a dopamine agonist

- Younger patients with bothersome tremor: anticholinergics may help
- For severe motor fluctuations and/or dyskinesias with good "on" time, functional neurosurgery is an option
- Amantadine may help suppress dyskinesias, although benefit is often short-lived
- Depression is common in PD and may respond to low-dose SSRIs
- Cognitive impairment/dementia is common in mid-late stage PD and may improve with acetylcholinesterase inhibitors

Tests
- None required

ADVERSE EFFECTS (AEs)

How the Drug Causes AEs
- COMT inhibition increases the level and duration of action of levodopa

Notable AEs
- (Entacapone alone) diarrhea (usually mild to moderate), dyspnea, weakness. May increase levodopa-related AEs such as dyskinesias, nausea, orthostatic hypotension, and hallucinations

Life-Threatening or Dangerous AEs
- Rare cases of rhabdomyolysis, unclear if related to entacapone. It is unclear if non-ergot medications such as entacapone that increase dopaminergic activity predispose to the fibrotic complications (e.g., pleural thickening, retroperitoneal fibrosis) seen with ergot agonists

Weight Gain
- Unusual

unusual   not unusual   common   problematic

Sedation
- Unusual

unusual   not unusual   common   problematic

What to Do About AEs
- Many AEs are related to increase in levodopa effect. Reduce levodopa dose.

Take after meals to reduce nausea. This may reduce the peak dose and AEs, but delays effect and reduces effectiveness

Best Augmenting Agents to Reduce AEs

- For nausea, increase dose of carbidopa relative to levodopa
- Lower levodopa dose and use amantadine or a dopamine agonist to reduce dyskinesias
- Orthostatic hypotension: adjust dose or stop antihypertensives, add dietary salt, and consider fludrocortisone or midodrine
- Urinary incontinence: reducing PM fluids, voiding schedules, oxybutynin, desmopressin nasal spray, hyoscyamine sulfate, urological evaluation

DOSING AND USE

Usual Dosage Range

- 600–1600 mg/day

Dosage Forms

- Entacapone tablets: 200 mg
- As carbidopa/levodopa/entacapone tablets (Stalevo): 12.5/50/200, 25/100/200, and 37.5/150/200 mg

How to Dose

- Add 200 mg to each dose of levodopa or change to combination carbidopa/levodopa/entacapone to maximum of 1600 mg (8 doses) per day

 Dosing Tips

- Food does not affect the absorption of entacapone, but since it is dosed with levodopa, take before meals for best effect. Distributing protein throughout the day may help avoid fluctuations in PD. Low protein meals may reduce "wearing-off"

Overdose

- Little clinical experience, but theoretically can produce inability to metabolize endogenous and exogenous catecholamines. Immediate gastric drug lavage and activated charcoal are recommended. Hemodialysis is unlikely to remove due to protein binding

Long-Term Use

- Safe for long-term use. Effectiveness may decrease over time

Habit Forming

- No

How to Stop

- Stopping abruptly may worsen symptoms of PD, especially if levodopa is also discontinued. This may cause confusion, rigidity, and hyperpyrexia, as seen in neuroleptic malignant syndrome

Pharmacokinetics

- Rapidly absorbed, with maximum effect in 1 hour and lasts about 8 hours. Hepatic metabolism and glucuronidation. Highly protein bound. Excreted through bile

 Drug Interactions

- MAOIs are also important in the metabolism of catecholamines. Do not use with non-selective MAOIs, but can use with the MAO-B selective inhibitors used in PD (rasagiline, selegiline)
- Drugs that interfere with biliary excretion or glucuronidation (probenecid, cholestyramine, erythromycin, rifampin, ampicillin, chloramphenicol) will increase the effect of entacapone
- Entacapone can increase the effect of all drugs metabolized by COMT, such as epinephrine, norepinephrine, dopamine, dobutamine, methyldopa, apomorphine, isoproterenol, isoetharine, bitolterol. This can lead to increased heart rates, arrhythmia, and increases in blood pressure

 Other Warnings/ Precautions

- Nephrotoxic and associated with renal tubular adenomas at high doses in mice, unknown if this occurs in humans

Do Not Use

- Patients with known hypersensitivity to the drug, non-selective MAOIs, patients with significant biliary disorders

Renal Impairment
• No known effects

Hepatic Impairment
• Effect of drug is approximately doubled in patients with alcoholism or hepatic impairment. Use with caution

Cardiac Impairment
• Use with caution in patients with known arrhythmias. Entacapone was not associated with an increased risk of acute myocardial infarction or stroke

Elderly
• Safe for use

 Children and Adolescents
• Not studied in children (PD is rare)

 Pregnancy
• Category C. Use only if benefit of medication may outweigh risks

Breast Feeding
• Concentration in breast milk unknown. Breast feeding is not recommended

THE ART OF NEUROPHARMACOLOGY

Potential Advantages
• Allows patients to lower dose or lengthen dosing intervals of levodopa. Fairly well

tolerated. Unlike tolcapone, it is not centrally acting and no risk of fulminant hepatic failure

Potential Disadvantages
• Not useful as monotherapy for PD. May increase levodopa AEs. Cost

Primary Target Symptoms
• PD: end-of-dose wearing-off

 Pearls
• Has effectively replaced tolcapone as the COMT inhibitor of choice for the treatment of PD
• Extends clinical effect of levodopa by 30–45 minutes and improves motor scores by about 16%
• A useful alternative to dopamine agonists for patients experiencing AEs, such as sudden-onset sleep or impulse control disorders. Less likely to cause hallucinations
• Entacapone does not augment antipsychotic treatment for negative symptoms in patients with residual schizophrenia
• Efficacious as an adjunct to levodopa in subjects with motor fluctuations
• Does not prevent or delay motor fluctuations and dyskinesia
• Combination of COMT inhibitor (entacapone) and droxidopa may improve freezing of gait in PD (typically unresponsive to subthalamic nucleus deep brain stimulation [STN-DBS])

Suggested Reading

Fox SH, Katzenschlager R, Lim S-Y, Ravina B, Seppi K, Coelho M, et al. The Movement Disorder Society Evidence-Based Medicine Review Update: Treatments for the motor symptoms of Parkinson's disease. *Mov Disord.* 2011;26 Suppl 3:S2–41.

Hauser RA, Zesiewicz TA. Advances in the pharmacologic management of early Parkinson disease. *Neurologist.* 2007;13(3):126–32.

Leegwater-Kim J, Waters C. Role of tolcapone in the treatment of Parkinson's disease. *Expert Rev Neurother.* 2007;7(12):1649–57.

Linazasoro G, Kulisevsky J, Hernández B; Spanish Stalevo Study Group. Should levodopa dose be reduced when switched to stalevo? *Eur J Neurol.* 2008;15(3):257–61.

Müller T, Kolf K, Ander L, Woitalla D, Muhlack S. Catechol-O-methyltransferase inhibition improves levodopa-associated strength increase in patients with Parkinson disease. *Clin Neuropharmacol.* 2008;31(3):134–40.

Olanow CW, Stern MB, Sethi K. The scientific and clinical basis for the treatment of Parkinson disease. *Neurology.* 2009;72(21 Suppl 4): S1–136.

Seeberger LC, Hauser RA. Levodopa/carbidopa/entacapone in Parkinson's disease. *Expert Rev Neurother.* 2009;9(7):929–40.

ESCITALOPRAM

THERAPEUTICS

Brands
- Lexapro

Generic?
- Yes

Class
- Selective serotonin reuptake inhibitor (SSRI)

Commonly Prescribed for
(FDA approved in bold)
- **Major depressive disorder (adolescent and adult)**
- **Generalized anxiety disorder**
- Obsessive-compulsive disorder
- Post-traumatic stress disorder
- Cataplexy
- Psychosis in dementia

How the Drug Works
- Both citalopram (50:50 S-,R-enantiomer) and escitalopram (S-enantiomer of citalopram) block serotonin reuptake pumps increasing their levels within hours, but antidepressant effect takes weeks. Escitalopram (Ki = 1.1 nM) is 100-fold more potent than the R-enantiomer in inhibiting serotonin reuptake transporter (SERT). No affinity for norepinephrine reuptake transporter (NET), serotonergic, adrenergic, muscarinic, H_1, dopamine, opiate, GABA receptors, and Ca^{2+}, Na^+, K^+, Cl^- channels

How Long Until It Works
- May start to see improvement in 1–2 weeks, but usually it takes longer period for full effect

If It Works
- Continue to use and monitor for AEs

If It Doesn't Work
- Increase to highest tolerated dose. Consider adding a second agent or changing to another one

Best Augmenting Combos for Partial Response or Treatment-Resistance
- For some patients, low-dose polytherapy with 2 or more drugs may be better tolerated and more effective than high-dose monotherapy

Tests
- Check ECG for QTc prolongation at baseline and when increasing dose, especially in those with a personal or family history of QTc prolongation, cardiac arrhythmia, heart failure, or recent myocardial infarction

ADVERSE EFFECTS (AEs)

How the Drug Causes AEs
- By increasing serotonin on non-therapeutic responsive receptors throughout the body. Most AEs are dose- and time-dependent

Notable AEs
- Incidence ≥ 5%: insomnia, nausea, fatigue, somnolence, hyperhidrosis, decreased libido, ejaculation delay, and anorgasmia

Life-Threatening or Dangerous AEs
- QTc prolongation, torsade de pointes, and rarely death
- Serotonin syndrome
- Rare activation of mania or suicidal ideation, especially during the initial few months
- Angle-closure glaucoma
- Rare worsening of existing seizure disorders
- Rare hyponatremia and abnormal bleeding

Weight Gain
- Not unusual

unusual   not unusual   common   problematic

Sedation
- Not unusual

unusual   not unusual   common   problematic

What to Do About AEs

- For minor AEs, lower dose, titrate more slowly, or switch to another agent. For serious AEs, lower dose and consider stopping, taper to avoid withdrawal symptoms

Best Augmenting Agents to Reduce AEs

- Cyproheptadine can be used for serotonin syndrome by blocking 5-HT receptors and SERT
- Sexual dysfunction (anorgasmia, impotence) may be reversed by agents with α_2-adrenergic antagonist activity (e.g., buspirone, amantadine, bupropion, mirtazapine, ginkgo biloba, etc.)

DOSING AND USE

Usual Dosage Range

- Escitalopram: 10–20 mg once daily

Dosage Forms

- Escitalopram: tablets (5, 10, 20 mg); oral solution (1 mg/mL)

How to Dose

- Escitalopram: initial 10 mg/day. Titrate 10 mg weekly. Maximum 20 mg/day (MDD, PTSD)

Dosing Tips

- Start at a low dose and titrate up every week as tolerated. Not affected by food

Overdose

- Often in combination with other drugs. Symptoms include convulsions, coma, dizziness, hypotension, insomnia, nausea, vomiting, sinus tachycardia, somnolence, and ECG changes (including QTc prolongation and very rare cases of torsade de pointes)
- Establish and maintain an airway. Gastric lavage with activated charcoal should be considered. Cardiac and vital sign monitoring are recommended, along with general symptomatic and supportive care. Due to the large volume of distribution of citalopram/escitalopram, forced diuresis, dialysis, hemoperfusion, and exchange transfusion are unlikely to be of benefit. There are no specific antidotes

Long-Term Use

- Safe for long-term use

Habit Forming

- No

How to Stop

- Taper slowly (no more than 50% reduction every 3–4 days until discontinuation) to avoid withdrawal symptoms (agitation, anxiety, confusion, dry mouth, dysphoria, etc.)

Pharmacokinetics

- Metabolized by CYP3A4, CYP2C19, and CYP2D6 (lesser extent). 20% eliminated by kidney. Bioavailability 80%. Half-life 20–40 hours. 80% protein bound

Drug Interactions

- Serotonin syndrome may occur with concomitant use of MAOIs or serotonergic drugs
- Concomitant use of CYP450 inhibitors typically does not significantly affect the pharmacokinetics of escitalopram due to the involvement of multiple enzyme systems
- Escitalopram has mild but clinically insignificant inhibitory effect on CYP2D6
- Abnormal bleeding: use caution in concomitant use with NSAIDs, aspirin, warfarin, or other drugs that affect coagulation

Other Warnings/Precautions

- May increase risk of seizure

Do Not Use

- Concurrently with MAOI; allow at least 14 days between discontinuation of an MAOI and initiation of escitalopram, or at least 7–14 days between discontinuation of escitalopram and initiation of an MAOI
- Concurrent use of serotonin precursors (e.g., tryptophan)
- In patients with uncontrolled narrow angle-closure glaucoma
- In patients treated with linezolid or methylene blue IV

Renal Impairment

- Use with caution in patients with severe impairment. No dosage adjustment for patients with mild or moderate renal impairment

Hepatic Impairment

- 10 mg/day for patients with hepatic function impairment

Cardiac Impairment

- Do not use in patients with cardiac structural lesions (e.g., myocardial infarction, severe heart failure), hypokalemia, hypomagnesemia, and history of QTc prolongation

Elderly

- 10 mg/day for most elderly

Children and Adolescents

- Safety and effectiveness not established in pediatric MDD patients < 12 years old

Pregnancy

- Category C. Neonates exposed to SNRIs or SSRIs late in the third trimester have developed complications necessitating extended hospitalizations, respiratory support, and tube feeding. Respiratory distress, cyanosis, apnea, seizures, temperature instability, feeding difficulty, vomiting, hypoglycemia, hypotonia, hyperreflexia, tremor, jitteriness, irritability, and constant crying consistent with a toxic effect of the drug or drug discontinuation syndrome have been reported

Breast Feeding

- Some drug is found in breast milk and use while breast feeding is not recommended

Potential Advantages

- Very effective SSRI. Indicated for adolescent MDD

Potential Disadvantages

- Requires gradual titration. Potential for sexual dysfunction

Primary Target Symptoms

- Depression and anxiety

Pearls

- Based on pooled and meta-analysis studies on depression, escitalopram demonstrates superior efficacy compared with citalopram and other SSRIs. Escitalopram shows similar efficacy to SNRI but the number of trials in these comparisons is limited
- Based on a Cochrane review, citalopram was more efficacious than paroxetine and reboxetine and more acceptable than TCAs, reboxetine, and venlafaxine; however, it seemed to be less efficacious than escitalopram
- In an animal study to investigate the normalization of sucrose solution consumption in stressed rats, escitalopram takes 1 week, citalopram takes 2 weeks, and TCAs and MAOIs take 3–5 weeks
- Limited evidence supporting citalopram/ escitalopram as preventives for migraine or tension-type headache
- No strong evidence supporting citalopram as treatment for fibromyalgia. However, it may help depressive symptoms in patients with fibromyalgia
- Limited evidence for its use in treating diabetic neuropathy
- May reduce binge eating and improve abstinence rates but does not lead to weight loss
- Only 2 SSRIs approved by FDA for treatment of depression in adolescents: escitalopram for 12–17 years of age and fluoxetine (gold standard) for 8–18 years of age
- Overall improves sleep quality in depressed patients (as most SSRIs). All SSRIs are associated with similar sleep architecture changes such as REM reduction, REM latency increase, slow wave sleep increase especially stages 1 and 2, and sleep fragmentation
- Overall decreases sleep quality in obsessive-compulsive disorder patients
- May be effective for cataplexy but not narcolepsy
- In a 6-week pilot study, both escitalopram (better tolerated) and risperidone (quicker onset) improved neuropsychiatric inventory in Alzheimer's disease patients

Suggested Reading

Ali MK, Lam RW. Comparative efficacy of escitalopram in the treatment of major depressive disorder. *Neuropsychiatr Dis Treat.* 2011;7:39–49.

Arnold LM. Duloxetine and other antidepressants in the treatment of patients with fibromyalgia. *Pain Med.* 2007;8 Suppl 2:S63–74.

Brownley KA, Berkman ND, Sedway JA, Lohr KN, Bulik CM. Binge eating disorder treatment: a systematic review of randomized controlled trials. *Int J Eat Disord.* 2007;40(4):337–48.

Cipriani A, Purgato M, Furukawa TA, Trespidi C, Imperadore G, Signoretti A, et al. Citalopram versus other anti-depressive agents for depression. *Cochrane Database Syst Rev.* 2012;7:CD006534.

Drago A. SSRIs impact on sleep architecture: guidelines for clinician use. *Clin Neuropsychiatry.* 2008;5:115–31.

Dworkin RH, O'Connor AB, Backonja M, Farrar JT, Finnerup NB, Jensen TS, et al. Pharmacologic management of neuropathic pain: evidence-based recommendations. *Pain.* 2007;132(3):237–51.

Smitherman TA, Walters AB, Maizels M, Penzien DB. The use of antidepressants for headache prophylaxis. *CNS Neurosci Ther.* 2010;17(5): 462–9.

ESLICARBAZEPINE ACETATE

Brands
- Aptiom

Generic?
- No

Class
- Antiepileptic drug (AED)

Commonly Prescribed for
(FDA approved in bold)
- **Adjunctive treatment of partial-onset seizures**
- Generalized tonic-clonic seizures

 How the Drug Works
- Eslicarbazepine acetate is a prodrug that is metabolized to its major active metabolite eslicarbazepine (S-licarbazepine), and to the minor active metabolites R-licarbazepine and oxcarbazepine
- Eslicarbazepine binds to the inactivated form of the voltage-gated sodium channel (VGSC) and prevents its reversion to the receptive resting or deactivated form. The mechanism is shared by carbamazepine and oxcarbazepine
- The affinity of S-licarbazepine for VGSC in the resting state was 5- to 15-fold lower than that of R-licarbazepine, oxcarbazepine, and carbamazepine. Thus, eslicarbazepine had enhanced inhibitory selectivity for rapidly firing neurons versus those displaying normal activity; i.e., eslicarbazepine binds preferentially to active neurons

How Long Until It Works
- Seizures: 2 weeks or less

If It Works
- The goal is seizure remission. Continue as long as effective and well tolerated. Consider tapering and slowly stopping after 2 years without seizures, depending on the type of epilepsy

If It Doesn't Work
- Increase to highest tolerated dose

- Consider changing to another agent, adding a second agent, using a medical device, or a referral for epilepsy surgery evaluation. When adding a second agent, keep drug interactions in mind

 Best Augmenting Combos for Partial Response or Treatment-Resistance
- Drug interactions can complicate multi-drug therapy

Tests
- Check sodium levels for symptoms of hyponatremia or in patients susceptible to hyponatremia

How the Drug Causes AEs
- CNS AEs are probably caused by sodium channel blockade effects

Notable AEs
- Sedation, dizziness, ataxia, headache, tremor, blurred vision, vertigo, cognitive dysfunction
- Nausea, vomiting, anorexia, dyspepsia

 Life-Threatening or Dangerous AEs
- Suicidal behavior and ideation
- Dermatological reactions uncommon and rarely severe but include erythema multiforme, toxic epidermal necrolysis, and Stevens-Johnson syndrome. Drug reaction with eosinophilia and systemic symptoms (DRESS)/multi-organ hypersensitivity
- Hyponatremia/SIADH (syndrome of inappropriate antidiuretic hormone secretion)
- Drug-induced liver injury

Weight Gain
- Not unusual

unusual | not unusual | common | problematic

Sedation
- Not unusual

unusual | not unusual | common | problematic

What to Do About AEs

- Use with caution in patients with low sodium at baseline, or those on medications that can lower sodium such as diuretics

Best Augmenting Agents to Reduce AEs

- Discontinuation. Correct underlying problems

DOSING AND USE

Usual Dosage Range

- 400–1200 mg daily

Dosage Forms

- Tablets: 200, 400, 600, 800 mg

How to Dose

- Start at 400 mg once daily. After 1 week, increase to 800 mg once daily (recommended maintenance dosage). Maximum 1200 mg once daily
- Patients with moderate to severe renal impairment: start at 200 mg once daily. After 2 weeks, increase to 400 mg once daily with maximum recommended maintenance dosage 600 mg once daily

 Dosing Tips

- Titrate slowly
- Can be taken with food or crushed
- Conversion to monotherapy: concomitant AEDs should be withdrawn over 3–6 weeks

Overdose

- Hyponatremia, dizziness, sedation, ataxia, diplopia
- Removal by gastric lavage or inactivation by activated charcoal. Hemodialysis may be considered

Long-Term Use

- Safe for long-term use

Habit Forming

- No

How to Stop

- Taper slowly
- Abrupt withdrawal can lead to status epilepticus

Pharmacokinetics

- Rapidly reduced by esterase in liver to the active form (S-licarbazepine) with 95% conversion efficiency (much greater than that of oxcarbazepine). T_{max} and C_{max} are lower in patients than in healthy subjects. Half-life 20–24 hours. Linear dose–response (400–2000 mg/day). Eliminated by kidney and 91% is in urine. Steady state reached in 4–5 days

 Drug Interactions

- Can inhibit CYP2C19, causing increase in phenytoin, phenobarbital, clobazam, omeprazole, etc.
- Can induce CYP3A4, causing decrease in statins, oral contraceptives, warfarin, etc.
- Phenytoin and phenobarbital can decrease eslicarbazepine concentration

 Other Warnings/ Precautions

- CNS AEs increase when used with other CNS depressants
- Risk of hyponatremia is highest in the first 3 months. Check sodium level for symptoms of hyponatremia (nausea, headache, lethargy, or worsening headache)

Do Not Use

- Hypersensitivity to eslicarbazepine acetate or oxcarbazepine

SPECIAL POPULATIONS

Renal Impairment

- Lower dose for patients with renal insufficiency (CrCl < 50 mL/min). Reduce initial dose by half and titrate slowly

Hepatic Impairment

- Safe for patients with mild to moderate disease at usual doses. Not recommended in patients with severe disease

Cardiac Impairment

- No known effects

Elderly

- Dose selection should take into consideration the greater frequency of renal impairment and other concomitant medical conditions and drug therapies in the elderly patient

 Children and Adolescents

- Safety and effectiveness in patients below 18 years of age have not been established

 Pregnancy

- Category C. Teratogenicity in animal studies
- Risks of stopping medication must outweigh risk to fetus for patients with epilepsy. Seizures and potential status epilepticus place the woman and fetus at risk and can cause reduced oxygen and blood supply to the womb
- Supplementation with 0.4 mg of folic acid before and during pregnancy is recommended

Breast Feeding

- Can be found in breast milk
- Generally recommendations are to discontinue drug or bottle feed
- Monitor infant for sedation, poor feeding, or irritability

THE ART OF NEUROPHARMACOLOGY

Potential Advantages

- Proven effectiveness as adjunctive agent for partial seizures. Generally fewer AEs than carbamazepine and oxcarbazepine

Potential Disadvantages

- Ineffective for absence and myoclonic seizures. Risk of hyponatremia

Primary Target Symptoms

- Seizure frequency and severity

 Pearls

- Effective for partial epilepsies. May improve generalized tonic-clonic epilepsy
- Not effective for absence or myoclonic seizures, infantile spasms
- Hyponatremia ($<$ 125 mEq/L) occurs in about 1–1.5% of patients. Typically dose related and generally appears within the first 8 weeks
- In one study, a dose-dependent decrease in seizure frequency was observed in children aged 2–7 years and adolescents aged 12–17 years but not in children aged 7–11 years

 Suggested Reading

Almeida L, Minciu I, Nunes T, Butoianu N, Falcão A, Magureanu S-A, et al. Pharmacokinetics, efficacy, and tolerability of eslicarbazepine acetate in children and adolescents with epilepsy. *J Clin Pharmacol.* 2008;48(8):966–77.

Brown ME, El-Mallakh RS. Role of eslicarbazepine in the treatment of epilepsy in adult patients with partial-onset seizures. *Ther Clin Risk Manag.* 2010;6:103–9.

Keating GM. Eslicarbazepine acetate: a review of its use as adjunctive therapy in refractory partial-onset seizures. *CNS Drugs.* 2014;28(7): 583–600.

Singh RP, Asconapé JJ. A review of eslicarbazepine acetate for the adjunctive treatment of partial-onset epilepsy. *J Cent Nerv Syst Dis.* 2011;3: 179–87.

ETHOSUXIMIDE

THERAPEUTICS

Brands
- Zarontin

Generic?
- Yes

Class
- Antiepileptic drug (AED)

Commonly Prescribed for
(FDA approved in bold)
- **Absence (petit mal) epilepsy**
- Intermittent explosive disorder

How the Drug Works
- There are multiple proposed mechanisms of action, and it is uncertain which of these give the drug its effectiveness
- Blocks or modulates low-voltage T-type calcium channels
- Modulates sodium channel function
- May alter glutamate or GABA levels
- Proven to suppress paroxysmal 3-hertz spike and slow wave discharges on EEG

How Long Until It Works
- Seizures: should decrease by 2 weeks

If It Works
- Seizures: goal is the remission of seizures. Continue as long as effective and well tolerated. Consider tapering and slowly stopping after 2 years without seizures, depending on the type of epilepsy

If It Doesn't Work
- Increase to highest tolerated dose
- Epilepsy: consider changing to another agent, adding a second agent, using a medical device, or a referral for epilepsy surgery evaluation. When adding a second agent, keep drug interactions in mind

Best Augmenting Combos for Partial Response or Treatment-Resistance
- Epilepsy: often used in combination when more than one type of epilepsy exists. Effective in combination with valproate or lamotrigine for absence seizures but this

can cause interactions and change levels of drug

Tests
- CBC, urinalysis, and liver function tests at baseline and on a periodic basis

ADVERSE EFFECTS (AEs)

How the Drug Causes AEs
- CNS AEs are probably caused by effects on calcium or sodium channels

Notable AEs
- Sedation, ataxia, dizziness, headache, blurred vision, insomnia
- Nausea, vomiting, cramps, anorexia, abdominal pain, constipation
- Increased urinary frequency, muscle weakness, periorbital edema, pruritus

Life-Threatening or Dangerous AEs
- Rare blood dyscrasias including leukopenia, eosinophilia, pancytopenia
- Rare cases of systemic lupus erythematosus
- Severe dermatological manifestations including Stevens-Johnson syndrome, erythema multiforme
- Suicidal behavior and ideation

Weight Gain
- Unusual

unusual | not unusual | common | problematic

Sedation
- Common

unusual | not unusual | common | problematic

What to Do About AEs
- Check CBC for any signs of systemic infection
- Lower dose or change to another agent

Best Augmenting Agents to Reduce AEs
- Most AEs cannot be reduced with the use of an augmenting agent

DOSING AND USE

Usual Dosage Range
- 250–1500 mg/day

Dosage Forms
- 250 mg capsule or syrup 250 mg/5 mL

How to Dose
- Start at 250 mg/day once daily or in 2 divided doses. Increase by 250 mg every 4–7 days to goal dose

 Dosing Tips
- If GI upset occurs take with food or milk
- Very young children (age 3 or less) are more likely to require twice-daily dosing

Overdose
- Acute: CNS depression with coma and respiratory depression. Confusion, hypotension, flaccid muscles, absent reflexes
- Chronic: skin rash, hematuria, confusion, ataxia, depression, dizziness

Long-Term Use
- Safe for long-term use

Habit Forming
- No

How to Stop
- Taper slowly
- Abrupt withdrawal can lead to seizures
- Patients with childhood absence epilepsy (onset before age 12) have a high rate of remission and little risk of grand mal seizures. Patients with juvenile absence (onset age 12 or later) have a higher risk of relapse with drug withdrawal

Pharmacokinetics
- Hepatic metabolism mostly by CYP3A system. Renal excretion
- Half-life is 30 hours in children, 40–60 hours in adults
- Bioavailability is 95–100%

 Drug Interactions
- Increases levels of phenytoin
- Decreases levels of primidone and phenobarbital

- Valproate can either increase or decrease ethosuximide levels
- Enzyme-inducing drugs including phenytoin, carbamazepine, phenobarbital, and rifampin lower ethosuximide levels

 Other Warnings/ Precautions
- CNS AEs increase when used with other CNS depressants
- Systemic symptoms such as fever, flu-like symptoms, swelling of eyelids, along with any dermatological changes require immediate evaluation
- Rare reports of psychiatric abnormalities including auditory hallucinations, depression, suicidal behavior, and psychosis

Do Not Use
- Patients with a proven allergy to succinimides

SPECIAL POPULATIONS

Renal Impairment
- Use with extreme caution

Hepatic Impairment
- Use with extreme caution

Cardiac Impairment
- No known effects

Elderly
- It is rarely used in the elderly. Elderly patients are more susceptible to AEs

 Children and Adolescents
- Approved for use in children 3 and older
- Ages 3–6: 250 mg/day
- Ages 6 and up: 500 mg/day
- Increase dose by 250 mg every 4–7 days until seizures are well controlled or side effects occur. Usual maximum dose 1500 mg/day

 Pregnancy
- Category C. Risks of stopping medication must outweigh risk to fetus for patients with epilepsy

- Supplementation with 0.4 mg of folic acid before and during pregnancy is recommended

Breast Feeding

- Breast milk contains 80–100% of mother's blood drug level
- Generally recommendations are to discontinue drug or bottle feed
- Monitor infant for sedation, poor feeding, or irritability

THE ART OF NEUROPHARMACOLOGY

Potential Advantages

- Effective for absence seizures. Avoids risk of hepatotoxicity

Potential Disadvantages

- Not effective for most types of epilepsy

Primary Target Symptoms

- Seizure frequency and severity

 Pearls

- Ethosuximide and valproic acid are more effective than lamotrigine in the treatment of childhood absence epilepsy. Valproate is slightly more effective but ethosuximide is associated with fewer adverse attentional effects
- One of 3 succinimides used in epilepsy. The others are phensuximide and methsuximide
- May increase risk of generalized tonic-clonic seizures in some individuals with absence seizures
- Useful in animal models for treating neuropathic pain and hyperalgesia

 Suggested Reading

Flatters SJ, Bennett GJ. Ethosuximide reverses paclitaxel- and vincristine-induced painful peripheral neuropathy. *Pain.* 2004;109(1–2):150–61.

Glauser TA, Cnaan A, Shinnar S, Hirtz DG, Dlugos D, Masur D, et al. Ethosuximide, valproic acid, and lamotrigine in childhood absence epilepsy. *N Engl J Med.* 2010;362(9):790–9.

Gomora JC, Daud AN, Weiergraber M, Perez-Reyes E. Block of cloned human T-type calcium channels by succinimide antiepileptic drugs. *Mol Pharm.* 2001;60(5):1121–32.

Sayer RJ, Brown AM, Schwindt PC, Crill WE. Calcium currents in acutely isolated human neocortical neurons. *J Neurophysiol.* 1993; 69(5):1596–606.

Schmitt B, Kovacevic-Preradovic T, Critelli H, Molinari L. Is ethosuximide a risk factor for generalized tonic-clonic seizures in absence epilepsy? *Neuropediatrics.* 2007;38(2):83–7.

EVEROLIMUS

THERAPEUTICS

Brands
- Afinitor, Afinitor Disperz, Zortress, Certican

Generic?
- No

Class
- Immunosuppressant, antineoplastic agent

Commonly Prescribed for
(FDA approved in bold)
- **Patients with subependymal giant cell astrocytoma (SEGA) associated with tuberous sclerosis complex (TSC) who require therapeutic intervention but are not candidates for curative surgical resection in adults or children 1 year and older (Afinitor or Afinitor Disperz only)**
- **Adults with renal angiomyolipoma and TSC not requiring immediate surgery. (Afinitor only)**
- **Adults with progressive neuroendocrine tumors of pancreatic origin (PNET) that are unresectable, locally advanced, or metastatic (Afinitor only)**
- **Advanced renal cell carcinoma (RCC), failure to sunitinib or sorafenib (Afinitor only)**
- **Prophylaxis of organ rejection in adult patients undergoing kidney or liver transplantation (Zortress only)**
- **Postmenopausal women with advanced hormone receptor-positive, HER2-negative breast cancer in combination with exemestane after failure of treatment with letrozole or anastrozole (Afinitor only)**
- Brainstem glioma

How the Drug Works
- A macrolide lactam that works as a mammalian target of rapamycin (mTOR) inhibitor by binding to the FK506 binding protein-12. It blocks the cell progression from G1 to S phase, causing apoptosis and cell death. It also inhibits hypoxia-inducible factor that subsequently decreases vascular endothelial growth factor. Overall, it inhibits cell proliferation, angiogenesis, and glucose uptake. Also, in TSC subjects, everolimus inhibits two regulators of mTORC$_1$ signaling

that are the oncogene suppressors harmatin (TSC1) and tuberin (TSC2)

How Long Until It Works
- Immunosuppression: usually within 1 week
- Tumor suppression: usually more than 1 month

If It Works
- Continue treatment if tolerated and effective. Monitor any adverse event

If It Doesn't Work
- Check drug concentration. Adjust dose if necessary. Consider surgical referral. Switch to other agents when needed

Best Augmenting Combos for Partial Response or Treatment-Resistance
- Combine with other immunosuppressive agents or antineoplastic agents

Tests
- Therapeutic drug concentration (trough 3–8 ng/mL), obtained 5 days after dose change or 2 weeks after a change in CYP3A4 or phosphoglycolate phosphatase inducer/inhibitor. Once stable, monitor trough concentration every 3–6 months in patients with changing body surface area or every 6–12 months in patients with stable body surface area
- Renal function, urinary protein, serum glucose, CBC, lipids, creatine kinase

ADVERSE EFFECTS (AEs)

How the Drug Causes AEs
- Interruption of cell cycles and angiogenesis

Notable AEs
- Stomatitis, infection (upper respiratory tract, urinary tract), rash, fatigue, diarrhea, anemia, leukopenia, edema, abdominal pain, nausea, fever, asthenia, cough, headache, decreased appetite

Life-Threatening or Dangerous AEs
- Angioedema: increased risk with concomitant use of ACE inhibitors

- Interstitial lung disease/non-infectious pneumonitis
- Hemolytic uremic syndrome: increased risk with concomitant use of cyclosporine
- Polyoma virus infection: activation of latent infection, virus-associated nephropathy
- Lymphoma and skin cancers

Weight Gain
- Unusual

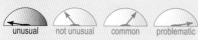
unusual   not unusual   common   problematic

Sedation
- Unusual

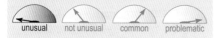
unusual   not unusual   common   problematic

What to Do About AEs
- Adjust dosage based on the severity of AEs
- Examine any potential drug interaction

Best Augmenting Agents to Reduce AEs
- Most AEs cannot be reduced with the use of an augmenting agent

DOSING AND USE

Usual Dosage Range
- SEGA: 4.5 mg/m^2
- RCC/PNET/renal angiomyolipoma/breast cancer: 10 mg once daily
- Transplantation: 0.75–1 mg twice daily

Dosage Forms
- Tablets (Afinitor): 2.5, 5, 7.5, 10 mg
- Tablets (Zortress): 0.25, 0.5, 0.75 mg
- Oral suspension (Afinitor Disperz): 2, 3, 5 mg

How to Dose
- SEGA: initial dose based on body surface area with subsequent titration to attain trough concentration of 5–10 ng/mL
- Advanced RCC: 10 mg daily
- Kidney transplant: 0.75 mg twice daily (12 hours apart). Use in combination with basiliximab, cyclosporine, and corticosteroid. Start as soon as possible after transplantation

- Liver transplant: 1 mg twice daily. Use in combination with tacrolimus and corticosteroid. Start 30 days after transplantation

 Dosing Tips
- Adjust dose based on the presence of CYP3A4 inhibitor/inducer, hepatic impairment, or adverse drug reactions
- Tablet should not be crushed or chewed

Overdose
- Reported experience very limited. In animal studies, it showed a low acute toxic potential

Long-Term Use
- Increased risk of AEs. See Other Warnings/Precautions

Habit Forming
- No

How to Stop
- No need to taper

Pharmacokinetics
- It is a substrate of CYP3A4 and phosphoglycolate phosphatase. T_{max} 1–2 hours. Steady state is reached in 2 weeks. Half-life is 30 hours. 80% excreted in feces and 5% in urine

 Drug Interactions
- Increase dose with concomitant use of strong CYP3A4 inducer (e.g., phenobarbital, phenytoin, carbamazepine, rifampin, St. John's wort)
- Decrease dose with concomitant use of strong CYP3A4 inhibitor (e.g., azole antifungals, nefazodone, antivirals, macrolides, grapefruit juice)

 Other Warnings/Precautions
- Increased susceptibility to infection and the possible development of malignancies resulting from immunosuppression

- An increased risk of kidney arterial and venous thrombosis mostly within the first 30 days post-transplantation
- Increased nephrotoxicity can occur when combined with use of cyclosporine
- Increased mortality, often associated with serious infection, within the first 3 months of heart transplantation
- Increases the risk of new-onset diabetes mellitus after transplant

Do Not Use

- Hypersensitivity to everolimus, to other sirolimus derivatives, or to any of the excipients
- It is not indicated for the treatment of patients with functional carcinoid tumors
- Any live vaccines (e.g., intranasal influenza, measles, mumps, rubella, oral polio, BCG, yellow fever, varicella, TY21a typhoid) during everolimus treatment

Renal Impairment

- No adjustment needed

Hepatic Impairment

- In mild or moderate impairment, a dose reduction is recommended. In severe impairment, use only if benefit outweighs the risk

Cardiac Impairment

- No known effects

Elderly

- No adjustment in initial dosing is required in elderly patients, but close monitoring and appropriate dose adjustments for adverse reactions are recommended

Children and Adolescents

- Afinitor is used for unresectable SEGA in patients 1 years or older. The long-term effects of Afinitor on growth and pubertal development are unknown. The safety of everolimus use in other disorders in children is not known

Pregnancy

- Category C (Zotress), D (Afinitor). Everolimus crossed the placenta and was toxic to the conceptus in rats and rabbits. The potential risk for humans is unknown

Breast Feeding

- It is not known whether everolimus is excreted in human milk. Patients taking everolimus should not breast feed

Potential Advantages

- Effective in some patients with TSC by decreasing tumor size and seizure frequency. Strong immunosuppressive agent

Potential Disadvantages

- Multiple AEs related to immunosuppression and kinase inhibition

Primary Target Symptoms

- TSC that regulates mTOR signaling. Immune reaction to transplants

Pearls

- $mTORC_1$-directed therapies may be most effective in cancer patients whose tumors harbor *TSC1* somatic mutations
- It not only reduces SEGA volume, but also improves seizure frequency
- The consensus recommendations for TSC surveillance and management guideline are available
- Under investigation for the treatment of pediatric brainstem glioma
- The effectiveness of Afinitor in the treatment of renal angiomyolipoma is based on an analysis of durable objective responses in patients treated for a median of 8.3 months. Further follow-up of patients is required to determine long-term outcomes
- In a meta-analysis of 14 randomized controlled trials comparing everolimus-eluting stents (EES) and sirolimus-eluting stents (SES), EES implantation was associated with lower risk for early stent thrombosis and target-lesion revascularization. No difference in the risk for all-cause death and myocardial infarction

- RADIANT-2 trial: everolimus plus octreotide long-acting repeatable (LAR), compared with placebo plus octreotide LAR, improved progression-free survival in patients with advanced neuroendocrine tumors associated with carcinoid syndrome

- Brain accumulation of everolimus was restricted by drug efflux transporter P-glycoprotein. Combining everolimus with P-glycoprotein inhibitors may be used to improve its therapeutic efficacy against brain tumor

 Suggested Reading

Franz DN, Belousova E, Sparagana S, Bebin EM, Frost M, Kuperman R, et al. Efficacy and safety of everolimus for subependymal giant cell astrocytomas associated with tuberous sclerosis complex (EXIST-1): a multicentre, randomised, placebo-controlled phase 3 trial. *Lancet*. 2013;381(9861):125–32.

Gurk-Turner C, Manitpisitkul W, Cooper M. A comprehensive review of everolimus clinical reports: a new mammalian target of rapamycin inhibitor. *Transplantation*. 2012; 94(7):659–68.

Krueger DA, Northrup H. Tuberous sclerosis complex surveillance and management: recommendations of the 2012 International Tuberous Sclerosis Complex Consensus Conference. *Pediatr Neurol*. 2013;49(4): 255–65.

Pavel ME, Hainsworth JD, Baudin E, Peeters M, Hörsch D, Winkler RE, et al. Everolimus plus octreotide long-acting repeatable for the treatment of advanced neuroendocrine tumours associated with carcinoid syndrome (RADIANT-2): a randomised, placebo-controlled, phase 3 study. *Lancet*. 2011;378(9808):2005–12.

Toyota T, Shiomi H, Morimoto T, Kimura T. Abstract 12022: Long-term clinical outcomes of everolimus-eluting stents versus sirolimus-eluting stents: systematic review and a meta-analysis of 14 randomized control trials, focused on stent thrombosis. *Circulation*. 2014;130(Suppl 2):A12022–2.

THERAPEUTICS

Brands
- Potiga

Generic?
- No

Class
- Antiepileptic drug (AED)

Commonly Prescribed for
(FDA approved in bold)
- **Adjunctive treatment of partial-onset seizures in patients ≥ 18 years old who have responded inadequately to several alternative treatments and for whom the benefits outweigh the risk of retinal abnormalities and potential decline in visual acuity**

How the Drug Works
- Ezogabine stabilizes the resting membrane potential and reduces brain excitability by keeping transmembrane potassium channels (KCNQ2, KCNQ3) open longer and delaying membrane repolarization (stabilizes M-current resting membrane potential). It may also potentiate GABA$_A$ receptors

How Long Until It Works
- T$_{max}$ 0.5–2 hours. Clinical effects may take weeks to months

If It Works
- Periodic ophthalmological and urological monitoring. May consider tapering after seizure free for 2 years, depending on the seizure type

If It Doesn't Work
- Consider changing to another agent, adding a second agent, using a medical device, or a referral for epilepsy surgery evaluation. When adding a second agent, keep drug interactions in mind

Best Augmenting Combos for Partial Response or Treatment-Resistance
- Not available

Tests
- No test required

ADVERSE EFFECTS (AEs)

How the Drug Causes AEs
- Affecting potassium channels in brain and bladder

Notable AEs
- Urinary retention (2%), skin discoloration (lips, nail beds, etc.), neuropsychiatric symptoms (confusion, psychosis, hallucination), dizziness, somnolence, QTc prolongation (7.7 ms at 1200 mg/day), withdrawal seizure, abuse potential

Life-Threatening or Dangerous AEs
- Retinal dystrophy (perivascular pigmentation, focal retinal epithelium clumping), vision loss, suicidal behavior

Weight Gain
- Common

unusual   not unusual   common   problematic

- Dose-related weight gain

Sedation
- Not unusual

unusual   not unusual   common   problematic

What to Do About AEs
- Discontinue and switch to another agent

Best Augmenting Agents to Reduce AEs
- Alcohol worsens the adverse reaction

DOSING AND USE

Usual Dosage Range
- 600–1200 mg 3 times daily, with or without food, swallowed whole

Dosage Forms
- Tablets: 50, 200, 300, and 400 mg

How to Dose
- Initial: 100 mg 3 times daily
- Titration: weekly with no more than 150 mg/day
- Maintenance: 600–1200 mg 3 times daily
- For elderly or moderate renal/hepatic impaired, use half dose during initiation, titration, and maintenance

 Dosing Tips
- Dosage adjustment based on clinical presentation, age, renal/hepatic conditions

Overdose
- Limited information. Standard overdose management

Long-Term Use
- May cause retinal abnormality. Test visual function at baseline and every 6 months during therapy

Habit Forming
- May have abuse potential

How to Stop
- Taper gradually over ≥ 3 weeks

Pharmacokinetics
- Average half-life is 7–11 hours. Ezogabine is extensively metabolized in liver via glucuronidation and acetylation (not CYP450 enzymes), and eliminated via renal excretion (85% urine, 12% feces)

 Drug Interactions
- Ezogabine serum concentration decreased by carbamazepine and phenytoin. Consider increase in dosage
- Ezogabine may increase digoxin serum level
- Alcohol may worsen ezogabine's adverse reaction
- May affect bilirubin lab assay (false elevation)

⚠ **Other Warnings/ Precautions**
- Urinary retention, skin discoloration, dizziness, somnolence
- Confusion, psychosis, hallucination, suicidal behavior
- QTc prolongation

Do Not Use
- If vision or retinal changes detected
- If no substantial benefit after adequate titration

SPECIAL POPULATIONS

Renal Impairment
- Dosage reduction for CrCl < 50 mL/min and for end-stage renal disease patients

Hepatic Impairment
- Dosage reduction in patients with moderate or severe hepatic impairment

Cardiac Impairment
- No known effects

Elderly
- Dosage adjustment in patients ≥ 65 years old
- Elderly men with symptomatic benign prostatic hyperplasia may be at risk for urinary retention

 Children and Adolescents
- Not studied in patients ≤ 18 years old. Increased neurotoxicity in young rats

 Pregnancy
- Category C. Developmental toxicity noted in animal studies

Breast Feeding
- Can be found in breast milk
- Generally recommendations are to discontinue drug or bottle feed
- Monitor infant for sedation, poor feeding, or irritability

THE ART OF NEUROPHARMACOLOGY

Potential Advantages
- First AED to control seizures by modulating potassium channels. Can be used in patients with severe renal/hepatic impairment. Not affected by CYP450 enzymes. Few drug interactions

Potential Disadvantages

- Retinal pigment dystrophy, vision loss, urinary retention

Primary Target Symptoms

- Seizure frequency and severity

 Pearls

- Ezogabine may be helpful for patients with partial epilepsy when other medications have failed

- Rapid titration may increase the risk of neuropsychiatric symptoms
- When urinary retention occurs, patients may require long-term intermittent self-catheterization even after ezogabine discontinuation
- May be useful in combination with sodium-blocking and GABA-facilitating drugs
- RESTORE 1 and RESTORE 2 provided Class II evidence that ezogabine is effective in adults with partial-onset seizures with or without secondary generalization

 Suggested Reading

Brodie MJ, Lerche H, Gil-Nagel A, Elger C, Hall S, Shin P, et al. Efficacy and safety of adjunctive ezogabine (retigabine) in refractory partial epilepsy. *Neurology.* 2010;75(20):1817–24.

French JA, Abou-Khalil BW, Leroy RF, Yacubian EMT, Shin P, Hall S, et al. Randomized, double-blind, placebo-controlled trial of ezogabine (retigabine) in partial epilepsy. *Neurology.* 2011;76(18):1555–63.

Gunthorpe MJ, Large CH, Sankar R. The mechanism of action of retigabine (ezogabine), a first-in-class K+ channel opener for the treatment of epilepsy. *Epilepsia.* 2012; 53(3):412–24.

FELBAMATE

THERAPEUTICS

Brands
- Fetbatol, Taloxa

Generic?
- Yes

 Class
- Antiepileptic drug (AED)

Commonly Prescribed for
(FDA approved in bold)
- **Complex partial seizures (adjunctive)**
- **Partial and generalized seizures associated with Lennox-Gastaut syndrome (children)**
- Infantile spasms (West syndrome)

 How the Drug Works
- The exact mechanism of action in epilepsy is unknown. Felbamate may reduce seizure spread or increase seizure threshold. Putative mechanisms include changes in binding at calcium (L-type) channel, sodium channel, GABA receptors and blockade of NMDA-activated glutamate receptors

How Long Until It Works
- Seizures: 2 weeks

If It Works
- Seizures: goal is the decrease or remission of seizures. Continue as long as effective and well tolerated

If It Doesn't Work
- Increase to highest tolerated dose. If not effective discontinue

 Best Augmenting Combos for Partial Response or Treatment-Resistance
- Epilepsy: generally used in combination with other agents for severe epilepsy. Keep drug interactions in mind

Tests
- Obtain liver function testing and CBC before starting, and monitor frequently – especially in the first months after initiating treatment
- Repeat liver function testing whenever new medications are added

ADVERSE EFFECTS (AEs)

How the Drug Causes AEs
- CNS AEs may be caused by binding changes at GABA, benzodiazepine, or NMDA receptors
- Aplastic anemia may be related to a reactive metabolite, 2-phenylpropenal

Notable AEs
- Most common: anorexia, weight loss, vomiting, insomnia, headache, dizziness, anxiety
- Less common: rash, acne, edema, rhinitis, otitis media, diplopia, abnormal taste or vision

 Life-Threatening or Dangerous AEs
- Liver failure, often with rapid onset (2–4 weeks)
- Aplastic anemia, often fatal and usually beginning 5–30 weeks after starting treatment

Weight Gain
- Unusual

unusual   not unusual   common   problematic

Sedation
- Common

unusual   not unusual   common   problematic

- Usually dose related

What to Do About AEs
- Most AEs resolve with reduction in dose
- For serious AEs discontinue drug

Best Augmenting Agents to Reduce AEs
- Most AEs do not respond to an augmenting agent

DOSING AND USE

Usual Dosage Range
- 2400–3600 mg/day

Dosage Forms
- Tablets: 400, 600 mg

• Suspension: 600 mg/5 mL

How to Dose

• Start at 400 mg 3 times daily. Increase dose every 2 weeks by 600 mg/day until taking 2400 mg/day 3–4 times daily and up to 3600 mg/day if tolerated and needed based on clinical response. Reduce dose of concomitant AEDs by 20–30% in the first week, then by one-third at 2 weeks

Dosing Tips

• Most AEs associated with felbamate resolve with lowering doses of concomitant AEDs
• Food does not affect absorption

Overdose

• GI distress and tachycardia have been reported with high doses

Long-Term Use

• Routine CBC and liver function testing are mandatory

Habit Forming

• No

How to Stop

• Taper slowly, as abrupt withdrawal can lead to seizures in patients with epilepsy

Pharmacokinetics

• Peak plasma levels at 1–4 hours with plasma half-life of 20–23 hours. About 50% of drug is metabolized, the remainder is excreted unchanged in urine. Bioavailabilty is 90%

Drug Interactions

• CYP2C19 inhibitor which may increase levels of many common medications (propranolol, warfarin, indomethacin, proton pump inhibitors)
• Phenytoin, phenobarbital, and carbamazepine increase clearance and lower levels
• Increases valproate and phenytoin levels and lowers carbamazepine levels
• May decrease effectiveness of oral contraceptives, but usually not to a relevant degree

Other Warnings/ Precautions

• Contains small amount of animal carcinogens

Do Not Use

• Hypersensitivity to drug, any active liver disease, or blood dyscrasias

SPECIAL POPULATIONS

Renal Impairment

• Clearance reduced and half-life prolonged. Lower dose and use with caution

Hepatic Impairment

• Do not use

Cardiac Impairment

• Prolongs QTc interval

Elderly

• No known effect

Children and Adolescents

• Approved for use in children with Lennox-Gastaut syndrome ages 2–14
• Start at 15 mg/kg/day in 3–4 divided doses daily and reduce dose of present AEDs by 20%. Increase by 15 mg/kg/day weekly until clinical effect or at 45 mg/kg/day

Pregnancy

• Risk category C
• Supplementation with 0.4 mg of folic acid before and during pregnancy is recommended

Breast Feeding

• Can be found in breast milk
• Generally recommendations are to discontinue drug or bottle feed
• Monitor infant for sedation, poor feeding, or irritability

THE ART OF NEUROPHARMACOLOGY

Potential Advantages

• Broad-spectrum and effective AED. Useful in refractory epilepsy

Potential Disadvantages
• Risk of aplastic anemia and liver failure

Primary Target Symptoms
• Seizure frequency and severity

Pearls
• Relatively well-tolerated, broad-spectrum, and effective AED, but idiosyncratic AE of liver failure and aplastic anemia have made it a drug only for refractory patients. The rate of aplastic anemia is about 100–250 times the risk for the disorder in the general population

• Flurofelbamate is a drug in development that may have similar efficacy to felbamate, with a lower risk of serious AEs
• The patient or guardian must read and sign an informed consent before felbamate can be prescribed
• From retrospective studies, felbamate seemed to be effective in the treatment of intractable seizures in children. However, based on a recent Cochrane review, no reliable evidence to support the use of felbamate as an add-on therapy in patients with refractory partial-onset epilepsy

Suggested Reading

Hancock EC, Cross HH. Treatment of Lennox-Gastaut syndrome. *Cochrane Database Syst Rev.* 2009;3:CD003277

Harden CL. Therapeutic safety monitoring: what to look for and when to look for it. *Epilepsia.* 2000;41 Suppl 8: S37–44.

Pellock JM. Felbamate. *Epilepsia.* 1999;40 Suppl 5:S57–62.

Rogawski MA. Diverse mechanisms of antiepileptic drugs in the development pipeline. *Epilepsy Res.* 2006;69(3):273–94.

Shi L, Dong J, Ni H, Geng J, Wu T. Felbamate as an add-on therapy for refractory epilepsy. *Cochrane Database Syst Rev* 2014;7:CD008295.

Tsao CY. Current trends in the treatment of infantile spasms. *Neuropsychiatr Dis Treat.* 2009;5:289–99.

FINGOLIMOD

THERAPEUTICS

Brands
- Gilenya

Generic?
- No

Class
- Immunomodulator

Commonly Prescribed for
(FDA approved in bold)
- **Relapsing types of multiple sclerosis (MS)**
- Amyotrophic lateral sclerosis (ALS)
- Heart failure and arrhythmia
- Prevention of rejection post-transplantation

How the Drug Works
- Modulates the sphingosine-1-phosphate receptor (S1PR), causing lymphocytes to sequester in lymph nodes. Sphingolipids and S1PR receptor are plentiful in the CNS and affect neurogenesis, neural cell function and migration. Fingolimod most likely acts at the S1PR1 receptor
- It may also stimulate glial cell repair and it may have cannabinoid receptor antagonism, and inhibit ceramide synthase

How Long Until It Works
- Typically takes months to determine clinical effects

If It Works
- May continue as long as needed for relapsing MS. Unclear if effective in progressive forms of MS

If It Doesn't Work
- May change to an alternative agent such as β-interferons, glatiramer acetate, or natalizumab

Best Augmenting Combos for Partial Response or Treatment-Resistance
- Generally not used along with other disease-modifying agents

Tests
- Before starting obtain CBC and liver function tests (within 6 months), ECG, ophthalmological examination, skin examination, and varicella serology. If varicella negative, give varicella zoster vaccination

ADVERSE EFFECTS (AEs)

How the Drug Causes AEs
- Sequestration of lymphocytes, as demonstrated by reduction in peripheral lymphocyte counts, likely explains the increased risk of infection. Release of sequestered lymphocytes after discontinuation may cause immediate clinical deterioration. The cause of cardiac events is unclear

Notable AEs
- Symptomatic bradycardia with initial dose, asymptomatic liver transaminase elevation, increased blood pressure, influenza, headache, back pain. These effects typically resolve in 6 hours or less
- Lymphocyte counts decreased to approximately 60% of baseline within 4–6 hours after the first dose and continue to decrease over a 2-week period to about 30% of baseline. CBC do not return to normal until 1–2 months

Life-Threatening or Dangerous AEs
- Varicella zoster infections, occasionally severe, after drug withdrawal
- Tumefactive MS lesions have been reported
- Dose-dependent reductions in forced expiratory volume
- Macular edema (0.4% of patients)
- Transient AV conduction delays and syncope (< 1% of patients)
- Four significant cardiac events were observed in clinical trials – it is unclear if these deaths were related to treatment or not

Weight Gain
- Unusual

unusual   not unusual   common   problematic

Sedation
- Unusual

unusual   not unusual   common   problematic

What to Do About AEs

- Due to risk of symptomatic bradycardia with the first dose, give the first dose in a monitored setting after obtaining a baseline pulse and blood pressure. In some cases, overnight monitoring may be needed. Milder effects on heart rate tend to dissipate over 2–4 weeks. The maximum effect usually occurs within 6 hours but may be delayed up to 20 hours
- Avoid live vaccines while on treatment
- Obtain ophthalmological evaluation within a few months after starting treatment
- Low BMI may be a risk factor for lymphopenia during treatment – monitor very thin patients more closely

Best Augmenting Agents to Reduce AEs

- Most AEs are not treatable with medications

DOSING AND USE

Usual Dosage Range
- 0.5 mg daily

Dosage Forms
- Capsules: 0.5 mg

How to Dose
- Take once daily

 Dosing Tips
- May take with or without food

Overdose
- Associated with bradycardia and AV block. Cannot be removed with hemodialysis or plasma exchange

Long-Term Use
- May be used as long as indicated and effective

Habit Forming
- No

How to Stop
- No need to taper, but monitor for worsening of MS or other clinical symptoms

Pharmacokinetics
- The clinical effects are actually caused by the active metabolite, fingolimod-phosphate

- Metabolized by mainly CYP4F2 and excreted in the urine as inactive metabolites
- T_{max} is 12–16 hours and oral bioavailability is 93%
- Steady state blood levels are reached by 1–2 months

 **Drug Interactions**
- Ketoconazole decreases drug metabolism and increases levels
- Use with immunosuppressant agents requires close monitoring for infection or other AEs
- Medications that prolong QTc interval (such as citalopram, chlorpromazine, haloperidol, methadone, erythromycin) may increase risk of torsade de pointes

 Other Warnings/ Precautions
- Multiple subjects developed skin cancers in clinical trials, although it was unclear if this was as a result of fingolimod

Do Not Use
- Known hypersensitivity to the drug or its components
- Recent (in the previous 6 months) myocardial infarction, unstable angina, stroke, transient ischemic attack, heart failure requiring hospitalization, or Class III/ IV heart failure
- Second- or third-degree AV block or sick sinus syndrome (unless patient has a functioning pacemaker), and if baseline QTc interval ≥ 500 ms
- In patients taking Class Ia or Class III antiarrhythmic drugs

SPECIAL POPULATIONS

Renal Impairment
- No contraindication: studies suggest only moderate increases in levels and no change in elimination half-life with severe renal failure

Hepatic Impairment
- Drug levels and effects are greater in those with severe, but not mild to moderate,

hepatic impairment and may increase AEs. Use with caution in those with severe impairment

Cardiac Impairment

- Given potential for adverse cardiac effects, do not use in those with significant heart failure, heart block, or arrhythmia

Elderly

- No known effect but limited experience in those over 65

Children and Adolescents

- Effectiveness and safety are unknown

Pregnancy

- Category C. Multiple malformations have been documented in fetuses exposed in the first trimester. Discontinue 2 months before attempting pregnancy. Otherwise use contraception during and 2 months after treatment

Breast Feeding

- Unknown if present in breast milk. Do not use if breast feeding

---

THE ART OF NEUROPHARMACOLOGY

Potential Advantages

- Oral medication that is highly effective in relapsing MS, even when compared to injectable therapies

Potential Disadvantages

- Potential AEs upon starting treatment and lack of long-term safety data

Primary Target Symptoms

- Preventing relapses and disability from MS

Pearls

- It is the first oral disease-modifying agent for relapsing-remitting MS (RRMS). It impacts the course of RRMS on relapses, MRI lesions, brain shrinkage, and disability progression
- Potential for AEs and need for monitoring may limit use. Home monitoring for initial use may be available through Novartis GILENYA Go program
- Reduces annual clinical relapses by greater than 50% compared to placebo (0.16/year vs. 0.33/year, $p < 0.001$) in clinical trials. Only 17% of the fingolimod-treated patients experienced relapses per year, compared with 30% of placebo
- Prevents new or enlarging T_2 MRI lesions (2.5 vs. 9.0 placebo, $p < 0.001$) and gadolinium-enhancing lesions (0.2 vs. 1.1, $p < 0.001$) over 24 months in clinical trial. Patients with diabetes were excluded from clinical trials
- In one study (the TRANSFORMS study), more effective than continuing interferon-β 1a treatment
- INFORMS study (phase III): fingolimod did not meet the primary endpoint in primary progressive MS
- In patients taking concurrent QTc prolonging medications, consider 24-hour monitoring after the first dose
- There are ongoing clinical trials of fingolimod for the treatment of ALS
- Not more effective than standard care for prevention of rejection post-transplant
- Effective in animal models for prevention of heart failure, cardiac hypertrophy, and arrhythmias
- Effective in 1 small study for improving outcomes after intracranial hemorrhage

Suggested Reading

Chun J, Hartung HP. Mechanism of action of oral fingolimod (FTY720) in multiple sclerosis. *Clin Neuropharmacol.* 2010;33(2): 91–101.

Cohen JA, Barkhof F, Comi G, et al. Oral fingolimod or intramuscular interferon for relapsing multiple sclerosis. *N Engl J Med.* 2010;362(5):402–15.

Kappos L, Radue EW, O'Connor P, et al. A placebo-controlled trial of oral ingolimod in relapsing multiple sclerosis. *N Engl J Med.* 2010;362(5):387–401.

Khatri B, Barkhof F, Comi G, et al. Comparison of fingolimod with interferon beta-1a in relapsing-remitting multiple sclerosis: a randomised extension of the TRANSFORMS study. *Lancet Neurol.* 2011;10(6):520–9.

THERAPEUTICS

Brands
- Sibelium

Generic?
- Yes

Class
- Calcium channel blocker, antihistamine

Commonly Prescribed for
(FDA approved in bold)
- Migraine prophylaxis
- Hemiplegic migraine prophylaxis
- Vasospasm in subarachnoid hemorrhage
- Adjunctive drug for epilepsy
- Vertigo
- Alternating hemiplegia of childhood
- Gilles de la Tourette syndrome
- Tinnitus

How the Drug Works
- Migraine/cluster: proposed prior mechanisms included inhibition of smooth muscle contraction preventing arterial spasm and hypoxia, prevention of vasoconstriction or platelet aggregation, and alterations of serotonin release and uptake.
- Prevention of cortical spreading depression may be one mechanism of action for all migraine preventives
- May also interact with other neurotransmitters, and may inhibit the synthesis and release of nitric oxide
- The drug also appears to act by blocking dopamine D_2 receptors in a manner similar to antipsychotics

How Long Until It Works
- Migraines may decrease in as little as 2 weeks, but can take up to 2 months to see full effect

If It Works
- Migraine: goal is a 50% or greater decrease in migraine frequency or severity. Consider tapering or stopping if headaches remit for more than 6 months or if patient considering pregnancy

If It Doesn't Work
- Increase to highest tolerated dose
- Migraine: address other issues, such as medication overuse, other coexisting medical disorders, such as anxiety, and consider changing to another agent or adding a second agent

Best Augmenting Combos for Partial Response or Treatment-Resistance
- Migraine: for some patients with migraine, low-dose polytherapy with 2 or more drugs may be better tolerated and more effective than high-dose monotherapy. May use in combination with AEDs, antidepressants, natural products, and non-medication treatments, such as biofeedback, to improve headache control

Tests
- Monitor ECG for PR interval

ADVERSE EFFECTS (AEs)

How the Drug Causes AEs
- Direct effects of calcium receptor antagonism and other CNS receptors. Antihistaminic properties likely cause weight gain and sedation. D_2 blockade can cause movement disorders

Notable AEs
- Sedation, depression, weight gain are most problematic
- Nausea, dry mouth, gingival hyperplasia, weakness, muscle aches, and abdominal pain can occur

Life-Threatening or Dangerous AEs
- Severe depression in a minority
- Extrapyramidal side effects and parkinsonism

Weight Gain
- Problematic

Sedation
- Common

What to Do About AEs
- Lower dose or switch to another agent. For serious AEs, do not use

Best Augmenting Agents to Reduce AEs
- Lower dose to 5mg

DOSING AND USE

Usual Dosage Range
- 5–10 mg/day

Dosage Forms
- Tablets: 5, 10 mg

How to Dose
- Migraine: initial dose is usually 10 mg at night. Start at 5 mg in sensitive patients. The dose is generally not increased for migraine prophylaxis

 Dosing Tips
- Take at night to minimize drowsiness

Overdose
- Sedation, weakness, confusion, or agitation may occur. Cardiac AEs, such as bradycardia or tachycardia, have been reported

Long-Term Use
- Safe for long-term use

Habit Forming
- No

How to Stop
- No need to taper, but migraine often returns after stopping

Pharmacokinetics
- Peak levels at 2–4 hours and more than 90% protein bound. Most metabolites are excreted in bile and elimination half-life is about 18 days

 Drug Interactions
- Enzyme inducers such as phenytoin, rifampin may increase clearance and lower levels

- Use with β-blockers can be synergistic and bradycardia, AV conduction disturbance may occur
- May increase risk of GI bleeding with NSAIDs
- May increase levels of carbamazepine
- Excess sedation with other CNS depressants (alcohol, barbiturates) can occur

 Other Warnings/ Precautions
- Similar to antipsychotics (D_2 receptor blockers) may increase prolactin levels

Do Not Use
- Sick sinus syndrome, second- or third-degree heart block
- Severe chronic heart failure, cardiogenic shock, severe left ventricular dysfunction, hypotension
- History of depression, parkinsonism, or porphyria

SPECIAL POPULATIONS

Renal Impairment
- No known effects

Hepatic Impairment
- Flunarizine is highly metabolized by the liver. Start with lower dose and use with caution

Cardiac Impairment
- Do not use in acute shock, severe chronic heart failure, hypotension, and greater than first-degree heart block

Elderly
- May be more likely to experience AEs (sedation)

 Children and Adolescents
- Appears to be effective in pediatric migraine at a dose of 5 mg daily

 Pregnancy
- Category C (all calcium channel blockers). Use only if potential benefit outweighs risk to the fetus

Breast Feeding
- Drug is found in breast milk at high concentrations. Do not breast feed on drug

THE ART OF NEUROPHARMACOLOGY

Potential Advantages
- Effective in both pediatric and adult migraine prophylaxis and possibly effective in epilepsy and schizophrenia

Potential Disadvantages
- Sedation and weight gain can limit use. Not available in the US

Primary Target Symptoms
- Headache frequency and severity
- Seizure frequency and severity
- Hemiplegic attacks

 Pearls
- Effective in reducing migraine frequency at rates comparable to other agents (propranolol, pizotifen)
- There have been investigations of using flunarizine for epilepsy, but the effect was weak and AEs were significant
- Unlike many calcium channel blockers, it does not alter heart rate and is a poor antihypertensive
- Generally more effective than other calcium channel blockers for migraine prophylaxis, but not available in many countries, including the US
- For hemiplegic migraine, flunarizine, verapamil, valproate, lamotrigine, and acetazolamide can be used

 Suggested Reading

Ciancarelli I, Tozzi-Ciancarelli MG, Di Massimo C, Marini C, Carolei A. Flunarizine effects on oxidative stress in migraine patients. *Cephalalgia.* 2004;24(7):528–32.

Hoppu K, Nergårdh AR, Eriksson AS, Beck O, Forssblad E, Boréus LO. Flunarizine of limited value in children with intractable epilepsy. *Pediatr Neurol.* 1995;13(2):143–7.

Lewis DW, Yonker M, Winner P, Sowell M. The treatment of pediatric migraine. *Pediatr Ann.* 2005;34(6):448–60.

Neville BG, Ninan M. The treatment and management of alternating hemiplegia of childhood. *Dev Med Child Neurol.* 2007;49 (10):777–80.

Pelzer N, Stam AH, Haan J, Ferrari MD, Terwindt GM. Familial and sporadic hemiplegic migraine: diagnosis and treatment. *Curr Treat Options Neurol.* 2013;15(1):13–27.

Silberstein SD. Preventive migraine treatment. *Neurol Clin.* 2009;27(2):429–43.

THERAPEUTICS

Brands
- Frova, Migard

Generic?
- Yes

 Class
- Triptan

Commonly Prescribed for
(FDA approved in bold)
- **Migraine**
- Menstrual migraine

 How the Drug Works
- Selective 5-HT$_{1B/1D/1F}$ receptor agonist. In addition to vasoconstriction of meningeal vessels, its antinociceptive effect is likely due to blocking the transmission of pain signals at trigeminal nerve terminals (preventing the release of inflammatory neuropeptides) and synapses of second-order neurons in trigeminal nucleus caudalis

How Long Until It Works
- 2 hours or less

If It Works
- Continue to take as needed. Patients taking acute treatment more than 2 days/week are at risk for medication-overuse headache, especially if they have migraine

If It Doesn't Work
- Treat early in the attack: triptans are less likely to work after the headache becomes moderate or severe, regardless of cutaneous allodynia, which is a marker of central sensitization
- Address life style issues (e.g., stress, sleep hygiene), medication use issues (e.g., compliance, overuse), and other underlying medical conditions
- Change to higher dosage, another triptan, another administration route, or combination of other medications. Add preventive medication when needed
- For patients with partial response or reoccurrence, other rescue medications include NSAIDs (e.g., ketorolac, naproxen), antiemetic (e.g., prochlorperazine, metoclopramide), neuroleptics (e.g., haloperidol, chlorpromazine), ergots, antihistamine, or corticosteroid

 Best Augmenting Combos for Partial Response or Treatment-Resistance
- NSAIDs or neuroleptics are often used to augment response

Tests
- None required

ADVERSE EFFECTS (AEs)

How the Drug Causes AEs
- Direct effect on serotonin receptors

Notable AEs
- Tingling, flushing, dizziness, palpitations, muscle pain, sensation of burning, vertigo, sensation of pressure, nausea. Transient increase in blood pressure

 Life-Threatening or Dangerous AEs
- Rare cardiac events including acute myocardial infaction, cardiac arrhythmias, and coronary artery vasospasm have been reported with frovatriptan

Weight Gain
- Unusual

unusual | not unusual | common | problematic

Sedation
- Unusual

unusual | not unusual | common | problematic

What to Do About AEs
- In most cases, only reassurance is needed. Lower dose, change to another triptan, or use an alternative headache treatment

Best Augmenting Agents to Reduce AEs
- Treatment of nausea with antiemetics is acceptable. Other AEs decrease with time

DOSING AND USE

Usual Dosage Range
• 2.5 mg

Dosage Forms
• Tablets: 2.5 mg

How to Dose
• Tablets: give 1 pill at the onset of an attack and repeat in 2 hours for a partial response or if headache returns. Maximum 7.5 mg/day (3 tablets). Limit 10 days/month

 Dosing Tips
• Treat early in attack

Overdose
• May cause hypertension, cardiovascular symptoms. Other possible symptoms include seizure, tremor, extremity erythema, cyanosis, or ataxia. For patients with angina, perform ECG and monitor for ischemia for at least 48 hours

Long-Term Use
• Monitor for cardiac risk factors with continued use

Habit Forming
• No

How to Stop
• No need to taper. Patients who overuse triptans often experience withdrawal headaches lasting up to several days

Pharmacokinetics
• Half-life about 25 hours. T_{max} 2–4 hours. Bioavailability is 30%. Metabolized by CYP1A2 isoenzymes. 15% protein binding

 Drug Interactions
• Concurrent propranolol use increases peak concentrations

 Other Warnings/ Precautions
• For patients with risk factors predictive of coronary artery disease, it is strongly recommended that administration of the first dose of frovatriptan take place in the setting of a physician's office or similar medically staffed and equipped facility unless the patient has previously received frovatriptan

Do Not Use
• Within 24 hours of ergot-containing medications such as dihydroergotamine
• Patients with proven hypersensitivity to frovatriptan, known cardiovascular disease, uncontrolled hypertension, or Prinzmetal's angina
• Frovatriptan was not studied in patients with hemiplegic and basilar migraine
• May worsen symptoms in ischemic bowel disease

SPECIAL POPULATIONS

Renal Impairment
• No change in pharmacokinetics in patients with moderate renal impairment (CrCl 16–70 mL/min). Use with caution. May be at increased cardiovascular risk

Hepatic Impairment
• Do not use with severe hepatic impairment

Cardiac Impairment
• Do not use in patients with known cardiovascular or peripheral vascular disease. May require cardiac stress test or cardiology clearance if triptans are necessary

Elderly
• May be at increased cardiovascular risk

 Children and Adolescents
• Safety and efficacy have not been established
• Triptan trials in children were negative, due to higher placebo response

 Pregnancy
• Category C. Use only if potential benefit outweighs risk to the fetus. Migraine often improves in pregnancy, and other acute agents (opioids, neuroleptics, prednisone) have more proven safety

Breast Feeding
- Frovatriptan is found in breast milk. Use with caution

THE ART OF NEUROPHARMACOLOGY

Potential Advantages
- Excellent tolerability and low rate of recurrence, even compared to other oral triptans. Less risk of abuse than opioids or barbiturate-containing treatments. Possible lower AEs rate

Potential Disadvantages
- Cost, potential for medication overuse headache. Less effective than other triptans

Primary Target Symptoms
- Headache pain, nausea, photo- and phonophobia

Pearls
- Early treatment of migraine is most effective
- Might have fewer AEs than sumatriptan
- Longer half-life than any other triptan but less effective
- May not be effective when taken during aura, before headache begins

- In patients with "status migrainosus" (migraine lasting more than 72 hours) neuroleptics and dihydroergotamine are more effective
- Triptans were not originally studied for use in the treatment of basilar or hemiplegic migraine
- Patients taking triptans more than 10 days/month are at increased risk of medication-overuse headache, which is less responsive to treatment
- Chest and throat tightness are usually benign and may be related to esophageal spasm rather than cardiac ischemia. These symptoms occur more commonly in patients without cardiac risk factors
- Useful for short-term prophylaxis of menstrual migraine at dose of 2.5 twice daily for up to 6 days
- Combination use of SNRI and triptans usually will not lead to serotonin syndrome, which requires activation of 5-HT_{2A} receptors and a possible limited role of 5-HT_{1A}. However, triptans are agonists at the $5\text{-HT}_{1B/1D/1F}$ receptor subtypes, with weak affinity for 5-HT_{1A} receptors and no activity at the 5-HT_2 receptors. Thus, given the seriousness of serotonin syndrome, caution is certainly warranted and clinicians should be vigilant for serotonin toxicity symptoms and signs to insure prompt treatment

Suggested Reading

Dodick D, Lipton RB, Martin V, Papademetriou V, Rosamond W, MaassenVanDenBrink A, et al. Consensus statement: cardiovascular safety profile of triptans (5-HT1B/1D agonists) in the acute treatment of migraine. *Headache.* 2004;44(5):414–25.

Evans RW, Tepper SJ, Shapiro RE, Sun-Edelstein C, Tietjen GE. The FDA alert on serotonin syndrome with use of triptans combined with selective serotonin reuptake inhibitors or selective serotonin-norepinephrine reuptake inhibitors: American Headache Society position paper. *Headache.* 2010;50(6):1089–99.

Ferrari MD, Roon KI, Lipton RB, Goadsby PJ. Oral triptans (serotonin 5-HT(1B/1D) agonists)

in acute migraine treatment: a meta-analysis of 53 trials. *Lancet.* 2001;358(9294):1668–75.

Gladstone JP, Gawel M. Newer formulations of the triptans: advances in migraine management. *Drugs.* 2003;63(21):2285–305.

Silberstein SD, Berner T, Tobin J, Xiang Q, Campbell JC. Scheduled short-term prevention with frovatriptan for migraine occurring exclusively in association with menstruation. *Headache.* 2009;49(9):1283–97.

Wenzel RG, Tepper S, Korab WE, Freitag F. Serotonin syndrome risks when combining SSRI/SNRI drugs and triptans: is the FDA's alert warranted? *Ann Pharmacother.* 2008;42(11):1692–6.

GABAPENTIN

THERAPEUTICS

Brands
- Neurontin, Gabarone, Neupentin, Neurostil, Gralise, Horizant (gabapentin enacarbil)

Generic?
- Yes

 Class
- Antiepileptic drug (AED)

Commonly Prescribed for
(FDA approved in bold)
- **Partial-onset seizures with and without secondary generalization (adjunctive for adults and children 3 years and older)**
- **Pain associated with post-herpetic neuralgia**
- **Moderate to severe primary restless legs syndrome (RLS) in adults (gabapentin enacarbil)**
- Diabetic neuropathic pain
- Allodynia and hyperalgesia
- Fibromyalgia
- Bipolar disorder
- Generalized anxiety disorder
- Alcohol and drug withdrawal
- Insomnia
- Migraine prophylaxis
- Back pain
- Hot flushes (cancer related, postmenopausal)
- Uremic pruritus

 How the Drug Works
- Structural analog of GABA that binds at the $\alpha_2\delta_1$ subunit of voltage-sensitive calcium channels (CACNA2D1) and reduces calcium influx. Modulates calcium channel function but not as a blocker
- Reduces release of excitatory neurotransmitters (glutamate, norepinephrine, calcitonin gene-related peptide [CGRP])
- Increased plasma serotonin levels
- Inactive at GABA receptors and does not affect GABA uptake or degradation

How Long Until It Works
- Seizures: 2 weeks
- Pain/anxiety: days to weeks

If It Works
- Seizures: goal is the remission of seizures. Continue as long as effective and well tolerated. Consider tapering and slowly stopping after 2 years without seizures, depending on the type of epilepsy
- Pain: goal is reduction of pain. Usually reduces but does not cure pain and there is recurrence off the medication. Consider tapering for conditions that may improve over time, i.e., post-herpetic neuralgia or migraine

If It Doesn't Work
- Increase to highest tolerated dose
- Epilepsy: consider changing to another agent, adding a second agent, using a medical device, or a referral for epilepsy surgery evaluation. When adding a second agent, keep drug interactions in mind
- Pain: if not effective in 2 months, consider stopping or using another agent

 Best Augmenting Combos for Partial Response or Treatment-Resistance
- Epilepsy: no major drug interactions with other AEDs. Using in combination may worsen CNS side effects
- Neuropathic pain: can use with TCAs, SNRIs, other AEDs, or opiates to augment treatment response. Gabapentin usually decreases opiate use
- Anxiety: usually used as an adjunctive agent with SSRIs, SNRIs, MAOIs, or benzodiazepines

Tests
- No regular blood tests are recommended

ADVERSE EFFECTS (AEs)

How the Drug Causes AEs
- CNS AEs are probably caused by interaction with calcium channel function

Notable AEs
- Sedation, dizziness, fatigue, ataxia, driving impairment
- In children: emotional lability, hostility, thought disorder, hyperkinesia
- Weight gain, nausea, constipation, dry mouth
- Blurred vision, peripheral edema

Life-Threatening or Dangerous AEs

- Suicidal behavior and ideation
- Drug reaction with eosinophilia and systemic symptoms (DRESS)

Weight Gain

- Not unusual

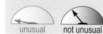

Sedation

- Common

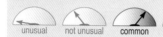

- May wear off with time but can limit titration

What to Do About AEs

- Decrease dose or take a higher dose at night to avoid sedation
- Switch to another agent

Best Augmenting Agents to Reduce AEs

- Adding a second agent unlikely to decrease AEs

DOSING AND USE

Usual Dosage Range

- Epilepsy: 900–1800 mg/day, but can use as much as 3600 mg/day
- Neuropathic pain: 300–1800 mg/day, but can use as much as 3600 mg/day
- RLS: 600 mg at about 5 PM (gabapentin enacarbil)

Dosage Forms

- Tablets: 100, 300, 400, 600, 800 mg
- Capsules: 100, 300, 400 mg
- Liquid: oral solution 250 mg/5 mL

How to Dose

- Epilepsy (ages 12 and older): 900 mg in 3 divided doses, then increase by 300 mg every few days until at goal dose. Maximum time between doses should not exceed 12 hours
- Neuropathic pain: start at 300 mg day 1 and increase by 300 mg every 1–3 days as tolerated to goal dose

 Dosing Tips

- Bioavailability decreases as dose increases, from 60% at 900 mg dose to 27% at 3600 mg dose
- Slow increase will improve tolerability. Increase evening dose first
- Use a slower titration for patients on other medications that can increase CNS side effects
- Twice-daily dosing may improve compliance and can be adequate for treatment of pain or anxiety. The need for 3 times a day dosing increases with higher daily doses
- Avoid taking until 2 hours after antacid administration

Overdose

- No reported deaths. Sedation, blurred vision, ataxia, slurred speech, diarrhea

Long-Term Use

- Safe for long-term use

Habit Forming

- No

How to Stop

- Taper slowly
- Abrupt withdrawal can lead to seizures in patients with epilepsy

Pharmacokinetics

- Renal excretion without being metabolized. Non-linear kinetics. Half-life 5–7 hours. Less than 3% is bound to plasma proteins. Gabapentin enacarbil, a prodrug, has greater bioavailability and linear kinetics

 Drug Interactions

- May increase CNS side effects of other medications
- Antacids decrease the bioavailability of gabapentin
- Cimetidine, naproxen, hydrocodone, and morphine increase the absorption of gabapentin and plasma levels

Other Warnings/ Precautions

- Adenocarcinomas found in male rats
- Emotional lability, hostility, and thought disorder in children ages 3–12

Do Not Use

- Patients with a proven allergy to pregabalin or gabapentin

SPECIAL POPULATIONS

Renal Impairment

- Renal excretion means that lower dose is needed and that hemodialysis will remove
- Adjust dose based on CrCl: < 15 mL/min: 100–300 mg/day once daily, 15–29 mL/min: 200–700 mg/day once daily, 30–59 mL/min: 400–1400 mg/day in 2 divided doses. Patients receiving hemodialysis may require supplemental doses

Hepatic Impairment

- No known effects

Cardiac Impairment

- No known effects

Elderly

- May tolerate lower doses better. More likely to experience AEs

Children and Adolescents

- Start at 10–15 mg/kg/day in 3 divided doses. Increase every 3 days to effective dose. In children aged 3–4 usually 40 mg/ kg/day and age 5 and up 25 mg/kg/day
- May be effective for benign rolandic epilepsy but not absence or generalized tonic-clonic seizures

Pregnancy

- Category C. Some teratogenicity in animal studies. Patients taking for pain or anxiety should generally stop before considering pregnancy
- Supplementation with 0.4 mg of folic acid before and during pregnancy is recommended

Breast Feeding

- Breast milk contains 70–130% of mother's blood drug level
- Generally recommendations are to discontinue drug or bottle feed
- Monitor infant for sedation, poor feeding, or irritability

THE ART OF NEUROPHARMACOLOGY

Potential Advantages

- Safe and wide therapeutic index
- Proven efficacy for multiple types of pain as well as epilepsy
- Relatively low side effects and drug interactions compared to older AEDs

Potential Disadvantages

- Dosing 3 times a day. Sedation. Difficult titration to therapeutic dose
- Non-linear kinetics means bioavailability decreases with dose; higher doses may be well tolerated but may not improve efficacy. Not effective for some primary generalized epilepsies

Primary Target Symptoms

- Seizure frequency and severity
- Pain
- Anxiety

Pearls

- As monotherapy for seizure: adults with partial-onset (Level of Evidence C), elderly with partial-onset (Level of Evidence A), adults with generalized-onset tonic-clonic (Level of Evidence D), benign epilepsy with centrotemporal spikes (Level of Evidence D)
- May be effective in the treatment of allodynia (pain in response to a normally non-painful stimulus) and hyperalgesia (exaggerated response to painful stimuli)
- Multiple potential uses for pain relief, such as pain after burn injury, postoperative pain, reducing opioid requirements in cancer, pain and spasticity in multiple sclerosis, and most forms of neuropathic pain
- 300 mg of gabapentin is about the same as 50 mg of pregabalin, but at higher doses this ratio often does not apply

- Appears to enhance slow-wave delta sleep – adding to effect in pain disorders
- The majority of gabapentin use is for off-label conditions
- Gabapentin enacarbil is effective for RLS and unlike dopamine agonists augmentation does not occur
- Can treat fibromyalgia at doses of 1200–2400 mg/day

- Not usually effective for trigeminal neuralgia
- Insufficient evidence to support its use for migraine prophylaxis. Maybe useful under larger dose
- Used off-label for bipolar disorder, but found ineffective in recent trials

 Suggested Reading

Attal N, Cruccu G, Baron R, Haanpää M, Hansson P, Jensen TS, et al. EFNS guidelines on the pharmacological treatment of neuropathic pain: 2010 revision. *Eur J Neurol.* 2010;17 (9):1113–88.

Bazil CW, Battista J, Basner RC. Gabapentin improves sleep in the presence of alcohol. *J Clin Sleep Med.* 2005;1(3):284–7.

Glauser T, Ben-Menachem E, Bourgeois B, Cnaan A, Guerreiro C, Kälviäinen R, et al. Updated ILAE evidence review of antiepileptic drug efficacy and effectiveness as initial monotherapy for epileptic seizures and syndromes. *Epilepsia.* 2013;54(3):551–63.

Mulleners WM, McCrory DC, Linde M. Antiepileptics in migraine prophylaxis: an updated Cochrane review. *Cephalalgia* 2015;35:51–62.

Silberstein SD, Holland S, Freitag F, Dodick DW, Argoff C, Ashman E. Evidence-based guideline update: pharmacologic treatment for episodic migraine prevention in adults: report of the Quality Standards Subcommittee of the American Academy of Neurology and the American Headache Society. *Neurology.* 2012;78(17):1337–45.

Tzellos TG, Toulis KA, Goulis DG, Papazisis G, Zampeli VA, Vakfari A, et al. Gabapentin and pregabalin in the treatment of fibromyalgia: a systematic review and a meta-analysis. *J Clin Pharm Ther.* 2010;35(6):639–56.

GALANTAMINE

THERAPEUTICS

Brands
• Razadyne, Razadyne ER, Reminyl

Generic?
• Yes

 Class
• Cholinesterase inhibitor

Commonly Prescribed for
(FDA approved in bold)
• **Alzheimer's dementia (AD) (mild or moderate)**
• Dementia with Lewy bodies (DLB)
• Vascular dementia

 How the Drug Works
• Increases the concentration of acetylcholine through reversible inhibition of metabolism by acetylcholinesterase enzyme, which increases availability of acetylcholine. A deficiency of cholinergic function is felt to be important in producing the signs and symptoms of AD
• May also modulate nicotine receptors thereby increasing acetylcholine release
• May interfere with amyloid deposition
• Although symptoms of AD can improve, galantamine does not prevent disease progression

How Long Until It Works
• Typically 2–6 weeks at a given dose, but effect is best observed over a period of months

If It Works
• Continue to use but symptoms of dementia usually worsen over time

If It Doesn't Work
• Consider adjusting dose
• Change to another cholinesterase inhibitor or NMDA antagonist (memantine)
• Non-pharmacological measures are the basis of dementia treatment. Maintain regular schedules and routines. Avoid prolonged travel, unnecessary medical procedures or emergency room visits, crowds, and large social gatherings
• Limit drugs with sedative properties such as opioids, hypnotics, AEDs, and TCAs

• Treat other disorders that can worsen symptoms, such as hyperglycemia or urinary difficulties

 Best Augmenting Combos for Partial Response or Treatment-Resistance
• Addition of the NMDA receptor antagonist memantine may be useful
• Treat depression or apathy with SSRIs but be cautious for increased risk of AEs (e.g., QTc prolongation, injurious falls). Avoid TCAs in demented patients due to risk of confusion. In dementia patients with severe depression, electroconvulsive therapy can be an option
• For significant confusion and agitation avoid neuroleptics (especially in DLB) because of the risk of neuroleptic malignant syndrome. Atypical antipsychotics (e.g., risperidone, clozapine, aripiprazole) or SSRIs can be used instead

Tests
• None required

ADVERSE EFFECTS (AEs)

How the Drug Causes AEs
• Acetylcholinesterase inhibition in the CNS and PNS

Notable AEs
• GI AEs (nausea/vomiting, diarrhea, anorexia and weight loss) are most common
• Fatigue, headache, and dizziness

 Life-Threatening or Dangerous AEs
• Rarely bradycardia or heart block causing syncope
• Generalized convulsions
• Increases gastric acid secretions, which can predispose to GI bleeding
• Exaggerates succinylcholine-type muscle relaxation during anesthesia

Weight Gain
• Unusual

| unusual | not unusual | common | problematic |

• Weight loss is more common

Sedation
- Unusual

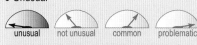

unusual | not unusual | common | problematic

What to Do About AEs
- In patients with dementia, determining if AEs are related to medication or another medical condition can be difficult. For CNS side effects, discontinuation of non-essential centrally acting medications may help. If a bothersome AE is clearly drug-related then lower the dose (especially for GI AEs), titrate more slowly, or discontinue

Best Augmenting Agents to Reduce AEs
- Most AEs do not respond to adding other medications

DOSING AND USE

Usual Dosage Range
- 16–24 mg/day in 2 divided doses for immediate-release formulations or once daily for extended-release capsules

Dosage Forms
- Tablets: 4, 8, 12 mg
- Oral solution: 4 mg/mL in a 100 mL pipette
- Capsules (extended release): 8, 16, and 24 mg

How to Dose
- Immediate release: start at 4 mg twice a day. Increase to 8 mg twice daily after a minimum of 4 weeks. After another 4 weeks can attempt to increase to 12 mg twice daily
- Extended release: start at 8 mg daily. Increase to 16 mg after a minimum of 4 weeks. After another 4 weeks can attempt to increase to 24 mg daily based on assessment of tolerability and clinical benefit

 Dosing Tips
- Slow titration can reduce AEs. Food delays time to peak effect

Overdose
- Symptoms of cholinergic crisis can occur: nausea/vomiting, salivation, hypotension, diaphoresis, convulsions, bradycardia/collapse. May cause muscle weakness and respiratory failure. Atropine with an initial dose of 1–2 mg IV is an antidote

Long-Term Use
- Safe for long-term use. Effectiveness may decrease over time as the dementing illness progresses

Habit Forming
- No

How to Stop
- Abrupt discontinuation can produce worsening of dementia symptoms, memory, and behavioral disturbances. Taper slowly

Pharmacokinetics
- Mainly hepatic metabolism via CYP2D6 and 3A4 isoenzymes. Half-life 7 hours. Maximum effect at 1 hour. About 7% of the population are 2D6 poor metabolizers. These patients excrete a larger percentage unchanged in urine and may need a lower dose. Bioavailability is 90% and plasma protein binding 18%

 Drug Interactions
- Increases the effect of anesthetics such as succinylcholine. Stop before surgery
- Anticholinergics interfere with effect of drug
- Cimetidine may increase bioavailability
- Other cholinesterase inhibitors and cholinergic agonists (bethanechol) may cause a synergistic effect
- CYP2D6 and 3A4 inhibitors, including ketoconazole, cimetidine, paroxetine, and erythromycin, may increase the concentration and effect of galantamine. Enzyme inducers (carbamazepine, phenobarbital, rifampin) may reduce concentration
- Bradycardia may occur when used with β-blockers

 Other Warnings/ Precautions
- Patients and caregivers should be advised to ensure adequate fluid intake during

treatment. If therapy has been interrupted for several days or longer, the patient should be restarted at the lowest dose and the dose escalated to the current dose

Do Not Use
• Hypersensitivity to the drug

Renal Impairment
• For patients with moderate impairment use 16 mg/day. If severe impairment do not use

Hepatic Impairment
• For moderate impairment use 16 mg/day. If severe impairment (Child-Pugh score 10–15), do not use

Cardiac Impairment
• Syncope has been reported. Use with caution in patients with bradyarrhythmias

Elderly
• Slightly higher concentrations than in younger subjects

 Children and Adolescents
• Not studied. AD does not occur in children

 Pregnancy
• Category B. Use only if benefits of medication outweigh risks

Breast Feeding
• Unknown if excreted in breast milk. Do not use

Potential Advantages
• Proven effectiveness for AD. Low risk of hepatotoxicity compared to other acetylcholinesterase inhibitors (tacrine). Relatively low non-GI AEs, even compared to other AD medications. Available as once daily in extended-release form

Potential Disadvantages
• Cost and minimal effectiveness. Does not prevent progression of AD or other dementia

Primary Target Symptoms
• Confusion, agitation, memory, performing activities of daily living

 Pearls
• May be used in combination with memantine with good effect, but combining with other cholinesterase inhibitors is not recommended
• In most clinical trials, all approved medications for AD had a similar rate of benefit
• May be useful for both behavioral problems in AD (delusion, anxiety, and apathy) as well as memory disturbance
• When changing from one cholinesterase inhibitor to another, avoid a washout period which could precipitate clinical deterioration
• May delay the need for nursing home placement
• Insufficient evidence for treating dementia in Parkinson's disease patients
• Actions at nicotinic receptors may enhance release of acetylcholine and other neurotransmitters, improving attention and behaviors
• The effect of galantamine is not dramatic, but patients with DLB might show more benefit
• A recent study shows that it may have slight benefit for vascular dementia
• May be useful for cognitive decline in Down's syndrome
• Via the vagal system, it can activate the efferent cholinergic arm of the anti-inflammatory reflex through a muscarinic receptor-dependent mechanism in the brain

Suggested Reading

Ballard CG, Chalmers KA, Todd C, McKeith IG, O'Brien JT, Wilcock G, et al. Cholinesterase inhibitors reduce cortical Abeta in dementia with Lewy bodies. *Neurology.* 2007;68(20):1726–9.

Bentué-Ferrer D, Tribut O, Polard E, Allain H. Clinically significant drug interactions with cholinesterase inhibitors: a guide for neurologists. *CNS Drugs.* 2003;17(13): 947–63.

Bhasin M, Rowan E, Edwards K, McKeith I. Cholinesterase inhibitors in dementia with Lewy bodies: a comparative analysis. *Int J Geriatr Psychiatry.* 2007;22(9):890–5.

Downey D. Pharmacologic management of Alzheimer disease. *J Neurosci Nurs.* 2008; 40(1):55–9.

Edwards K, Royall D, Hershey L, Lichter D, Hake A, Farlow M, et al. Efficacy and safety of galantamine in patients with dementia with Lewy bodies: a 24-week open-label study. *Dement Geriatr Cogn Disord.* 2007;23(6):401–5.

Levine DA, Langa KM. Vascular cognitive impairment: disease mechanisms and therapeutic implications. *Neurotherapeutics.* 2011;8(3):361–73.

Olin J, Schneider L. Galantamine for Alzheimer's disease. *Cochrane Database Syst Rev.* 2002;3: CD001747.

Seppi K, Weintraub D, Coelho M, Perez-Lloret S, Fox SH, Katzenschlager R, et al. The Movement Disorder Society Evidence-Based Medicine Review Update: Treatments for the non-motor symptoms of Parkinson's disease. *Mov Disord.* 2011;26 Suppl 3:S42–80.

Stahl SM. The new cholinesterase inhibitors for Alzheimer's disease, Part 1: their similarities are different. *J Clin Psychiatry.* 2000;61(10): 710–11.

GLATIRAMER ACETATE

THERAPEUTICS

Brands
- Copaxone, Copolymer 1

Generic?
- No

Class
- Immunomodulator

Commonly Prescribed for
(FDA approved in bold)
- **For reduction of relapses in patients with relapsing-remitting multiple sclerosis (RRMS)**
- Clinically isolated syndromes (CIS)

How the Drug Works
- By modifying the immune processes responsible in part for the development of MS. Glatiramer is a mixture of 4 amino acids thought to approximate the antigenic structure of myelin basic protein (MBP). Experimentally competes with CNS MBP for presentation to T cells
- Induces specific type 2 helper T cells that express anti-inflammatory cytokines

How Long Until It Works
- At least 6 months

If It Works
- Continue to use until RRMS becomes progressive

If It Doesn't Work
- Change to an interferon, reconsider the diagnosis of RRMS, and consider using natalizumab or mitoxantrone, especially for secondary progressive MS

Best Augmenting Combos for Partial Response or Treatment-Resistance
- Acute attacks are often treated with glucocorticoids, especially if there is functional impairment due to vision loss, weakness, or cerebellar symptoms
- Treat common clinical symptoms with appropriate medication for spasticity

(baclofen, tizanidine), neuropathic pain, and fatigue (modafinil)
- For patients with RRMS refractory to glatiramer (measured by clinical relapses and MRI accumulation of lesions), consider changing to interferon-β (INFβ), natalizumab, or newer oral agents

Tests
- None required

ADVERSE EFFECTS (AEs)

How the Drug Causes AEs
- Except for injection site reactions, the causes of AEs (i.e., chest pain) seen with glatiramer use are unclear

Notable AEs
- Chest pain, usually immediately post-injection, is common and typically lasts less than a minute, with no associated ECG changes or adverse consequences. This usually starts about 1 month after initiation of treatment
- About 10% of patients experience immediate post-injection reactions, including anxiety, flushing, dyspnea, throat constriction, and urticaria
- Injection site reactions including erythema, induration, pain, pruritus, welts, inflammation, or hemorrhage
- Fever, neck pain, migraine, agitation, anxiety, sweating, and weight gain are slightly more common in treated patients

Life-Threatening or Dangerous AEs
- None

Weight Gain
- Not unusual

unusual | not unusual | common | problematic

Sedation
- Unusual

unusual | not unusual | common | problematic

What to Do About AEs
- The chest pain and post-injection reactions do not require any specific treatment and

are self-limiting but may cause distress for the patient. If AEs are bothersome enough, consider changing to another disease-modifying agent

Best Augmenting Agents to Reduce AEs

- Most AEs cannot be reduced with an augmenting agent

 Other Warnings/ Precautions

- In theory, can interfere with normal immune function. No evidence of this to date

Do Not Use

- Known hypersensitivity to the drug or to mannitol

DOSING AND USE

Usual Dosage Range

- 20 mg daily or 40 mg 3 times weekly

Dosage Forms

- Injection: 20, 40 mg/mL (prefilled syringe)

How to Dose

- Self-inject at a site in the arms, abdomen, hips, or thighs
- Also available as an autoinjector

 Dosing Tips

- Remove from refrigerator for 20 minutes to allow solution to warm to room temperature before injecting

Overdose

- No information available

Long-Term Use

- Safe for long-term use

Habit Forming

- No

How to Stop

- No need to taper

Pharmacokinetics

- Some drug metabolized locally and some enters the lymphatic circulation and regional lymph nodes. It is unclear how much drug reaches the systemic circulation

 Drug Interactions

- In general, do not combine with other immunosuppressant medications

SPECIAL POPULATIONS

Renal Impairment

- No known effects

Hepatic Impairment

- No known effects

Cardiac Impairment

- No known effects

Elderly

- No known effects

 Children and Adolescents

- Not studied in initial trials, but has been used since with AEs similar to those of adults. Disease-modifying therapy appears to have benefit in reducing long-term cognitive and physical disability from RRMS; it is reasonable to offer treatment early in the disease course

 Pregnancy

- Category B. Use in pregnancy only if clearly needed. In most cases, it is discontinued and corticosteroids are used for acute relapses during pregnancy

Breast Feeding

- Unknown if excreted in breast milk. Use with caution

THE ART OF NEUROPHARMACOLOGY

Potential Advantages

- Excellent initial treatment option for RRMS. Lower incidence of AEs compared to interferons (including flu-like symptoms, depression, fever, myalgias, and liver function abnormalities). Neutralizing antibodies do not occur. Likely safe in pregnancy

Potential Disadvantages

- Probably not effective for most progressive forms of MS and not always effective in RRMS. Injection site reactions

Primary Target Symptoms

- Decrease in relapse rates, delay/prevention of disability, and slower accumulation of lesions on MRI

 Pearls

- It reduces RRMS activity, relapse rate, and MRI progression. Similar efficacy to INFβ-1a or INFβ-1b in RRMS. It delays the conversion of CIS to clinically definite MS. Benefits can be sustained up to 15 years so far. It may promote remyelination
- One large study suggested that glatiramer is ineffective for primary progressive MS

- Glatiramer and INFβ probably have greater safety profile but lesser efficacy than natalizumab and fingolimod
- Combination therapy may have a role. However, combination of glatiramer and INFβ was not superior to glatiramer alone in RRMS
- MRI studies and clinical experience demonstrate that RRMS usually changes over time into secondary progressive MS, which has a more degenerative than inflammatory course. There is no evidence for using glatiramer in any progressive form of MS, but it could be useful for some patients who have an inflammatory component and acute relapses
- Early treatment of RRMS with disease-modifying therapies is superior to placebo. Given that early intervention leads to better outcome in RRMS, consider using glatiramer for patients with clearly defined, clinically isolated syndromes, especially if there is MRI evidence of progression
- Newer dosing regimen, with injections 3 times weekly, appears to reduce injection site reactions and erythema compared to daily injections

 ## Suggested Reading

La Mantia L, Munari LM, Lovati R. Glatiramer acetate for multiple sclerosis. *Cochrane Database Syst Rev*. 2010;5:CD004678.

Lublin FD, Cofield SS, Cutter GR, Conwit R, Narayana PA, Nelson F, et al. Randomized study combining interferon and glatiramer acetate in multiple sclerosis. *Ann Neurol*. 2013;73(3): 327–40.

Patten SB, Williams JV, Metz LM. Anti-depressant use in association with interferon and glatiramer acetate treatment in multiple sclerosis. *Mult Scler*. 2008;14(3):406–11.

Perumal J, Filippi M, Ford C, Johnson K, Lisak R, Metz L, et al. Glatiramer acetate therapy for multiple sclerosis: a review. *Expert Opin Drug Metab Toxicol*. 2006;2(6): 1019–29.

Scott LJ. Glatiramer acetate: a review of its use in patients with relapsing-remitting multiple sclerosis and in delaying the onset of clinically definite multiple sclerosis. *CNS Drugs*. 2013; 27(11):971–88.

Stuart WH. Combination therapy for the treatment of multiple sclerosis: challenges and opportunities. *Curr Med Res Opin*. 2007;23(6): 1199–208.

Wingerchuk DM. Current evidence and therapeutic strategies for multiple sclerosis. *Semin Neurol*. 2008;28(1):56–68.

Ytterberg C, Johansson S, Andersson M, Olsson D, Link H, Holmqvist LW, et al. Combination therapy with interferon-beta and glatiramer acetate in multiple sclerosis. *Acta Neurol Scand*. 2007;116(2):96–9.

THERAPEUTICS

Brands
- Tenex, Intuniv

Generic?
- Yes

 ### Class
- α_2-adrenergic agonist

Commonly Prescribed for
(FDA approved in bold)
- **Attention deficit hyperactivity disorder (ADHD)**
- **Hypertension**
- Gilles de la Tourette syndrome (GTS)
- Tics
- Neuropathic pain
- Opioid detoxification
- Alcohol withdrawal
- Hypertensive "urgency"
- Post-traumatic stress disorder

 ### How the Drug Works
- A centrally acting α_{2A}-adrenergic agonist. Reduces sympathetic output from CNS, which decreases cardiac output, peripheral vascular resistance, and blood pressure
- Specifically targets α_{2A} receptors in the brainstem vasomotor center, decreasing presynaptic calcium levels and the release of norepinephrine

How Long Until It Works
- ADHD: after 1 week
- Hypertension, withdrawal: less than 2 hours
- GTS: weeks to months

If It Works
- In neurological disorders, such as tics, continue to assess effect of the medication to see if it is still needed

If It Doesn't Work
- GTS/tics: neuroleptics are often effective, but their use should be reserved for patients with significant social isolation or embarrassment

 ### Best Augmenting Combos for Partial Response or Treatment-Resistance
- In hypertension, combine with treatments less likely to cause orthostasis (ACE inhibitors, diuretics)
- Tics and GTS symptoms may change over time. Many patients improve with age. Behavioral and psychological therapies are useful and education and reassurance are all that is needed in mild cases
- Indentify and treat comorbid conditions such as ADHD or obsessive-compulsive disorder

Tests
- Monitor blood pressure and pulse

ADVERSE EFFECTS (AEs)

How the Drug Causes AEs
- Related to α_{2A}-adrenergic agonist effect – hypotension and sedation

Notable AEs
- Dry mouth, drowsiness, dizziness, constipation, weakness, headache, depression, paresthesia, dermatitis, impotence, and syncope

 ### Life-Threatening or Dangerous AEs
- Hypotension, bradycardia, and syncope
- Rapid withdrawal can cause rebound hypertension with increased catecholamine levels

Weight Gain
- Unusual

unusual | not unusual | common | problematic

Sedation
- Common

unusual | not unusual | common | problematic

What to Do About AEs
- Lower the dose and take the highest dose in the evening. Many AEs (especially sedation) decrease with time

Best Augmenting Agents to Reduce AEs

- Most AEs cannot be reduced by an augmenting agent

DOSING AND USE

Usual Dosage Range

- 0.5–2mg/day at night or in 2 divided doses
- ADHD: 1–7mg (0.05–0.12mg/kg target dose range)

Dosage Forms

- Tablets: 1, 2mg
- Tablet, extended release: 1, 2, 3, 4mg

How to Dose

- Hypertension: start with 1mg at night. If effect less than desired, increase to 1mg twice daily or 2mg at night
- ADHD: start with 1mg once daily than adjust in increments of no more than 1mg/week
- GTS/tics: start at 0.5mg/day. Increase by 0.5mg every 3–4 days as needed and tolerated. Average dose is 1.5mg/day. Most patients take the entire dose at night

Dosing Tips

- Start at bedtime only, and if well tolerated (little sedation) can divide doses
- Rebound hypertension usually occurs 2–4 days after discontinuation
- For extended-release tablet, do not crush or chew before swallowing
- Do not substitute for immediate-release tablets on a mg-per-mg basis due to differing pharmacokinetic profiles

Overdose

- Hypotension, bradycardia, drowsiness, and lethargy have been reported. Consider gastric lavage for large quantities. Low dialysis clearance

Long-Term Use

- Safe, but tolerance to antihypertensive effects is common

Habit Forming

- No

How to Stop

- Taper slowly (1mg every 3–7 days) to avoid rebound tachycardia and hypertension. Other withdrawal symptoms may include nervousness and anxiety

Pharmacokinetics

- Half-life is 17 hours, but shorter in younger patients. T_{max} 3 hours (6 hours for extended-release tablet). Bioavailability is 80% (50% for extended-release tablet), with about half of the drug metabolized by CYP3A4/5 into inactive metabolites and the other excreted unchanged in urine

Drug Interactions

- Use with other CNS depressants increases sedation
- Strong CYP3A4 inhibitor (e.g., protease inhibitors, macrolides, azole antifungals, nefazodone) can increase guanfacine concentration
- Strong CYP3A4 inducer (e.g., carbamazepine, phenytoin, phenobarbital, rifampin, glucocorticoid, St. John's wort) can decrease guanfacine concentration

⚠ Other Warnings/ Precautions

- Do not discontinue perioperatively and monitor blood pressure closely
- Skin rash (exfoliative) has been reported

Do Not Use

- Known hypersensitivity to guanfacine or its excipients

SPECIAL POPULATIONS

Renal Impairment

- It may be necessary to reduce the dosage in patients with significant impairment of renal function

Hepatic Impairment

- It may be necessary to reduce the dosage in patients with significant impairment of hepatic function

Cardiac Impairment

- Avoid using in patients with known coronary artery disease, conduction disturbances, recent myocardial infarction, or cerebrovascular events. May worsen sinus node dysfunction and AV block, especially in patients taking other sympatholytic drugs. It does not prolong QTc interval

Elderly

- No known effects

Children and Adolescents

- Children may be more sensitive to CNS AEs than adults. Doses for GTS and tics are similar to those for adults, but titrate more slowly. Consider giving the entire oral dose at night

Pregnancy

- Category B. There are no adequate and well-controlled studies of Intuniv in pregnant women. No fetal harm was observed in rats and rabbits with administration of guanfacine at 4 and 2.7 times, respectively, the maximum recommended human dose. Use only if there is a clear need

Breast Feeding

- It is not known whether guanfacine is excreted in human milk; however, guanfacine is excreted in rat milk. Observe breast-fed infants for sedation and somnolence. Discontinue if possible

---

THE ART OF NEUROPHARMACOLOGY

Potential Advantages

- Fewer AEs than neuroleptics in the treatment of GTS and tic disorders. Less somnolence than clonidine

Potential Disadvantages

- Less effective than neuroleptics for GTS or tics. Hypotension and rebound hypertension may limit use. High discontinuation rate

Primary Target Symptoms

- Tics, ADHD, hypertension

Pearls

- In adolescent patients with severe ADHD, stimulants are more effective. Among non-stimulants, guanfacine has similar efficacy to atomoxetine and modafinil, and superior to bupropion and clonidine
- Small ADHD cohorts ranging from 13 to 17 years of age did not show significant improvement. Guanfacine XR was therefore only approved for patients 6–12 years of age in Canada; FDA approves 6–17 years of age
- Coadministration of guanfacine XR with methylphenidate or amphetamine-based stimulants does not produce unique adverse effects other than from psychostimulants or guanfacine XR alone
- For GTS, only classical antipsychotics are approved by FDA. Centrally acting α_2-adrenergic agonist (clonidine, guanfacine), although being less effective than antipsychotics, has been used as first-line treatment due to lower extrapyramidal side effects, as well as for patients with GTS and ADHD. Guanfacine XR is preferred due to less sedation, longer half-life, and slower rebound hypertension
- Not an imidazoline ligand, which explains the lower incidence of somnolence compared to clonidine and tizanidine
- In children, case reports exist of guanfacine-related behavioral changes, including mania and aggression

Suggested Reading

Elbe D, Reddy D. Focus on guanfacine extended-release: a review of its use in child and adolescent psychiatry. *J Can Acad Child Adolesc Psychiatry.* 2014;23(1):48–60.

Faraone SV. Using meta-analysis to compare the efficacy of medications for attention-deficit/hyperactivity disorder in youths. *P&T.* 2009; 34(12):678–94.

Kurlan RM. Treatment of Tourette syndrome. *Neurotherapeutics.* 2014; 11(1):161–5.

Smith H, Elliott J. Alpha(2) receptors and agonists in pain management. *Curr Opin Anaesthesiol.* 2001;14(5): 513–18.

HALOPERIDOL

THERAPEUTICS

Brands
- Haldol, Haldol Decanoate, Dozic, Serenace

Generic?
- Yes

 Class
- Antipsychotic

Commonly Prescribed for
(FDA approved in bold)
- **Tics in Gilles de la Tourette syndrome (GTS) in adults and children**
- **Psychotic disorders**
- **Refractory severe behavioral problems in children with combative explosive hyperexcitability (oral only)**
- **Short-term treatment in children of excessive motor activity with conduct disorder (oral only)**
- **Schizophrenia (Decanoate only)**
- Acute mania
- Nausea and vomiting
- Acute migraine
- Hiccup
- Delirium
- Behavioral disturbances in dementia
- Augmentation for refractory obsessive-compulsive disorder

 How the Drug Works
- It is a butyrophenone derivative that exerts its function at multiple levels of the CNS
- It is a D_{2-4} inverse agonist (for positive symptoms), 5-HT_{2A} antagonist (for negative symptoms), and α_{1A} antagonist
- Due to negligible affinity for H_1 and M_1 receptors, it has relatively lower risk for sedation, weight gain, and orthostatic hypotension but with more dyskinesia
- Antiemetic action is probably through blocking the dopamine receptors in the chemoreceptor trigger zone

How Long Until It Works
- Psychosis: usually within a week
- GTS: weeks to months
- Acute migraine: usually within hours

If It Works
- Use at lowest effective dose
- Monitor QTc interval
- Continue to assess effect of the medication and if it is still needed

If It Doesn't Work
- Psychosis: increase dose or change to another agent
- GTS: discontinue or change to another agent

 Best Augmenting Combos for Partial Response or Treatment-Resistance
- Tics and GTS symptoms may change over time. Many patients improve with age. Behavioral and psychological therapies are useful. Education and reassurance are all that is needed in mild cases
- Indentify and treat comorbid conditions, such as ADHD or obsessive-compulsive disorder
- In GTS, α_2 agonists such as clonidine, guanfacine, reserpine, and other neuroleptics are also useful
- For intractable migraine, often combined with NSAIDs or dihydroergotamine

Tests
- Monitor weight, blood pressure, lipids, and fasting glucose with chronic use. Obtain blood pressure and pulse before initial IV use and monitor QTc with ECG. Therapeutic level 4–25 mcg/L

ADVERSE EFFECTS (AEs)

How the Drug Causes AEs
- Motor AEs and prolactinemia: blocking of D_2 receptors
- Hypotension: blocking of α_1-adrenergic receptors

Notable AEs
- Most common: dizziness, sedation, dry mouth, constipation, weight gain
- Tachycardia, hypotension, or hypertension
- Akathisia, parkinsonism

Life-Threatening or Dangerous AEs

- Tardive dyskinesias
- Neuroleptic malignant syndrome

Weight Gain

- Not unusual

Sedation

- Common

What to Do About AEs

- Take at night to avoid sedation. For severe AEs, change to another agent
- Rarely causes ECG changes. Use with caution in patients if QTc is above 450 (females) or 440 (males) and do not administer with QTc greater than 500
- If excessive sedation, use only as a rescue agent for intractable migraine in hospitalized patients or when patients can lie down or sleep

Best Augmenting Agents to Reduce AEs

- Give fluids to avoid hypotension, tachycardia, and dizziness
- Give anticholinergics (diphenhydramine or benztropine) or benzodiazepines for extrapyramidal reactions

DOSING AND USE

Usual Dosage Range

- GTS: 0.25–4 mg/day
- Migraine: 2–5 mg 3–4 times daily

Dosage Forms

- Tablets: 0.5, 1, 2, 5, 10, 20 mg
- Solution: 2 mg/mL; 15, 120 mL
- Injection: 5 mg/mL; 1, 10 mL
- Decanoate injection (extended release): 50 or 100 mg/mL; 1, 2, 5 mL

How to Dose

- GTS: Start at 0.25–0.5 mg/day and increase slowly as needed to 3–4 mg/day if tolerated, depending on symptom relief

- Migraine: Give IV/IM or oral. Up to 5 mg 3–4 times daily for acute headache

 Dosing Tips

- Low doses are often effective in GTS and can be given as a once-daily dose at night
- For migraine, use often in hospitalized patients while monitoring blood pressure, pulse, and daily ECG

Overdose

- CNS depression, hypotension, and extrapyramidal reactions are most common. Respiratory suppression or death is rare

Long-Term Use

- Safe for long-term use but may cause irreversible AEs (tardive dyskinesias)

Habit Forming

- No

How to Stop

- No need to taper, but GTS/tics often recur

Pharmacokinetics

- Metabolized by liver via glucuronidation and P450 system (CYP3A4, 2D6). Half-life 3 weeks, 92% protein bound

 Drug Interactions

- Use with CNS depressants (barbiturates, opiates, general anesthetics) potentiates CNS AEs
- Strong CYP3A4 inhibitor (e.g., protease inhibitor, macrolide, azole antifungals, nefazodone) and moderate CYP3A4 inhibitor (e.g., aprepitant, verapamil, grapefruit juice) can increase drug levels
- Strong CYP2D6 inhibitor (e.g., fluoxetine, paroxetine, bupropion, quinidine) and moderate CYP2D6 inhibitor (e.g., sertraline, duloxetine) can increase drug levels
- CYP enzyme inducer (e.g., dexamethasone, rifampin, carbamazepine, phenytoin, barbiturate, St. John's wort) can lower drug level
- Haloperidol and lithium together may produce encephalopathy similar to neuroleptic malignant syndrome
- May enhance effects of antihypertensives
- Use with alcohol or diuretics may increase hypotension

- May decrease effectiveness of dopaminergic agents
- Reduces effectiveness of anticoagulants
- Greater risk for QTc prolongation, especially if concomitant use of ziprasidone, zuclopenthixol

 Other Warnings/ Precautions

- Use cautiously in patients with Parkinson's disease (PD) or dementia with Lewy bodies (DLB)
- Neuroleptic malignant syndrome is characterized by fever, rigidity, confusion, and autonomic instability, and is more common with typical neuroleptics, such as haloperidol, given IV
- Increased mortality from haloperidol use in elderly patients with dementia-related psychosis

Do Not Use

- Hypersensitivity to drug, CNS depression/ coma, or QTc greater than 500

Renal Impairment

- No dose adjustment needed

Hepatic Impairment

- Use with caution

Cardiac Impairment

- May worsen orthostatic hypotension. Particularly IV form, risk of QTc prolongation and torsade de pointes

Elderly

- Start with lower doses and monitor for hypotension

 Children and Adolescents

- Efficacy and safety unknown for children under age 3. Start at 0.05 mg/kg/day for GTS. Not a first-line agent in migraine

 Pregnancy

- Category C. Limb deformities have been reported. Use only if benefit outweighs risks

Breast Feeding

- Use while breast feeding is generally not recommended

Potential Advantages

- Perhaps the most effective drug in the treatment of GTS and tics

Potential Disadvantages

- Potential for long-term AEs (tardive dyskinesias). Risk of torsade de pointes

Primary Target Symptoms

- Tics, headache, and nausea

 Pearls

- In acute migraine, greater risk of abnormal movement AEs than metoclopramide or prochlorperazine, but less sedation and hypotension than chlorpromazine
- Pretreat or combine with diphenhydramine, 25–50 mg, to reduce rate of akathisia and dystonic reactions. Benztropine is also useful and may be given orally or IM
- Avoid in patients with PD or DLB, but can be used as a one-time dose in patients with florid psychosis (i.e., in emergency room setting)
- Non-pharmacological approaches or clozapine are preferred for chronic psychosis or hallucinations in PD/DLB patients. Olanzapine is not efficacious for psychosis in PD/DLB; long-term use has a greater risk of mortality and cerebrovascular event. Quetiapine has insufficient evidence
- Based on a recent Cochrane review, antipsychotics might be used as an add-on therapy in the treatment of painful conditions. Nevertheless, extrapyramidal and sedating side effects have to be considered before using antipsychotics for treating pain
- Associated with greater infection and mortality risk than risperidone or quetiapine in treating aggression or psychosis in dementia patients

Suggested Reading

Marmura MJ. Use of dopamine antagonists in treatment of migraine. *Curr Treat Options Neurol.* 2012;14(1):27–35.

Schwarz S, Froelich L, Burns A. Pharmacological treatment of dementia. *Curr Opin Psychiatry.* 2012;25(6):542–50.

Seidel S, Aigner M, Ossege M, Pernicka E, Wildner B, Sycha T. Antipsychotics for acute and chronic pain in adults. *Cochrane Database Syst Rev.* 2013;8:CD004844.

Seppi K, Weintraub D, Coelho M, Perez-Lloret S, Fox SH, Katzenschlager R, et al. The Movement Disorder Society Evidence-Based Medicine Review Update: Treatments for the non-motor symptoms of Parkinson's disease. *Mov Disord.* 2011;26 Suppl 3:S42–80.

HEPARIN

THERAPEUTICS

Brands
- Hep-lock, Hepflush

Generic?
- Yes

Class
- Anticoagulant

Commonly Prescribed for
(FDA approved in bold)
- **Deep venous thrombosis (DVT)/pulmonary embolism (PE)**
- **Atrial fibrillation with embolization**
- **Prevention of evolving thrombosis in acute ischemic stroke (AIS)**
- **Coagulopathies (acute and chronic)**
- **Prophylaxis against postoperative DVT/PE in at-risk patients**
- **Clotting prevention (i.e., during procedures)**
- Prophylaxis of left ventricular thrombi and cerebrovascular accidents post-myocardial infarction (MI)
- Cerebral venous sinus thrombosis (CVST)
- During percutaneous coronary intervention (PCI), to mitigate plaque rupture and reduce thrombosis
- Unstable angina

How the Drug Works
- Inhibits multiple sites in the coagulation system, preventing normal clotting of blood and formation of fibrin clots. Heparin, in combination with antithrombin III, inactivates activated Factor X and prevents the conversion of prothrombin to thrombin
- Larger doses inhibit further coagulation by inactivating thrombin and preventing conversion of fibrinogen to fibrin and inhibiting the activation of fibrin stabilizing factor

How Long Until It Works
- IV bolus: anticoagulant effect is immediate but increases in proportion to dose and duration of use. SC: peak levels occur at 2–4 hours

If It Works
- Monitor for bleeding complications and check activated partial thromboplastin time (aPTT)

If It Doesn't Work
- Patients can still have DVT/PE or IS despite treatment. Check aPTT to determine effectiveness

Best Augmenting Combos for Partial Response or Treatment-Resistance
- Often used with aspirin adjunctively in the setting of acute MI and coronary occlusion
- Usually used in acute setting after cardioembolic IS. Warfarin is usually used for long-term prophylaxis

Tests
- Monitor aPPT to determine effectiveness. Periodically monitor platelet counts and test for occult blood in stool

ADVERSE EFFECTS (AEs)

How the Drug Causes AEs
- Anticoagulation increases bleeding risk, hypersensitivity accounts for most of the other AEs

Notable AEs
- Generalized hypersensitivity (chills, fever, urticaria, rhinitis, headache). Mild thrombocytopenia. Osteoporosis with extended use

Life-Threatening or Dangerous AEs
- Heparin can cause retroperitoneal, adrenal, ovarian, GI, urinary tract, or intracranial bleeding. Complications can be life-threatening. Patients at increased risk include those with liver or renal disease, severe hypertension, bacterial endocarditis, ulcerative colitis, and diverticulitis
- Heparin-induced thrombocytopenia: 5% of patients, 20% mortality. Antibody directed against platelet factor 4 (PF4) causing catastrophic arterial and venous thrombosis. Treat with non-heparin anticoagulant (e.g., agatroban, fondaparinux). New oral anticoagulants (rivaroxaban, apixaban, dabigatran) do not interact with PF4 antibody but have not been studied

- Vasospasm in limbs, up to 6 hours, may occur 6–10 days after initiating therapy
- Hypersensitivity reactions, including asthma, shock, or anaphylaxis

Weight Gain

- Unusual

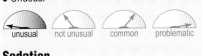

unusual | not unusual | common | problematic

Sedation

- Unusual

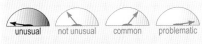

unusual | not unusual | common | problematic

What to Do About AEs

- Stop infusion for serious AEs. Thrombocytopenia is not necessarily dose related. Stop if platelets are below 100 000/mm^3 or if recurrent thrombosis develops. Consider alternative anticoagulants, if patients require them

Best Augmenting Agents to Reduce AEs

- Most AEs cannot be reduced by an augmenting agent

DOSING AND USE

Usual Dosage Range

- 5000–20 000 units (u)/m^2/24 h (as continuous IV infusion)
- 8000–20 000 u every 8–12 hours (SC)

Dosage Forms

- Injection: 1000 u in 500 mL or 2000 u in 1000 mL with 0.9% sodium chloride. With 0.45% sodium chloride, 12 500 u in 250 mL or 25 000 units in 250 or 500 mL
- Multiple-dose vials: 1000, 2000, 2500, 5000, 10 000, 20 000, or 40 000 u/mL
- Single-dose ampules and vials: 1000, 5000, 10 000, 20 000, 40 000 u per mL or 1000, 2500, 5000, 7500, 10 000, or 20 000 u per dose
- Lock flush: 1, 10, or 100 u/mL in 1, 2, 5, or 10 mL syringes

How to Dose

IV infusion: start at 800–1000 u/hour (low dose) for prevention of cardioembolic IS. Goal

aPTT is usually higher for treatment of acute DVT or PE (see below). Perform coagulation tests every 4–6 hours in initial stages and adjust dose based on results

- aPTT < 45, increase by 250 u/hour
- aPTT 45–64, increase by 159 u/hour
- aPTT 65–85, no change
- aPTT 86–110, decrease by 150 u/hour
- aPTT > 110, decrease by 250 u/hour

SC injection for DVT prevention: 5000 u every 8–12 hours for 7 days or until ambulatory

 Dosing Tips

- Note that heparin may increase PT as well as aPTT. This can cause confusion when starting oral anticoagulation. To ensure continuous anticoagulation, continue heparin for a few days after reaching therapeutic INR

Overdose

- Bleeding complications such as nosebleeds, hematuria, and GI bleeding are common. Protamine sulfate can reverse heparin effect

Long-Term Use

- Usually warfarin is preferred

Habit Forming

- No

How to Stop

- No need to taper, but patients will be at increased risk of thromboembolic complications after discontinuation

Pharmacokinetics

- Average half-life is 30–180 minutes but is non-linear and highly dose-dependent: increased with higher doses. Heparin is partially metabolized by the liver and reticuloendothelial system, but up to 50% is excreted unchanged in urine

 Drug Interactions

- Cephalosporins and penicillins may have additive effects and increase bleeding
- Platelet inhibitors including aspirin, NSAIDs, dipyridamole, hydroxychloraquine, dextran, and phenylbutazone interfere with platelet aggregation and may increase bleeding

- Digitalis, nicotine, tetracyclines, and antihistamines may partially counteract the anticoagulant effect of heparin
- Streptokinase administration before initiation may cause resistance to heparin
- May increase PT up to 5 hours after stopping drug. This may cause confusion when using with warfarin

⚠ Other Warnings/ Precautions

- May increase free fatty acid levels by induction of lipoprotein lipase
- Hyperkalemia, probably due to induced hypoaldosteronism, has been reported
- Elevation of hepatic transaminases is common but is unclear if this is related to heparin

Do Not Use

- Hypersensitivity to the drug, active bleeding, and severe thrombocytopenia

Renal Impairment

- Prolongs half-life, patients are more likely to experience bleeding complications. Use with caution

Hepatic Impairment

- Increased risk of bleeding complications due to increased half-life and decreased synthesis of clotting factors

Cardiac Impairment

- No known effects

Elderly

- Women over 60 have a higher rate of bleeding complications

Children and Adolescents

- Start with 50 u/kg bolus followed by 100 u/kg per dose every 4 hours or as continuous infusion 20 000 u/m²/24 h. Safety in newborns is unknown. Low-birth-weight infants are at risk of germinal matrix hemorrhage

Pregnancy

- Category C. Stillbirths and prematurity may occur, but complications are fewer than with warfarin. Heparin (or low molecular weight heparin [LMWH]) is preferred in pregnant patients who require anticoagulation

Breast Feeding

- Not found in breast milk

Potential Advantages

- Immediate effectiveness. Useful for prophylaxis of IS in patients with mechanical heart valves, cardiac thrombus, or atrial fibrillation

Potential Disadvantages

- Not a treatment for acute stroke. Generally used in hospital setting only. Serious bleeding and thrombocytopenia risks require frequent monitoring

Primary Target Symptoms

- Prevention of complications resulting from deep vein thrombosis, pulmonary embolism, or IS

Pearls

- SC heparin 5000 units twice daily appeared to help prevent stroke recurrence with relatively low AEs after IS, but 6-month outcomes were not improved
- Higher doses of heparin are associated with greater AEs, including intracranial hemorrhage
- Delay anticoagulation in the setting of large IS or uncontrolled hypertension due to risk of hemorrhagic transformation
- Heparin does not have fibrinolytic activity; use alteplase for AIS in the treatment window
- When using after cardioembolic IS, monitor patients for changes in exam that may indicate hemorrhagic conversion of stroke
- Large ventricular thrombus is a relative indication to begin heparin shortly after AIS

- LMWH, such as enoxaparin, are an alternative to SC heparin for DVT prophylaxis and can be used at higher weight-based doses for acute DVT or PE. No role for LMWH in the treatment of ischemic stroke
- Stroke/transient ischemic attack and extracranial carotid or vertebral arterial dissection, either antiplatelet or anticoagulant for at least 3–6 months

is reasonable (Class IIa; Level of Evidence B)
- Anticoagulation is reasonable for patients with acute CVST, even in selected patients with intracranial hemorrhage (Class IIa; Level of Evidence B)
- A recent randomized trial on cerebral venous sinus thrombosis, LMWH outperforms unfractionated heparin in hospital mortality

Suggested Reading

Bakchoul T, Greinacher A. Recent advances in the diagnosis and treatment of heparin-induced thrombocytopenia. *Ther Adv Hematol.* 2012; 3(4):237–51.

Kernan WN, Ovbiagele B, Black HR, Bravata DM, Chimowitz MI, Ezekowitz MD, et al. Guidelines for the prevention of stroke in patients with stroke and transient ischemic attack: a guideline for healthcare professionals from the American Heart Association/American Stroke Association. *Stroke.* 2014;45(7):2160–236.

Misra UK, Kalita J, Chandra S, Kumar B, Bansal V. Low molecular weight heparin versus unfractionated heparin in cerebral venous sinus thrombosis: a randomized controlled trial. *Eur J Neurol.* 2012;19(7):1030–6.

INDOMETHACIN

THERAPEUTICS

Brands
- Indocin, Indocin IV, Indocid, Indochron E-R, Indocin-SR, Tivorbex, Indo-Lemmon

Generic?
- Yes

Class
- Non-steroidal anti-inflammatory drug (NSAID)

Commonly Prescribed for
(FDA approved in bold)
- **Relief of mild to moderate acute pain of osteoarthritis, rheumatoid arthritis, ankylosing spondylitis, gout, trauma, fractures, bursitis, tendinitis, renal colic, surgery**
- Migraine, tension-type, and cluster headache
- Indomethacin-responsive headache disorders
- Suppression of uterine activity to prevent premature labor
- Patent ductus arteriosus

How the Drug Works
- Like other NSAIDs, inhibits cyclo-oxygenase (predominantly COX-1) thus inhibiting synthesis of proinflammatory thromboxane (TXA_2) and prostaglandins (PGE_2)
- The reason indomethacin is more effective than other NSAIDs for many headache disorders is unclear, but could be due to its structural similarities to serotonin, central vasoconstrictive and analgesic properties, or lowering of intracranial pressure. It also inhibits the metabolism of an active progesterone metabolite

How Long Until It Works
- Acute migraine: less than 2 hours
- Indomethacin-responsive headache disorders: (preventive) less than a week after starting a given daily dose
- Pain: within 30 minutes

If It Works
- Continue to use

If It Doesn't Work
- Migraine: add triptan, dihydroergotamine, antiemetic, or another NSAID
- Indomethacin-responsive headache disorders: reconsider the diagnosis

Best Augmenting Combos for Partial Response or Treatment-Resistance
- Migraine: combine with triptan or antiemetic

Tests
- None required

ADVERSE EFFECTS (AEs)

How the Drug Causes AEs
- COX-1 is required for maintaining production of prostanoids, including prostacyclin (PGI_2), for GI mucosal protection and platelet aggregation inhibition

Notable AEs
- Dyspepsia, dizziness, nausea, diarrhea most common
- Inhibition of platelet aggregation is usually mild
- Elevation in hepatic transaminases (usually borderline)

Life-Threatening or Dangerous AEs
- GI ulcers and bleeding, increasing with duration of therapy
- May worsen depression, psychiatric disturbances, and parkinsonism
- May increase risk of fluid retention and edema, cardiovascular events, including myocardial infarction and stroke
- Renal insufficiency, proteinuria, and hyperkalemia
- Aseptic meningitis (rare)
- Hypersensitivity reactions: most common in patients with asthma

Weight Gain
- Unusual

unusual   not unusual   common   problematic

Sedation

- Not unusual

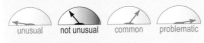

unusual   not unusual   common   problematic

What to Do About AEs

- For significant GI or intracranial bleeding, stop drug. Some AEs respond to lowering dose

Best Augmenting Agents to Reduce AEs

- Proton pump inhibitors may reduce risk of GI ulcers

DOSING AND USE

Usual Dosage Range

- Acute pain: 25–75 mg
- Headache preventive: 25–300 mg daily

Dosage Forms

- Capsules: 25, 50 mg
- Sustained-release capsules: 75 mg
- Oral suspension: 25 mg/5 mL
- Suppository: 50 mg
- Injection (IV): 1 mg/vial

How to Dose

- Acute migraine: give 25–50 mg orally or as suppository for acute pain
- Indomethacin-responsive headaches: start at 75 mg/day (once daily sustained release or 25 mg 3 times daily with meals). If headache does not remit in 48 hours, increase dose in 3 days to 150 mg/day for another 3–10 days. Increase to 225 mg/day (75 mg 3 times daily) if no response. If there is no benefit in less than 2 weeks discontinue drug. Occasional patients will require a higher dose (up to 300 mg/day) or 4 weeks of treatment to improve. For maintenance, slowly reduce to lowest effective dose

 Dosing Tips

- Taking with food decreases absorption and reduces GI AEs

Overdose

- GI distress, drowsiness, paresthesias, and numbness are most common. Severe overdose may cause hypertension, metabolic acidosis, hepatic or renal failure, and cardiac arrest. Consider multiple doses of activated charcoal or hemodialysis for severe cases

Long-Term Use

- Safe for long-term use. In patients with indomethacin-responsive headache disorders, periodically attempt to lower dose

Habit Forming

- No

How to Stop

- No need to taper

Pharmacokinetics

- T_{max} 2 hours. Minimal hepatic metabolism. Half-life is 4.5 hours. Renal excretion 60% and fecal 33%. Bioavailability 100% (oral) and 89–90% (rectal). 97% protein bound. Strong inhibitor of CYP2C9

 Drug Interactions

- Use with alcohol, bisphosphonates, corticosteroids, anticoagulants, and other NSAIDs increases GI bleeding risk
- Cyclosporine and NSAIDs increase risk of nephrotoxicity
- Cholestyramine may decrease absorption
- Aspirin use may decrease NSAID serum levels and increases risk of GI AEs
- May blunt effectiveness of β-blockers and ACE inhibitors
- May decrease effect of loop diuretics and spironolactone
- May increase drug levels of warfarin, amitriptyline, sulfonylureas, NSAIDs, digoxin, aminoglycosides, methotrexate, lithium, and phenytoin

 Other Warnings/ Precautions

- Risk factors for GI bleeding include smoking, alcoholism, older age, poor health status, and treatment with anticoagulants or corticosteroids
- May cause photosensitivity

Do Not Use

- Known hypersensitivity to diclofenac, its excipients, or other NSAIDs
- Treatment with anticoagulants, renal or hepatic disease, age under 12, rectal bleeding, or proctitis (suppositories)
- Use during the perioperative period in the setting of coronary artery bypass graft (CABG) surgery

SPECIAL POPULATIONS

Renal Impairment

- Use with caution in chronic renal insufficiency as may worsen renal function. Use low dose and monitor frequently

Hepatic Impairment

- Use with caution in patients with significant disease. May have increase risk of GI bleeding and toxicity

Cardiac Impairment

- May cause fluid retention and decompensation in patients with cardiac failure. May cause hypertension or lower effectiveness of antihypertensives

Elderly

- More likely to experience GI bleeding or CNS AEs

Children and Adolescents

- Safety in children 14 and under is not established. Do not exceed 150–200 mg/day or 4 mg/kg/day

Pregnancy

- Category B, except category D in third trimester. May prolong pregnancy and increase risk of septal heart defects, incidence of dystocias, and delivery time. May cause premature closure of ductus arteriosus and pulmonary hypertension. Do not use, especially in third trimester

Breast Feeding

- Most NSAIDs are excreted in breast milk. Do not breast feed due to effects on infant cardiovascular system

THE ART OF NEUROPHARMACOLOGY

Potential Advantages

- Fairly effective in many primary headache disorders and the drug of choice for many uncommon primary headache disorders

Potential Disadvantages

- More AEs than other NSAIDs. More COX-1 specific than other NSAIDs such as diclofenac. GI AEs increase with extended use

Primary Target Symptoms

- Headache pain severity with acute use, headache frequency and severity with chronic use

 Pearls

- Indomethacin-responsive headache disorders: hemicrania continua (HC), paroxysmal hemicrania, Valsalva-induced headache (primary cough headache, primary exertional headache, primary headache associated with sexual activity), primary stabbing, hypnic headache
- Indomethacin suppositories are useful for severe migraine with nausea and vomiting
- HC is a continuous unilateral headache disorder, often with autonomic symptoms, that may be confused with migraine or cluster headache. HC responds absolutely to indomethacin, often at low doses (less than 100 mg/day). Patients with constant unilateral headache should receive a trial of indomethacin, which will usually improve HC in a few weeks. Because unilateral headache is common in migraine and other headache disorders, it may be difficult to diagnose HC without an appropriate trial
- Unilateral photophobia may distinguish HC from migraine
- Indomethacin injection may be a more efficient way to diagnose indomethacin-responsive headaches. HC patients usually respond absolutely in a few hours
- Hypnic headache, a disorder of headache during sleep usually occurring later in life, may respond to a bedtime dose of indomethacin
- Indomethacin may lower intracranial pressure for Valsalva-induced headache. It may inhibit trigeminal nociceptive firing and trigeminoautonomic activation for trigeminal autonomic cephalalgias

Suggested Reading

Dodick DW. Indomethacin-responsive headache syndromes. *Curr Pain Headache Rep.* 2004; 8(1):19–26.

Dodick DW, Jones JM, Capobianco DJ. Hypnic headache: another indomethacin-responsive headache syndrome? *Headache.* 2000; 40(10):830–5.

Marmura MJ, Silberstein SD, Gupta M. Hemicrania continua: who responds to indomethacin? *Cephalalgia.* 2009;29(3): 300–7.

Peres MF, Silberstein SD, Nahmias S, Shechter AL, Youssef I, Rozen TD, Young WB. Hemicrania continua is not that rare. *Neurology.* 2001; 57(6):948–51.

VanderPluym J. Indomethacin-responsive headaches. *Curr Neurol Neurosci Rep.* 2015; 15(2):516.

INTERFERON-β (1A AND 1B)

THERAPEUTICS

Brands
- Avonex (1a), Rebif (1a), CinnoVex (1a), Plegridy (1a), Betaseron (1b), Extavia (1b)

Generic?
- No

Class
- Immunomodulator

Commonly Prescribed for
(FDA approved in bold)
- **Reduction of relapses in patients with relapsing forms of multiple sclerosis (MS) (relapsing-remitting [RRMS] or secondary progressive with relapses)**
- Clinically isolated syndromes (CIS)

How the Drug Works
- By modifying the immune processes believed responsible in part for the development of MS. Interferon-β (INFβ) has antiviral and immunomodulatory activities. Produces multiple gene products and markers, including β2-microglobulin, which affect immune function
- It may promote the nerve growth factor for regeneration

How Long Until It Works
- At least 6 months

If It Works
- Continue to use if effective. Monitor AEs

If It Doesn't Work
- Repeat brain MRI, check for neutralizing antibodies, reconsider the diagnosis of relapsing MS, and consider changing to another disease-modifying agent, such as natalizumab, glatiramer, or other newer agents depending on the clinical situation

Best Augmenting Combos for Partial Response or Treatment-Resistance
- Acute attacks are often treated with glucocorticoids, especially if there is functional impairment such as vision loss, weakness, or cerebellar symptoms

- Treat common clinical symptoms in MS with appropriate medication for spasticity (baclofen, tizanidine), neuropathic pain, and fatigue (modafinil)
- For patients with relapsing MS refractory to INFβ, as measured by clinical outcome and MRI accumulation of lesions, consider changing to other agents, such as natalizumab, fingolimod, or other newer agents depending on the clinical situation
- Combined use of INFβ and natalizumab is more effective but may increase the risk of progressive multifocal leukoencephalopathy

Tests
- None required

ADVERSE EFFECTS (AEs)

How the Drug Causes AEs
- Except for injection site reactions, AEs are from INF component of drug

Notable AEs
- Flu-like symptoms, fatigue, weakness or myalgias, chest pain, and headache can occur within hours after starting drug. Long-term use may cause elevation of hepatic enzymes, leukopenia, photosensitivity, or injection site necrosis. Monitor for depression or worsening of existing psychiatric disorders

Life-Threatening or Dangerous AEs
- Hepatic injury, occasionally severe
- Rarely pancytopenia, thrombocytopenia, or autoimmune disorders, such as thyroid disease
- Rarely worsens existing cardiac disease such as angina, congestive heart failure, or arrhythmia

Weight Gain
- Unusual

unusual | not unusual | common | problematic

Sedation
- Not unusual

unusual | **not unusual** | common | problematic

What to Do About AEs

- Most reactions are self-limiting and do not require any specific treatment but may cause some distress for the patient. Some patients have benefited from using anti-inflammatory medications (ibuprofen and naproxen) at the time of injection to decrease the AEs. If AEs are bothersome enough, change to another disease-modifying agent. For more serious AEs, discontinue drug

Best Augmenting Agents to Reduce AEs

- Most AEs cannot be reduced with an augmenting agent

DOSING AND USE

Usual Dosage Range

- INFβ-1a: Avonex: 30 mcg. Plegridy: 125 mcg. Rebif: 22–44 mcg
- INFβ-1b: Betaseron: 250 mcg

Dosage Forms

- Avonex: 30 mcg lyophilized powder or 0.5 mL single-use prefilled syringe or autoinjector
- Plegridy: 63, 94, 125 mcg per 0.5 mL in single-use prefilled syringe or pen
- Rebif: 8.8 mcg in 0.2 mL, 22 or 44 mcg in 0.5 mL prefilled syringe or autoinjector
- Betaseron: 300 mcg lyophilized powder

How to Dose

- Avonex: IM only, inject in the thigh or upper arm once weekly. Start with 7.5 mcg weekly then increase 7.5 mcg weekly until reach 30 mcg
- Plegridy: SC only, inject at different sites every 2 weeks. Start with 63 mcg on day 1, 94 mcg on day 15, 125 mcg on day 29. Then 125 mcg every 14 days
- Rebif: SC only, inject at different sites 3 times weekly, with more than 48 hours between doses. Start at 20% of final dose for 2 weeks, then increase to 50% of dose for 2 weeks. At week 5, start the maintenance dose (either 22 or 44 mcg)
- Betaseron: SC only, inject at different site every other day. Start at 62.5 mcg every other day. Increase over 6 weeks to 250 mcg every other day

 Dosing Tips

- Avonex, Plegridy, Rebif have autoinjectors
- Betaseron comes as a powder (no refrigeration needed), which must be reconstituted in saline before use

Overdose

- No information available

Long-Term Use

- Safe for long-term use

Habit Forming

- No

How to Stop

- No need to taper

Pharmacokinetics

- Clearance mechanism includes catabolism and excretion. Half-life: Avonex 19 hours, Plegridy 78 hours, Rebif 69 hours, Betaseron 8 minutes to 4 hours

 Drug Interactions

- In general, do not combine with other immunosuppressant medications

 Other Warnings/ Precautions

- May worsen existing seizure disorders

Do Not Use

- Hypersensitivity to the drug or human albumin

SPECIAL POPULATIONS

Renal Impairment

- No known effects

Hepatic Impairment

- Use with caution in patients with significant disease

Cardiac Impairment

- No known effects

Elderly

- No known effects

Children and Adolescents

- Not studied in initial trials, but has been used since with AEs similar to those of adults. Disease-modifying therapy appears to have benefit in reducing long-term cognitive and physical disability from RRMS; it is reasonable to offer treatment early in the disease course

Pregnancy

- Category C. Use in pregnancy only if clearly needed. In most cases, it is discontinued and corticosteroids are used for acute relapses during pregnancy

Breast Feeding

- Unknown if excreted in breast milk. Do not breast feed while on drug

THE ART OF NEUROPHARMACOLOGY

Potential Advantages

- Excellent treatment option for relapsing forms of MS. Multiple dosing schedule options. Less chest pain and fewer post-injection reactions than glatiramer

Potential Disadvantages

- Not effective for primary progressive MS. Many AEs, including some that are serious. Flu-like symptoms, depression, fever, myalgias, and liver function abnormalities are more common than with glatiramer. Risk of neutralizing antibodies

Primary Target Symptoms

- Decrease in relapse rates, delay/prevention of disability, and slower accumulation of lesions on MRI

Pearls

- INFβ reduces annual relapse rate and delays the progression of CIS to clinically definite MS. The benefit is dose dependent. However, about 40% of MS patients are non-responders. It is ineffective for primary progressive MS. It also does not prevent the development of permanent physical disability in secondary progressive MS
- SENTINEL study: natalizumab added to INFβ-1a was significantly more effective than INFβ-1a alone in RRMS
- REGARD study: similar efficacy between Rebif and glatiramer acetate in RRMS
- CombiRx study: combining INFβ-1a and glatiramer did not produce significant clinical benefit over 3 years in RRMS. Glatiramer may be superior to INF in reducing the risk of exacerbation
- BENEFIT trial 11-year data suggest favorable outcome in those using INFβ after diagnosis of CIS
- MRI studies and clinical experience demonstrate that relapsing MS usually changes over time into progressive MS, which has a more degenerative than inflammatory course. There is no evidence for using INFβ in non-relapsing forms of MS. Disease-modifying therapy reduces MRI lesions but not brain atrophy
- Neutralizing antibodies are a subset of binding antibodies that can inhibit the activity of INFβ. The incidence of neutralizing antibodies with INFβ therapy varies widely in clinical trials. The prevalence is highest with INFβ-1b and lowest with IM INFβ-1a
- Most patients develop antibodies within the first 3–18 months of treatment. Patients with proven neutralizing antibodies have about double the risk of relapses and have more new lesions on MRI. Check neutralizing antibodies in patients who experience clinical deterioration while being treated with INFβ. Because these antibodies are cross-reactive among the different forms, if patient has neutralizing antibodies, change to a disease-modifying agent that does not contain INFβ
- Plegridy has the longest injection interval due to larger molecule design. Prolonged treatment with Plegridy may induce therapeutic effects that go beyond the immunomodulatory action of INFβ. Has the advantage (compared to Avonex) of less frequent injections (every 2 weeks compared to 1) and SC rather than IM administration

Suggested Reading

Annibali V, Mechelli R, Romano S, Buscarinu MC, Fornasiero A, Umeton R, et al. IFN-β and multiple sclerosis: From etiology to therapy and back. *Cytokine Growth Factor Rev.* 2015;26(2): 221–8.

Cohen JA, Calabresi PA, Chakraborty S, Edwards KR, Eikenhorst T, Felton WL 3rd, et al; ACT Investigators. Avonex Combination Trial in relapsing–remitting MS: rationale, design and baseline data. *Mult Scler.* 2008;14(3):370–82.

Kinkel RP, Dontchev M, Kollman C, Skaramagas TT, O'Connor PW, et al. Association between immediate initiation of intramuscular interferon beta-1a at the time of a clinically isolated syndrome and long-term outcomes: a 10-year follow-up of the Controlled High-Risk Avonex Multiple Sclerosis Prevention Study in Ongoing Neurological Surveillance. *Arch Neurol.* 2012; 69(2):183–90.

La Mantia L, Vacchi L, Di Pietrantonj C, Ebers G, Rovaris M, Fredrikson S, et al. Interferon beta for secondary progressive multiple sclerosis. *Cochrane Database Syst Rev.* 2012;1: CD005181.

Lublin FD, Cofield SS, Cutter GR, Conwit R, Narayana PA, Nelson F, et al. Randomized study combining interferon and glatiramer acetate in multiple sclerosis. *Ann Neurol.* 2013;73(3): 327–40.

Mikol DD, Barkhof F, Chang P, Coyle PK, Jeffery DR, Schwid SR, et al. Comparison of subcutaneous interferon beta-1a with glatiramer acetate in patients with relapsing multiple sclerosis (the REbif vs Glatiramer Acetate in Relapsing MS Disease [REGARD] study): a multicentre, randomised, parallel, open-label trial. *Lancet Neurol.* 2008;7(10):903–14.

Pachner AR, Cadavid D, Wolansky L, Skurnick J. Effect of anti-IFN{beta} antibodies on MRI lesions of MS patients in the BECOME study. *Neurology.* 2009;73(18):1485–92.

Panitch H, Miller A, Paty D, Weinshenker B; North American Study Group on Interferon beta-1b in Secondary Progressive MS. Interferon beta-1b in secondary progressive MS: results from a 3-year controlled study. *Neurology.* 2004;63(10):1788–95.

Rudick RA, Stuart WH, Calabresi PA, Confavreux C, Galetta SL, Radue E-W, et al. Natalizumab plus interferon beta-1a for relapsing multiple sclerosis. *N Engl J Med.* 2006;354(9): 911–23.

INTRAVENOUS IMMUNOGLOBULIN (IVIg)

Brands
- Gamunex, Polygam, Gammagard S/D, Gammagard liquid, Iveegam, Octagam, Flebogamma, Carimune, Panglobulin, Privigen, Gammaked, Bivigam

Generic?
- No

Class
- Immunomodulator

Commonly Prescribed for
(FDA approved in bold)
- **Chronic inflammatory demyelinating polyneuropathy (CIDP) (Gamunex-C, Gammaked only)**
- **Multifocal motor neuropathy (MMN) (Gammagard liquid only)**
- **Primary humoral immunodeficiency (PHI) in adults or children 2 years and older**
- **Immune thrombocytopenic purpura (ITP)**
- **Prevention of bacterial infection associated with B-cell chronic lymphocytic leukemia (Gammagard S/D only)**
- **Prevention of coronary artery aneurysms associated with Kawasaki syndrome in pediatric patients (Gammagard S/D only)**
- **Kidney transplant with a high antibody recipient or with an ABO incompatible donor**
- **Prevention of bacterial infection in pediatric HIV**
- Guillain-Barré syndrome (GBS)
- Myasthenia gravis (MG)
- Inflammatory myopathies: dermatomyositis (DM) and polymyositis (PM)
- Stiff-person syndrome
- Adrenoleukodystrophy
- Paraneoplastic syndromes
- Paraproteinemic immunoglobulin M demyelinating polyneuropathy
- Intractable childhood epilepsy including West syndrome, Lennox-Gastaut and Rasmussen syndromes
- Multiple myeloma
- Acute demyelinating encephalomyelitis (ADEM)
- Optic neuritis and multiple sclerosis (MS)
- Central pontine myelinolysis
- Diabetic amyotrophy
- Peripheral polyneuropathy
- Myelopathy associated with human T-cell lymphotropic virus-1 (HTLV-1) infection
- Wegener's granulomatosis
- Churg-Strauss syndrome
- Amyotrophic lateral sclerosis (ALS)
- Alzheimer's dementia

How the Drug Works
- IVIg preparations are derived from a pool of at least 1000 donors. They contain anti-idiotypic antibodies that bind to and neutralize pathogenic autoantibodies. The infused Ig may downregulate production of endogenous Ig. The Ig from IVIg may block Fc receptors on immune cells
- IVIg contains high-affinity neutralizing antibodies against interleukin (IL)-1a, IL-6, and tumor necrosis factor-α (TNF-α), which may downregulate synthesis of cytokines by T cells
- It forms complexes with products of complement activation, preventing the formation and deposition of attack complexes on target cells
- IVIg also causes transient lymphopenia and reduces the number of natural killer cells

How Long Until It Works
- Days. Usually there is some effect within a week

If It Works
- CIDP and GBS: improves strength and sensory symptoms. In GBS improves prognosis and prevents residual disability
- MG: may allow improvement in symptoms and prevent acute deterioration. Often initiated at the time of a clinical flare, before starting long-term disease-modifying therapy
- MMN: symptoms and conduction block improve, but GM1 antibody titers may remain elevated

If It Doesn't Work
- CIDP and GBS: consider corticosteroids for CIDP. In GBS, plasma exchange (PE) is an alternative
- MG: start or change disease-modifying therapies (usually at the same time as initiating IVIg)

- MMN: if no effect, reconsider the diagnosis, as treatment options for MMN are limited. If the effect of IVIg wears off, consider a short course of PE before repeating dose

 Best Augmenting Combos for Partial Response or Treatment-Resistance

- CIDP and GBS: most patients require corticosteroids for long-term treatment of CIDP. There are small studies that suggest a combination with 500 mg methylprednisolone improves outcomes in GBS
- MG: usually used with symptomatic treatment such as pyridostigmine. Often combined with other disease-modifying agents such as prednisone, azathioprine, cyclophosphamide, mycophenolate mofetil, or cyclosporine
- MMN: cyclophosphamide may be useful in refractory cases

Tests

- Check renal function, CBC before starting treatment and monitor renal function periodically during therapy

ADVERSE EFFECTS (AEs)

How the Drug Causes AEs

- The cause of most AEs, except for hypersensitivity in patients with IgA deficiency, is unknown

Notable AEs

- Headache is the most common AE
- Chest tightness, edema, chills, fever, myalgia, nausea
- Hypotension
- Increased erythrocyte sedimentation rate for 2–3 weeks
- Hyponatremia due to assay error from high protein concentration

 Life-Threatening or Dangerous AEs

- Renal tubular necrosis, renal failure
- Pulmonary edema
- Congestive heart failure
- Serum viscosity (increase up to 0.5 centipoise) and venous thrombosis

- Myocardial infarction
- Posterior reversible encephalopathy syndrome
- Aseptic meningitis
- Anaphylaxis (especially in patients with IgA deficiency)

Weight Gain

- Unusual

Sedation

- Unusual

What to Do About AEs

- Administer at a slower rate
- Change to an alternative formulation of IVIg (individuals have variable AEs to different formulations)

Best Augmenting Agents to Reduce AEs

- NSAIDs are generally effective for headache
- Hydrate and give aspirin before administration in patients with vascular disease or diabetes
- Antihistamines may help prevent hypersensitivity reactions
- Epinephrine should be available to treat anaphylaxis or severe hypotension

DOSING AND USE

Usual Dosage Range

- 1–2 g/kg each dose

Dosage Forms

Powder

- Carimune: powder with sodium chloride/sucrose. 3, 6, 12 g (3%: 498 mOsm/kg)
- Gammagard S/D: powder with glycine/PEG/polysorbate 80. 5, 10 g (5%: 636 mOsm/kg)
- Iveegam: 5 g freeze dried powder for solution

Solution

- Bivigam: 10% (100 mg/mL in polysorbate 80 solution; < 510 mOSM/kg) in 50 and 100 mL vials

- Flebogamma: 5% (50 mg/mL in sorbital/PEG solution; 240–370 mOsm/kg) in 10, 50, 100, 200, 400 mL vials
- Flebogamma: 10% (100 mg/mL in sorbital/PEG solution) in 50, 100, 200 mL vials
- Gamunex-C, Gammaked: 10% (100 mg/mL in glycine solution; 256 mOsm/kg) in 10, 25, 50, 100, 200 mL vials
- Gammagard liquid: 10% (100 mg/mL in glycine solution; 240–300 mOsm/kg) in 10, 25, 50, 100, 200, 300 mL vials
- Gammaplex: 5% (50 mg/mL in glycine/polysorbate 80 solution; 420–500 mOsm/kg) in 50, 100, 200 mL vials
- Octagam: 5% (50 mg/mL in maltose solution; 310–380 mOsm/kg) in 20, 50, 100, 200, 500 mL vials
- Privigen: 10% (100 mg/mL; 240–440 mOsm/kg) in 50, 100, 200, 400 mL vials

How to Dose

- The rate of infusion is based on the formulation. Start at a slow rate (varies; typically < 5 mL/kg/h) and increase after 30 minutes if tolerated and vital signs are normal. The infusions are generally given over 2–5 days
- CIDP: loading: 2 g/kg in divided doses. Maintenance: 1 g/kg in divided doses every 3 weeks
- MMN: 0.5–2.4 g/kg in divided doses per month
- GBS: 2 g/kg in divided doses
- MG: 1–2 g/kg in divided doses
- ITP: 1 g/kg in divided doses
- PHI: 300–600 mg/kg in divided doses every 3–4 weeks. Adjust dose based on target IgG trough level

 Dosing Tips

- Administer more slowly in chronically ill patients or those with renal insufficiency
- IVIg brands differ in their sodium and glucose content

Overdose

- Fluid overload and edema are most common

Long-Term Use

- Appears safe for long-term use

Habit Forming

- No

How to Stop

- No need to taper but monitor for recurrence of neurological disorder

Pharmacokinetics

- Peak action in a few days and half-life of about 3 weeks. 100% bioavailability after IV administration. IgG levels decline to about 40% of peak after 1 week

 Drug Interactions

- Do not give live vaccines within 3 months of IVIg administration

 Other Warnings/Precautions

- Thrombosis may occur
- Renal dysfunction, osmotic nephrosis, acute renal failure, and death may occur

Do Not Use

- Known hypersensitivity to drug or its components, severe renal insufficiency, IgA deficiency, or presence of anti-immunoglobulin antibodies. Privigen is contraindicated in patients with hyperprolinemia

SPECIAL POPULATIONS

Renal Impairment

- Renal dysfunction more common with IVIg products containing sucrose. Use an iso-osmolar brand of IVIg to avoid worsening of renal function. Avoid volume depletion

Hepatic Impairment

- No known effects

Cardiac Impairment

- Use with caution in patients with diabetes or known vascular disease

Elderly

- May be more likely to experience complications. Use a low sodium and glucose brand

Children and Adolescents

- Appears safe and effective in GBS, although experience is limited

Pregnancy

- Category C. Probably safe in pregnancy

Breast Feeding

- Unknown if excreted in breast milk

THE ART OF NEUROPHARMACOLOGY

Potential Advantages

- Rapid onset of action in MG, CIDP, GBS, and many other neurological disorders. Relatively well tolerated, with few long-term AEs

Potential Disadvantages

- Need for repeated IV administration and cost. Effectiveness varies depending on the disorder

Primary Target Symptoms

- Preventive treatment of complications from CIDP, MG, and GBS

Pearls

- Often used as an alternative to PE for similar clinical situations (GBS, MG). In contrast to PE, it does not require large-bore catheters or special equipment, and is safer in the setting of sepsis
- When compared to PE, outcomes in MG and GBS are similar with IVIg. One randomized controlled trial reported similar response between 1g/kg and 2g/kg for MG exacerbation
- It is unclear if a second course of IVIg is beneficial in GBS for patients with suboptimal response to treatment. Low deltaIgG seems to associate with poor outcome
- Unlike GBS, CIDP requires long-term treatment. The use of monthly infusions (usually 1g) for maintenance therapy may be

beneficial, especially if corticosteroids are contraindicated
- MMN usually does not respond to corticosteroids or PE, so IVIg is the first-line treatment. Patients without clear clinical or laboratory features of MMN (i.e., other lower motor neuron syndromes without conduction block) do not usually improve with IVIg
- In a case series examining DM refractory to corticosteroids, IVIg was effective after multiple infusions
- Inclusion body myositis does not typically respond to immunotherapy but open-label and controlled trials report functional improvement with IVIg in a minority of patients
- IVIg is a relatively rapid-acting disease-modifying treatment in MG. Small studies demonstrate effectiveness similar to PE. The role of maintenance infusions is unclear
- Paraproteinemic IgM demyelinating polyneuropathy (MGUS-associated neuropathy) patients showed modest benefit in open-label studies but antibody levels were unchanged
- Intractable childhood epilepsies may respond to treatment with IVIg, based on the assumption that seizures are related to postviral encephalitis. Rasmussen syndrome with glutamate receptor antibodies is one example and 8 of 9 IVIg-treated patients improved in 1 series
- Small series suggest IVIg is effective in stiff-person syndrome, producing clinical improvement and lower antibody titers
- Case reports suggest IVIg is useful for ADEM cases refractory to corticosteroids
- Clinical trials are underway to assess the effect of various IVIg regimens in relapsing-remitting MS
- IVIg appears ineffective in the treatment of ALS and adrenoleukodystrophy
- It is ineffective for Alzheimer's disease but was superior to placebo in apolipoprotein E4 carriers
- Flebogamma DIF, Gammagard S/D, Gammaplex have low IgA ($<$ 10mcg/mL)
- Flebogamma DIF, Gamunex, Gammagard liquid, Gammaked, Privigen contain no sugar and minimal sodium
- Gammagard liquid, Gamunex-C, Gammaked can also be used SC. SC IVIg is under investigation for treating neuromuscular diseases

Suggested Reading

Dalakas MC. The role of IVIg in the treatment of patients with stiff person syndrome and other neurological diseases associated with anti-GAD antibodies. *J Neurol.* 2005;252 Suppl 1:I19–25.

Dalakas MC. Role of IVIg in autoimmune, neuroinflammatory and neurodegenerative disorders of the central nervous system: present and future prospects. *J Neurol.* 2006;253 Suppl 5:V25–32.

Gajdos P, Chevret S, Toyka KV. Intravenous immunoglobulin for myasthenia gravis. *Cochrane Database Syst Rev.* 2012;12: CD002277.

Granata T, Fusco L, Gobbi G, Freri E, Ragona F, Broggi G, Mantegazza R, Giordano L, Villani F, Capovilla G, Vigevano F, Bernardina BD, Spreafico R, Antozzi C. Experience with immunomodulatory treatments in Rasmussen's encephalitis. *Neurology.* 2003;61(12):1807–10.

Léger JM, Viala K, Cancalon F, Maisonobe T, Gruwez B, Waegemans T, Bouche P. Intravenous immunoglobulin as short- and long-term therapy of multifocal motor neuropathy: a retrospective study of response to IVIg and of its predictive criteria in 40 patients. *J Neurol Neurosurg Psychiatry.* 2008;79(1):93–6.

Lünemann JD, Nimmerjahn F, Dalakas MC. Intravenous immunoglobulin in neurology – mode of action and clinical efficacy. *Nat Rev Neurol.* 2015;11(2):80–9.

Simon NG, Ayer G, Lomen-Hoerth C. Is IVIg therapy warranted in progressive lower motor neuron syndromes without conduction block? *Neurology.* 2013;81(24):2116–20.

Tasdemir HA, Dilber C, Kanber Y, Uysal S. Intravenous immunoglobulin for Guillain-Barré syndrome: how effective? *J Child Neurol.* 2006;21(11):972–4.

THERAPEUTICS

Brands
- Vimpat

Generic?
- No

 Class
- Antiepileptic drug (AED)

Commonly Prescribed for
(FDA approved in bold)
- **Partial seizures in patients 17 years or older (monotherapy and adjunctive therapy)**
- Status epilepticus
- Myoclonus
- Diabetic neuropathic pain

 How the Drug Works
- Lacosamide likely acts by enhancing slow inactivation of voltage-gated sodium channels, resulting in stabilization of hyperexcitable neuronal membranes and inhibition of repetitive neuronal firing
- It also binds to collapsin response mediator protein-2 (CRMP-2), which causes changes in axon outgrowth
- Unlike many AEDs, does not appear to affect AMPA, kainate, NMDA, or GABA receptors and does not block potassium or calcium currents

If It Works
- Seizures: goal is the remission of seizures. Continue as long as effective and well tolerated. Consider tapering and slowly stopping after 2 years without seizures, depending on the type of epilepsy

If It Doesn't Work
- Increase to highest tolerated dose
- Epilepsy: consider changing to another agent, adding a second agent, using a medical device, or a referral for epilepsy surgery evaluation. When adding a second agent, keep drug interactions in mind

 Best Augmenting Combos for Partial Response or Treatment-Resistance
- Epilepsy: designed for use with other AEDs. No interactions with AEDs in terms of levels but risk of AEs and hepatic dysfunction increase with polytherapy

Tests
- No regular blood tests are recommended

ADVERSE EFFECTS (AEs)

How the Drug Causes AEs
- CNS AEs are mostly related to changes in sodium channel function

Notable AEs
- Dizziness, ataxia, vomiting, diplopia, nausea, vertigo, blurry vision, and tremor are most common. Palpitations, dry mouth, tinnitus, paresthesias are less common. Injection site pain and erythema with IV administration
- Increase in hepatic transaminases in about 0.7% of patients. More common in patients on multiple AEDs

 Life-Threatening or Dangerous AEs
- Hepatitis, neutropenia (both rare)
- Risk of behavioral or mood effects including depression, suicidal ideation
- Rare PR prolongation and first-degree AV block, atrial fibrillation or flutter. Does not affect QTc interval
- Multi-organ hypersensitivity reactions

Weight Gain
- Unusual

unusual | not unusual | common | problematic

Sedation
- Not unusual

unusual | not unusual | common | problematic

What to Do About AEs
- A small dose decrease may improve most AEs. Titrate more slowly

Best Augmenting Agents to Reduce AEs

- Most AEs can not be reduced by use of augmenting agents

DOSING AND USE

Usual Dosage Range

- Epilepsy: 200–400 mg/day

Dosage Forms

- Tablets: 50, 100, 150, 200 mg
- Injection: 10 mg/mL

How to Dose

- Start at 100 mg/day (50 mg twice a day) for 1 week, then increase by 100 mg/day every week until reaching goal dose of 200–400 mg/day in 2 divided doses

 Dosing Tips

- The IV dose is equal to oral dose and only used in patients unable to take oral medications
- Food does not affect absorption

Overdose

- Little information is available. Hemodialysis would theoretically be useful

Long-Term Use

- Safe for long-term use

Habit Forming

- A Schedule V controlled substance. No physical dependence, but a small minority of patients (less than 1%) report euphoria with doses of 200 mg or more

How to Stop

- Taper slowly (over 1 week) in patients with epilepsy to prevent withdrawal seizures. No need to taper in patients with neuropathy without epilepsy

Pharmacokinetics

- Bioavailability almost 100%. Maximum concentrations at 1–4 hours, with steady state reached after 3 days of twice daily dosing. Elimination half-life is 13 hours.

Metabolized by hepatic P450 system, primarily CYP2C19. Eliminated by renal excretion

 Drug Interactions

- Omeprazole, a CYP2C19 substrate and inhibitor, can theoretically decrease metabolism. Other AEDs (carbamazepine, phenytoin, phenobarbital) may lower serum concentration. These are not clinically significant in studies

 Other Warnings/ Precautions

- May cause syncope

Do Not Use

- Patients with a proven allergy to lacosamide

SPECIAL POPULATIONS

Renal Impairment

- No adjustment is needed except in patients with severe or end-stage renal disease. In patients with severe disease, use maximum of 300 mg/day and give a supplemental 50% of daily dose after hemodialysis sessions

Hepatic Impairment

- Titrate with caution. Usual maximum dose 300 mg/day

Cardiac Impairment

- May cause arrhythmias (AV block, atrial fibrillation, syncope), use with caution

Elderly

- Pharmacokinetics appear fairly similar to other adults with minor difference in drug levels. Monitor for AEs

 Children and Adolescents

- Not studied in children under age 17. The bind of drug to CRMP-2, a phosphoprotein important in neuronal differentiation and control of axonal outgrowth, is poorly understood. Its effect on CNS development is uncertain

Pregnancy

- Risk category C. Relatively low rate of teratogenicity in animal studies compared to other AEDs. Patients taking for pain should generally stop before considering pregnancy
- Supplementation with 0.4 mg of folic acid before and during pregnancy is recommended

Breast Feeding

- Some drug is found in mother's breast milk
- Generally recommendations are to discontinue drug or bottle feed
- Monitor infant for sedation, poor feeding, or irritability

THE ART OF NEUROPHARMACOLOGY

Potential Advantages

- Effective as an adjunctive agent with 2 new mechanisms of action and no significant interactions with other AEDs. Interchangeable dosing during oral–IV

replacement therapy. Generally well tolerated and available IV

Potential Disadvantages

- Less is known about usefulness in many common types of epilepsy

Primary Target Symptoms

- Seizure frequency and severity

 Pearls

- AEs appear to be dose related. The 600 mg dose in clinical trials was associated with much higher rates of tremor, dizziness, fatigue, vomiting, and ataxia
- Potentially useful treatment (200–400 mg) of partial-onset status epilepticus in humans
- New mechanism. Lacosamide: enhances slow inactivation of sodium channel. Carbamazepine: blocks sodium channels in the fast inactivated state
- Dizziness may be increased when combined with other sodium channel blockers
- Limited efficacy in the treatment of diabetic neuropathy

 Suggested Reading

Doty P, Rudd GD, Stoehr T, Thomas D. Lacosamide. *Neurotherapeutics.* 2007;4(1): 145–8.

Harris JA, Murphy JA. Lacosamide: an adjunctive agent for partial-onset seizures and potential therapy for neuropathic pain. *Ann Pharmacother.* 2009;43(11):1809–17.

Hearn L, Derry S, Moore RA. Lacosamide for neuropathic pain and fibromyalgia in adults. *Cochrane Database Syst Rev.* 2012;2: CD009318.

Höfler J, Trinka E. Lacosamide as a new treatment option in status epilepticus *Epilepsia.* 2013 Jan 7;54(3):393–404.

THERAPEUTICS

Brands
- Lamictal, Lamictin

Generic?
- Yes

 Class
- Antiepileptic drug (AED)

Commonly Prescribed for
(FDA approved in bold)
- **Adjunctive therapy in patients ≥ 2 years of age: partial seizure, primary generalized tonic-clonic seizures, Lennox-Gastaut syndrome**
- **Conversion to monotherapy for partial seizures in patients ≥ 16 years of age**
- **Maintenance of bipolar II disorder in patients ≥ 18 years of age**
- Generalized tonic-clonic seizures including juvenile myoclonic epilepsy
- Absence seizures (children and adults)
- Temporal lobe epilepsy (children and adults)
- Migraine with aura
- SUNCT (short-lasting unilateral neuralgiform headache with conjunctival injection and tearing)
- Post-stroke pain
- Trigeminal neuralgia
- Bipolar depression or mania
- Psychosis/schizophrenia (adjunctive)
- Obesity

 How the Drug Works
- Inhibits voltage-sensitive sodium channels and calcium (N, P/Q, R, T types) channels
- Suppresses NMDA, AMPA receptors and GABA$_A$ receptors
- Weakly inhibits serotonin 5-HT$_3$ receptors

How Long Until It Works
- Seizures: should decrease by 2 weeks at a specific dose, but slow titration can delay time to effective dose
- Headaches: weeks to months
- Mania: may take weeks to months

If It Works
- Seizures: goal is the remission of seizures. Continue as long as effective and well tolerated. Consider tapering and slowly stopping after 2 years without seizures, depending on the type of epilepsy
- Headache: goal is a 50% or greater decrease in frequency or severity of pain or aura

If It Doesn't Work
- Increase to highest tolerated dose
- Epilepsy: consider changing to another agent, adding a second agent, using a medical device, or a referral for epilepsy surgery evaluation. When adding a second agent, keep drug interactions in mind
- Headache: if not effective in 2 months, consider stopping or using another agent

 Best Augmenting Combos for Partial Response or Treatment-Resistance
- Epilepsy: drug interactions complicate multi-drug therapy. Increase dose if using with enzyme-inducing drugs and lower when using with valproate. May be particularly effective in combination with valproate
- Headache: consider β-blockers, antidepressants, natural products, other AEDs, and non-medication treatments such as biofeedback to improve headache control

Tests
- No regular blood tests are recommended

ADVERSE EFFECTS (AEs)

How the Drug Causes AEs
- CNS AEs are probably caused by sodium channel blockade effects

Notable AEs
- Rash (usually benign) in about 10%
- Sedation, diplopia, ataxia, headache, tremor, insomnia
- Nausea, vomiting, abdominal pain, constipation
- In children, pharyngitis associated with flu syndrome

Life-Threatening or Dangerous AEs

- Severe dermatological reactions include Stevens-Johnson syndrome, angioedema, toxic epidermal necrolysis, and hypersensitivity. May include fever or multi-organ abnormalities
- Severe reaction in about 1/1000 adults but 8/1000 in children
- Drug reaction with eosinophilia and systemic symptoms (DRESS)
- Rare blood dyscrasias
- Suicidal ideation and behavior
- Aseptic meningitis

Weight Gain

- Unusual

unusual   not unusual   common   problematic

Sedation

- Unusual

unusual   not unusual   common   problematic

What to Do About AEs

- A small dose decrease may improve CNS AEs
- Rashes much more common with high initial dose, rapid dose increases, coadministration with valproate
- Should be discontinued at the first sign of rash, unless the rash is clearly not drug related. Discontinuation of treatment may not prevent a rash from becoming life-threatening. May require hospitalization

Best Augmenting Agents to Reduce AEs

- Topical corticosteroids or antihistamines for rash
- Initially dose at night to avoid sedation

DOSING AND USE

Usual Dosage Range

- Epilepsy: 100–500 mg/day. For patients on valproate, 100–150 mg/day
- Bipolar maintenance: 100–200 mg/day, with lower dose for patients on valproate and higher if on enzyme-inducing AEDs

Dosage Forms

- Tablets: 25, 100, 150, 200 mg
- Chewable dispersion tablets: 2, 5, 25 mg
- Oral disintegrating tablets: 25, 50, 100, 200 mg
- Extended-release tablets: 25, 50, 100, 200 mg

How to Dose

- Monotherapy: start at 25 mg/day (usually at night) for 2 weeks, then increase to 50 mg/day for 2 weeks, then 100 mg and continue to increase as needed by 100 mg/day every 2 weeks until goal dose. On lower dose (50 mg or less) administer once daily at bedtime but on higher doses (over 100 mg) dose twice daily
- With valproate (DPX): start 25 mg every other day, week 3 increase to 25 mg/day, week 5 increase to 50 mg/day, week 6 increase to 100 mg/day if no side effects. If/when DPX dose is lowered then will need to increase dose of lamotrigine
- With enzyme-inducing AEDs (carbamazepine, phenytoin, primidone, phenobarbital): start at 50 mg/day (25 mg twice daily), week 3 increase to 100 mg/day, then increase by 100 mg/day every 1–2 weeks to usual dose of 300–500 mg/day

 ### Dosing Tips

- Slow increase will avoid complication of serious rash
- Patients may need to repeat slow titration when off lamotrigine for more than a few days
- For patients on both lamotrigine and VDPX who are stopping DPX decrease DPX dose by 250/500 mg/day per week. This usually requires increasing lamotrigine dose by about 50%
- For patients on both lamotrigine and enzyme-inducing AEDs, decrease that AED dose slowly and only once the patient is on goal dose of lamotrigine

Overdose

- Coma, ataxia, nystagmus, dizziness in patients with overdoses > 4g. Intraventricular conduction delay. Supportive care and gastric lavage. Hemodialysis may help in severe cases

Long-Term Use
- Safe for long-term use

Habit Forming
- No

How to Stop
- Taper slowly over 2 weeks or more
- Abrupt withdrawal can lead to seizures in patients with epilepsy

Pharmacokinetics
- Metabolized by glucuronic acid conjugation, not via CYP450 system. Bioavailability is 98%. Half-life is 33 hours in adults on single-dose lamotrigine, but 59 hours in epilepsy patients on DPX and 14 hours when used with enzyme-inducing AEDs. May reduce folate by inhibiting dihydrofolate reductase. Renal excretion

Drug Interactions
- DPX increases lamotrigine levels
- Enzyme-inducing AEDs (phenobarbital, phenytoin, carbamazepine) and rifampin decrease levels
- Oral contraceptives (estrogen, not progestin) significantly decrease levels. Use intrauterine system (with or without hormone) instead
- Does not interact with antidepressants, antipsychotics, or lithium

⚠ Other Warnings/ Precautions
- Rash is the most common serious reaction. Avoid starting lamictal at the same time as other medications and discontinue for serious rash. Risk of rash increases with rapid dose increases and in children
- CNS AEs increase when used with other CNS depressants
- Systemic symptoms such as fever, flu-like symptoms, swelling of eyelids along with any dermatological changes require immediate evaluation
- May cause photosensitivity

Do Not Use
- Patients with a proven allergy to lamotrigine

Renal Impairment
- Renal excretion of drug requires lowering of dose. About 55% protein bound. Give supplemental doses after dialysis

Hepatic Impairment
- Patients with moderate to severe disease may need lower dose or slower titration

Cardiac Impairment
- No known effects

Elderly
- May need lower dose. More likely to experience AEs (except rash)

Children and Adolescents
- Lamotrigine extended release: adjunctive therapy for primary generalized tonic-clonic seizure and partial seizure in 13 years or older
- Lamotrigine immediate release: adjunctive therapy for 2 years or older with partial seizures, Lennox-Gastaut syndrome, and primary generalized tonic-clonic seizure
- Children have an increased risk of complicated rash
- With enzyme-inducing AEDs: start 2 mg/kg/ day in 2 divided doses, week 3 increase to 5 mg/kg/day, then increase by 2–3 mg/kg/ day every 1–2 weeks until at goal; usual therapeutic dose 5–15 mg/kg/day in 2 doses
- With DPX: start at 0.15 mg/kg/day, week 3 0.3 mg/kg/day, then increase by 0.3 mg/kg/ day every 1–2 weeks until at goal, typically 1–14 mg/kg/day
- Monotherapy: 0.6 mg/kg/day, week 3 increase to 1.2 mg/kg/day, then increase by 1.2 mg/kg/day every 1–2 weeks until at goal, usually 5–15 mg/kg/day in 2 doses

Pregnancy
- Risk category C. Relatively low rate of teratogenicity in animal studies compared to other AEDs. Patients taking for headache or pain should generally stop before considering pregnancy. For patients with bipolar disorder, risks of relapse may outweigh risks of drug

- Levels usually decrease during pregnancy. Check levels before and periodically during pregnancy to ensure therapeutic dose
- Supplementation with 0.4mg of folic acid before and during pregnancy is recommended

Breast Feeding

- 40–80% of mother's blood drug level found in breast milk
- Generally recommendations are to discontinue drug or bottle feed
- Monitor infant for sedation, poor feeding, or irritability

THE ART OF NEUROPHARMACOLOGY

Potential Advantages

- Effective for multiple types of epilepsy due to broad spectrum of action
- Treats generalized seizures as well as partial and useful in myoclonic epilepsies
- Useful for patients with more than one condition such as epilepsy and mania
- Less likely to cause weight changes than other agents

Potential Disadvantages

- Risk of rash requires a slow titration

Primary Target Symptoms

- Seizure frequency and severity
- Pain
- Recurrent depression or mania in bipolar disorder; impulsivity and aggression

 Pearls

- Effective for most patients with generalized and partial epilepsies and fairly well tolerated
- Effective in about 85% of patients with myoclonic epilepsy, but a minority may worsen
- Not superior to placebo in migraine trials, but multiple case series demonstrated utility for treating bothersome auras in patients with migraine. Consider as a prophylactic agent for migraine with aura in patients who do not respond to or cannot tolerate other agents
- Lamotrigine can help treat SUNCT (short-lasting unilateral neuralgiform headache with conjunctival injection and tearing)
- Effective in maintaining bipolar depression patients, not proven for acute mania
- Most trials using lamotrigine for the treatment of neuropathic and central pain have been negative
- Rash is most common during titration phase, but can be delayed up to a year

 Suggested Reading

Culy CR, Goa KL. Lamotrigine. A review of its use in childhood epilepsy. *Paediatr Drugs.* 2000;2(4):299–330.

Goa KL, Ross SR, Chrisp P. Lamotrigine. A review of its pharmacological properties and clinical efficacy in epilepsy. *Drugs.* 1993;46(1): 152–76.

Harden CL, Pennell PB Koppel BS, Hovinga CA, Gidal B, Meador KJ, et al; American Academy of Neurology; American Epilepsy Society. Practice parameter update: management issues for women with epilepsy – focus on pregnancy (an evidence-based review): vitamin K, folic acid, blood levels, and breastfeeding: report of the Quality Standards Subcommittee and Therapeutics and Technology Assessment Subcommittee of the American Academy of Neurology and American Epilepsy Society. *Neurology.* 2009;73(2):142–9.

Lampl C, Katsarava Z, Diener HC, Limmroth V. Lamotrigine reduces migraine aura and migraine attacks in patients with migraine with aura. *J Neurol Neurosurg Psychiatry.* 2005;76(12):1730–2.

Rosselli JL, Karpinski JP. The role of lamotrigine in the treatment of short-lasting unilateral neuralgiform headache attacks with conjunctival injection and tearing syndrome. *Ann Pharmacother.* 2011;45(1):108–13.

Sabers A, Petrenaite V. Seizure frequency in pregnant women treated with lamotrigine monotherapy. *Epilepsia.* 2009;50(9):2163–6.

Silberstein SD. Preventive migraine treatment. *Neurol Clin.* 2009;27(2):429–43.

LEVETIRACETAM

Brands
- Keppra, Kopodex, Keppra XR

Generic?
- Yes

Class
- Antiepileptic drug (AED)

Commonly Prescribed for
(FDA approved in bold)
- **Adjunctive therapy for partial seizure (≥ 1 month of age), myoclonic seizure (≥ 12 years of age), and primary general tonic-clonic seizures (≥ 6 years of age)**
- Status epilepticus
- Headache prophylaxis
- Seizure prophylaxis after severe traumatic brain injury
- Mania

How the Drug Works
- Binds to synaptic vesicle protein isoform SV2A in the brain, a unique mechanism of action compared with other AEDs. SV2A is involved in synaptic vesicle exocytosis
- Does not appear to affect GABA transmission, sodium channel or potassium channel function. Modulation of N-type calcium and glycine-gated currents
- Effective in rat kindling models

How Long Until It Works
- Seizures: effective within 48 hours at starting dose, and should reduce seizures by 2 weeks

If It Works
- Seizures: goal is the remission of seizures. Continue as long as effective and well tolerated. Consider tapering and slowly stopping after 2 years without seizures, depending on the type of epilepsy
- Headache/pain: goal is a 50% or greater decrease in frequency or severity

If It Doesn't Work
- Increase to highest tolerated dose
- Epilepsy: consider changing to another agent, adding a second agent, using a medical device, or a referral for epilepsy surgery evaluation. When adding a second agent, keep drug interactions in mind

Best Augmenting Combos for Partial Response or Treatment-Resistance
- Epilepsy: commonly used in combination with other AEDs

Tests
- No regular blood tests are recommended

How the Drug Causes AEs
- CNS AEs are probably caused by effects on SV2A synaptic vesicle proteins

Notable AEs
- Sedation, asthenia, nausea, dizziness, headache
- Behavioral symptoms: agitation, hostility, emotional lability, and depression. More common when used in combination with other AEDs or history of a preexisting behavioral disorder

Life-Threatening or Dangerous AEs
- Rare psychotic symptoms or suicidal ideation

Weight Gain
- Unusual

unusual   not unusual   common   problematic

Sedation
- Common

unusual   not unusual   common   problematic

- May wear off with time

What to Do About AEs
- A small dose decrease may improve CNS AEs
- Titrate slowly and start at low dose (500 mg/day)
- Behavioral AEs resolve when medication stopped

Best Augmenting Agents to Reduce AEs

- No treatment for AEs other than lowering dose or stopping drug

DOSING AND USE

Usual Dosage Range

- Epilepsy: 1000–3000 mg/day
- Status epilepticus: 500–1500 mg over 15 minutes

Dosage Forms

- Tablets: 250, 500, 750, 1000 mg
- Oral solution: 100 mg/mL
- Injection: 500 mg/mL diluted in 100 mL. Give over 15 minutes
- Extended release: 500, 750 mg

How to Dose

- Start at 1000 mg/day in twice-daily dosing. Titrate to effective dose by 500–1000 mg/day every 2 weeks
- Start at lower dose (250 mg twice a day or 500 mg extended release) in elderly or chronically ill patients
- For patients with myoclonic seizures, the 3000 mg/day dose is recommended

 Dosing Tips

- Increase PM dose first to avoid daytime sedation
- Effectiveness improves at higher doses up to 3000 mg/day

Overdose

- Somnolence. May worsen seizures at very high doses

Long-Term Use

- Safe for long-term use

Habit Forming

- No

How to Stop

- Taper slowly
- Abrupt withdrawal can lead to seizures in patients with epilepsy

Pharmacokinetics

- Some drug metabolized by enzymatic hydrolysis of acetamide group
- No P450 metabolism. Most excreted renally unchanged
- Low protein binding ($< 10\%$). Half-life is 6–8 hours in healthy patients

 Drug Interactions

- May increase risk of carbamazepine toxicity, unrelated to plasma concentration

 Other Warnings/ Precautions

- Uncommon minor but statistically significant decreases in WBC and neutrophils

Do Not Use

- Patients with a proven allergy to levetiracetam

SPECIAL POPULATIONS

Renal Impairment

- Renal excretion of drug requires lowering of dose
- Mild (CrCl 50–80 mL/min): 500–1500 mg twice daily
- Moderate (CrCl 30–50 mL/min): 500–1000 mg twice daily
- Severe (CrCl < 30 mL/min): 250–500 mg twice daily
- Dialysis patients: 500–1000 mg once a day with 250–500 mg supplemental dose after dialysis

Hepatic Impairment

- No dose adjustment needed

Cardiac Impairment

- No known effects

Elderly

- May need lower dose. More likely to experience AE

Children and Adolescents

Partial seizures:
- 1 month to < 6 months: 7 mg/kg twice daily, titrate 7 mg/kg twice daily every 2 weeks to 21 mg/kg twice daily
- 6 months to < 4 years: 10 mg/kg twice daily, titrate 10 mg/kg twice daily every 2 weeks to 25 mg/kg twice daily
- 4 years to < 16 years: 10 mg/kg twice daily, titrate 10 mg/kg twice daily every 2 weeks to 30 mg/kg twice daily
- The most common AEs in children are behavioral (20% of children)

 Pregnancy

- Risk category C. Teratogenicity in animal studies. Patients taking for pain should generally stop before considering pregnancy
- Levels often change during pregnancy. Check levels periodically during pregnancy to ensure therapeutic dose
- Supplementation with 0.4 mg of folic acid before and during pregnancy is recommended

Breast Feeding

- 80–130% of mother's blood drug level is found in breast milk
- Generally recommendations are to discontinue drug or bottle feed
- Monitor infant for sedation, poor feeding, or irritability

THE ART OF NEUROPHARMACOLOGY

Potential Advantages

- Broad-spectrum AED effective for multiple types of epilepsy. Unique mechanism of action. Safe, easy to combine with other AEDs, lack of significant drug interactions

Potential Disadvantages

- Limited evidence for pain or mood disorders. Rare but bothersome psychiatric symptoms

Primary Target Symptoms

- Seizure frequency and severity

 Pearls

- For patients with excess sedation, or history of AEs on other AEDs, start at lower dose (250 mg twice a day)
- IV form useful in refractory status epilepticus, especially in patients with contraindications to other agents
- Studies suggest particularly useful for photosensitive epilepsies and myoclonic seizures
- May be used for seizure prophylaxis after severe brain injury if treated early
- Unique mechanism of action suggests utility for patients with poor response to other AEDs (such as sodium channel modulators) or in combination with other agents
- Can treat post-myoclonic and post-encephalitic myoclonus
- In patients with preexisting psychotic or severe affective disorders, symptom fluctuation can be hard to differentiate from a potential levetiracetam effect. Given potential for confusion with these symptoms, consider levetiracetam a second-line drug for these patients
- In 1 controlled trial on chronic daily headache treatment, levetiracetam showed insignificant increase in headache-free rate but significant reduction in pain severity and disability than placebo
- In 1 controlled trial on migraine prophylaxis, levetiracetam orally 1000 mg/day for 3 months reduced migraine frequency and severity more than placebo
- Not effective for neuropathic pain

Suggested Reading

Beran RG, Spira PJ. Levetiracetam in chronic daily headache: a double-blind, randomised placebo-controlled study. (The Australian KEPPRA Headache Trial [AUS-KHT]). *Cephalalgia.* 2011;31(5):530–6.

Brophy GM, Bell R, Claassen J, Alldredge B, Bleck TP, Glauser T, Laroche SM, Riviello JJ, Shutter L, Sperling MR, et al. Guidelines for the evaluation and management of status epilepticus. *Neurocrit Care.* 2012;17:3–23.

Glauser T, Ben-Menachem E, Bourgeois B, Cnaan A, Guerreiro C, Kälviäinen R, Mattson R, French JA, Perucca E, Tomson T, *et al.* Updated ILAE Evidence Review of Antiepileptic Drug Efficacy and Effectiveness as Initial Monotherapy for Epileptic Seizures and Syndromes. *Epilepsia.* 2013;54:551–63.

Krauss GL, Bergin A, Kramer RE, Cho YW, Reich SG. Suppression of post-hypoxic and post-encephalitic myoclonus with levetiracetam. *Neurology.* 2001;56(3):411–12.

Lynch BA, Lambeng N, Nocka K, Kensel-Hammes P, Bajjalieh SM, Matagne A, Fuks B. The synaptic vesicle protein SV2A is the binding site for the antiepileptic drug levetiracetam. *Proc Natl Acad Sci USA.* 2004;101(26):9861–6.

Rowe AS, Goodwin H, Brophy GM, Bushwitz J, Castle A, Deen D, Johnson D, Lesch C, Liang N, Potter E, et al. Seizure prophylaxis in neurocritical care: a review of evidence-based support. *Pharmacotherapy.* 2014;34:396–409.

Verma A, Srivastava D, Kumar A, Singh V. Levetiracetam in migraine prophylaxis. *Clin Neuropharmacol.* 2013;36(6):193–7.

Wiffen PJ, Derry S, Moore RA, Lunn MPT. Levetiracetam for neuropathic pain in adults. *Cochrane Database Syst Rev.* 2014;7: CD010943.

LEVODOPA AND CARBIDOPA

Brands
- Sinemet, Sinemet CR, Parcopa, Laradopa (levodopa), Lodosyn (carbidopa), Atamet, Caramet, Co-careldopa, Rytary, Duopa

Generic?
- Yes

Class
- Antiparkinson agent

Commonly Prescribed for
(FDA approved in bold)
- **Treating symptoms of idiopathic Parkinson's disease (PD), post-encephalitic parkinsonism, symptomatic parkinsonism**
- Dopa-responsive dystonia (DRD)
- Restless legs syndrome (RLS)

How the Drug Works
- Levodopa, the metabolic precursor of dopamine, crosses the BBB and is converted by dopa decarboxylase to dopamine in the brain
- Carbidopa is a peripheral decarboxylase inhibitor that prevents levodopa from being metabolized in the gut, increasing CNS dopamine
- In PD, there is a loss of dopaminergic neurons in the substantia nigra and relative excess of cholinergic input. In DRD, there is a deficiency of tetrahydrobiopterin, a cofactor for tyrosine hydroxylase, the rate-limiting enzyme in dopamine synthesis

How Long Until It Works
- PD: hours, but may take 4–8 weeks to receive maximal benefit from a particular dose level when starting
- DRD: usually improves within days or weeks
- RLS: days to weeks

If It Works
- PD: may require dose adjustments over time or augmentation with other agents
- DRD: effective at low doses

If It Doesn't Work
- PD: bradykinesia, gait, and tremor should improve. Non-motor symptoms, including autonomic symptoms such as postural hypotension, depression, and bladder dysfunction, do not improve with carbidopa/levodopa. If the response is poor, reconsider the diagnosis of idiopathic PD and consider drug-induced parkinsonism or atypical parkinsonism syndromes
- RLS: rule out peripheral neuropathy, iron deficiency, thyroid disease. Change to dopamine agonist or another drug

Best Augmenting Combos for Partial Response or Treatment-Resistance
- For end-of-dose failure (wearing-off), early morning or nocturnal akinesia, and end-of-dose dystonia: increase frequency and decrease amount of each dose of medication, add a dopamine agonist with a longer half-life, add a monoamine oxidase (MAO)-B or catechol-*O*-methyltransferase (COMT) inhibitor
- Amantadine may help suppress dyskinesias, although benefit is often short-lived
- For severe motor fluctuations and/or dyskinesias with good "on" time, functional neurosurgery is an option
- For patients with DRD, anticholinergic drugs are also helpful
- For RLS, can change to a different dopamine agonist (pramipexole, ropinirole) or add another drug such as a clonazepam. Gabapentin enacarbil may be beneficial. In severe cases consider opioids

Tests
- May cause elevation of liver enzymes or anemia. Regular blood work may be needed

How the Drug Causes AEs
- Direct effect of levodopa systemically and dopamine in CNS. Carbidopa does not have AEs but can reduce systemic AE (nausea) and increase CNS AE (hallucinations)

Notable AEs
- Nausea/vomiting, orthostatic hypotension, urinary retention, psychosis, depression, insomnia, dry mouth, dysphagia, nightmares, edema, change in urine color, muscle twitching, and blepharospasm.

Rare GI bleeding, hypertension, and hemolytic anemia

 Life-Threatening or Dangerous AEs

- May cause somnolence or sudden-onset sleep, often without warning

Weight Gain

- Unusual

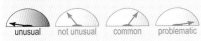

unusual · not unusual · common · problematic

Sedation

- Common

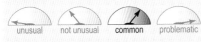

unusual · not unusual · common · problematic

What to Do About AEs

- Nausea can be problematic when starting. Taking after meals will reduce the peak dose and AEs, but delays effect and reduces effectiveness
- For severe peak-dose dyskinesias, use extended-release form, use a dopamine agonist, lower the amount of each levodopa dose, and shorten the dosing interval

Best Augmenting Agents to Reduce AEs

- For nausea, increase dose of carbidopa relative to levodopa
- Memantine and amantadine may help suppress dopa-induced dyskinesias, although long-term benefit is uncertain
- Dopamine agonists are less likely to cause dyskinesias
- Orthostatic hypotension: adjust dose or stop antihypertensives, add dietary salt, and consider droxidopa, fludrocortisone, or midodrine
- Urinary incontinence: reduce PM fluids, voiding schedules, oxybutynin, desmopressin nasal spray, hyoscyamine sulfate, urological evaluation

DOSING AND USE

Usual Dosage Range

- PD: 300–800 mg levodopa with at least 75 mg carbidopa per day

- DRD: lower doses may be effective. 50–200 mg levodopa per day, max 400 mg/day

Dosage Forms

- Carbidopa tablets: 25 mg
- Levodopa tablets: 100, 250, and 500 mg
- Carbidopa/levodopa tablets: 25/100 mg, 10/100 mg, 25/250 mg
- Carbidopa/levodopa controlled release (CR): 25/100 mg, 50/200 mg
- Carbidopa/levodopa orally disintegrating tablets (Parcopa): 10/100 mg, 25/100 mg, 25/250 mg
- Carbidopa/levodopa extended-release capsule (Rytary): 23.75/95, 36.25/145, 48.75/195, 61.25/245 mg
- Carbidopa/levodopa enteral suspension (Duopa): 4.63/20 mg/mL

How to Dose

- Immediate release: start 25/100 3 times per day. Dosage may be increased by 1 tablet every other day up to a dosage of 8 tablets. Provide carbidopa 75–100 mg/day. Maximum 200/2000 mg/day
- Extended release: 50/200 twice a day. Increase by ½ to 1 tablet every other day, up to a dosage of 8 tablets, with interval 4–8 hours while awake. Typically levodopa 400–1600 mg
- Give extra carbidopa for patients with AEs such as nausea or orthostatic hypotension. This will increase CNS dopamine and may require lowering levodopa dose. Watch for worsening hallucinations and dyskinesias
- For RLS: take extended-release form before bedtime

 Dosing Tips

- Take before meals for best effect. Distributing protein throughout the day may help avoid fluctuations. Low protein meals may reduce "wearing-off." CR tablets should be swallowed whole

Overdose

- Monitor for cardiac arrhythmias. Gastric lavage and IV fluids. Pyridoxine may help

Long-Term Use

- Safe for long-term use. Effectiveness may decrease over time in PD (years) and RLS (months)

Habit Forming
- No

How to Stop
- Stopping abruptly will worsen symptoms of PD and lead to confusion, rigidity, and hyperpyrexia similar to neuroleptic malignant syndrome

Pharmacokinetics
- Dopamine is metabolized to dopamine and homovanillic acid in the brain. The peak effect is at 0.5 hours for the immediate-release tablets. Levodopa has a half-life of 50 minutes alone but 90 minutes when taken with carbidopa. The extended-release form has decreased systemic bioavailability (70–75%), decreased maximum concentration, and longer half-life, with peak effect at 2 hours. Absorbed by large neutral amino acid transporter in large intestine and BBB so absorption through gut and across BBB can be affected by protein loads

 Drug Interactions
- Pyridoxine (vitamin B6), benzodiazepines, phenytoin, methionine, papaverine can impair effectiveness of levodopa
- Anticholinergics and TCAs may decrease bioavailability and absorption
- Non-selective MAOIs can cause hypertensive crisis
- Antacids increase bioavailability
- Levodopa may decrease effectiveness of metoclopramide
- Use levodopa with caution in patients on antihypertensive medications due to orthostatic hypotension
- Dopamine receptor antagonists may reduce therapeutic response

⚠ Other Warnings/ Precautions
- May worsen intraocular pressure in patients with chronic wide-angle glaucoma
- Leukopenia, increased incidence of melanoma in PD with or without levodopa treatment have been reported
- May worsen existing peptic ulcers

Do Not Use
- Patients on non-selective MAOIs, narrow angle-closure glaucoma, or known hypersensitivity to the drug

Renal Impairment
- Use with caution but no known effects

Hepatic Impairment
- Use with caution but no known effects

Cardiac Impairment
- Use with caution in patients with known arrhythmias

Elderly
- Safe for use

 Children and Adolescents
- Not studied in children (PD is rare in children)
- Children with DRD usually tolerate well, and dyskinesias are rare

 Pregnancy
- Category C. Teratogenic in some animal studies. Benefit of medication may outweigh risks in some patients

Breast Feeding
- Concentration in breast milk unknown. Breast feeding is not recommended

Potential Advantages
- The most effective symptomatic treatment for PD. Less postural hypotension and fewer hallucinations than dopamine agonists

Potential Disadvantages
- Risk for motor complications, dyskinesias, and response fluctuations after 3–5 years of therapy. Not indicated by FDA for RLS. Need for frequent dosing, especially in late-stage PD

Primary Target Symptoms

- PD: bradykinesia, hand function, gait and rest tremor
- RLS: pain, insomnia

 Pearls

- Levodopa, when given alone, causes severe anorexia and nausea. In clinical practice it is almost always used with carbidopa. Carbidopa has no therapeutic benefit without levodopa
- For patients with mildly symptomatic disease, dopamine agonists are also appropriate for initial therapy, but for patients with significant disability, use carbidopa/levodopa early. For patients with significant symptoms, consider levodopa as a first-line agent
- For elderly, where the risk of dyskinesia is lower, start levodopa early. There is no evidence that delaying the use of levodopa postpones the development of motor complications, especially in the elderly
- Both immediate-release and CR levodopa are effective, although some measures suggest CR is more likely to improve quality of life. Motor complications and dyskinesias can occur with either form
- Carbidopa/levodopa extended-release capsule seems to achieve greater improvement in "off" time than carbidopa/levodopa immediate release or carbidopa/levodopa plus entacapone

- Changing from immediate release to CR does not require changing the daily dose
- For younger patients with bothersome tremor: anticholinergics may help
- Depression is common in PD and may respond to TCAs, pramipexole, or agomelatine
- Cognitive impairment/dementia is common in mid-late stage PD and may improve with cholinesterase inhibitors
- For patients with late-stage PD experiencing hallucinations or delusions, withdraw dopamine agonists and consider oral atypical neuroleptics (quetiapine, olanzapine, clozapine). Acute psychosis is a medical emergency that may require hospitalization
- Not effective for insomnia in PD
- For RLS, carbidopa/levodopa is usually effective but often patients develop tolerance or rebound symptoms in the morning. This phenomenon, called "augmentation," is why dopamine agonists are generally preferred for RLS
- The use of levodopa may be most advantageous for those patients with intermittent RLS symptoms that do not require daily therapy. Vigilance for secondary impulsive behavior as an adverse reaction is needed
- Carbidopa (without levodopa) may have a role in the prevention of hyperdopaminergic crises including nausea and vomiting in familial dysautonomia

Suggested Reading

Aurora RN, Kristo DA, Bista SR, Rowley JA, Zak RS, Casey KR, et al. The treatment of restless legs syndrome and periodic limb movement disorder in adults – an update for 2012: practice parameters with an evidence-based systematic review and meta-analyses: an American Academy of Sleep Medicine Clinical Practice Guideline. *Sleep.* 2012;35(8): 1039–62.

Fox SH, Katzenschlager R, Lim S-Y, Ravina B, Seppi K, Coelho M, et al. The Movement Disorder Society Evidence-Based Medicine Review Update: Treatments for the motor symptoms of Parkinson's disease. *Mov Disord.* 2011;26 Suppl 3:S2–41.

Koller WC, Hutton JT, Tolosa E, Capilldeo R. Immediate-release and controlled-release carbidopa/levodopa in PD: a 5-year randomized multicenter study. Carbidopa/ Levodopa Study Group. *Neurology.* 1999; 53(5):1012–19.

Lang AE. When and how should treatment be started in Parkinson disease? *Neurology.* 2009;72(7 Suppl):S39–43.

Manyam BV, Hare TA, Robbs R, Cubberley VB. Evaluation of equivalent efficacy of sinemet and sinemet CR in patients with Parkinson's disease applying levodopa dosage conversion formula. *Clin Neuropharmacol.* 1999;22(1):33–9.

Olanow CW, Stern MB, Sethi K. The scientific and clinical basis for the treatment of Parkinson disease. *Neurology.* 2009;72(21 Suppl 4): S1–136.

Robbottom BJ, Weiner WJ. Dementia in Parkinson's disease. *Int Rev Neurobiol.* 2009;84:229–44.

Trenkwalder C, Hening WA, Montagna P, Oertel WH, Allen RP, Walters AS, et al. Treatment of restless legs syndrome: an evidence-based review and implications for clinical practice. *Mov Disord.* 2008;23(16):2267–302.

LEVOMILNACIPRAN

THERAPEUTICS

Brands
- Levomilnacipran: Fetzima

Generic?
- No

 Class
- Serotonin and norepinephrine reuptake inhibitor (SNRI)

Commonly Prescribed for
(FDA approved in bold)
- **Major depressive disorder**
- Fibromyalgia
- Post-stroke depression
- Migraine prophylaxis
- Stress urinary incontinence

 How the Drug Works
- Both milnacipran and levomilnacipran (levo-enantiomer of milnacipran) are potent balanced inhibitors of serotonin and norepinephrine reuptake transporters (SERT, NET), increasing serotonin and norepinephrine levels within hours, but antidepressant effects take weeks. Effect is more likely related to adaptive changes in serotonin and norepinephrine receptor systems over time
- No affinity for serotonergic, adrenergic, muscarinic, dopamine, opiate, GABA receptors, and Ca^{2+}, Na^+, K^+, Cl^- channels
- It may modulate NMDA receptors in the superficial dorsal horn for antinociceptive effect
- Unlike venlafaxine or duloxetine where SERT effect dominates, milnacipran exerts a relatively equal influence on SERT and NET whereas levomilnacipran demonstrates a slightly greater NET inhibition than SERT inhibition

How Long Until It Works
- 2 weeks to 2 months for full effect

If It Works
- Continue to use and monitor for AEs

If It Doesn't Work
- Increase to highest tolerated dose. Consider adding a second agent or changing to another one

 Best Augmenting Combos for Partial Response or Treatment-Resistance
- For some patients, low-dose polytherapy with 2 or more drugs may be better tolerated and more effective than high-dose monotherapy

Tests
- Check blood pressure, at baseline and when increasing dose
- Monitor sodium, intraocular pressure, suicidality, and unusual change in behavior

ADVERSE EFFECTS (AEs)

How the Drug Causes AEs
- By increasing serotonin and norepinephrine on non-therapeutic responsive receptors throughout the body. Most AEs are dose- and time-dependent

Notable AEs
- Incidence $\geq$ 5%: nausea, vomiting, headache, constipation, dizziness, insomnia, hot flush, hyperhidrosis, elevated blood pressure, palpitation, urinary hesitancy/retention, and erectile dysfunction

 Life-Threatening or Dangerous AEs
- Serotonin syndrome
- Rare hepatotoxicity
- Rare activation of mania/hypomania or suicidal ideation
- Rare worsening of coexisting seizure disorders
- Abnormal bleeding
- Angle-closure glaucoma

Weight Gain
- Unusual

unusual   not unusual   common   problematic

Sedation
- Unusual

unusual   not unusual   common   problematic

What to Do About AEs

- For minor AEs, lower dose, titrate more slowly, or switch to another agent. For serious AEs, lower dose and consider stopping, taper to avoid withdrawal symptoms

Best Augmenting Agents to Reduce AEs

- Try magnesium for constipation
- Cyproheptadine can be used for serotonin syndrome by blocking 5-HT receptors and SERT
- Sexual dysfunction (anorgasmia, impotence) may be reversed by agents with α_2-adrenergic antagonist activity (e.g., buspirone, amantadine, bupropion, mirtazapine, ginkgo biloba, etc.)

DOSING AND USE

Usual Dosage Range

- 40–120 mg daily

Dosage Forms

- Capsule (extended release); 20, 40, 80, 120 mg

How to Dose

- Starting at 20 mg daily for 2 days, increase to 40 mg daily for 2 days. Based on the tolerability, increase at 40 mg daily every 2 or more days until 120 mg maximum dose
- Food does not affect bioavailability

 Dosing Tips

- Levomilnacipran capsule should be swallowed whole, and not chewed or crushed

Overdose

- In postmarketing experience of milnacipran, the most common signs and symptoms included increased blood pressure, cardio-respiratory arrest, changes in the level of consciousness (ranging from somnolence to coma), confusional state, dizziness, and increased hepatic enzymes. No specific antidote. If serotonin syndrome ensues, cyproheptadine and/or temperature control may be considered

Long-Term Use

- Safe for long-term use with monitoring of blood pressure and suicidality

Habit Forming

- No

How to Stop

- Taper slowly (no more than 50% reduction every 3–4 days until discontinuation) to avoid withdrawal symptoms (agitation, anxiety, confusion, dry mouth, dysphoria, etc.)

Pharmacokinetics

- C_{max} reached in 6–8 hours. Bioavailability 92%. It is metabolized by desethylation, hydroxylation, and conjugation, and eliminated primarily by renal excretion. No stereoisomer interconversion

 Drug Interactions

- Milnacipran
- Dose should be reduced when coadministered with strong CYP3A4 inhibitors (e.g., ketoconazole)
- Alcohol interacts with the capsule. Coadministration of alcohol may lead to accelerated drug release
- The release of serotonin by platelets is important for maintaining hemostasis. Combined use of SSRIs or SNRIs and NSAIDs, and/or drugs that affect platelets or coagulation have been associated with an increased risk of bleeding

 Other Warnings/ Precautions

- May increase risk of seizure
- Patients should be observed closely for clinical worsening, suicidality, and changes in behavior in known or unknown bipolar disorder

Do Not Use

- Proven hypersensitivity to drug
- Concurrently with MAOI; allow at least 14 days between discontinuation of an MAOI and initiation of levomilnacipran, or at least 7–14 days between discontinuation of levomilnacipran and initiation of an MAOI
- Concurrent use of serotonin precursors (e.g., tryptophan)

- In patients with uncontrolled narrow angle-closure glaucoma
- In patients treated with linezolid or methylene blue IV

SPECIAL POPULATIONS

Renal Impairment
- Use with caution in moderate or severe renal impairment. Decrease usual dose by 25–50%

Hepatic Impairment
- No adjustment needed

Cardiac Impairment
- Dose-dependent effect on blood pressure and heart rate. No effect on QTc

Elderly
- No adjustment necessary. At greater risk for hyponatremia

 Children and Adolescents
- Safety and efficacy not established. Use with caution. Observe closely for clinical worsening, suicidality, and changes in behavior in known or unknown bipolar disorder. Parents should be informed and advised of the risks

 Pregnancy
- Category C. Generally not recommended for the treatment of headaches or neuropathic pain during pregnancy. Neonates exposed to SNRIs or SSRIs late in the third trimester have developed complications necessitating extended hospitalizations, respiratory support, and tube feeding. Respiratory distress, cyanosis, apnea, seizures, temperature instability, feeding difficulty, vomiting, hypoglycemia, hypotonia, hyperreflexia, tremor, jitteriness, irritability, and constant crying consistent with a toxic effect of the drug or drug discontinuation syndrome have been reported

Breast Feeding
- Some drug is found in breast milk and use while breast feeding is not recommended

THE ART OF NEUROPHARMACOLOGY

Potential Advantages
- A novel balanced SNRI for fibromyalgia and depression

Potential Disadvantages
- May cause or worsen hypertension. Requires gradual titration

Primary Target Symptoms
- Fibromyalgia syndrome (sleep, fatigue, pain, mood)
- Depression

 Pearls
- Levomilnacipran is superior to conventional SSRIs in treating anhedonia and lack of energy in depression patients
- In theory may work as other SNRIs for headache, fibromyalgia, and neuropathic pain but remains to be determined
- May work for stress urinary incontinence
- Short-term (6 months) weight loss is normalized at 30 months

Suggested Reading

Derry S, Gill D, Phillips T, Moore RA. Milnacipran for neuropathic pain and fibromyalgia in adults. *Cochrane Database Syst Rev.* 2012;3:CD008244.

Engel ER, Kudrow D, Rapoport AM. A prospective, open-label study of milnacipran in the prevention of headache in patients with episodic or chronic migraine. *Neurol Sci.* 2014;35(3):429–35.

Häuser W, Petzke F, Sommer C. Comparative efficacy and harms of duloxetine, milnacipran, and pregabalin in fibromyalgia syndrome. *J Pain.* 2010;11(6):505–21.

Kohno T, Kimura M, Sasaki M, Obata H, Amaya F, Saito S. Milnacipran inhibits glutamatergic N-methyl-D-aspartate receptor activity in spinal dorsal horn neurons. *Mol Pain.* 2012;8:45.

Mansuy L. Antidepressant therapy with milnacipran and venlafaxine. *Neuropsychiatr Dis Treat.* 2010;6(Suppl I):17.

Matsuzawa-Yanagida K, Narita M, Nakajima M, Kuzumaki N, Niikura K, Nozaki H, et al. Usefulness of antidepressants for improving the neuropathic pain-like state and pain-induced anxiety through actions at different brain sites. *Neuropsychopharmacology.* 2008;33(8): 1952–65.

Sansone RA, Sansone LA. Serotonin norepinephrine reuptake inhibitors: a pharmacological comparison. *Innov Clin Neurosci.* 2014;11(3–4):37–42.

LIDOCAINE

THERAPEUTICS

Brands
- Xylocaine, Akten, Alphacaine, Anestacon, Dentipatch, Glydo, Lidocaton, Zingo

Generic?
- Yes

Class
- Antiarrhythmic

Commonly Prescribed for
(FDA approved in bold)
- **Regional anesthesia**
- **Ventricular arrhythmias**
- Post-herpetic neuralgia (patch only)
- Intractable headache
- Trigeminal autonomic cephalalgia
- Symptomatic myotonia
- Pain after spinal cord injury
- Tinnitus

How the Drug Works
- Class 1b antiarrhythmic agent. It blocks fast voltage-gated sodium channels on neuronal cell membrane, resulting in inhibition of the ionic flow required for initiation and conduction of action potentials and thus creating the anesthetic effect
- It also reduces the effective refractory period in Purkinje fibers in the heart and raises the depolarization threshold of the ventricle during diastole

How Long Until It Works
- Anesthetic and antiarrhythmic effects will occur within minutes
- May take more time (days or weeks) to see relief and determine the most effective dose in myotonia or pain disorders

If It Works
- Continue to use with appropriate monitoring

If It Doesn't Work
- Check serum levels and if not effective change to an alternative agent

Best Augmenting Combos for Partial Response or Treatment-Resistance
- Bupivacaine for long-acting local anesthesia

Tests
- Obtain ECG at baseline and for any new symptoms. Check a serum lidocaine level to guide therapy (1.5–6 mcg/mL) and for any AEs

ADVERSE EFFECTS (AEs)

How the Drug Causes AEs
- Drug effect blocking sodium channels

Notable AEs
- Dizziness, bradycardia, paresthesias, perioral numbness, hypo or hypertension, and tremor. Convulsions, visual disturbances (including hallucinations), depression, euphoria, agitation, or paranoid ideation

Life-Threatening or Dangerous AEs
- New or worsening cardiac arrhythmias
- Methemoglobinemia

Weight Gain
- Unusual

Sedation
- Unusual

What to Do About AEs
- Check serum level and ECG. For serious AEs, discontinue drug

Best Augmenting Agents to Reduce AEs
- Most AEs cannot be reduced by an augmenting agent

DOSING AND USE

Usual Dosage Range
- Headache therapeutic plasma level: 1.5–6 mcg/mL
- Cardiac arrhythmias: 200–300mg in 1 hour

Dosage Forms
- Injection: 0.5, 1, 1.5, 2, 4%
- Patch: 5%
- Topical: 0.5, 2, 3, 4, 5%

How to Dose
- For headache, adjust the rate of continuous infusion gradually until effective. Slow adjustment reduces the risk of AEs. Monitor serum level daily

Dosing Tips
- Discontinue the infusion if severe AEs develop. Restart at lower dose after 10–15 minutes

Overdose
- Nausea, hypotension, sinus bradycardia, paresthesia, seizures, AV heart block, and ventricular tachycardias

Long-Term Use
- Usually for short-term use

Habit Forming
- No

How to Stop
- No need to taper for the treatment of neurological disorders

Pharmacokinetics
- Hepatic metabolism via CYP1A2/3A4 to less potent metabolites. Half-life 1–2 hours. Protein binding 50–60%. Eliminated in 15 minutes in urine

Drug Interactions
- Lidocaine inhibits CYP1A2/2D6/3A4
- Propranolol and metoprolol may decrease its clearance
- Strong CYP1A2 inhibitors (e.g., fluoroquinolones, fluvoxamine, verapamil) and moderate CYP1A2 inhibitors (e.g., St. John's wort) can increase levels
- Strong CYP3A4 inhibitors (e.g., protease inhibitors, macrolide antibiotics, azole antifungals, nefazodone) and moderate CYP3A4 inhibitors (e.g., aprepitant, verapamil, grapefruit juice) can increase its serum concentration
- Enzyme inducers (e.g., hydantoins, rifampin, dexamethasone) can increase drug clearance and lower levels

Other Warnings/Precautions
- All antiarrhythmic agents can worsen or cause new arrhythmias. These may include increase in premature ventricular arrhythmias to life-threatening tachycardias

Do Not Use
- Known hypersensitivity to the drug; patients with Stokes-Adams syndrome, Wolff-Parkinson-White syndrome; severe degrees of sinoatrial, atrioventricular, or intraventricular block; concomitant use of other class I antiarrhythmic agents; acute intermittent porphyria; methemoglobinemia

SPECIAL POPULATIONS

Renal Impairment
- Likely no effect on dose

Hepatic Impairment
- Use with caution. Patients with severe disease may need a lower dose

Cardiac Impairment
- Dose adjustment in patients with heart failure

Elderly
- No known effects

Children and Adolescents
- Not studied in children. Not for treating tooth pain in children and infants

Pregnancy
- Category B. Only use in pregnancy if clearly needed

Breast Feeding
- Excreted in breast milk. Do not use

THE ART OF NEUROPHARMACOLOGY

Potential Advantages
- Useful for intractable headache

Potential Disadvantages
- Multiple AEs and need for monitoring complicate use

Primary Target Symptoms
- Headache, arrhythmia, pain

 Pearls

- Occasionally used for refractory headache. Successful treatment with IV lidocaine, if practical, may predict response to mexiletine, an oral analog of lidocaine
- Due to potential for significant interactions, including neurotoxicity, mexiletine should not be given to patients while receiving IV lidocaine
- For patients with SUNCT (short-lasting unilateral neuralgiform headache with conjunctival injection and tearing) or SUNA (short-lasting unilateral neuralgiform headache attacks with cranial autonomic symptoms), lidocaine (1–4 mg/kg/h) can be used for a short-term while initiating lamotrigine (100–300 mg/day) or others
- When delivered through a subarachnoid lumbar catheter, it provides more short-term neuropathic pain relief than placebo in patients with spinal cord injury
- Intranasal lidocaine (4%) 0.5 mL can be used for acute cluster headache or migraine treatment
- Lidocaine patch can be used for post-herpetic neuralgia

 Suggested Reading

Attal N, Cruccu G, Baron R, Haanpää M, Hansson P, Jensen TS, et al. EFNS guidelines on the pharmacological treatment of neuropathic pain: 2010 revision. *Eur J Neurol.* 2010;17(9): 1113–88.

Finnerup NB, Sindrup SH, Jensen TS. The evidence for pharmacological treatment of neuropathic pain. *Pain.* 2010;150(3):573–81.

den Hartigh J, Hilders CG, Schoemaker RC, Hulshof JH, Cohen AF, Vermeij P. Tinnitus suppression by intravenous lidocaine in relation to its plasma concentration. *Clin Pharmacol Ther.* 1993;54(4):415–20.

Marmura MJ. Intravenous lidocaine and mexiletine in the management of trigeminal autonomic cephalalgias. *Curr Pain Headache Rep.* 2010;14(2):145–50.

Marmura M, Rosen N, Abbas M, Silberstein S. Intravenous lidocaine in the treatment of refractory headache: a retrospective case series. *Headache.* 2009;49(2): 286–91.

Pareja JA, Álvarez M, Montojo T. SUNCT and SUNA: recognition and treatment. *Curr Treat Options Neurol.* 2013;15(1):28–39.

Teasell RW, Mehta S, Aubut J-AL, Foulon B, Wolfe DL, Hsieh JTC, et al. A systematic review of pharmacologic treatments of pain after spinal cord injury. *Arch Phys Med Rehabil.* 2010;91(5): 816–31.

LITHIUM (CARBONATE OR CITRATE)

THERAPEUTICS

Brands
- Carbolith, Eskalith, Priadel, Litarex, Lithicarb, Lithotab, Camcolit, Quilonum

Generic?
- Yes

Class
- Mood stabilizer

Commonly Prescribed for
(FDA approved in bold)
- **Manic episodes in bipolar disorder**
- **Maintenance treatment in bipolar disorder**
- Cluster headache prophylaxis
- Hypnic headache
- Major depressive disorder
- Bipolar depression
- Borderline personality disorder
- Anorexia nervosa
- Hypersomnia

How the Drug Works
- Lithium exhibits mood-stabilizing effect by modulating pre and postsynaptic neurotransmission of dopamine, glutamate (NMDA), nitric oxide, and GABA. It also exhibits neuroprotective effect by modulating oxidative metabolism, glycogen synthase kinase 3β promotor, brain-derived neurotrophic factor, and autophagy. In mania, where the levels of neurotransmitters are high, lithium stabilizes the neurotransmission. In the absence of pathology, lithium increases the level of these neurotransmitters
- It influences the circadian clock by increasing BMAL1 expression, disrupting the natural cycle
- The exact mechanism for preventing cluster headache is unknown

How Long Until It Works
- Cluster headache prophylaxis: usually effective in 2–3 weeks
- Acute mania: normalization of symptomatology within 1–3 weeks

If It Works
- Produces reduction in the severity or frequency of attacks. Consider tapering or stopping if headaches remit (more than 2 weeks in episodic cluster patients) or if considering pregnancy

If It Doesn't Work
- Increase to highest tolerated dose
- Cluster/hypnic headache: address other issues, such as medication overuse, other coexisting medical disorders, such as anxiety, and consider changing to another agent or adding a second agent

Best Augmenting Combos for Partial Response or Treatment-Resistance
- Cluster: at the start of the cycle can use a corticosteroid slam and taper. Verapamil is effective in cluster but may cause fluctuations in lithium levels. Valproate, topiramate, triptans, and methysergide are effective for many cluster patients

Tests
- Obtain baseline renal function, thyroid function, weight/BMI, and ECG before starting
- Repeat renal function every 6–12 months, monitor lithium levels, thyroid function, and weight
- Trough lithium levels (immediately before the next dose) should be between 0.6 and 1.2 mEq/L for acute and chronic treatment. Patients sensitive to lithium may exhibit toxic signs at level 1–1.5 mEq/L

ADVERSE EFFECTS (AEs)

How the Drug Causes AEs
- The cause of CNS AEs is unknown, but renal AEs are due to changes in ion transport

Notable AEs
- Bradycardia, hypotension
- Dizziness, vertigo, psychomotor retardation, tremor, restlessness, muscle hyperexcitability
- Anorexia, nausea, diarrhea, weight gain
- Polyuria, edema, metallic taste, fever, alopecia

Life-Threatening or Dangerous AEs
- Lithium toxicity, especially at levels above 1.5 mEq/L. Diarrhea, vomiting, drowsiness,

weakness occur early. Ataxia, polyuria, tinnitus, blurred vision, seizures, cardiac arrhythmias, ECG changes, syncope, or hallucinations may be seen in severe cases
• Thyroid disease, including hypothyroidism with myxedema or hyperthyroidism
• Nephrogenic diabetes insipidus
• Movement disorders, such as chorea, rigidity, and acute dystonia
• Rarely intracranial hypertension

Weight Gain
• Common

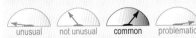

Sedation
• Common

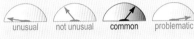

What to Do About AEs
• Check serum levels and reduce dose or stop drug for signs of toxicity
• Dose in the evening and take with food
• Maintain adequate hydration

Best Augmenting Agents to Reduce AEs
• For tremor, combine with propranolol. Most AEs cannot be reduced with an augmenting agent

DOSING AND USE

Usual Dosage Range
• Cluster headache: 600–1200mg/day in divided doses
• Bipolar: 600–1800mg/day in divided doses

Dosage Forms
• Tablets: 300mg. Extended release 300, 450mg
• Capsules: 150, 300, 600mg
• Syrup: 8mEq (300mg/5mL) (citrate)

How to Dose
• Headache: start at 150mg daily. Increase dose after a few days until headaches improve. Usually effective at doses of 600–1200mg/day or less

 Dosing Tips
• Dosing with extended-release tablets taken at night may reduce GI and other AEs

Overdose
• Tremor, dysarthria, delirium, coma, seizures, and death have been reported

Long-Term Use
• Safe for long-term use with monitoring

Habit Forming
• No

How to Stop
• Taper at 2 weeks after cessation of cluster attacks. Taper much more slowly in patients with bipolar disorder

Pharmacokinetics
• Elimination half-life about 24 hours. Mostly excreted unchanged in urine

 Drug Interactions
• Osmotic diuretics, theophyllines, urinary alkalinizers, and acetazolamide increase renal excretion and decrease levels
• Loop diuretics, ACE inhibitors, and thiazide diuretics increase levels
• NSAIDs decrease renal clearance of lithium
• Topiramate decreases lithium levels
• Fluoxetine may increase levels
• Methyldopa, carbamazepine, phenytoin, haloperidol, and phenothiazines may increase neurotoxic effects, even with normal serum levels
• May increase effects of neuromuscular blocking drugs
• Verapamil may either reduce levels or cause toxicity
• Metronidazole may increase toxicity
• Use with SSRIs may cause diarrhea, tremor, dizziness, agitation (rare), and serotonin syndrome

 Other Warnings/ Precautions
• Increases sodium excretion – maintain normal diet and consider salt supplementation

- Encephalopathy with irreversible brain damage may occur in patients taking lithium with haloperidol

Do Not Use

- Hypersensitivity to drug, cardiac arrhythmia, severe dehydration or hyponatremia, or severe kidney disease

SPECIAL POPULATIONS

Renal Impairment

- Chronic use is associated with glomerular and interstitial fibrosis. Avoid using in patients with significant disease or those developing abnormalities on treatment

Hepatic Impairment

- No known effects

Cardiac Impairment

- Do not use in patients with arrhythmias or heart failure

Elderly

- Require lower doses to achieve therapeutic levels and more likely to experience AEs

 Children and Adolescents

- Appears safe in children over age 12. Monitor more closely

 Pregnancy

- Category D. May increase cardiac abnormalities, such as Ebstein's anomaly. Do not use for headache disorders

Breast Feeding

- Not recommended. Lithium is found in breast milk, and hypertonia, cyanosis, and ECG changes have been reported

THE ART OF NEUROPHARMACOLOGY

Potential Advantages

- Effective in cluster and hypnic headache at levels below those needed for mood disorders

Potential Disadvantages

- Potential AEs with long-term therapy and narrow therapeutic window

Primary Target Symptoms

- Headache frequency and severity
- Mania

 Pearls

- Effective in cluster headache, even in patients with chronic cluster headache with no headache-free months. Most patients will require a relatively low dose (1200 mg/day or less) when compared with doses used for acute mania (often 1800 mg/day), but higher doses can be used if needed, with monitoring of serum levels
- For patients with episodic cycles of cluster headache, taper off starting 2 weeks after last attack. For chronic cluster, periodically taper medication every 6–12 months to detect remissions
- Patients with hypnic or "alarm-clock" headache may respond to doses of 300–600 mg at night. Hypnic headache is more common in elderly patients
- For hypnic headache, caffeine is an effective acute treatment and lithium is one of the few preventive treatments
- Limited if any efficacy in migraine
- CNS manifestations of lithium toxicity often persist for days after serum levels return to normal levels
- May work best in euphoric mania rather than mixed states or rapid cycling
- Lithium-related weight gain may be more common in women
- Lithium may be effective for recurrent hypersomnia but can also increase somnambulism

Suggested Reading

Ashkenazi A, Schwedt T. Cluster headache – acute and prophylactic therapy. *Headache*. 2011;51(2):272–86.

Cohen AS, Matharu MS, Goadsby PJ. Trigeminal autonomic cephalalgias: current and future treatments. *Headache*. 2007;47(6):969–80.

Geddes JR, Burgess S, Hawton K, Jamison K, Goodwin GM. Long-term lithium therapy for bipolar disorder: systematic review and meta-analysis of randomized controlled trials. *Am J Psychiatry*. 2004;161(2):217–22.

Liang J-F, Wang S-J. Hypnic headache: a review of clinical features, therapeutic options and outcomes. *Cephalalgia*. 2014;34(10): 795–805.

Malhi GS, Tanious M, Das P, Coulston CM, Berk M. Potential mechanisms of action of lithium in bipolar disorder. *CNS Drugs*. 2013; 27(2):135–53.

Silberstein SD. Preventive migraine treatment. *Neurol Clin*. 2009;27(2): 429–43.

MANNITOL

Brands
- Osmitrol

Generic?
- Yes

Class
- Osmotic diuretic

Commonly Prescribed for
(FDA approved in bold)
- **Reduction of elevated intracranial pressure (ICP)**
- **Reduction of elevated intraocular pressure**
- **Diuresis (prophylaxis in acute renal failure)**
- **Increased excretion of urinary toxins**
- **Urological irrigation**

How the Drug Works
- Mannitol induces diuresis by elevating the osmolarity of the glomerular filtrate, which decreases tubular reabsorption of water

How Long Until It Works
- 15 minutes

If It Works
- Assess effectiveness and need for continued use. Usually used as a short-term measure before more definitive treatment

If It Doesn't Work
- Usually mannitol is a temporary measure for acute increases in ICP before more definitive treatment

Best Augmenting Combos for Partial Response or Treatment-Resistance
- Treatment of increased ICP depends on the etiology
- Causes of increased ICP due to general swelling include liver failure, hypertensive encephalopathy, and hypercarbia. Intervention should consist of treating the underlying medical problem
- In some cases, meningitis can cause increased production of CSF or obstruction of CSF flow

- Increased ICP due to mass effect from stroke (ischemic or hemorrhagic) may require neurosurgical intervention such as an intraventricular catheter, craniotomy, or craniectomy
- Permitting hypertension may increase perfusion and reduce swelling, but calcium channel blockers may also be useful (especially in subarachnoid hemorrhage)
- Analgesia and sedation may be useful
- Hyperventilation, hypothermia, and barbiturate coma are occasionally used, usually in refractory cases
- Hypertonic saline is an alternative to mannitol for acutely increased ICP
- Corticosteroids are often used to reduce vasogenic edema, i.e., brain tumors

Tests
- Carefully monitor serum sodium, potassium, BUN, and urine output during therapy

How the Drug Causes AEs
- Most are related to changes in electrolytes and diuresis

Notable AEs
- Pulmonary edema, hypo- or hypertension, tachycardia
- Headache, thirst, nausea, diarrhea, blurred vision, rhinitis, chills, fever

Life-Threatening or Dangerous AEs
- Severe hypernatremia or renal failure

Weight Gain
- Unusual

unusual   not unusual   common   problematic

Sedation
- Unusual

unusual   not unusual   common   problematic

What to Do About AEs
- Hold infusion for any significant AEs. Discontinue infusion if urine output is low

Best Augmenting Agents to Reduce AEs

- Most AEs cannot be reduced by augmenting agents

DOSING AND USE

Usual Dosage Range

- 100–200 g/kg/day

Dosage Forms

- Infusion: 5% in 1000 mL, 10% in 500 or 1000 mL, 15% in 150 or 500 mL, 20% in 250 or 500 mL, 25% in 50 mL vials and 5 g/100 mL solution

How to Dose

- The 20% or 25% solution is the most efficient. Give 0.25 to 2 g/kg body weight over 30 to 60 minutes. Adjust to maintain a urine flow between 30 and 50 mL/h

 Dosing Tips

- Effect of treatment should be apparent by 15 minutes, and peak effect occurs from 30–60 minutes

Overdose

- May result in increased renal excretion of sodium, potassium, or chloride. Risks include orthostatic tachycardia, hypotension, weakness, intestinal dilation, ileus, and pulmonary edema

Long-Term Use

- Unknown

Habit Forming

- No

How to Stop

- No need to taper. Monitor neurological status after discontinuation

Pharmacokinetics

- Only slightly metabolized. Excreted by kidney. About 80% of a dose renally excreted in 3 hours. Peak effect at 30–60 minutes

 Drug Interactions

- Many additives are incompatible with mannitol
- Do not give with blood products (may cause clumping of erythrocytes)

 Other Warnings/ Precautions

- May increase blood flow and the risk of postoperative neurosurgical bleeding

Do Not Use

- Anuria due to renal failure
- Pulmonary congestion or edema, congestive heart failure
- Active intracranial bleeding
- Progressive renal disease or dysfunction after mannitol
- Known hypersensitivity

SPECIAL POPULATIONS

Renal Impairment

- Do not use in anuric patients or worsening renal functioning after mannitol. In those with renal impairment, give a test dose of 0.2 g/kg body weight as a 15% to 25% solution over a period of 3 to 5 minutes. If urine output dose not increase, give a second test dose. If no effect, discontinue use

Hepatic Impairment

- No known effects

Cardiac Impairment

- Do not use with severe congestive heart failure

Elderly

- No known effects

 Children and Adolescents

- As in adults, use 0.25 to 2 g/kg as a 15% to 20% solution. Give over a longer period – up to 6 hours

 Pregnancy

- Category B. Use only if clearly needed

Breast Feeding

• Unknown if excreted in breast milk

THE ART OF NEUROPHARMACOLOGY

Potential Advantages

• Rapid onset of action for treatment of increased ICP. No central line access needed for administration

Potential Disadvantages

• Does not address the cause of increased ICP and not always effective

Primary Target Symptoms

• Symptoms of increased ICP which may include nausea/vomiting, headache, papilledema, extraocular palsies, pupillary dilation, hypertension, bradycardia, or changes in breathing pattern (hyperventilation or Cheyne-Stokes respiration)

Pearls

• Long-standing first-line drug for increased ICP, but new available medical therapies have challenged this. Mannitol actually has little evidence for improving outcomes
• Based on a meta-analysis, hypertonic saline may be slightly more effective than mannitol in lowering the ICP, especially in patients with traumatic brain injury, for improving short-term (not long-term) neurological outcome

Suggested Reading

Davis SM. Medical management of haemorrhagic stroke. *Crit Care Resusc.* 2005;7(3):185–8.

Forsyth LL, Liu-DeRyke X, Parker D Jr, Rhoney DH. Role of hypertonic saline for the management of intracranial hypertension after stroke and traumatic brain injury. *Pharmacotherapy.* 2008;28(4):469–84.

Rickard AC, Smith JE, Newell P, Bailey A, Kehoe A, Mann C. Salt or sugar for your injured brain? A meta-analysis of randomised controlled trials of mannitol versus hypertonic sodium solutions to manage raised intracranial pressure in traumatic brain injury. *Emerg Med J.* 2014; 31(8):679–83.

White H, Cook D, Venkatesh B. The use of hypertonic saline for treating intracranial hypertension after traumatic brain injury. *Anesth Analg.* 2006;102(6): 1836–46.

THERAPEUTICS

Brands
- Antivert, Bonine

Generic?
- Yes

Class
- Antiemetic

Commonly Prescribed for
(FDA approved in bold)
- **Motion sickness**
- **Vertigo**

How the Drug Works
- Antihistamine and anticholinergic drug

How Long Until It Works
- 30 minutes

If It Works
- Continue to use as needed, especially in short-term disorders, such as viral labyrinthitis

If It Doesn't Work
- Treat the underlying disorder with appropriate agents for that disorder
- Benzodiazepines (Valium) may be effective for vertigo; antiemetics, such as promethazine, help also treat motion sickness

Best Augmenting Combos for Partial Response or Treatment-Resistance
- Benzodiazepines (Valium) may be effective for vertigo
- Meniere's disease: diuretics, antiemetics, and low-salt diet
- Vestibular rehabilitation may be helpful

Tests
- None

ADVERSE EFFECTS (AEs)

How the Drug Causes AEs
- Antihistamine and anticholinergic actions

Notable AEs
- Dry mouth, sedation are most common
- Paradoxical excitation (nervousness, agitation), blurred vision, rash, tinnitus
- Hypotension, tachycardia

 ### Life-Threatening or Dangerous AEs
- May precipitate narrow-angle glaucoma
- Risk of heat stroke, especially in elderly patients
- Can precipitate tachycardia, cardiac arrhythmias, and hypotension
- May cause urinary retention in patients with prostate hypertrophy

Weight Gain
- Common

unusual   not unusual   common   problematic

Sedation
- Common

unusual   not unusual   common   problematic

What to Do About AEs
- Sedation: give at night or lower dose
- Dry mouth: chewing gum or water

Best Augmenting Agents to Reduce AEs
- Most AEs cannot be reduced with the use of an augmenting agent

DOSING AND USE

Usual Dosage Range
- Vertigo: 25–100 mg/day

Dosage Forms
- Tablets: 12.5, 25, 50 mg
- Chewable: 25 mg
- Capsules: 25 mg

How to Dose
- Motion sickness: 25–50 mg 1 hour before travel
- Vertigo: 25–50 mg 2–3 times daily (maximum 100 mg/day)

Dosing Tips

• Taking with meals may reduce AEs

Overdose

• Large overdoses may cause convulsions, hallucinations, or respiratory depression

Long-Term Use

• Unknown, usually a short-term medication

Habit Forming

• No

How to Stop

• No need to taper

Pharmacokinetics

• Onset of action in 30–60 minutes, duration of action 4–24 hours depending on dose

 Drug Interactions

• Increases AEs of CNS depressants

 Other Warnings/ Precautions

• Use with caution in hot weather – may increase risk of heat stroke
• Tablets contain tartrazine, which may precipitate allergic-type reactions in asthmatic patients

Do Not Use

• Known hypersensitivity to the drug, severe asthma, glaucoma (especially angle-closure type), prostate hypertrophy or bladder neck obstructions, severe dyspnea

SPECIAL POPULATIONS

Renal Impairment

• No known effects

Hepatic Impairment

• Eliminated more slowly in patients with severe disease

Cardiac Impairment

• Use with caution in patients with orthostatic hypotension

Elderly

• Use with caution. More susceptible to AEs

 Children and Adolescents

• Appears safe in children over 12

 Pregnancy

• Category B. No known teratogenicity

Breast Feeding

• Use if benefits outweigh risk

THE ART OF NEUROPHARMACOLOGY

Potential Advantages

• Useful in the treatment of acute vertigo and motion sickness

Potential Disadvantages

• Often ineffective for long-term disorders associated with vertigo, such as migraine or Meniere's disease

Primary Target Symptoms

• Vertigo, nausea

 Pearls

• Usually used for the short-term management of viral labyrinthitis
• Antihistamine and anticholinergic AEs often limit use

Suggested Reading

Baloh RW. Approach to the dizzy patient. *Baillieres Clin Neurol.* 1994;3(3):453–65.

Horak FB, Jones-Rycewicz C, Black FO, Shumway-Cook A. Effects of vestibular rehabilitation on dizziness and imbalance. *Otolaryngol Head Neck Surg.* 1992;106(2): 175–80.

Newman-Toker DE, Camargo CA Jr, Hsieh YH, Pelletier AJ, Edlow JA. Disconnect between charted vestibular diagnoses and emergency department management decisions: a cross-sectional analysis from a nationally representative sample. *Acad Emerg Med.* 2009;16(10):970–7.

MEMANTINE

THERAPEUTICS

Brands
- Namenda, Namenda XR, Ebixa, Namzaric (memantine + donepezil)

Generic?
- Yes (except XR)

Class
- NMDA receptor antagonist

Commonly Prescribed for
(FDA approved in bold)
- **Alzheimer's dementia (AD) (moderate or severe)**
- Parkinson's disease-related dementia
- Dementia with Lewy bodies (DLB)
- Vascular dementia
- HIV dementia
- Migraine prophylaxis
- Attention deficit hyperactivity disorder
- Binge-eating disorder

How the Drug Works
- An uncompetitive NMDA receptor antagonist that prevents the tonic pathological influx of Ca^{2+} (caused by amyloid-β binding on NMDA receptors) but permits the transient strong physiological glutamatergic signal
- It also reduces oxidative stress in postsynaptic neurons and targets extracellular NR2B subunits ("death" receptors), which may be related to the pathological process of AD
- It is also a $5\text{-}HT_3$ antagonist of similar potency
- Although symptoms of AD can improve, memantine does not prevent disease progression

How Long Until It Works
- Weeks to months

If It Works
- Continue to use but symptoms of dementia usually continue to worsen

If It Doesn't Work
- Non-pharmacological measures are the basis of dementia treatment. Maintain regular schedules and routines. Avoid prolonged travel, unnecessary medical procedures or emergency room visits, crowds, and large social gatherings
- Limit drugs with sedative properties such as opioids, hypnotics, AEDs, and TCAs
- Treat other underlying disorders that can worsen symptoms, such as hyperglycemia or urinary difficulties

Best Augmenting Combos for Partial Response or Treatment-Resistance
- Addition of cholinesterase inhibitors may be beneficial. In one study donepezil plus memantine reduced the rate of progression compared to that in those taking donepezil alone
- Treat depression or apathy with SSRIs but be cautious for increased risk of AEs (e.g., QTc prolongation, injurious falls). Avoid TCAs in demented patients due to risk of confusion. In dementia patients with severe depression, electroconvulsive therapy can be an option
- For significant confusion and agitation avoid neuroleptics (especially in DLB) because of the risk of neuroleptic malignant syndrome. Atypical antipsychotics (e.g., risperidone, clozapine, aripiprazole) or SSRIs can be used instead

Tests
- None required

ADVERSE EFFECTS (AEs)

How the Drug Causes AEs
- Direct effect on NMDA receptors

Notable AEs
- Hypertension, dizziness, constipation, diarrhea, coughing, dyspnea, fatigue, pain, ataxia, vertigo, confusion

Life-Threatening or Dangerous AEs
- Syncope or cardiac arrhythmia can occur although it is unclear that these events are related to memantine

Weight Gain

• Unusual

Sedation

• Unusual

What to Do About AEs

• In patients with dementia, determining if AEs are related to medication or another medical condition can be difficult. For CNS side effects, discontinuation of non-essential centrally acting medications may help. If a bothersome AE is clearly drug-related then discontinue memantine

Best Augmenting Agents to Reduce AEs

• Most AEs do not respond to additional medications

DOSING AND USE

Usual Dosage Range

• 5–20 mg/day. XR: 14–28 mg/day

Dosage Forms

• Tablets: 5, 10 mg
• XR capsules: 7, 14, 21, 28 mg
• Oral solution: 2 mg/mL
• Capsules (memantine XR/donepezil): 14/10, 28/10 mg

How to Dose

• Start at 5 mg in the evening. Increase by 5 mg/week until taking 10 mg twice daily or until reaching desired effect. Do not increase dose faster than intervals of 1 week. If AEs occur, titrate more slowly. Dose used when there is renal impairment is 5 mg twice daily
• For XR form, start at 7 mg daily. Increase by 7 mg/week until 28 mg daily. Dose used when there is renal impairment is 14 mg daily

 Dosing Tips

• Slow titration can reduce AEs. Food does not affect absorption. Can sprinkle content of capsule on food

Overdose

• Symptoms may include restlessness, psychosis, hallucinations, and stupor. Treatment: acidification of urine will enhance urinary excretion of memantine

Long-Term Use

• Safe for long-term use. Effectiveness may decrease over time as the dementing illness progresses

Habit Forming

• No

How to Stop

• Abrupt discontinuation is unlikely to produce AEs except worsening of dementia symptoms

Pharmacokinetics

• T_{max} 3–7 hours (9–12 hours for XR). Protein binding 45%. Partial hepatic metabolism (not through CYP450) to inactive metabolites; most drug is secreted in urine unchanged (48%) with an elimination half-life of 60–80 hours. Renal clearance involves active tubular secretion moderated by pH-dependent tubular reabsorption

 Drug Interactions

• Use with caution with other drugs which are NMDA antagonists (amantadine, ketamine, dextromethorphan)
• Use with caution with drugs that also utilize renal mechanisms of excretion such as ranitidine, cimetidine, hydrochlorothiazide, or nicotine
• No interaction between cholinesterase inhibitor and memantine

 Other Warnings/ Precautions

• Alkaline urine (carbonic anhydrase inhibitors, sodium bicarbonate, thiazide, or in patients with renal tubular acidosis or urinary tract infection) reduces memantine clearance. Use with caution

Do Not Use
- Hypersensitivity to the drug

Renal Impairment
- Drug is renally excreted. Consider dose reduction with severe impairment

Hepatic Impairment
- No dose adjustment in patients with mild and moderate hepatic impairment. Not studied in patients with severe hepatic impairment

Cardiac Impairment
- No significant change in ECG observed in trials compared to placebo. No known effects

Elderly
- There is reduced drug clearance, but no dose adjustment needed as the dose used is the lowest that provides clinical improvement

 Children and Adolescents
- Not studied in children. AD does not occur in children

 Pregnancy
- Category B. Decreased birth weight in animal studies. Use only if benefits of medication outweigh risks

Breast Feeding
- Unknown if excreted in breast milk. Use with caution

Potential Advantages
- Proven effectiveness for AD, even with severe dementia. Fewer cholinergic or GI AEs than cholinesterase inhibitors

Potential Disadvantages
- Cost and minimal effectiveness. Does not prevent progression of AD or other dementias. May be less effective for DLB than cholinesterase inhibitors

Primary Target Symptoms
- Confusion, agitation, performing activities of daily living

 Pearls
- Although it is generally not effective for mild AD, it is frequently prescribed
- When combined with cholinesterase inhibitors, it may further reduce short-term (at least 24 weeks) decline (cognition, function, behavior, global status) in moderate (Mini Mental State Examination [MMSE] 10–19) to severe (MMSE < 10) AD patients
- It may improve Clinical Global Impression of Change Scale and behavioral symptoms but not cognitive function in patients with mild to moderate DLB (not in Parkinson's disease). It may minimize agitation, delusion, and irritability hence reducing the need for atypical antipsychotics. Cholinesterase inhibitors enhance cognitive function and possibly mood symptoms
- Not proven for use in frontal lobe dementia, dementia in Down's syndrome, or fragile X-associated dementia
- Effective for migraine prophylaxis in open-label studies at doses of 10–20 mg/day. It also showed a trend (non-significant) toward efficacy in chronic tension-type headache prophylaxis
- Other NMDA receptor antagonists (ketamine, dextromethorphan) might exert more analgesic effects than memantine
- Structurally related to amantadine, a weak NMDA antagonist
- More tolerable than cholinesterase inhibitors

Suggested Reading

Danysz W, Parsons CG. Alzheimer's disease, β-amyloid, glutamate, NMDA receptors and memantine – searching for the connections. *Br J Pharmacol.* 2012;167(2):324–52.

Downey D. Pharmacologic management of Alzheimer disease. *J Neurosci Nurs.* 2008; 40(1):55–9.

Emre M, Tsolaki M, Bonuccelli U, Destée A, Tolosa E, Kutzelnigg A, et al. Memantine for patients with Parkinson's disease dementia or dementia with Lewy bodies: a randomised, double-blind, placebo-controlled trial. *Lancet Neurol.* 2010;9(10):969–77.

Grossberg GT, Edwards KR, Zhao Q. Rationale for combination therapy with galantamine and memantine in Alzheimer's disease. *J Clin Pharmacol.* 2006;46(7 Suppl 1):17S–26S

Huang L, Bocek M, Jordan JK, Sheehan AH. Memantine for the prevention of primary headache disorders. *Ann Pharmacother.* 2014;48(11):1507–11.

Krymchantowski A, Jevoux C. Memantine in the preventive treatment for migraine and refractory migraine. *Headache.* 2009;49(3): 481–2.

McKeage K. Memantine: a review of its use in moderate to severe Alzheimer's disease. *CNS Drugs.* 2009;23(10):881–97.

Porsteinsson AP, Grossberg GT, Mintzer J, Olin JT; Memantine MEM-MD-12 Study Group. Memantine treatment in patients with mild to moderate Alzheimer's disease already receiving a cholinesterase inhibitor: a randomized, double-blind, placebo-controlled trial. *Curr Alzheimer Res.* 2008;5(1):83–9.

Schmitt FA, van Dyck CH, Wichems CH, Olin JT; for the Memantine MEM-MD-02 Study Group. Cognitive response to memantine in moderate to severe Alzheimer disease patients already receiving donepezil: an exploratory reanalysis. *Alzheimer Dis Assoc Disord.* 2006;20(4): 255–62.

THERAPEUTICS

Brands
- Skelaxin

Generic?
- Yes

 Class
- Muscle relaxant

Commonly Prescribed for
(FDA approved in bold)
- **Musculoskeletal conditions (adjunct to rest and physical therapy for relief of acute pain)**
- Spasticity

 How the Drug Works
- Unclear but might be related to general CNS depression effect

How Long Until It Works
- Pain: hours

If It Works
- Slowly titrate to most effective tolerated dose

If It Doesn't Work
- Increase to highest tolerated dose and consider alternative treatments

 Best Augmenting Combos for Partial Response or Treatment-Resistance
- Use other centrally acting muscle relaxants with caution due to potential CNS depressant effect
- Can combine with NSAIDs for acute pain

Tests
- None

ADVERSE EFFECTS (AEs)

How the Drug Causes AEs
- CNS depression

Notable AEs
- Nausea, drowsiness, dizziness, headache, irritability, rash

 Life-Threatening or Dangerous AEs
- Hemolytic anemia and leukopenia have been reported

Weight Gain
- Unusual

unusual · not unusual · common · problematic

Sedation
- Common

unusual · not unusual · common · problematic

What to Do About AEs
- Lower the dose or discontinue drug

Best Augmenting Agents to Reduce AEs
- Most AEs cannot be reduced by an augmenting agent

DOSING AND USE

Usual Dosage Range
- 800–3200 mg/day

Dosage Forms
- Tablets: 800 mg

How to Dose
- In children over 12 and adults, give 400–800 mg 3–4 times daily

 Dosing Tips
- Taking with food increases CNS depression

Overdose
- Overdose with alcohol can lead to death. Reports of serotonin syndrome. Treat with gastric lavage and supportive therapy

Long-Term Use
- Not well studied

Habit Forming
- No

How to Stop
- Taper not required

Pharmacokinetics
- Peak effect at 3 hours and half-life 9 hours. Hepatic metabolism to metabolites excreted in urine

 Drug Interactions
- May enhance effect of other CNS depressants, such as alcohol, barbiturates, or benzodiazepines

Other Warnings/ Precautions
- May impair mental or physical abilities when driving or performing hazardous tasks

Do Not Use
- Known hypersensitivity to the drug, hemolytic anemia, or severe renal or hepatic disease

Renal Impairment
- Not studied – use with caution. Risk of renal toxicity

Hepatic Impairment
- Not studied – use with caution. Risk of hepatotoxicity

Cardiac Impairment
- No known effects

Elderly
- Drug metabolism is slower in elderly patients. Use with caution

 Children and Adolescents
- Not studied in children under age 12

 Pregnancy
- Not categorized due to lack of data but likely category B. Use only if there is a clear need

Breast Feeding
- Unknown if excreted in breast milk but likely, due to drug structure

THE ART OF NEUROPHARMACOLOGY

Potential Advantages
- Quick onset for pain and muscle spasm

Potential Disadvantages
- Not effective for most pain symptoms related to neurological disorders, such as spasticity due to multiple sclerosis, migraine, or neuropathic pain disorders

Primary Target Symptoms
- Spasticity, pain

 Pearls
- Patients with spasticity due to multiple sclerosis or spinal cord disease are more likely to respond to baclofen or tizanidine

 Suggested Reading

Chou R, Peterson K, Helfand M. Comparative efficacy and safety of skeletal muscle relaxants for spasticity and musculoskeletal conditions: a systematic review. *J Pain Symptom Manage.* 2004;28(2):140–75.

See S, Ginzburg R. Choosing a skeletal muscle relaxant. *Am Fam Physician.* 2008;78(3):365–70.

Toth PP, Urtis J. Commonly used muscle relaxant therapies for acute low back pain: a review of carisoprodol, cyclobenzaprine hydrochloride, and metaxalone. *Clin Ther.* 2004;26(9):1355–67. Review

METHOCARBAMOL

THERAPEUTICS

Brands
- Robaxin, Robaxin 750, Delaxin, Forbaxin

Generic?
- Yes

 **Class**
- Muscle relaxant

Commonly Prescribed for
(FDA approved in bold)
- **Musculoskeletal conditions (adjunct to rest and physical therapy for relief of acute pain)**
- Muscle spasm
- Tetanus

 How the Drug Works
- It is structurally similar to guaifenesin. Its mode of action is unclear but might be related to general CNS depression effect. It has no direct relaxant effect on muscle, nerve, or neuromuscular junction

How Long Until It Works
- Spasm pain: 30 minutes or less

If It Works
- Slowly titrate to most effective tolerated dose

If It Doesn't Work
- Increase to highest tolerated dose and consider alternative treatments

 Best Augmenting Combos for Partial Response or Treatment-Resistance
- Use other centrally acting muscle relaxants with caution due to potential additive CNS depressant effect
- Can combine with NSAIDs for acute pain

Tests
- None

ADVERSE EFFECTS (AEs)

How the Drug Causes AEs
- Most AEs are due to CNS depression

Notable AEs
- Confusion, amnesia, dizziness, drowsiness, sedation, blurred vision, nystagmus, bradycardia, hypotension, pruritus, nasal congestion. Urine discoloration. Jaundice has been reported

 Life-Threatening or Dangerous AEs
- Leukopenia, seizures, and anaphylactic reactions have been reported

Weight Gain
- Unusual

unusual   not unusual   common   problematic

Sedation
- Common

unusual   not unusual   common   problematic

What to Do About AEs
- Lower the dose or discontinue drug

Best Augmenting Agents to Reduce AEs
- Most AEs cannot be reduced by an augmenting agent

DOSING AND USE

Usual Dosage Range
- 4–8 g/day in divided doses

Dosage Forms
- Tablets: 500, 750 mg
- Injection: 100 mg/mL

How to Dose
- For acute muscle spasm, start 1500 mg 4 times daily (max 8 g/day). Decrease dose to 1000 mg 4 times daily or 1500 mg 3 times daily after a few days

 Dosing Tips
- Crushed tablets in water or saline can be given through a nasogastric tube

Overdose

- Overdose is most dangerous when combined with alcohol or other CNS depressants. Symptoms include nausea, drowsiness, hypotension, seizures, and coma. Treat with gastric lavage and supportive therapy

Long-Term Use

- Not well studied

Habit Forming

- No

How to Stop

- Taper not required

Pharmacokinetics

- Peak effect at 2 hours and half-life 1–2 hours. Metabolized by dealkylation and hydroxylation to metabolites excreted in urine

 Drug Interactions

- May enhance effect of other CNS depressants such as alcohol, barbiturates, or benzodiazepines
- Can inhibit the effect of pyridostigmine in myasthenia gravis
- Causes color interference in screening tests for 5-hydroxindoleacetic acid and urinary vanillylmandelic acid

 Other Warnings/ Precautions

- May impair mental or physical abilities when driving or performing hazardous tasks

Do Not Use

- Hypersensitivity to the drug, severe renal or hepatic disease

Renal Impairment

- Clearance reduced by 40% in end-stage renal disease. Use with caution. Do not use injection in patients with renal failure

Hepatic Impairment

- Clearance reduced by about 70% in patients with alcoholic cirrhosis. Reduce dose and use with caution

Cardiac Impairment

- No known effects

Elderly

- Drug metabolism is slightly slower in elderly patients. Use with caution. Increased risk of injury

 Children and Adolescents

- Not studied in children under age 16 except in tetanus. For the treatment of tetanus, give 15 mg/kg IV and repeat every 6 hours as needed

 Pregnancy

- Category C. Use only if there is a clear need

Breast Feeding

- Likely excreted in human milk, do not use

Potential Advantages

- Relatively safe for the short-term treatment of pain with few drug interactions. Useful in the treatment of tetanus

Potential Disadvantages

- Not effective for most pain symptoms related to neurological disorders such as spasticity due to multiple sclerosis, migraine, or neuropathic pain disorders

Primary Target Symptoms

- Spasticity, pain

 Pearls

- Patients with spasticity due to multiple sclerosis or spinal cord diseases are more likely to respond to baclofen or tizanidine
- May be helpful as an injection in helping to control the neuromuscular manifestations of tetanus in addition to usual treatments
- May exacerbate symptoms of myasthenia gravis

Suggested Reading

Chou R, Peterson K, Helfand M. Comparative efficacy and safety of skeletal muscle relaxants for spasticity and musculoskeletal conditions: a systematic review. *J Pain Symptom Manage.* 2004; 28(2):140–75.

See S, Ginzburg R. Choosing a skeletal muscle relaxant. *Am Fam Physician.* 2008;78(3):365–70.

Valtonen EJ. A double-blind trial of methocarbamol versus placebo in painful muscle spasm. *Curr Med Res Opin.* 1975;3(6):382–5.

METHOTREXATE

THERAPEUTICS

Brands
- Amethopterin, Emthexate, Ledertrexate, Maxtrex, Mexate, MTX, Otrexup, Trexall, Rheumatrex, Metoject

Generic?
- Yes

Class
- Antineoplastic agent, immunosuppressant

Commonly Prescribed for
(FDA approved in bold)
- **Treatment of malignancies, including non-Hodgkin lymphoma, gestational choriocarcinoma, head and neck epidermoid cancer, and lung and breast cancer**
- **Psoriasis**
- **Rheumatoid arthritis**
- Inflammatory myopathies: polymyositis (PM) and dermatomyositis (DM)
- Vasculitis, including Wegener's granulomatosis
- Relapsing-remitting or chronic progressive multiple sclerosis (MS)
- Primary CNS lymphoma
- Ulcerative colitis or Crohn's disease
- Systemic lupus erythematosus
- Psoriatic arthritis

How the Drug Works
- Inhibits dihydrofolic acid reductase. Prevents synthesis of purine nucleotides and thymidylate. This interferes with DNA synthesis, repair, and replication

How Long Until It Works
- Within a week, but effect on neurological diseases may take months

If It Works
- DM/PM: improves strength, and may allow discontinuation or reduced dose of corticosteroids. Corticosteroids are tapered first. Taper slowly over 6 months if clinical remission occurs
- MS: may reduce relapses and new lesions on MRI

- Other disorders: Improves symptoms and clinical markers of the disease

If It Doesn't Work
- DM/PM: question the diagnosis (inclusion-body myositis, hypothyroidism, muscular dystrophy), rule out corticosteroid-induced myopathy, and evaluate for undiagnosed malignancy (especially in DM). Change to azathioprine
- MS: if clearly not helpful, change to another agent

Best Augmenting Combos for Partial Response or Treatment-Resistance
- Usually used in combination with corticosteroids (to reduce corticosteroid dose) in DM and PM. Occasionally combined with other treatments for the treatment of MS

Tests
- Obtain CBC, liver and renal function tests, and chest x-ray at baseline and at dosage adjustments, or for any clinical symptoms. Use serum level and WBC to assess response to treatment

ADVERSE EFFECTS (AEs)

How the Drug Causes AEs
- Folic acid antagonism

Notable AEs
- Ulcerative stomatitis, nausea, abdominal distress
- Malaise, fatigue, chills and fever, dizziness
- Headache, speech impairment, convulsions, encephalopathy
- Rash or photosensitivity
- Elevated liver function tests (up to 15%)

Life-Threatening or Dangerous AEs
- Leukopenia, anemia, aplastic anemia, thrombocytopenia
- Thrombotic events, such as cerebral thrombosis and pulmonary embolus
- Respiratory fibrosis and failure, renal failure
- Leukoencephalopathy, stroke-like symptoms (usually with high doses IV only)

Weight Gain
- Unusual

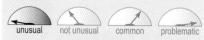

Sedation
- Unusual

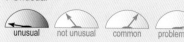

What to Do About AEs
- Renal failure: stop drug and ensure adequate hydration and urine alkalinization
- Hepatic failure: transient abnormalities are common. For persistently abnormal tests, perform liver biopsy and discontinue if moderate to severe changes. For significant disease, stop drug
- Pulmonary symptoms: cough or dyspnea could indicate significant disease. Stop drug and evaluate with chest x-ray

Best Augmenting Agents to Reduce AEs
- Leucovorin (a folate analog that is able to participate in reactions utilizing folates) is used after high-dose therapy as a rescue drug. Give 15 mg orally, IM, or IV every 6 hours for 10 doses

DOSING AND USE

Usual Dosage Range
- DM/PM: 7.5–30 mg/week
- Rheumatoid arthritis, MS: 7.5 mg/week

Dosage Forms
- Tablets: 2.5, 5, 7.5, 10, 15 mg
- Injection: 2.5 mg/mL or 25 mg/mL, powder for injection (20 mg, 50 mg, 100 mg, and 1 g)
- Injection, SC: autoinjector (0.4 mL) 7.5, 10, 15, 20, 25 mg

How to Dose
- DM/PM: 2.5 mg 3 times a day, 1 day/week initially. Increase dose based on clinical response and creatine kinase levels as long as WBC is 3000/mm^3 or greater every 2 weeks or greater
- MS: 7.5 mg once weekly, or 2.5 mg 3 times a day, 1 day/week. Dose is generally not increased

 Dosing Tips
- Food delays absorption and reduces peak concentration

Overdose
- GI bleeding or ulceration, mucositis, and oral ulceration are common
- Hematological reactions are common. Rarely renal failure, aplastic anemia, sepsis, shock, or death. Often occur as a consequence of daily dosing (instead of weekly)

Long-Term Use
- Usually used on a short-term basis for refractory disorders

Habit Forming
- No

How to Stop
- No need to taper but monitor for recurrence of neurological disorder

Pharmacokinetics
- Oral absorption is dose- and patient-dependent (lower percentage with higher dose). Peak serum levels in 1–2 hours. Terminal half-life is 3–10 hours at low doses but 8–15 hours with high doses. Mostly (about 90%) renal excretion

 Drug Interactions
- NSAIDs or salicylates may elevate levels and increase GI and hematological toxicity
- Salicylates, phenylbutazone, phenytoin, and sulfonamides may displace methotrexate from albumin and increase toxicity
- Probenecid reduces renal tubular transport and increases levels
- Oral antibiotics such as aminoglycosides, chloramphenicol may decrease absorption
- May increase hepatotoxicity when used with other hepatotoxic agents, such as azathioprine
- May decrease clearance of theophylline, increasing levels
- Folic acid vitamins may reduce response to methotrexate, and folate deficiency may increase toxicity

Other Warnings/ Precautions

- Methotrexate given concomitantly with radiotherapy may increase the risk of soft tissue necrosis and osteonecrosis
- Diarrhea and ulcerative stomatitis require interruption of therapy: otherwise, hemorrhagic enteritis and death from intestinal perforation may occur

Do Not Use

- Known hypersensitivity, pregnancy or breast feeding, preexisting blood dyscrasias, chronic liver disease, or alcoholism

SPECIAL POPULATIONS

Renal Impairment

- At greater risk for toxicity and renal function may worsen. Use with caution

Hepatic Impairment

- Do not use. Alcoholism, obesity, advanced age, and diabetes are risk factors for hepatotoxicity

Cardiac Impairment

- No known effects

Elderly

- Monitor closely. Bone marrow suppression, thrombocytopenia, and pneumonitis are more common

 Children and Adolescents

- In the treatment of cancer and rheumatoid arthritis, AEs are similar to adults. Not well studied in children with DM or MS

 Pregnancy

- Category X. Causes abortion, embryotoxicity, and fetal defects. Avoid pregnancy after use for 3 months in men and at least 1 ovulatory cycle in women

Breast Feeding

- Do not breast feed

THE ART OF NEUROPHARMACOLOGY

Potential Advantages

- Useful corticosteroid-sparing agent in PM/DM. Once-weekly dosing. Effective in the treatment of CNS lymphoma

Potential Disadvantages

- Multiple AEs complicate use

Primary Target Symptoms

- Preventive treatment of complications from PM, DM, or MS

 Pearls

- In DM or PM, use azathioprine instead of methotrexate as a corticosteroid-sparing agent in patients with interstitial lung disease, liver disease, or in those that refuse to abstain from alcohol
- Improvement in muscle strength a better predictor of improvement in PM or DM than a decrease in creatine kinase
- Anti-Jo-1 antibodies are predictive of worsening response in PM and DM
- PM in general is less likely to respond to corticosteroids (about 50%) than DM (over 80%), but DM patients may have a more difficult time tapering corticosteroids
- In 1 trial, lowered serum creatine kinase levels in subjects with inclusion body myositis but did not prevent progression of illness
- In relapsing-remitting MS, clinical studies demonstrated preservation of upper extremity function with low-dose weekly methotrexate at a dose of 7.5 mg/day once weekly (2.5 mg 3 times a day for 1 day). One study showed effectiveness in reducing the rate of progression in chronic progressive MS
- Established as effective for primary CNS lymphoma. Requires rapid infusion. Often used in combination with other agents such as temozolomide or rituximab. The potential benefit of intrathecal or intraventricular administration for CNS lymphomas is unclear
- A recent trial of IV vincristine, oral procarbazine, and intraventricular methotrexate for CNS lymphoma did show prolonged survival

Suggested Reading

Badrising UA, Maat-Schieman ML, Ferrari MD, Zwinderman AH, Wessels JA, Breedveld FC, et al. Comparison of weakness progression in inclusion body myositis during treatment with methotrexate or placebo. *Ann Neurol.* 2002; 51(3):369–72.

Gray OM, McDonnell GV, Forbes RB. A systematic review of oral methotrexate for multiple sclerosis. *Mult Scler.* 2006;12 (4):507–10.

Hengstman GJ, van den Hoogen FH, van Engelen BG. Treatment of the inflammatory myopathies: update and practical recommendations. *Expert Opin Pharmacother.* 2009;10(7):1183–90.

Roth P, Korfel A, Martus P, Weller M. Pathogenesis and management of primary CNS lymphoma. *Expert Rev Anticancer Ther.* 2012; 12(5):623–33.

Tsuji G, Maekawa S, Saigo K, Nobuhara Y, Nakamura T, Kawano S, et al. Dermatomyositis and myelodysplastic syndrome with myelofibrosis responding to methotrexate therapy. *Am J Hematol.* 2003;74(3): 175–8.

Vencovský J, Jarosová K, Machácek S, Studýnková J, Kafková J, Bartůnková J, et al. Cyclosporine A versus methotrexate in the treatment of polymyositis and dermatomyositis. *Scand J Rheumatol.* 2000;29(2):95–102.

White ES, Lynch JP. Pharmacological therapy for Wegener's granulomatosis. *Drugs.* 2006; 66(9):1209–28.

METHYLERGONOVINE

THERAPEUTICS

Brands
- Methergine

Generic?
- Yes

Class
- Ergot

Commonly Prescribed for
(FDA approved in bold)
- **Prevention and control of post-partum hemorrhage**
- Migraine prophylaxis
- Cluster headache

How the Drug Works
- $5\text{-HT}_{2A/B/C}$ receptor antagonist and $5\text{-HT}_{1B/D}$ agonist
- Used to prevent or control excessive bleeding following childbirth and spontaneous or elective abortion. Causes uterine contractions to aid in expulsion of retained products of conception after miscarriage and to help deliver the placenta after childbirth
- Migraine/cluster: proposed mechanisms include vasoconstrictive actions or inhibition of the release of inflammatory neuropeptides, such as calcitonin gene-related peptide. Prevention of cortical spreading depression may be one mechanism of action for all migraine preventatives. An active metabolite of methysergide

How Long Until It Works
- Obstetrical: hours, or minutes as an injection
- Migraines: within 2 weeks, but can take up to 2 months on a stable dose to see full effect

If It Works
- In migraine, the goal is a 50% or greater decrease in migraine frequency or severity. Consider tapering or stopping if headaches remit for more than 6 months or if considering pregnancy

If It Doesn't Work
- Increase to highest tolerated dose
- Migraine: address other issues, such as medication overuse, other coexisting medical disorders, such as anxiety, and consider changing to another drug or adding a second drug

Best Augmenting Combos for Partial Response or Treatment-Resistance
- Migraine: usually used in refractory cases of migraine and cluster headache, usually as an adjunctive agent. May use in combination with AEDs, antidepressants, natural products, and non-pharmacological treatments, such as biofeedback, to improve headache control

Tests
- Monitor blood pressure. In patients on long-term continuous therapy, consider screening for fibrotic disorders

ADVERSE EFFECTS (AEs)

How the Drug Causes AEs
- Actions on serotonin receptors, including vasoconstriction. Fibrotic complications are related to 5-HT_{2B} actions

Notable AEs
- Muscle aching, claudication, nausea, vomiting, weight gain
- Dizziness, giddiness, drowsiness, paresthesias
- Hypertension
- Rarely hallucinations

Life-Threatening or Dangerous AEs
- Severe hypertension
- Ergots and related drugs are associated with the development of retroperitoneal, pulmonary, or endocardial fibrosis. Long-term continuous use appears to be the biggest risk factor

Weight Gain
- Unusual

unusual | not unusual | common | problematic

Sedation

- Unusual

unusual   not unusual   common   problematic

What to Do About AEs

- Lower dose for nausea, stop for serious AEs

Best Augmenting Agents to Reduce AEs

- Most AEs cannot be treated with an augmenting agent

DOSING AND USE

Usual Dosage Range

- 0.4–1.2 mg/day

Dosage Forms

- Tablets: 0.2 mg
- Injection: 0.2 mg/mL

How to Dose

- Obstetrical: 1 tablet 3–4 times daily, or injection (IM or IV) 0.2 mg every 2–4 hours
- Migraine: 1 tablet twice a day, increase by 1–2 tablets every week in 2–3 divided doses to maximum of 6 tablets per day

 Dosing Tips

- Parenteral drug products should be inspected visually for particulate matter and discoloration prior to administration

Overdose

- Abdominal pain, nausea, numbness, vomiting, paresthesias, and hypertension are most common. Convulsions, coma, hypotension, and respiratory depression have been reported

Long-Term Use

- Long-term, continuous use of methysergide (methylergonovine is a metabolite) is associated with the development of retroperitoneal, pulmonary, or endocardial fibrosis

Habit Forming

- No

How to Stop

- In migraine prophylaxis, reduce/taper dose over 2–4 weeks, as stopping quickly may trigger headache

Pharmacokinetics

- Mean elimination half-life 3–4 hours. Bioavailability is 60%. Hepatic metabolism and excretion

 Drug Interactions

- Use with caution with other vasoconstrictive agents, ergot alkaloids, or triptans
- Do not administer with potent CYP3A4 inhibitors, including macrolide antibiotics (erythromycin, clarithromycin), HIV protease or reverse transcriptase inhibitors (delaviridine, ritonavir, nelfinavir, indinavir), or azole antifungals (ketoconazole, itraconazole, voriconazole). Less potent 3A4 inhibitors include saquinavir, nefazodone, fluconazole, fluoxetine, fluvoxamine, grapefruit juice, and clotrimazole. Concomitant use may lead to cerebral or limb ischemia

 Other Warnings/ Precautions

- Use with caution in the setting of sepsis

Do Not Use

- With CYP3A4 inhibitors
- Hypertension, toxemia, pregnancy
- Proven hypersensitivity to drug

SPECIAL POPULATIONS

Renal Impairment

- Safety and effect of significant disease on drug metabolism unknown. Use with caution

Hepatic Impairment

- Safety and effect of significant disease on drug metabolism unknown. Avoid using in patients with severe disease

Cardiac Impairment

- Do not use in patients with hypertension or significant vascular disease

Elderly

- Use with caution, especially in those with known hypertension

 Children and Adolescents

- Not studied in children. The pediatric dose is unknown

 Pregnancy

- Category C, but contraindicated due to uterotonic effects

Breast Feeding

- A small amount is found in breast milk. Use with caution

THE ART OF NEUROPHARMACOLOGY

Potential Advantages

- Believed effective and well-tolerated prophylactic agent in refractory migraine

Potential Disadvantages

- Potential for serious AEs, including fibrosis. Limited clinical trial evidence

Primary Target Symptoms

- Migraine frequency and severity

 Pearls

- Not a first-line drug, but may be used as a rescue preventive for very frequent migraines. Well tolerated but long-term AEs of ergots may raise concerns. Most frequently used in tertiary headache clinics
- Metabolite of methysergide, an FDA-approved migraine prophylactic agent no longer available in the US
- Safety with other potentially vasoconstrictive drugs (i.e., triptans) is unknown
- Because methylergonovine and methysergide are weak vasoconstrictors compared with oral ergots, they are occasionally used for patients using triptans for acute attacks. In early clinical studies of sumatriptan many patients were on 5-HT$_2$ agonists, such as methysergide or pizotifen. Consider the risks and benefit of treatment
- Perhaps most effective in cluster headache
- Reportedly effective in post-dural puncture headache

 Suggested Reading

Dodick DW, Silberstein SD. Migraine prevention. *Pract Neurol.* 2007;7(6):383–93.

Gaiser R. Postdural puncture headache. *Curr Opin Anaesthesiol.* 2006;19(3):249–53.

Graff-Radford SB, Bittar GT. The use of methylergonovine (Methergine) in the initial control of drug induced refractory headache. *Headache.* 1993;33(7):390–3.

Mueller L, Gallagher RM, Ciervo CA. Methylergonovine maleate as a cluster headache prophylactic: a study and review. *Headache.* 1997;37(7):437–42.

Silberstein SD. Preventive migraine treatment. *Neurol Clin.* 2009;27(2):429–43.

METOCLOPRAMIDE

THERAPEUTICS

Brands
- Reglan, Maxolon, Clopra

Generic?
- Yes

Class
- Antiemetic

Commonly Prescribed for
(FDA approved in bold)
- **Diabetic gastroparesis**
- **Symptomatic gastroesophageal reflux (short-term therapy)**
- Nausea and vomiting (postoperative, chemotherapy, pregnancy)
- Small bowel intubation
- Migraine (acute)
- Tics in Gilles de la Tourette syndrome (GTS)
- Hiccup

How the Drug Works
- Antagonism at dopamine receptor (specifically D_2) and 5-HT$_3$ (at higher dose) decreases nausea. It may also increase absorption of coadministered drugs. May stimulate GI motility by sensitizing tissues to the actions of muscarinic activity, D_2 antagonism, and 5-HT$_4$ receptor agonism

How Long Until It Works
- 30–60 minutes with oral dose for nausea. Gastroparesis improves maximally by 3 weeks

If It Works
- Use at lowest effective dose
- Continue to assess effect of the medication and if it is still needed

If It Doesn't Work
- Increase dose, or discontinue and change to another agent
- Migraine: change to another antiemetic (prochlorperazine, droperidol, chlorpromazine) or combine with other agents
- Gastroparesis: domperidone (where available) is an alternative. Smaller, more frequent meals with low fat and fiber might improve symptoms

Best Augmenting Combos for Partial Response or Treatment-Resistance
- Migraine: often combined with NSAIDs, triptans, or ergots. Usually not used as monotherapy
- Gastroparesis: may be combined with erythromycin, botulinum toxin, electrical gastric stimulation

Tests
- None required

ADVERSE EFFECTS (AEs)

How the Drug Causes AEs
- Motor AEs and prolactinemia: blocking of D_2 receptors

Notable AEs
- Most common: sedation, CNS depression
- Fluid retention, bradycardia or superventricular tachycardia, hypo or hypertension, rash, galactorrhea, urinary frequency or incontinence
- Akathisia, parkinsonism (bradykinesia, tremor, rigidity), acute dystonic reactions

Life-Threatening or Dangerous AEs
- Tardive dyskinesias
- Neuroleptic malignant syndrome (rare)
- Hepatotoxicity (rare)

Weight Gain
- Unusual

unusual not unusual common problematic

Sedation
- Not unusual

unusual not unusual common problematic

What to Do About AEs
- Excessive sedation: lower dose or use only as a rescue agent when patient can lie down or sleep
- Movement disorders: lower dose or stop

Best Augmenting Agents to Reduce AEs

- Give fluids to avoid hypotension, tachycardia, and dizziness
- Give anticholinergics (diphenhydramine or benztropine) or benzodiazepines for extrapyramidal reactions

DOSING AND USE

Usual Dosage Range

- Migraine: 5–30 mg per dose
- Gastroparesis: 10–15 mg 3–4 times daily before meals

Dosage Forms

- Tablets: 5, 10 mg
- Syrup: 5 mg/5 mL
- Injection: 5 mg/mL
- Oral disintegrating tablet: 5, 10 mg

How to Dose

- Migraine/vertigo: IV, IM, or oral. Non-oral routes are useful for severe vomiting. IV/IM: 10–30 mg 3–4 times daily. Oral: 10–20 mg, usually as adjunctive treatment

 Dosing Tips

- Give before meals for gastroparesis, and 10–20 minutes (oral or IM) before other medications for migraine. To reduce risk of motor AEs including akathisia, administer IV formulation more slowly (over 10–15 minutes)

Overdose

- Drowsiness, confusion, and extrapyramidal reactions may occur

Long-Term Use

- Risk of movement AEs (tardive dyskinesias, parkinsonism) with frequent use

Habit Forming

- No

How to Stop

- No need to taper

Pharmacokinetics

- Half-life 5–6 hours. Peak effect 1–2 hours. 85% eliminated in urine

 Drug Interactions

- Increases bioavailability of levodopa due to increased absorption, which in turn decreases metoclopramide effect on gastric emptying
- Anticholinergics and opioids decrease effects on GI motility
- Releases catecholamines and may increase effect of MAOIs
- May increase absorption and enhance effects of alcohol and cyclosporine
- May decrease effectiveness of cimetidine and digoxin because of decreased absorption due to faster transit time
- Increases the neuromuscular blocking effects of succinylcholine

 Other Warnings/ Precautions

- May precipitate hypertensive crisis in patients with pheochromocytoma
- Parkinsonism may occur, usually within 6 months of starting, and may persist for 2–3 months after discontinuation

Do Not Use

- Hypersensitivity to drug, known pheochromocytoma, or any condition where GI stimulation could be dangerous (bowel obstruction, hemorrhage, or perforation)

SPECIAL POPULATIONS

Renal Impairment

- Clearance decreased. Use lower doses

Hepatic Impairment

- Use with caution

Cardiac Impairment

- May alter blood pressure or cause fluid retention in patients with heart failure

Elderly

- More likely to experience movement AEs

 Children and Adolescents

- Efficacy and safety unknown. Poorly studied, but a dose of 0.15 mg/kg in acute migraine has been studied. In GTS, give 10–60mg/day in divided doses. May have greater risk of AEs

Pregnancy

- Category B. Metoclopramide use in pregnancy not associated with increased risk of major congenital malformation

Breast Feeding

- Found in breast milk. Monitor infant for sedation

THE ART OF NEUROPHARMACOLOGY

Potential Advantages

- Effective medication for intractable migraine, vomiting, or vertigo. Less sedation and orthostasis than most antiemetics and no risk of QTc changes

Potential Disadvantages

- Usually not effective as monotherapy in oral form. Potential for movement disorders, especially with long-term use

Primary Target Symptoms

- Headache, vertigo, and nausea

Pearls

- In the treatment of status migrainosus, combining metoclopramide and dihydroergotamine for up to 1 week is usually effective. Give the metoclopramide first
- Pretreat or combine with diphenhydramine, 25–50mg, to reduce rate of akathisia and dystonic reactions. Benztropine is also useful and may be given orally or IM
- Restlessness can be treated by lorazepam or propranolol
- In outpatients with severe or daily headache, may be used daily for short periods of time (3–10 days) as a bridge treatment in conjunction with NSAIDs before preventive medication becomes effective. May be especially helpful in persons with gastroparesis
- Prochlorperazine 10mg IV is comparable to metoclopramide 20mg IV in acute migraine treatment; the former has better pain outcome, the latter has less akathisia
- Combination of dihydroergotamine and metoclopramide is particularly effective for migraine treatment
- Higher dose (20 or 40mg IV) may not increase efficacy above that of 10mg IV
- May use 10mg orally during migraine prodrome to prevent acute attack
- Appears safe for migraine treatment during pregnancy
- Originally thought to be peripherally acting, but CNS AEs including parkinsonism, tardive dyskinesias, or dystonias are common with prolonged use
- In GTS, less weight gain or sedation compared to neuroleptics, but less evidence of effectiveness

Suggested Reading

Friedman BW, Esses D, Solorzano C, Dua N, Greenwald P, Radulescu R, Chang E, Hochberg M, Campbell C, Aghera A, Valentin T, Paternoster J, Bijur P, Lipton RB, Gallagher EJ. A randomized controlled trial of prochlorperazine versus metoclopramide for treatment of acute migraine. *Ann Emerg Med.* 2008;52(4):399–406.

Kelley NE, Tepper DE. Rescue therapy for acute migraine, part 2: neuroleptics, antihistamines, and others. *Headache.* 2012; 52(2):292–306.

Marmura MJ. Silberstein SD. Migraine: essentials of patient evaluation and acute treatment. *Pract Neurol.* 2009;8(3):12–17.

Pasternak B, Svanstrom H, Molgaard-Nielsen D, Melbye M, Hviid A. Metoclopramide in pregnancy and risk of major congenital malformations and fetal death. *JAMA.* 2013;310(15):1601–11.

Regan LA, Hoffman RS, Nelson LS. Slower infusion of metoclopramide decreases the rate of akathisia. *Am J Emerg Med.* 2009;27(4):475–80.

Silberstein SD, Ruoff G. Combination therapy in acute migraine treatment: the rationale behind the current treatment options. *Postgrad Med.* 2006;Spec No:20–6.

Skidmore F, Reich SG. Tardive dystonia. *Curr Treat Options Neurol.* 2005;7(3):231–6.

MEXILETINE

THERAPEUTICS

Brands
- Mexitil

Generic?
- Yes

Class
- Antiarrhythmic

Commonly Prescribed for
(FDA approved in bold)
- **Ventricular arrhythmias**
- Symptomatic myotonia (myotonia congenita, myotonic dystrophy)
- Intractable headache
- Trigeminal autonomic cephalalgia

How the Drug Works
- An oral analog of lidocaine. Class 1b antiarrhythmic agent that depresses phase 0; it reduces the rate of rise of the action potential (not the duration) by inhibiting the inward sodium current but not affecting resting membrane potential. It acts more on faster than slower heart rates. It has actions on surfaces and membranes of skeletal muscle and neuronal sodium-channel blocking properties. It also reduces the effective refractory period in Purkinje fibers in the heart

How Long Until It Works
- Antiarrhythmic effect will occur within hours, although it may take time to find optimal dose. May take more time (days or weeks) to see relief and determine most effective dose in myotonia or pain disorders

If It Works
- Continue to use with appropriate monitoring

If It Doesn't Work
- Check serum levels and if not effective change to an alternative agent

Best Augmenting Combos for Partial Response or Treatment-Resistance
- Myotonia: quinine and other AEDs are occasionally used. Phenytoin is also effective but has similar antiarrhythmic properties and may interact with mexiletine

Tests
- Monitor hepatic enzymes and CBC during therapy. Obtain ECG at baseline and for any new symptoms. Check a serum mexiletine level to guide therapy and for any AEs

ADVERSE EFFECTS (AEs)

How the Drug Causes AEs
- Drug effect blocking sodium channels

Notable AEs
- GI AEs (nausea, vomiting, heartburn) are most common. CNS AEs (tremor, nervousness, coordination difficulties, blurred vision, confusion) are much more common when serum levels exceed 2 mcg/mL

Life-Threatening or Dangerous AEs
- New or worsening cardiac arrhythmias
- Acute hepatic injury (usually in the first few weeks of therapy)
- Blood dyscrasias, including leukopenia (rare)

Weight Gain
- Unusual

unusual not unusual common problematic

Sedation
- Not unusual

unusual not unusual common problematic

What to Do About AEs
- Check serum level and ECG. For serious AEs, discontinue drug

Best Augmenting Agents to Reduce AEs
- Most AEs cannot be improved by an augmenting agent

DOSING AND USE

Usual Dosage Range
- Usual dose: 300–1200 mg/day in divided doses

Dosage Forms
- Tablets: 150, 200, 250 mg

How to Dose
- In patients on lidocaine infusion, stop lidocaine before starting mexiletine. Start at 200 mg every 8 hours. Adjust daily dose by 50–100 mg based on clinical effect every 3 or more days. Base dose on serum levels. Consider changing patients on a stable dose to twice-daily dosing

 Dosing Tips
- Take with food to reduce AEs

Overdose
- Nausea, hypotension, sinus bradycardia, paresthesia, seizures, AV heart block, and ventricular tachycardias

Long-Term Use
- Safe for long-term use with appropriate monitoring

Habit Forming
- No

How to Stop
- No need to taper for the treatment of neurological disorders

Pharmacokinetics
- Hepatic metabolism via CYP2D6 and 1A2 to less potent metabolites. Half-life 10–12 hours. Protein binding 50–60%. Bioavailability 90%. T_{max} 2–3 hours

 Drug Interactions
- Mexiletine may decrease clearance and increase levels of caffeine and theophylline
- Cimetidine may affect (increase or decrease) mexiletine levels
- Atropine, opioids, aluminum-magnesium hydroxide may slow absorption and decrease effect

- Metoclopramide increases absorption and increases levels
- Strong CYP1A2 inhibitors (e.g., fluoroquinolones, fluvoxamine, verapamil) and moderate CYP1A2 inhibitors (e.g., St. John's wort) can increase levels
- Strong CYP2D6 inhibitors (e.g., fluoxetine, paroxetine, buproprion, quinidine, ritonavir) and moderate CYP2D6 inhibitors (e.g., sertraline, duloxetine) can increase levels
- Enzyme inducers (e.g., carbamazepine, phenytoin, rifampin, dexamethasone) can increase drug clearance and lower levels
- Urinary pH affects renal clearance of mexiletine. Acidifiers increase clearance; alkalinizers decrease clearance

 Other Warnings/ Precautions
- All antiarrhythmic agents can worsen or cause new arrhythmias. These may include increase in premature ventricular arrhythmias to life-threatening tachycardias

Do Not Use
- Known hypersensitivity to the drug, cardiogenic shock, or preexisting second or third degree AV block (without pacemaker)

SPECIAL POPULATIONS

Renal Impairment
- Likely no effect on dose

Hepatic Impairment
- Use with caution. Patients with severe disease may need a lower dose

Cardiac Impairment
- Right-sided congestive heart failure can reduce hepatic metabolism and increase blood level and patients may require a reduced dose. Cardiac patients with existing disease are more prone to life-threatening arrhythmias

Elderly
- No known effects

 Children and Adolescents
- Not studied in children

Pregnancy

- Category C but not studied. Only use in pregnancy if clearly needed

Breast Feeding

- Excreted in breast milk. Do not use

THE ART OF NEUROPHARMACOLOGY

Potential Advantages

- Useful treatment for myotonia and refractory pain disorders

Potential Disadvantages

- Multiple AEs and need for monitoring complicate use

Primary Target Symptoms

- Symptoms of myotonia (muscle pain, stiffness, weakness, dysphagia), pain

Pearls

- Many patients with myotonia (delayed relaxation of muscles after activity) do not require pharmacological treatment of their symptoms

- Weakness in myotonia is usually in the arms or hands
- In non-dystrophic myotonia caused by mutation of *SCN4A* or *CLCN1*, patients with latter mutation seem to experience greater reduction in handgrip myotonia than patients with former mutation
- Other medications of putative usefulness in myotonia include other sodium channel blockers, such as phenytoin, procainamide, TCAs, benzodiazepines, calcium channel blockers, taurine, and prednisone. There are no large controlled drug trials for myotonia treatment
- Physical therapy may be of some benefit in myotonia
- Mexiletine is occasionally used for refractory headache. Successful treatment with IV lidocaine, if practical, may predict response to mexiletine
- Due to potential for significant interactions, including neurotoxicity, mexiletine should not be given to patients receiving IV lidocaine
- For patients with SUNCT (short-lasting unilateral neuralgiform headache with conjunctival injection and tearing) or SUNA (short-lasting unilateral neuralgiform headache attacks with cranial autonomic symptoms), mexiletine can be used short term while initiating lamotrigine or others
- May not be effective for neuropathic pain

Suggested Reading

Finnerup NB, Sindrup SH, Jensen TS. The evidence for pharmacological treatment of neuropathic pain. *Pain*. 2010;150(3): 573–81.

Marmura MJ. Intravenous lidocaine and mexiletine in the management of trigeminal autonomic cephalalgias. *Curr Pain Headache Rep*. 2010;14(2):145–50.

Marmura MJ, Passero FC Jr, Young WB. Mexiletine for refractory chronic daily headache: a report of nine cases. *Headache*. 2008;48 (10):1506–10.

Statland JM, Bundy BN, Wang Y, Rayan DR, Trivedi JR, Sansone VA, et al. Mexiletine for symptoms and signs of myotonia in nondystrophic myotonia: a randomized controlled trial. *JAMA*. 2012;308(13):1357–65.

Trip J, Drost G, van Engelen BG, Faber CG. Drug treatment for myotonia. *Cochrane Database Syst Rev*. 2006;1:CD004762.

Wright JM, Oki JC, Graves L 3rd. Mexiletine in the symptomatic treatment of diabetic peripheral neuropathy. *Ann Pharmacother*. 1997;31(1): 29–34.

MILNACIPRAN

THERAPEUTICS

Brands
- Savella

Generic?
- No

Class
- Serotonin and norepinephrine reuptake inhibitor (SNRI)

Commonly Prescribed for
(FDA approved in bold)
- **Fibromyalgia**
- Major depressive disorder
- Post-stroke depression
- Migraine prophylaxis
- Stress urinary incontinence

How the Drug Works
- Both milnacipran and levomilnacipran (levo-enantiomer of milnacipran) are potent balanced inhibitors of serotonin and norepinephrine reuptake transporters (SERT, NET), increasing serotonin and norepinephrine levels within hours, but antidepressant effects take weeks. Effect is more likely related to adaptive changes in serotonin and norepinephrine receptor systems over time
- No affinity for serotonergic, adrenergic, muscarinic, dopamine, opiate, GABA receptors, and Ca^{2+}, Na^+, K^+, Cl^- channels
- It may modulate NMDA receptors in the superficial dorsal horn for antinociceptive effect
- Unlike venlafaxine or duloxetine where SERT effect dominates, milnacipran exerts a relatively equal influence on SERT and NET whereas levomilnacipran demonstrates a slightly greater NET inhibition than SERT inhibition

How Long Until It Works
- 2 weeks to 2 months for full effect

If It Works
- Continue to use and monitor for AEs

If It Doesn't Work
- Increase to highest tolerated dose. Consider adding a second agent or changing to another one

Best Augmenting Combos for Partial Response or Treatment-Resistance
- For some patients, low-dose polytherapy with 2 or more drugs may be better tolerated and more effective than high-dose monotherapy

Tests
- Check blood pressure, at baseline and when increasing dose
- Monitor sodium, intraocular pressure, suicidality, and unusual change in behavior

ADVERSE EFFECTS (AEs)

How the Drug Causes AEs
- By increasing serotonin and norepinephrine on non-therapeutic responsive receptors throughout the body. Most AEs are dose- and time-dependent

Notable AEs
- Incidence $\geq 5\%$: nausea, vomiting, headache, constipation, dizziness, insomnia, hot flush, hyperhidrosis, elevated blood pressure, palpitation, urinary hesitancy/retention, and erectile dysfunction

Life-Threatening or Dangerous AEs
- Serotonin syndrome
- Rare hepatotoxicity
- Rare activation of mania/hypomania or suicidal ideation
- Rare worsening of coexisting seizure disorders
- Abnormal bleeding
- Angle-closure glaucoma

Weight Gain
- Unusual

unusual   not unusual   common   problematic

Sedation
- Unusual

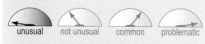

unusual   not unusual   common   problematic

What to Do About AEs
- For minor AEs, lower dose, titrate more slowly, or switch to another agent. For serious AEs, lower dose and consider stopping, taper to avoid withdrawal symptoms

Best Augmenting Agents to Reduce AEs
- Try magnesium for constipation
- Cyproheptadine can be used for serotonin syndrome by blocking 5-HT receptors and SERT
- Sexual dysfunction (anorgasmia, impotence) may be reversed by agents with α_2-adrenergic antagonist activity (e.g., buspirone, amantadine, bupropion, mirtazapine, ginkgo biloba, etc.)

DOSING AND USE

Usual Dosage Range
- 50 mg twice daily. Maximum 100 mg

Dosage Forms
- Tablet; 12.5, 25, 50, 100 mg

How to Dose
- Day 1: 12.5 mg daily. Days 2–3: 12.5 mg twice daily. Days 4–7: 25 mg twice daily. After day 7: 50 mg twice daily

 Dosing Tips
- Food does not affect bioavailability

Overdose
- In postmarketing experience of milnacipran, the most common signs and symptoms included increased blood pressure, cardio-respiratory arrest, changes in the level of consciousness (ranging from somnolence to coma), confusional state, dizziness, and increased hepatic enzymes. No specific antidote. If serotonin syndrome ensues, cyproheptadine and/or temperature control may be considered

Long-Term Use
- Safe for long-term use with monitoring of blood pressure and suicidality

Habit Forming
- No

How to Stop
- Taper slowly (no more than 50% reduction every 3–4 days until discontinuation) to avoid withdrawal (agitation, anxiety, confusion, dry mouth, dysphoria, etc.)

Pharmacokinetics
- C_{max} reached in 2–4 hours. Bioavailability 85–90%. Low protein binding (13%). Eliminated primarily by renal excretion (55% unchanged)

 Drug Interactions
- Levomilnacipran
- No need for adjustment on CYP450 system
- Concomitant use of catecholamines may be associated with paroxysmal hypertension and possible arrhythmia
- When switching from clomipramine, an increase in euphoria and postural hypotension was observed
- Postural hypotension and tachycardia have been reported in combination therapy with IV administered digoxin
- The release of serotonin by platelets is important for maintaining hemostasis. Combined use of SSRIs or SNRIs and NSAIDs, and/or drugs that affect platelets or coagulation has been associated with an increased risk of bleeding

 Other Warnings/ Precautions
- May increase risk of seizure
- Patients should be observed closely for clinical worsening, suicidality, and changes in behavior in known or unknown bipolar disorder

Do Not Use
- Proven hypersensitivity to drug
- Concurrently with MAOI; allow at least 14 days between discontinuation of an MAOI and initiation of milnacipran, or at

least 7–14 days between discontinuation of milnacipran and initiation of an MAOI
- Concurrent use of serotonin precursors (e.g., tryptophan)
- In patients with uncontrolled narrow angle-closure glaucoma
- In patients treated with linezolid or methylene blue IV

hyperreflexia, tremor, jitteriness, irritability, and constant crying consistent with a toxic effect of the drug or drug discontinuation syndrome have been reported

Breast Feeding
- Some drug is found in breast milk and use while breast feeding is not recommended

SPECIAL POPULATIONS

Renal Impairment
- Use with caution in moderate or severe renal impairment. Decrease usual dose by 25–50%

Hepatic Impairment
- No adjustment needed

Cardiac Impairment
- Dose-dependent effect on blood pressure and heart rate. No effect on QTc

Elderly
- No adjustment necessary. At greater risk for hyponatremia

Children and Adolescents
- Safety and efficacy not established. Use with caution. Observe closely for clinical worsening, suicidality, and changes in behavior in known or unknown bipolar disorder. Parents should be informed and advised of the risks

Pregnancy
- Category C. Generally not recommended for the treatment of headaches or neuropathic pain during pregnancy. Neonates exposed to SNRIs or SSRIs late in the third trimester have developed complications necessitating extended hospitalizations, respiratory support, and tube feeding. Respiratory distress, cyanosis, apnea, seizures, temperature instability, feeding difficulty, vomiting, hypoglycemia, hypotonia,

THE ART OF NEUROPHARMACOLOGY

Potential Advantages
- A novel, balanced SNRI for fibromyalgia and depression

Potential Disadvantages
- May cause or worsen hypertension. Requires gradual titration

Primary Target Symptoms
- Reduction in fibromyalgia syndrome (sleep, fatigue, pain, mood)
- Reduction in depression

 Pearls
- In a recent comparative study on treating fibromyalgia syndrome, milnacipran was superior to duloxetine in reducing fatigue but inferior in reducing sleep disturbance and depressed mood
- Based on a Cochrane review, milnacipran 100 mg or 200 mg is effective for a minority in the treatment of pain due to fibromyalgia. There were no data for the use of milnacipran for other chronic neuropathic pain conditions
- May work as other SNRIs for anxiety and neuropathic pain but remain to be determined
- Milnacipran (200 mg/day) may be as effective antidepressant as venlafaxine (200 mg/day)
- May work for stress urinary incontinence
- In an open-label study, milnacipran 100 mg is effective in reducing migraine days and disability
- Short-term (6 months) weight loss is normalized at 30 months

MILNACIPRAN (continued)

Suggested Reading

Derry S, Gill D, Phillips T, Moore RA. Milnacipran for neuropathic pain and fibromyalgia in adults. *Cochrane Database Syst Rev.* 2012;3:CD008244.

Engel ER, Kudrow D, Rapoport AM. A prospective, open-label study of milnacipran in the prevention of headache in patients with episodic or chronic migraine. *Neurol Sci.* 2014;35(3):429–35.

Häuser W, Petzke F, Sommer C. Comparative efficacy and harms of duloxetine, milnacipran, and pregabalin in fibromyalgia syndrome. *J Pain.* 2010;11(6):505–21.

Kohno T, Kimura M, Sasaki M, Obata H, Amaya F, Saito S. Milnacipran inhibits glutamatergic N-methyl-D-aspartate receptor activity in spinal dorsal horn neurons. *Mol Pain.* 2012;8:45.

Mansuy L. Antidepressant therapy with milnacipran and venlafaxine. *Neuropsychiatr Dis Treat.* 2010;6(Suppl I):17.

Matsuzawa-Yanagida K, Narita M, Nakajima M, Kuzumaki N, Niikura K, Nozaki H, et al. Usefulness of antidepressants for improving the neuropathic pain-like state and pain-induced anxiety through actions at different brain sites. *Neuropsychopharmacology.* 2008;33(8):1952–65.

Sansone RA, Sansone LA. Serotonin norepinephrine reuptake inhibitors: a pharmacological comparison. *Innov Clin Neurosci.* 2014;11(3–4):37–42.

MIRTAZAPINE

THERAPEUTICS

Brands
- Remeron, Remeron SolTab

Generic?
- Yes

Class
- Tetracyclic antidepressant

Commonly Prescribed for
(FDA approved in bold)
- **Major depressive disorder**
- Tension-type headache prophylaxis
- Post-traumatic stress disorder (PTSD)
- Panic disorder
- Fibromyalgia
- Neuropathic pain
- Phantom limb pain
- Antiemetic

How the Drug Works
- Mirtazapine enhances central noradrenergic and serotonergic activity via presynaptic α_2-receptor blockade. Mirtazapine is an antagonist of 5-HT$_2$, 5-HT$_3$, H$_1$, α_1-, α_2-adrenergic, and muscarinic receptors. Mirtazapine has no significant affinity for the 5-HT$_{1A}$ and 5-HT$_{1B}$ receptors

How Long Until It Works
- Depression: 2 weeks but up to 2 months for full effect

If It Works
- Continue to use and monitor for AEs. May continue for 1 year following first depression episode or indefinitely if > 1 episode of depression

If It Doesn't Work
- Increase to highest tolerated dose. Change to another agent or add a second agent

Best Augmenting Combos for Partial Response or Treatment-Resistance
- For some patients, low-dose polytherapy with 2 or more drugs may be better tolerated and more effective than high-dose monotherapy

Tests
- Monitor transaminase, serum sodium, and CBC

ADVERSE EFFECTS (AEs)

How the Drug Causes AEs
- Through serotonin, histamine, adrenergic, muscarinic receptor antagonism throughout the body. Most AEs are dose- and time-dependent

Notable AEs
- Somnolence, dizziness, constipation, dry mouth, increased appetite, weight gain, increased cholesterol, akathisia

Life-Threatening or Dangerous AEs
- Serotonin syndrome
- Rare hepatitis
- Rare activation of mania or suicidal ideation
- Rare worsening of coexisting seizure disorders
- Hyponatremia
- Agranulocytosis

Weight Gain
- Problematic

unusual   not unusual   common   problematic

Sedation
- Common

unusual   not unusual   common   problematic

What to Do About AEs
- For minor AEs, lower dose, titrate more slowly, or switch to another agent. For serious AEs, lower dose and consider stopping, taper to avoid withdrawal symptoms

Best Augmenting Agents to Reduce AEs
- Try magnesium for constipation
- Cyproheptadine can be used for serotonin syndrome by blocking 5-HT receptors and SERT

DOSING AND USE

Usual Dosage Range
- 15–45 mg/day

Dosage Forms
- Tablet: 7.5, 15, 30, 45 mg
- Oral disintegrating tablet: 15, 30, 45 mg

How to Dose
- Initial dose 15 mg/day prior to sleep. Increase 15 mg/day at no less than 1–2 week interval until 45 mg/day

 Dosing Tips
- Can be taken with food. For SolTab, place it on tongue immediately after removal from the package

Overdose
- Disorientation, drowsiness, impaired memory, and tachycardia. No antidote. Standard overdose management

Long-Term Use
- Safe for long-term use with monitoring of suicidality

Habit Forming
- No

How to Stop
- Taper slowly (no more than 50% reduction every 1–2 weeks until discontinuation) to avoid withdrawal symptoms (agitation, abnormal dreams, anxiety, confusion, headache, tremor, nausea, vomiting, dysphoria, sensory disturbance, etc.)

Pharmacokinetics
- Metabolized by CYP1A2, 2D6, 3A4. Half-life 20–40 hours. C_{max} in 2 hours. Bioavailability 50%. Eliminated via urine (75%) and feces (15%). 85% protein bound

 Drug Interactions
- Potential serotonin syndrome with concomitant use of MAOIs and serotonergic drugs
- Increase dose if used with CYP enzyme inducers (phenytoin, carbamazepine, rifampin)
- Reduce dose if used with CYP enzyme inhibitors (cimetidine, ketoconazole, protease inhibitors, erythromycin, nefazodone)
- Cautious on CNS depressant (alcohol, diazepam)

 Other Warnings/ Precautions
- May increase risk of seizure
- Patients should be observed closely for clinical worsening, suicidality, and changes in behavior in known or unknown bipolar disorder

Do Not Use
- Proven hypersensitivity to drug
- Concurrently with MAOI; allow at least 14 days between discontinuation of an MAOI and initiation of mirtazapine or at least 7–14 days between discontinuation of mirtazapine and initiation of an MAOI
- Concurrent use of serotonin precursors (e.g., tryptophan)
- In patients with uncontrolled narrow angle-closure glaucoma
- In patients treated with linezolid or methylene blue IV

SPECIAL POPULATIONS

Renal Impairment
- Use with caution. Decrease usual dose by 25–50%

Hepatic Impairment
- Use with caution. Decrease usual dose by 50%

Cardiac Impairment
- No significant QTc prolongation

Elderly
- May have decreased renal clearance

 Children and Adolescents
- Safety and efficacy not established. Use with caution

Pregnancy

- Category C. Generally not recommended during pregnancy

Breast Feeding

- Some drug is found in breast milk and use while breast feeding is not recommended

THE ART OF NEUROPHARMACOLOGY

Potential Advantages

- Antidepressant without sleep disturbance and sexual dysfunction

Potential Disadvantages

- Somnolence. Weight gain

Primary Target Symptoms

- Reduction in depression, anxiety
- Reduction in headache frequency, duration, and/or intensity
- Reduction in neuropathic pain

 Pearls

- Unlike TCAs or SSRIs, it does not affect REM sleep. It decreases sleep latency and increases slow wave sleep
- Can be used to ameliorate nausea (via 5-HT$_3$ antagonism) and increase appetite
- May improve PTSD symptoms
- It may be useful for anxiety symptoms in depressed patients but has no role in generalized social anxiety disorder
- It may be more cost-effective than placebo for treating depressed demented patients by ameliorating sleep disturbances and anxiety but probably not depression
- It increases pain tolerance
- Mirtazapine 30 mg/day is recommended for prophylaxis of tension-type headache but not migraine
- Combining mirtazapine and pregabalin may be more effective than pregabalin alone in managing post-herpetic neuralgia
- It has been used for phantom limb pain in a case series

 Suggested Reading

Alexander W. Pharmacotherapy for post-traumatic stress disorder in combat veterans: focus on antidepressants and atypical antipsychotic agents. *P & T.* 2012;37(1): 32–8.

Arnold P, Vuadens P, Kuntzer T, Gobelet C, Deriaz O. Mirtazapine decreases the pain feeling in healthy participants. *Clin J Pain.* 2008; 24(2):116–19.

Bendtsen L, Evers S, Linde M, Mitsikostas DD, Sandrini G, Schoenen J, et al. EFNS guideline on the treatment of tension-type headache – report of an EFNS task force. *Eur J Neurol.* 2010; 17(11):1318–25.

Bomholt SF, Mikkelsen JD, Blackburn-Munro G. Antinociceptive effects of the antidepressants amitriptyline, duloxetine, mirtazapine and citalopram in animal models of acute, persistent and neuropathic pain. *Neuropharmacology.* 2005;48(2):252–63.

McCormick Z, Chang-Chien G, Marshall B, Huang M, Harden RN. Phantom limb pain: a systematic neuroanatomical-based review of pharmacologic treatment. *Pain Med.* 2013; 15(2):292–305.

Schutters SIJ, Van Megen HJGM, Van Veen JF, Denys DAJP, Westenberg HGM. Mirtazapine in generalized social anxiety disorder: a randomized, double-blind, placebo-controlled study. *Int Clin Psychopharmacol.* 2010;25(5):302–4.

Yeephu S, Suthisisang C, Suttiruksa S, Prateepavanich P, Limampai P, Russell IJ. Efficacy and safety of mirtazapine in fibromyalgia syndrome patients: a randomized placebo-controlled pilot study. *Ann Pharmacother.* 2013;47(7–8):921–32.

MITOXANTRONE

THERAPEUTICS

Brands
- Novantrone

Generic?
- Yes

Class
- Antineoplastic agent

Commonly Prescribed for
(FDA approved in bold)
- **Reducing neurological disability or relapses in patients with secondary progressive, progressive relapsing, or worsening relapsing-remitting multiple sclerosis (MS)**
- **Acute non-lymphocytic leukemia in adults**
- **Pain related to advanced hormone-refractory prostate cancer**
- Breast cancer
- Non-Hodgkin's lymphoma

How the Drug Works
- A DNA-reactive agent that causes crosslinks and strand breaks, interferes with DNA uncoiling and repair, and has a cytocidal effect on cells. In MS, it appears to blunt the immune processes believed to be responsible in part for the disease
- It suppresses B-cell, T-cell, and macrophage function, impairs antigen proliferation, and decreases the secretion of inflammatory cytokines, including tumor necrosis factor-α, interleukin 2, and interferon-γ, that mediate demyelination
- Due to its slow release from sequestered tissue into blood it is a long-acting immunosuppressant

How Long Until It Works
- MS: months to years. In trials treated patients had fewer relapses at 1 and 2 years

If It Works
- Continue to use until ineffective or a total of 140 mg/m^2 then discontinue because of cardiotoxicity risk

If It Doesn't Work
- For patients failing first-line agents in MS (interferons, glatiramer) and mitoxantrone

with frequent relapses (measured by clinical outcome and MRI accumulation of lesions) consider using natalizumab, alemtuzumab, fingolimod, or other newer agents

Best Augmenting Combos for Partial Response or Treatment-Resistance
- Acute attacks in MS are often treated with glucocorticoids, especially if there is functional impairment due to vision loss, weakness, or cerebellar symptoms
- Treat common clinical symptoms with appropriate medication for spasticity (baclofen, tizanidine), neuropathic pain, and fatigue (modafinil)
- Generally not combined with most other MS disease-modifying treatments (natalizumab, interferons, glatiramer) but 1 study showed that adding monthly mitoxantrone to monthly doses of 1 g methylprednisolone improved outcomes

Tests
- Assess cardiac left ventricular (LV) function using ECG or MUGA (multigated acquisition scan) at baseline and before each dose of mitoxantrone. Obtain a baseline blood count and recheck if symptoms of infection occur

ADVERSE EFFECTS (AEs)

How the Drug Causes AEs
- Most AEs are likely related to effect on DNA synthesis and function and its immunosuppressive effect

Notable AEs
- Arrhythmias or ECG changes, leukopenia, anemia, thrombocytopenia, hepatic enzyme elevations, amenorrhea, nausea, urinary tract infections, anorexia, malaise/fatigue, alopecia, weakness, pharyngitis, extravasation at IV sites, peripheral edema, dyspnea, chills, infection. Urine may turn blue-green color

Life-Threatening or Dangerous AEs
- Suppression of LV ejection fraction can lead to heart failure and death
- Serious infections have occurred in patients developing neutropenia on mitoxantrone

Weight Gain
- Unusual

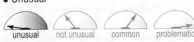

Sedation
- Common

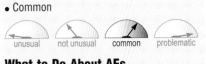

What to Do About AEs
- Significant changes in LV ejection fraction or < 50%: discontinue
- Neutropenia (< 1500 cells/mm^3): discontinue

Best Augmenting Agents to Reduce AEs
- Pretreat to prevent nausea before first infusion. Topical corticosteroids for IV extravasation

DOSING AND USE

Usual Dosage Range
- 12 mg/m^2 is the standard dose in MS

Dosage Forms
- Injection: 2 mg/mL in 10, 12.5, and 15 mL vials

How to Dose
- Give 12 mg/m^2 every 3 months as an infusion. Infusing slowly (over 30 minutes) may reduce risk of cardiotoxicity

 Dosing Tips
- Should be given in specialty infusion center

Overdose
- Some patients died a result of leukopenia and infection

Long-Term Use
- Use is limited to 2–3 years (a total of 140 mg/body surface area in m^2) due to cardiac toxicity

Habit Forming
- No

How to Stop
- No need to taper

Pharmacokinetics
- Drug has a wide distribution into tissue, exceeding the concentrations in the blood. The drug is slowly released into the bloodstream from tissue. The elimination half-life is 23–215 hours (mean 75). 78% of drug is protein bound. Excreted in urine or feces as unchanged or inactive metabolites

 Drug Interactions
- No known drug interactions

 Other Warnings/ Precautions
- Risk of acute myeloblastic leukemia even years after stopping the medication

Do Not Use
- Known hypersensitivity to the drug. Known liver or heart failure

SPECIAL POPULATIONS

Renal Impairment
- No known effects

Hepatic Impairment
- Do not use for treatment of MS

Cardiac Impairment
- Do not use in patients with LV ejection fraction of 50% or less, or in patients experiencing significant decrease after starting treatment

Elderly
- Clearance of drug might be slower

 Children and Adolescents
- Safety and efficacy are not established

 Pregnancy
- Category D. Considered teratogenic based on mechanism of action. Do not use, and do

a pregnancy test in women with MS of childbearing potential before starting treatment

Breast Feeding

• Drug is excreted in breast milk. Do not breast feed on drug

THE ART OF NEUROPHARMACOLOGY

Potential Advantages

• Effective treatment for rapidly advancing MS including those failing first-line agents

Potential Disadvantages

• Potential for multiple AEs, including irreversible heart failure, limits use. Not effective for primary progressive MS. Needs to be infused by physicians familiar with chemotherapeutic agents. Risk of acute myeloblastic leukemia, even years after stopping the medication. Role in treatment lessened by emergence of newer therapies

Primary Target Symptoms

• Decrease in relapse rate, prevention of disability, and slower accumulation of lesions on MRI

Pearls

• Not indicated for primary progressive MS
• Partial efficacy in reducing the risk of MS progression in patients with worsening relapsing-remitting MS (RRMS), progressive relapsing MS, secondary progressive MS in the 2-year follow-up. Long-term use was associated with systolic dysfunction and therapy-related acute leukemia (0.8–12%)
• Appropriate patient selection is important. Patients with an aggressive form of RRMS with a need to preserve ambulation and independence. Effective in decreasing disability for 2–3 years while on the medication
• In clinical trials, decreased disability based on expanded disability status scores by about 60% or more compared to placebo. Increase in T_2 MRI lesions was 80% less than placebo
• Hematological effects are more common at the higher doses used in leukemia treatment
• Some suggest a minority (about 25%) of MS patients have subclinical ventricular dysfunction, making monitoring of LV ejection fraction even more essential
• Cardiac events may occur at lower doses than previously thought

Suggested Reading

Cohen BA, Mikol DD. Mitoxantrone treatment of multiple sclerosis: safety considerations. *Neurology.* 2004;63(12 Suppl 6):S28–32.

Kingwell E, Koch M, Leung B, Isserow S, Geddes J, Rieckmann P, et al. Cardiotoxicity and other adverse events associated with mitoxantrone treatment for MS. *Neurology.* 2010;74(22): 1822–6.

Krapf H, Morrissey SP, Zenker O, Zwingers T, Gonsette R, Hartung HP; MIMS Study Group. Effect of mitoxantrone on MRI in progressive MS: results of the MIMS trial. *Neurology.* 2005;65(5):690–5.

Le Page E, Leray E, Taurin G, Coustans M, Chaperon J, Morrissey SP, et al. Mitoxantrone as induction treatment in aggressive relapsing remitting multiple sclerosis: treatment response factors in a 5 year follow-up observational study of 100 consecutive patients. *J Neurol Neurosurg Psychiatry.* 2008;79(1):52–6.

Martinelli Boneschi F, Vacchi L, Rovaris M, Capra R, Comi G. Mitoxantrone for multiple sclerosis. *Cochrane Database Syst Rev.* 2013;5: CD002127.

Zipoli V, Portaccio E, Hakiki B, Siracusa G, Sorbi S, Amato MP. Intravenous mitoxantrone and cyclophosphamide as second-line therapy in multiple sclerosis: an open-label comparative study of efficacy and safety. *J Neurol Sci.* 2008;266(1–2):25–30.

MODAFINIL

Brands
- Provigil, Alertec, Modiodal

Generic?
- Yes

Class
- Psychostimulant

Commonly Prescribed for
(FDA approved in bold)
- **Reducing excessive sleepiness in patients with narcolepsy or shift work disorder**
- **Reducing excessive sleepiness in patients with obstructive sleep apnea (OSA)/ hypopnea syndrome**
- Treatment of fatigue in multiple sclerosis (MS)
- Fatigue in depression
- Attention deficit hyperactivity disorder
- Fatigue in cancer, HIV, fibromyalgia, or post-stroke patients
- Bipolar depression

How the Drug Works
- Unlike traditional stimulants which act directly via dopaminergic pathways, it may also act in the hypothalamus by stimulating wake-promoting areas, or inhibiting sleep-promoting areas
- It may also have effects on dopamine transporter pathways similar to other stimulants, hypothetically inhibiting the dopamine transporter
- Increases neuronal activity selectively in the hypothalamus and activates tuberomammillary nucleus neurons that release histamine
- It also activates hypothalamic neurons that release orexin/hypocretin

How Long Until It Works
- Typically 1–2 hours, although maximal benefit may take days to weeks

If It Works
- Continue to use indefinitely as long as symptoms persist. Complete resolution of symptoms is unusual. Does not cause insomnia when dosed correctly

If It Doesn't Work
- Change to most effective dose or alternative agent. Re-evaluate treatment of underlying cause (i.e., OSA) of fatigue. Consider other causes of fatigue (i.e., anemia, heart disease) as appropriate. Screen for use of CNS depressants that can interfere with sleep, i.e., opioids or alcohol

 Best Augmenting Combos for Partial Response or Treatment-Resistance
- In treating OSA, modafinil is an adjunct to standard treatments such as continuous positive airway pressure (CPAP), weight loss, and treatment of obstruction when possible
- In MS change drug regimen, i.e., antispasticity or disease-modifying agents when possible if they are significantly contributing to fatigue. Amantadine is an alternative treatment for MS-related fatigue.
- Treat coexisting medical illnesses such as HIV, depression, or chronic pain disorders with appropriate agents

Tests
- None required

How the Drug Causes AEs
- Unknown but most AEs are likely related to drug actions on CNS neurotransmitters

Notable AEs
- Nervousness, insomnia, headache, nausea, anorexia, palpitations, dry mouth, diarrhea, hypertension

 Life-Threatening or Dangerous AEs
- Transient ECG changes have been reported in patients with preexisting heart disease
- Rare psychiatric reactions (activation of mania, anxiety)
- Rare severe dermatological reactions

Weight Gain
- Unusual

unusual | not unusual | common | problematic

Sedation
- Unusual

unusual not unusual common problematic

What to Do About AEs
- Try lowering the dose or dividing doses. If insomnia, do not take later in the day

Best Augmenting Agents to Reduce AEs
- Most AEs do not respond to adding other medications

DOSING AND USE

Usual Dosage Range
- 100–400 mg daily

Dosage Forms
- Tablets: 100, 200 mg (scored)

How to Dose
- Start at 200 mg in the morning
- In patients sensitive to medications, start at 100 mg in the morning
- When dividing dose, give the first dose in the morning, the second 4–6 hours later (i.e., at noon)
- If sleepiness does not improve on 200 mg/day dose, increase to 400 mg if no AEs

 Dosing Tips
- Dose requirements can escalate over time due to autoinduction. A drug holiday may restore effectiveness of lower dose
- In general, patients with sleepiness do better with higher doses (200 mg or more) and patients with fatigue or inability to concentrate may do well at lower doses
- In patients with shift work disorder, take 1 hour prior to beginning a shift

Overdose
- No reported deaths. Agitation, anxiety, and hypertension are common

Long-Term Use
- Although most initial trials were only a few months, appears safe. Periodically re-evaluate need for use

Habit Forming
- Class IV medication, but rarely abused in clinical practice

How to Stop
- Withdrawal is not problematic, unlike traditional stimulants. Symptoms of sleepiness may recur

Pharmacokinetics
- Metabolized by CYP450 system including isoenzymes 2C19, 3A4, among others. Peak concentrations at 2 hours and elimination half-life is 10–12 hours. About 10% of drug is excreted unchanged in urine. Mild CYP3A4 induction

 Drug Interactions
- Can increase plasma levels and effect of many drugs metabolized by 2C19 or 2D6 including phenytoin, diazepam, propranolol, TCAs, and SSRIs
- Can induce CYP450 3A4, reducing plasma levels of triazolam, and many steroidal contraceptives
- Carbamazepine can lower modafinil plasma levels and fluvoxamine and fluoxetine can increase levels
- Modafinil can affect warfarin effectiveness, requiring closer monitoring of PTs
- May interact with MAOIs

 Other Warnings/Precautions
- May adversely affect mood. Can cause activation of psychosis or mania

Do Not Use
- Known hypersensitivity to the drug, severe hypertension or cardiac arrhythmias

SPECIAL POPULATIONS

Renal Impairment
- No known effects. May require lower dose

Hepatic Impairment
- Reduce dose in patients with severe impairment

Cardiac Impairment

- Do not use in patients with ischemic ECG changes, chest pain, left ventricular hypertrophy, or recent myocardial infarction

Elderly

- No known effects

Children and Adolescents

- Not studied in children under 16. Not a first-line agent in ADHD

Pregnancy

- Category C. Generally not used in pregnancy

Breast Feeding

- Unknown if excreted in breast milk. Do not use

THE ART OF NEUROPHARMACOLOGY

Potential Advantages

- Less risk of addiction, withdrawal, and abuse compared to other stimulants

Potential Disadvantages

- Cost. May be less effective than other stimulants

Primary Target Symptoms

- Sleepiness, fatigue, concentration difficulties

Pearls

- The Epworth sleepiness scale is a reliable way to measure daytime sleepiness and response to treatment. It is a self-administered 8-item questionnaire with scores of 0–24. A score of 10 or greater indicates excessive daytime sleepiness. A reduction of 4 or more points on the Epworth is considered a good response to treatment
- Narcolepsy is characterized by excessive daytime sleepiness, uncontrollable sleep, and observed cataplexy. Hypnagogic or hypnopompic hallucinations or sleep paralysis suggest the diagnosis. In sleep studies, a sleep latency of 8 minutes or less and quick onset of REM sleep confirms the diagnosis. The maintenance of wakefulness test can monitor response to treatment or be used to document safety in patients in which wakefulness is important for public safety (e.g., pilots). An increase of 1–2 minutes in maintenance of wakefulness is considered a good response to treatment
- Dividing doses and giving a second dose at noon does not appear to affect sleep architecture
- For MS-related fatigue, amantadine is another commonly used treatment. Modafinil is usually most effective at the 200 mg/day dose
- May be effective in treating excessive sleepiness in Parkinson's disease (at 200 mg/day dose) but does not usually improve motor scores
- Technically not a psychostimulant and minimal abuse potential

Suggested Reading

Gerrard P, Malcolm R. Mechanisms of modafinil: a review of current research. *Neuropsychiatr Dis Treat.* 2007;3(3):349–64.

Keating GM, Raffin MJ. Modafinil: a review of its use in excessive sleepiness associated with obstructive sleep apnoea/hypopnoea syndrome and shift work sleep disorder. *CNS Drugs.* 2005;19(9):785–803.

Kumar R. Approved and investigational uses of modafinil: an evidence-based review. *Drugs.* 2008;68(13):1803–39.

Parmentier R, Anaclet C, Guhennec C, Brousseau E, Bricout D, Giboulot T, Bozyczko-Coyne D, Spiegel K, Ohtsu H, Williams M, Lin JS. The brain H3-receptor as a novel therapeutic target for vigilance and sleep-wake disorders. *Biochem Pharmacol.* 2007;73(8):1157–71.

Stankoff B, Waubant E, Confavreux C, Edan G, Debouverie M, Rumbach L, Moreau T, Pelletier J, Lubetzki C, Clanet M; French Modafinil Study Group. Modafinil for fatigue in MS: a randomized placebo-controlled double-blind study. *Neurology.* 2005;64(7):1139–43.

MYCOPHENOLATE MOFETIL

THERAPEUTICS

Brands
- CellCept, Myfortic

Generic?
- Yes

Class
- Immunosuppressant

Commonly Prescribed for
(FDA approved in bold)
- **Prophylaxis of organ rejection in patients with allogenic renal, cardiac, or hepatic transplants**
- Myasthenia gravis (MG)
- Chronic inflammatory demyelinating polyneuropathy
- Neurosarcoidosis
- Multiple sclerosis (MS)
- Refractory uveitis
- Churg-Strauss syndrome
- Diffuse proliferative lupus nephritis
- Psoriasis

How the Drug Works
- Prodrug that is actively metabolized to mycophenolic acid, a selective inhibitor of inosine monophosphate dehydrogenase, an important enzyme in de novo synthesis of guanine nucleotide. This alters purine metabolism, which preferentially affects T and B lymphocytes, which depend on this pathway
- Inhibits proliferation of T and B lymphocytes and suppresses antibody formation
- May inhibit recruitment of leukocytes into sites of inflammation and graft rejection
- Does not affect production of interleukins

How Long Until It Works
- In as little as 2–3 weeks, and usually within 6 months

If It Works
- Usually used as a corticosteroid-sparing agent. May allow reduction in dose or discontinuation of corticosteroids. Most MG patients require long-term treatment, but occasionally may remit, allowing careful discontinuation

If It Doesn't Work
- Usually used as an adjunctive agent in conjunction with corticosteroids in MG. Azathioprine, cyclosporine, cyclophosphamide, plasma exchange, and IV immune globulin are alternative long-term treatments. Thymectomy may also be effective for selected patients

Best Augmenting Combos for Partial Response or Treatment-Resistance
- Generally combined with prednisone or other corticosteroids for treatment of MG, allowing eventual decrease in dose, and occasionally combined with other immunosuppressive agents

Tests
- Obtain a CBC when initiating treatment, then weekly in the first month, twice monthly in months 2–3, and monthly through the first year

ADVERSE EFFECTS (AEs)

How the Drug Causes AEs
- Serious AEs are related to immunosupression and neutropenia

Notable AEs
- Diarrhea is most common. Other frequent AEs include abdominal pain, insomnia, nausea, peripheral edema, anxiety, back pain or headache, cough, and mild leukopenia. GI bleeding can also occur

Life-Threatening or Dangerous AEs
- Increased risk of lymphomas or other malignancies, including skin cancers. Increased risk of infection or sepsis, severe neutropenia

Weight Gain
- Unusual

unusual   not unusual   common   problematic

Sedation
- Unusual

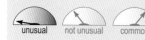

unusual   not unusual   common   problematic

What to Do About AEs
- Decrease dose or change to another agent. Diarrhea may decrease if taken with food or use lower doses taken more frequently (3 times daily)

Best Augmenting Agents to Reduce AEs
- Diarrhea: loperamide or diphenoxylate hydrochloride-atropine. Most other AEs do not respond to augmenting agents

DOSING AND USE

Usual Dosage Range
- MG: 1–3 g/day in 2 divided doses

Dosage Forms
- Capsules: 250 mg
- Tablets: 500 mg
- Powder for oral suspension: 200 mg/mL
- Powder for injection: 500 mg in 20 mL vials

How to Dose
- Start at 500 mg twice a day for 1–2 weeks
- Increase by 1 g a day if CBC stable up to 1500 mg twice daily

 Dosing Tips
- Take with food to reduce GI AEs

Overdose
- Little clinical experience, but GI AEs are more common at higher doses. Bile acid sequestrants, such as cholestyramine, may increase excretion of drug

Long-Term Use
- Safe for long-term use with appropriate monitoring

Habit Forming
- No

How to Stop
- No need to taper but monitor for recurrence of MG complications

Pharmacokinetics
- Rapidly metabolized to active metabolite mycophenolic acid. 97% protein bound. T_{max} less than 1 hour in healthy patients. Oral doses are 94% of IV dose. Metabolites are excreted in urine

 Drug Interactions
- Decreases protein binding and increases free levels of phenytoin and theophylline
- Decreases levels of oral contraceptives
- Competes for tubular secretion when used with acyclovir or ganciclovir, resulting in increased levels of both drugs
- Iron, antacids, and cholestyramine decrease levels of mycophenolate
- Probenecid increases levels of mycophenolate and salicylates can increase free drug level
- Calcium supplements inhibit absorption of mycophenolate. Take calcium supplements 1 hour before or 2 hours after mycophenolate

 Other Warnings/ Precautions
- Oral suspension contains aspartame and should not be used in phenylketonurics. Live attenuated vaccines may be less effective and should be avoided. Patients with hereditary defects in purine metabolism, such as Lesch-Nyhan syndrome, should avoid

Do Not Use
- Known hypersensitivity to the drug or its components

SPECIAL POPULATIONS

Renal Impairment
- Concentration of metabolites can be dramatically increased in renal insufficiency. Monitor closely and use with caution. In renal transplant patients, a daily dose of 2 g/day is recommended, unlike liver or cardiac transplant patients, who usually take 3 g/day

Hepatic Impairment
- Appears safe in many disorders, including alcoholic cirrhosis. Its safety in patients with

hepatic failure related to primary biliary cirrhosis is unknown

Cardiac Impairment

- No known effects

Elderly

- Use with caution, may be more prone to AEs

Children and Adolescents

- Mostly used in transplant patients. Dose based on surface area, usually $600 \, mg/m^2$ twice a day, up to a maximum of 2g/day

Pregnancy

- Category D. Do not use within 6 weeks of considering pregnancy. High rate of first trimester pregnancy loss and congenital malformations. Women with childbearing potential must have a negative pregnancy test before starting drug. Use 2 forms of contraception while on drug if sexually active

Breast Feeding

- Excreted in breast milk. Choose between discontinuing breast feeding or the drug

THE ART OF NEUROPHARMACOLOGY

Potential Advantages

- Relatively fewer AEs than many other immunosuppressive agents and relatively rapid onset of effect compared to some corticosteroid-sparing drugs, such as azathioprine

Potential Disadvantages

- May be less effective than other treatments. May take over 6 months to see improvement. Diarrhea

Primary Target Symptoms

- Long-term preventive treatment of MG complications, such as weakness, visual problems, respiratory difficulties

Pearls

- An attractive treatment based on tolerability and rapid effect, but not always effective in MG. It is considered as third-line treatment in MG based on clinical impression of effect
- Observational case reports suggest effective in the long-term treatment of chronic inflammatory demyelinating polyneuropathy (CIDP)
- Effective in one study in replacing long-term corticosteroid use in neurosarcoidosis
- Avoid using telithromycin, aminoglycosides, interferon-α, pencillamine, IV magnesium, and IV lidocaine in MG patients
- Use β-blockers, fluoroquinolones, and CNS depressants such as opioids or muscle relaxants with caution in MG
- Recent phase III placebo-controlled studies of 2g/day mycophenolate do not demonstrate superiority to placebo in allowing MG patients to taper off corticosteroids, or in the initial treatment of MG when combined with prednisone 20mg
- In clinical trials, appears to have benefit in relapsing-remitting forms of MS. One study suggested its use as combination therapy with interferon-β may be superior to interferon-β alone

Suggested Reading

Androdias G, Maillet D, Marignier R, Pinède L, Confavreux C, et al. Mycophenolate mofetil may be effective in CNS sarcoidosis but not in sarcoid myopathy. *Neurology.* 2011;76(13): 1168–72.

Benatar M, Rowland LP. The muddle of mycophenolate mofetil in myasthenia. *Neurology.* 2008;71(6):390–1.

Hanisch F, Wendt M, Zierz S. Mycophenolate mofetil as second line immunosuppressant in myasthenia gravis – a long-term prospective open-label study. *Eur J Med Res.* 2009;14(8): 364–6.

Heatwole C, Ciafaloni E. Mycophenolate mofetil for myasthenia gravis: a clear and present controversy. *Neuropsychiatr Dis Treat.* 2008; 4(6):1203–9.

Remington GM, Treadaway K, Frohman T, Salter A, Stüve O, et al. A one-year prospective, randomized, placebo-controlled, quadruple-blinded, phase II safety pilot trial of combination therapy with interferon beta-1a and mycophenolate mofetil in early relapsing-remitting multiple sclerosis (TIME MS). *Ther Adv Neurol Disord.* 2010;3(1): 3–13.

Sanders DB, Hart IK, Mantegazza R, Shukla SS, Siddiqi ZA, et al. An international, phase III, randomized trial of mycophenolate mofetil in myasthenia gravis. *Neurology.* 2008;71(6): 400–6.

Sathasivam S. Current and emerging treatments for the management of myasthenia gravis. *Ther Clin Risk Manag.* 2011;7: 313–23.

Villarroel MC, Hidalgo M, Jimeno A. Mycophenolate mofetil: an update. *Drugs Today (Barc).* 2009;45(7):521–32.

NABIXIMOLS

THERAPEUTICS

Brands
- Sativex

Generic?
- No

Class
- Cannabinoid

Commonly Prescribed for
(FDA approved in bold)
- Spasticity and spastic pain in multiple sclerosis (MS)
- Neuropathic pain
- Advanced cancer pain
- Pain in fibromyalgia, rheumatoid arthritis

How the Drug Works
- It is composed of 1:1 mixture of 2 cannabinoids: cannabidiol (CBD) and 9-δ-tetrahydrocannabinol (THC)
- THC, a partial agonist of both cannabinoid receptors (CB_1, CB_2) in brain and spinal cord, reduces spasticity but causes sedation and psychotropic side effects. Its action also involves analgesia, muscle relaxation, anti-inflammation, neuroprotection, and anxiolysis
- CBD reduces sedation and psychotropic side effects

How Long Until It Works
- Minutes to hours

If It Works
- Takes weeks to months for full effect. Usually within 4 weeks

If It Doesn't Work
- Treat underlying conditions. Consider addition of other agents

Best Augmenting Combos for Partial Response or Treatment-Resistance
- For spasticity, may consider use of other centrally acting muscle relaxant or botulinum toxin

- For neuropathic pain, many consider use of TCAs, SNRIs, AEDs, and opioids

Tests
- None

ADVERSE EFFECTS (AEs)

How the Drug Causes AEs
- Related to CB_1 and CB_2 agonist effect in peripheral tissues, such as sympathetic ganglia, adrenal gland, heart, lung, reproductive tissues, urinary bladder, GI tract, immune cells

Notable AEs
- Sedation, dizziness, dry mouth, nausea, headache. Administration site irritation

 ### Life-Threatening or Dangerous AEs
- Cardiac arrhythmia, myocardial infarction
- Operational hazard (driving, heavy machinery)
- Psychosis and dependence

Weight Gain
- Not unusual

unusual not unusual common problematic

Sedation
- Common

unusual not unusual common problematic

What to Do About AEs
- Lower the dose and titrate more slowly

Best Augmenting Agents to Reduce AEs
- Most AEs cannot be reduced by an augmenting agent

DOSING AND USE

Usual Dosage Range
- 5–12 sprays per day

Dosage Forms
- Buccal spray: THC 27 mg/mL and CBD 25 mg/mL

How to Dose
- First day: 1 spray every 4 hours, maximum 4 sprays
- Titrate: spread out the doses throughout the day. Watch for adverse reactions. Titrate to a tolerated dosage with acceptable pain relief
- Maximum: 12 sprays per day

 Dosing Tips
- Spray directly below the tongue or inside of the cheeks. It must not be sprayed into the nose

Overdose
- Rarely. Symptomatic treatment for altered mental status, psychosis, agitation, hypotension, etc.

Long-Term Use
- Not well studied

Habit Forming
- Slight abuse potential. Schedule yet to be defined

How to Stop
- No need to taper. Minimal withdrawal symptoms. Reported temporary changes in sleeping patterns, mood, or appetite

Pharmacokinetics
- Metabolized by CYP2C9 and CYP3A4. Half-life 1–2 hours. Extensively distributed in body fat and takes several days for complete elimination. 30% in urine and 70% in feces

 Drug Interactions
- Increased risk of falls when combined with other antispasticity medication
- Use with other CNS depressants (e.g., alcohol, sleeping pills) increases sedation
- Strong CYP2C9 inhibitor (azoles, St. John's wort, valproic acid) may increase its concentration
- Strong CYP2C9 inducer (rifampin) may decrease its concentration

- It is a weak inhibitor of multiple CYP450 enzymes, especially CYP2C19 and CYP3A4. Drugs at risk of increased concentration are amitriptyline, citalopram, proton pump inhibitors, some AEDs

 Other Warnings/ Precautions
- At risk for developing psychosis
- Cautious in patients with history of drug abuse, epilepsy, and heart problems

Do Not Use
- Known hypersensitivity to cannabinoids, propylene glycol, ethanol
- Patients with significant hepatic, renal, cardiovascular disorder
- Patients with schizophrenia or other psychotic disorder
- Pregnant or nursing women

Renal Impairment
- Not fully studied. Use with caution in patients with severe renal impairment

Hepatic Impairment
- Not fully studied. Use with caution in patients with severe hepatic impairment

Cardiac Impairment
- Caution in patients with cardiovascular disease

Elderly
- Drug metabolism is slower in elderly patients. Use with caution. Risk of falls

 Children and Adolescents
- Not studied in children

 Pregnancy
- Category C. It crosses placenta. Use only if there is a clear need

Breast Feeding
- It is excreted in breast milk. Do not use

THE ART OF NEUROPHARMACOLOGY

Potential Advantages
- Novel pathway for pain and spasticity management

Potential Disadvantages
- Abuse potential

Primary Target Symptoms
- Spasticity, pain

 Pearls

- For spasticity in MS, smoked marijuana has uncertain efficacy. Nabiximols, when measured at 6 weeks, is probably effective for reducing patient-reported symptoms but probably ineffective for reducing objective measures. The actual effect may last longer
- It improves pain and urinary symptoms due to MS. However, there is conflicting evidence for reducing spastic pain in patients with spinal cord injury

- Deficiency of endocannabinoids has been hypothesized in the pathophysiology of migraine. Cannabinoids may block nitroglycerin-induced c-Fos expression in nucleus trigeminalis caudalis. However, at the moment, there is no evidence for its use in migraine management. It is also not effective for acute management of cluster headache
- It may improve neuropathic pain related to chemotherapy and malignancy. Its role in diabetic, post-herpetic, and other causes of neuropathic pain remains to be studied. Inhaled cannabinoid can be used for post-traumatic, HIV, and mixed neuropathic pain
- No head-to-head comparison against other pharmacological agents for neuropathic pain
- The active ingredient of dronabinol is THC. It is currently approved for appetite stimulation in AIDS, and nausea/vomiting associated with cancer chemotherapy in patients who fail to respond to conventional antiemetics

 Suggested Reading

Aggarwal SK. Cannabinergic pain medicine: a concise clinical primer and survey of randomized-controlled trial results. *Clin J Pain.* 2013;29(2):162–71.

Finnerup NB, Sindrup SH, Jensen TS. The evidence for pharmacological treatment of neuropathic pain. *Pain.* 2010;150(3): 573–81.

Koppel BS, Brust JCM, Fife T, Bronstein J, Youssof S, Gronseth G, et al. Systematic review: efficacy and safety of medical marijuana in selected neurologic disorders: report of the Guideline Development Subcommittee of the American Academy of Neurology. *Neurology.* 2014;82(17):1556–63.

Lynch ME, Cesar-Rittenberg P, Hohmann AG. A double-blind, placebo-controlled, crossover pilot trial with extension using an oral mucosal cannabinoid extract for treatment of

chemotherapy-induced neuropathic pain. *J Pain Symptom Manage.* 2014;47(1):166–73.

McGeeney BE. Cannabinoids and hallucinogens for headache. *Headache.* 2013;53(3):447–58.

Snedecor SJ, Sudharshan L, Cappelleri JC, Sadosky A, Mehta S, Botteman M. Systematic review and meta-analysis of pharmacological therapies for painful diabetic peripheral neuropathy. *Pain Pract.* 2013;14(2):167–84.

Teasell RW, Mehta S, Aubut J-AL, Foulon B, Wolfe DL, Hsieh JTC, et al. A systematic review of pharmacologic treatments of pain after spinal cord injury. *Arch Phys Med Rehabil.* 2010;91(5): 816–31.

Wade DT, Collin C, Stott C, Duncombe P. Meta-analysis of the efficacy and safety of Sativex (nabiximols), on spasticity in people with multiple sclerosis. *Mult Scler.* 2010;16(6): 707–14.

NARATRIPTAN

THERAPEUTICS

Brands
- Amerge, Naramig

Generic?
- Yes

Class
- Triptan

Commonly Prescribed for
(FDA approved in bold)
- **Acute treatment of migraine with or without aura in adults**

 How the Drug Works
- Selective 5-HT$_{1B/1D/1F}$ receptor agonist. In addition to vasoconstriction of meningeal vessels, its antinociceptive effect is likely due to blocking the transmission of pain signals at trigeminal nerve terminals (preventing the release of inflammatory neuropeptides) and synapses of second-order neurons in trigeminal nucleus caudalis

How Long Until It Works
- 1–3 hours or less

If It Works
- Continue to take as needed. Patients taking acute treatment more than 2 days/week are at risk for medication-overuse headache, especially if they have migraine

If It Doesn't Work
- Treat early in the attack: triptans are less likely to work after the headache becomes moderate or severe, regardless of cutaneous allodynia, which is a marker of central sensitization
- Address life style issues (e.g., stress, sleep hygiene), medication use issues (e.g., compliance, overuse), and other underlying medical conditions
- Change to higher dosage, another triptan, another administration route, or combination of other medications. Add preventive medication when needed
- For patients with partial response or reoccurrence, other rescue medications include NSAIDs (e.g., ketorolac, naproxen),

antiemetic (e.g., prochlorperazine, metoclopramide), neuroleptics (e.g., haloperidol, chlorpromazine), ergots, antihistamine, or corticosteroid

 Best Augmenting Combos for Partial Response or Treatment-Resistance
- NSAIDs or neuroleptics are often used to augment response

Tests
- None required

ADVERSE EFFECTS (AEs)

How the Drug Causes AEs
- Direct effect on serotonin receptors

Notable AEs
- Tingling, flushing, warm/cold temperature sensations, palpitations, sensation of burning, vertigo, sensation of pressure, nausea

 Life-Threatening or Dangerous AEs
- Rare cardiac events including acute myocardial infarction, cardiac arrhythmias, and coronary artery vasospasm have been reported with naratriptan

Weight Gain
- Unusual

unusual   not unusual   common   problematic

Sedation
- Unusual

unusual   not unusual   common   problematic

What to Do About AEs
- In most cases, only reassurance is needed. Lower dose, change to another triptan, or use an alternative headache treatment

Best Augmenting Agents to Reduce AEs
- Treatment of nausea with antiemetics is acceptable. Other AEs decrease with time

DOSING AND USE

Usual Dosage Range
- 1–2.5 mg

Dosage Forms
- Tablets: 1 and 2.5 mg

How to Dose
- Tablets: most patients respond best with 2.5 mg oral dose. Give 1 pill at the onset of an attack and repeat in 4 hours for a partial response or if the headache returns. Maximum 5 mg/day. Limit 10 days/month

 Dosing Tips
- Treat early in attack

Overdose
- May cause hypertension, cardiovascular symptoms. Other possible symptoms include seizure, tremor, extremity erythema, cyanosis, or ataxia. For patients with angina, perform ECG and monitor for ischemia for at least 24 hours

Long-Term Use
- Monitor for cardiac risk factors with continued use

Habit Forming
- No

How to Stop
- No need to taper. Patients who overuse triptans often experience withdrawal headaches up to several days

Pharmacokinetics
- Half-life 5–6 hours. T_{max} 1–3 hours. Bioavailability is 74%. Metabolized by CYP3A4 and monoamine oxidase (MAO)-A. 28% protein binding

 Drug Interactions
- Use with sibutramine, a weight loss drug, can cause serotonin syndrome including weakness, irritability, myoclonus, and confusion
- From population pharmacokinetic analyses, coadministration of naratriptan and fluoxetine, β-blockers, or TCAs did not affect the clearance of naratriptan
- Hormone replacement therapy had no effect on pharmacokinetics in older female patients

 Other Warnings/ Precautions
- Perform cardiac evaluation in patients with multiple cardiovascular risk factors

Do Not Use
- Within 24 hours of ergot-containing medications such as dihydroergotamine
- Patients with proven hypersensitivity to naratriptan, known cardiovascular disease, uncontrolled hypertension, or Prinzmetal's angina
- Naratriptan was not studied in patients with hemiplegic and basilar migraine
- May worsen symptoms in ischemic bowel disease

SPECIAL POPULATIONS

Renal Impairment
- Concentration increases in those with moderate renal impairment (CrCl < 39 mL/min). Use half-dose. Do not use if CrCl < 15 mL/min. May be at increased cardiovascular risk

Hepatic Impairment
- Drug metabolism is decreased with moderate disease; use half-dose. Do not use with severe hepatic impairment

Cardiac Impairment
- Do not use in patients with known cardiovascular or peripheral vascular disease. May require cardiac stress test or cardiology clearance if tripans are necessary

Elderly
- May be at increased cardiovascular risk

 Children and Adolescents
- Safety and efficacy have not been established
- Triptan trials in children were negative, due to higher placebo response

Pregnancy

- Category C. Use only if potential benefit outweighs risk to the fetus. Pregnancy registries are ongoing. Migraine often improves in pregnancy, and other acute agents (opioids, neuroleptics, prednisone) have more proven safety

Breast Feeding

- Naratriptan is found in breast milk. Use with caution

THE ART OF NEUROPHARMACOLOGY

Potential Advantages

- Excellent tolerability and low rate of recurrence even compared to other oral triptans. Less risk of abuse than opioids or barbiturate-containing treatments

Potential Disadvantages

- Cost, potential for medication-overuse headache. Not as effective as other triptans

Primary Target Symptoms

- Headache pain, nausea, photo and phonophobia

 Pearls

- Early treatment of migraine is most effective
- Fewer AEs and longer half-life than most triptans but less effective (2-hour pain-free rate 18%, number needed to treat 15)

- May not be effective when taking during aura, before headache begins
- In patients with "status migrainosus" (migraine lasting more than 72 hours) neuroleptics and dihydroergotamine are more effective
- Triptans were not originally studied for use in the treatment of basilar or hemiplegic migraine
- Patients taking triptans more than 10 days/ month are at increased risk of medication-overuse headache, which is less responsive to treatment
- Chest and throat tightness are usually benign and may be related to esophageal spasm rather than cardiac ischemia. These symptoms occur more commonly in patients without cardiac risk factors
- Combination use of SNRI and triptans usually will not lead to serotonin syndrome, which requires activation of 5-HT$_{2A}$ receptors and a possible limited role of 5-HT$_{1A}$. However, triptans are agonists at the 5-HT$_{1B/1D/1F}$ receptor subtypes, with weak affinity for 5-HT$_{1A}$ receptors and no activity at the 5-HT$_2$ receptors. Thus, given the seriousness of serotonin syndrome, caution is certainly warranted and clinicians should be vigilant to serotonin toxicity symptoms and signs to insure prompt treatment
- The site of pharmacological action, whether central or peripheral, remains to be studied. Although triptans generally do not penetrate BBB, it has been postulated that transient BBB breakdown may occur during a migraine attack

Suggested Reading

Evans RW, Tepper SJ, Shapiro RE, Sun-Edelstein C, Tietjen GE. The FDA Alert on Serotonin syndrome with use of triptans combined with selective serotonin reuptake inhibitors or selective serotonin-norepinephrine reuptake inhibitors: American Headache Society position paper. *Headache.* 2010;50(6):1089–99.

Ferrari MD, Roon KI, Lipton RB, Goadsby PJ. Oral triptans (serotonin 5-HT(1B/1D) agonists) in acute migraine treatment: a meta-analysis of 53 trials. *Lancet.* 2001;358(9294):1668–75.

Gladstone JP, Gawel M. Newer formulations of the triptans: advances in migraine management. *Drugs.* 2003;63(21):2285–305.

Mannix LK, Savani N, Landy S, Valade D, Shackelford S, Ames MH, Jones MW. Efficacy and tolerability of naratriptan for short-term prevention of menstrually related migraine: data from two randomized, double-blind, placebo-controlled studies. *Headache.* 2007; 47(7):1037–49.

Pringsheim T, Davenport WJ, Dodick D. Acute treatment and prevention of menstrually related migraine headache: evidence-based review. *Neurology.* 2008;70(17):1555–63.

Silberstein SD, Berner T, Tobin J, Xiang Q, Campbell JC. Scheduled short-term prevention with frovatriptan for migraine occurring exclusively in association with menstruation. *Headache.* 2009;49(9): 1283–97.

Wenzel RG, Tepper S, Korab WE, Freitag F. Serotonin syndrome risks when combining SSRI/SNRI drugs and triptans: is the FDA's alert warranted? *Ann Pharmacother.* 2008;42(11): 1692–6.

NATALIZUMAB

THERAPEUTICS

Brands
- Tysabri, Antegren

Generic?
- No

Class
- Immunosuppressant

Commonly Prescribed for
(FDA approved in bold)
- **As monotherapy for reducing neurological disability or relapses in patients with progressive relapsing, or worsening relapsing-remitting multiple sclerosis (MS)**
- **Crohn's disease (adults)**

How the Drug Works
- Natalizumab is a monoclonal antibody that binds to the α4 integrin chain of the very late activation antigen (VLA)-4 adhesion molecule and blocks T-cell migration and costimulatory activating signals. These receptors include vascular cell adhesion molecule-1 (VCAM-1), which is expressed on activated vascular endothelium
- Disruption of these interactions prevents migration of leukocytes across the BBB and reduces plaque formation as measured by MRI. It does not affect the absolute neutrophil count

How Long Until It Works
- Months to years. In trials treated patients had fewer relapses up to 2 years

If It Works
- Continue to use until ineffective. Screen for AEs and consider periodic (3–6 months) monitoring of JC virus antibody status in patients continuing treatment

If It Doesn't Work
- For patients failing first-line agents (interferons, glatiramer) and with frequent relapses (measured by clinical outcome and MRI accumulation of lesions), consider using mitoxantrone or new oral agents such

as fingolimod, monthly methylprednisolone, or pulse cyclophosphamide

Best Augmenting Combos for Partial Response or Treatment-Resistance
- Acute attacks are often treated with glucocorticoids, especially if there is functional impairment due to vision loss, weakness, or cerebellar symptoms
- Treat common clinical symptoms with appropriate medication for spasticity (baclofen, tizanidine), neuropathic pain, and fatigue (modafinil)
- The SENTINEL study showed that adding natalizumab to interferon-β (INFβ)-1a decreases clinical relapses, MRI measures of disease severity and disability compared to INFβ alone, but did not compare this combination to natalizumab alone. Given that combination therapy may increase risk of adverse events, combination therapy is not recommended at this time

Tests
- MRI and serial exams to monitor disease activity. Anti-JC virus antibody prior to therapy and periodically during treatment

ADVERSE EFFECTS (AEs)

How the Drug Causes AEs
- Most AEs are likely related to immunosuppression or hypersensitivity

Notable AEs
- Headache, fatigue, abdominal discomfort, depression, dermatitis, rash, pruritus, menstrual irregularities, weight changes, urinary tract infection, and vaginitis

Life-Threatening or Dangerous AEs
- Progressive multifocal leukoencephalopathy (PML) is a neurological infection seen in immunosuppressed patients related to activation of the JC virus. PML can cause weakness (usually unilateral), clumsiness, or changes in cognition, personality, and memory. This can progress to severe disability or death over a period of weeks to months. Occurs in 1/1000 patients receiving natalizumab

- Opportunistic infections are also uncommon, but there have been cases of acute cytomegalovirus infection, pulmonary aspergillosis, *Mycobacterium avium-intracellulare*, and *Pneumocystis jiroveci* pneumonia in patients treated with natalizumab. It is unclear if drug increases the risk of infection in patients receiving short courses of corticosteroids for acute relapses

Weight Gain
- Unusual

unusual not unusual common problematic

Sedation
- Common

unusual not unusual common problematic

- Usually not related to drug

What to Do About AEs
- For milder infections, such as upper respiratory or urinary tract infection, treat with appropriate agents. In cases of PML or opportunistic infection, discontinue drug

Best Augmenting Agents to Reduce AEs
- Most AEs will not respond to augmenting agents

DOSING AND USE

Usual Dosage Range
- 300 mg is the standard dose

Dosage Forms
- Injection: 300 mg in 15 mL single-use vial

How to Dose
- Give 300 mg over 1 hour every 4 weeks
- It is available only through TOUCH prescription program

 Dosing Tips
- Not applicable

Overdose
- Unknown

Long-Term Use
- Drug is available only under a restricted distribution program called the TOUCH prescribing program. These centers are responsible for reporting serious infections, evaluating patients no less than every 6 months, and determining the effectiveness of treatment. Treatment must be authorized every 6 months

Habit Forming
- No

How to Stop
- No need to taper. There is no evidence to date of "rebound" from stopping drug

Pharmacokinetics
- Approximate time to steady state is about 24 weeks after q4-week dosing. The mean half-life is 11 days and mean clearance 16 days

 Drug Interactions
- Increases risk of serious infection when used with other immunosuppressants, especially in those on concomitant immunosuppressants (such as azathioprine, cyclosporine, methotrexate, and 6-mercaptopurine) or inhibitors of tumor necrosis factor-α

⚠️ **Other Warnings/ Precautions**
- PML is a rare complication of treatment with natalizumab. PML is more likely in patients with positive anti-JC virus antibody
- For suspected cases, stop drug, obtain MRI with gadolinium and CSF fluid analysis for JC virus DNA

Do Not Use
- Hypersensitivity to drug. Patients who have or have had PML. Patients treated with other immunosuppressants

---

SPECIAL POPULATIONS

Renal Impairment
- No known effects

Hepatic Impairment
• No known effects

Cardiac Impairment
• No known effects

Elderly
• No known effects

Children and Adolescents
• Safety and efficacy are not established. Initial retrospective studies suggest similar benefit to in adults, but with a significant risk of infectious complications

Pregnancy
• Category C. Pregnancy registry is ongoing. Use only if benefit of preventing MS relapse outweighs risk

Breast Feeding
• Unknown if excreted in breast milk. Do not breast feed on drug

THE ART OF NEUROPHARMACOLOGY

Potential Advantages
• Effective treatment for some of the most disabled MS patients including those failing first-line agents. Efficacy may be superior to other disease-modifying agents. Once a month treatment

Potential Disadvantages
• Rare but potentially fatal AE of PML or opportunistic infection. Only available through specific infusion centers as IV infusion

Primary Target Symptoms
• Decrease in relapse rate, prevention of disability, and slower accumulation of lesions on MRI

Pearls
• Monotherapy decreases annual relapse rate, lowers disability progression rate, and reduces MRI progression and gadolinium-enhancing lesions. It improves visual function and quality of life
• Generally one of the most effective treatments for severe MS but insurers may require a trial of an alternative agent first
• Based on clinical trials and effectiveness, can consider using as first-line agent, especially in tough cases
• It shows synergistic effect when used as adjunct with INFβ-1a or glatiramer acetate
• After initial launch, 3 cases of PML resulted in the drug being pulled from the market. Only a few subsequent cases have been reported in the thousands of patients treated since drug approval
• A CSF JC virus antibody index > 1.5 may predict potential cases of natalizumab-associated PML
• In theory, because natalizumab blocks immune cells from entering the CNS, there could be rebound progression with drug discontinuation. It is unknown if the immune cells die or remain sequestered in blood
• Due to possible sequestration of immune cells, stopping natalizumab in theory would acutely increase the risk of MS relapse.
• A study evaluating patients switching from natalizumab to fingolimod did not confirm this idea. It is unclear if fingolimod prevented the relapses or if the risk relapse from natalizumab discontinuation is overstated
• Patients who do not respond to other disease-modifying agents or with a particularly aggressive disease course are candidates for natalizumab. In studies there was a reduction in mean attack rate of 68%
• There is an increased risk of PML in MS patients who have anti-JC virus antibodies and prior use of immunosuppressants (natalizumab > 2 years). It should probably be used before immunosuppressant
• CSF osteopontin, a biomarker of intrathecal inflammation, may be used to assess treatment effect in MS
• Although not established as effective to date, may decrease markers of inflammation in progressive forms of MS

- Alemtuzumab (CD-52 antibody) is also approved for relapsing-remitting MS (RRMS) with superior 2-year relapse-free rate to INFβ-1a (not disability) but greater side effects (infection, malignancy, thyroid disorder, thrombocytopenic purpura). It is typically reserved as third-line treatment for RRMS patients who fail to respond to INFβ or galatiramer

 Suggested Reading

Dale RC, Brilot F, Duffy LV, Twilt M, Waldman AT, Narula S, et al. Utility and safety of rituximab in pediatric autoimmune and inflammatory CNS disease. *Neurology.* 2014;83(2):142–50.

Fox R, Cree B, Seze J, Gold R, Hartung HP, Jeffery D, et al. MS disease activity in RESTORE. *Neurology.* 2014;82:1491–8.

Gold R. Combination therapies in multiple sclerosis. *J Neurol.* 2008;255 Suppl 1:51–60.

Jokubaitis VG, Li V, Kalincik T, Izquierdo G, Hodgkinson S et al. Fingolimod after natalizumab and the risk of short-term relapse. *Neurology.* 2014;82(14):1204–11.

Kappos L, Bates D, Edan G, Eraksoy M, Garcia-Merino A, Grigoriadis N, et al. Natalizumab treatment for multiple sclerosis: updated recommendations for patient selection and monitoring. *Lancet Neurol.* 2011;10(8):745–58.

Lindå H, von Heijne A, Major EO, Ryschkewitsch C, Berg J, Olsson T, et al. Progressive multifocal leukoencephalopathy after natalizumab monotherapy. *N Engl J Med.* 2009;361(11):1081–7.

Romme Christensen J, Ratzer R, Bornsen L, Lyksborg M, Garde E, Dyrby TB, et al. Natalizumab in progressive MS: results of an open-label, phase 2A, proof-of-concept trial. *Neurology.* 2014;82(17):1499–507.

Schwab N, Schneider-Hohendorf T, Wiendl H. Therapeutic uses of anti-4-integrin (anti-VLA-4) antibodies in multiple sclerosis. *Int Immunol.* 2014;27(1):47–53.

Stuart WH. Combination therapy for the treatment of multiple sclerosis: challenges and opportunities. *Curr Med Res Opin.* 2007;23(6):1199–208.

Tavazzi E, Rovaris M, La Mantia L. Drug therapy for multiple sclerosis. *CMAJ.* 2014;186(11):833–40.

NETUPITANT/PALONOSETRON

Brands
- Akynzeo

Generic?
- No

Class
- Antiemetic

Commonly Prescribed for
(FDA approved in bold)
- **Prevention of chemotherapy-induced nausea and vomiting (CINV)**
- Nausea and vomiting (gastroenteritis, postoperative)
- Pruritus

How the Drug Works
- Netupitant: selectively inhibits substance P (vomit inducer) at neurokinin 1 (NK$_1$) receptors with long-lasting brain receptor (brainstem, area postrema) saturation after single dose
- Palonosetron: second-generation 5-HT$_3$ antagonist with higher binding affinity and longer plasma half-life. It may trigger 5-HT$_3$ receptor internalization and prolong receptor inhibition

How Long Until It Works
- Typically less than an hour

If It Works
- Use at lowest effective dose

If It Doesn't Work
- Increase dose, or discontinue and change to another agent

Best Augmenting Combos for Partial Response or Treatment-Resistance
- May add D$_2$ antagonist, antihistamine, benzodiazepine, or corticosteroid

Tests
- None required

ADVERSE EFFECTS (AEs)

How the Drug Causes AEs
- Not known

Notable AEs
- Headache, asthenia, dyspepsia, fatigue, constipation, and erythema

Life-Threatening or Dangerous AEs
- Serotonin syndrome
- Hypersensitivity reactions such as angioedema and Stevens-Johnson syndrome have been reported

Weight Gain
- Unusual

unusual / not unusual / common / problematic

Sedation
- Unusual

unusual / not unusual / common / problematic

What to Do About AEs
- Reduce dose or discontinuation

Best Augmenting Agents to Reduce AEs
- Symptomatic management

DOSING AND USE

Usual Dosage Range
- 1 capsule

Dosage Forms
- Capsule: 300 mg netupitant and 0.5 mg palonosetron

How to Dose
- One capsule 1 hour and dexamethasone 12 mg 30 minutes prior to chemotherapy on day 1. Dexamethasone 8 mg orally once daily on days 2 to 4 if under highly emetogenic chemotherapy (cisplatin)

Dosing Tips
- Can be taken with or without food. Only for short-term use

Overdose
- May develop drowsiness or headache

Long-Term Use
- Not been studied

Habit Forming
- No

How to Stop
- No need to taper

Pharmacokinetics
- Netupitant: T_{max}: 5 hours. Half-life: 80 hours. > 99.5% protein bound. Metabolized by CYP3A4 and inhibits CYP3A4
- Palonosetron: T_{max}: 5 hours. Half-life: 44 hours. Bioavailability 97%. 60% protein bound. Metabolized by CYP2D6, and less by CYP3A4 and CYP1A2

 Drug Interactions
- Increased level by CYP3A4 inhibitors (e.g., azole antifungals, macrolides, antivirals, nefazodone)
- Decreased level by CYP3A4 inducers (e.g., rifampin, carbamazepine, phenytoin, barbiturates)
- As a CYP3A4 moderate inhibitor, it increases the concentration of many drugs
- It does not affect levonorgestrel or ethinyl estradiol-based oral contraceptives

 Other Warnings/ Precautions
- May lead to serotonin syndrome when combined with serotonergic drugs

Do Not Use
- Known hypersensitivity

SPECIAL POPULATIONS

Renal Impairment
- Avoid use in patients with severe renal impairment

Hepatic Impairment
- Avoid use in patients with severe hepatic impairment

Cardiac Impairment
- Typically needs no adjustment. No effect on QTc interval

Elderly
- Typically needs no adjustment

 Children and Adolescents
- Safety and effectiveness have not been established

 Pregnancy
- Category C. Use only if the potential benefit justifies the potential risk to the fetus

Breast Feeding
- It is not known whether Akynzeo is present in human milk. Bottle feed if possible

THE ART OF NEUROPHARMACOLOGY

Potential Advantages
- Novel dual mechanisms for severe nausea

Potential Disadvantages
- Drug interaction with CYP3A4 inhibitors/ inducers. Cost

Primary Target Symptoms
- Nausea and vomiting

 Pearls
- Combined treatment is superior in response rate to monotherapy
- Compared with aprepitant and ondansetron, which are both pregnancy category B, it may not be suitable for pregnant women
- Commonly used in combination with dexamethasone for CINV
- It may be as effective as aprepitant plus palonosetron in CINV

Suggested Reading

Basch E, Prestrud AA, Hesketh PJ, Kris MG, Feyer PC, Somerfield MR, et al. Antiemetics: American Society of Clinical Oncology clinical practice guideline update. *J Clin Oncol.* 2011;29 (31):4189–98.

Navari RM. Profile of netupitant/palonosetron (NEPA) fixed dose combination and its potential in the treatment of chemotherapy-induced nausea and vomiting (CINV). *Drug Des Devel Ther.* 2015;9:155–61.

Brands
- Nymalize, Nimotop

Generic?
- Yes

Class
- Calcium channel blocker

Commonly Prescribed for
(FDA approved in bold)
- **Reduce the incidence and severity of ischemic deficits in adult patients with subarachnoid hemorrhage (SAH) from ruptured intracranial berry aneurysms regardless of their post-ictus neurological condition (i.e., Hunt and Hess Grades I–V)**
- Hypertension
- Traumatic brain injury
- Reversible cerebral vasoconstrictive syndromes (RCVS)

How the Drug Works
- Cardiac and vascular smooth muscle contraction depends on movement of calcium through L-type calcium channels, which is inhibited by nimodipine. In animals, nimodipine has a greater effect on cerebral arteries compared with other calcium channel blockers, probably because it is more lipophilic. There is no angiographic evidence that this is correct

How Long Until It Works
- Within hours for both SAH vasospasm and hypertension

If It Works
- Prevents delayed ischemic complications after SAH caused by vasospasm, improves recovery time, and reduces disability
- Typically used for 3 weeks

If It Doesn't Work
- Continue supportive care

Best Augmenting Combos for Partial Response or Treatment-Resistance
- Treatment of SAH should take place in a medical center with experience and 24-hour physician availability

- Occlude the aneurysm in SAH by surgery or coiling
- Do not treat hypertension aggressively
- Normovolemia is preferred
- Treat hyperglycemia and use measures to avoid deep vein thrombosis

Tests
- Monitor blood pressure and heart rate

How the Drug Causes AEs
- Direct effects of L-type calcium receptor antagonism on cardiac and smooth muscle

Notable AEs
- Hypotension, bradycardia
- Flushing, headache, constipation, nausea, myalgia, edema

Life-Threatening or Dangerous AEs
- Rare elevation of hepatic transaminases or thrombocytopenia
- May slow AV conduction or worsen symptoms of heart failure

Weight Gain
- Unusual

unusual   not unusual   common   problematic

Sedation
- Unusual

unusual   not unusual   common   problematic

What to Do About AEs
- Complications of SAH are more serious than significant AEs due to nimodipine. Continue or lower dose

Best Augmenting Agents to Reduce AEs
- Constipation can be treated by usual agents such as magnesium

Usual Dosage Range
- For SAH: 60mg every 4 hours

Dosage Forms

- Liquid-filled capsule: 30 mg
- Oral solution: 60 mg/20 mL

How to Dose

- Start within 4 days of SAH. Give 2 capsules (60 mg) or 20 mL every 4 hours for 21 days

Dosing Tips

- If patients are unable to take orally, the liquid content extracted from the capsule should be emptied via nasogastric tube and flush with saline. Food decreases absorption. Administer 1 hour before meal or 2 hours after meal. It should not be administered IV

Overdose

- There are no reports of overdose. Bradycardia, hypotension, and low-output heart failure are among the risks with calcium channel blocker overdose

Long-Term Use

- Unknown

Habit Forming

- No

How to Stop

- No need to taper. Less risk of rebound tachycardia than β-blockers

Pharmacokinetics

- Hepatic metabolism mainly by CYP3A4. Elimination half-life 8–9 hours. T_{max} 1 hour. Oral bioavailability 13% with > 95% protein binding

Drug Interactions

- Use with caution with other antihypertensives, especially other calcium channel blockers
- H_2 antagonists (cimetidine, ranitidine) increase nimodipine levels
- Use with β-blockers can be synergistic or additive, use with caution
- CYP3A4 inhibitors (ketoconazole, clarithromycin, indinavir) increase nimodipine levels

- CYP3A4 inducers (carbamazepine, rifampin, phenytoin, St. John's wort) should be avoided

Other Warnings/ Precautions

- Do not administer nimodipine IV or by other parenteral routes

Do Not Use

- Proven hypersensitivity to nimodipine or other calcium channel blockers

Renal Impairment

- Unknown. Use with caution

Hepatic Impairment

- Decrease dose to 30 mg every 4 hours in patients with cirrhosis

Cardiac Impairment

- Do not use in acute shock. Use with caution in severe chronic heart failure, hypotension, and greater than first-degree heart block

Elderly

- Use with caution

Children and Adolescents

- Little is known about efficacy or safety

Pregnancy

- Category C (all calcium channel blockers). Use only if potential benefit outweighs risk to the fetus

Breast Feeding

- Not recommended. Nimodipine is probably excreted in breast milk

Potential Advantages

- Multiple studies show efficacy for the treatment of vasospasm after SAH

Potential Disadvantages
- Outcomes are still often poor in SAH

Primary Target Symptoms
- Prevention of delayed ischemic complications from vasospasm after SAH

 Pearls
- Oral nimodipine should be administered to all patients with aneurysmal SAH (to improve neurological outcomes but not cerebral vasospasm) (Class I, Level of Evidence A)
- No beneficial effect on outcome in patients with traumatic SAH or traumatic brain injury
- No longer available in IV form. Studies failed to show that IV administration was superior and serious AEs including cardiac arrest and dramatic blood pressure drop were greater
- May be useful in the treatment of RCVS, a potential cause of "thunderclap headache." No definitive benefit in outcome. The best dose and duration of use is unknown

 Suggested Reading

Connolly ES, Rabinstein AA, Carhuapoma JR, Derdeyn CP, Dion J, Higashida RT, et al. Guidelines for the management of aneurysmal subarachnoid hemorrhage: a guideline for healthcare professionals from the American Heart Association/American Stroke Association. *Stroke.* 2012;43(6):1711–37.

Ducros A. Reversible cerebral vasoconstriction syndrome. *Lancet Neurol.* 2012;11(10):906–17.

Kramer DR, Winer JL, Pease BAM, Amar AP, Mack WJ. Cerebral vasospasm in traumatic brain injury. *Neurol Res Int.* 2013;2013: 415813.

Vergouwen MD, Vermeulen M, Roos YB. Effect of nimodipine on outcome in patients with traumatic subarachnoid haemorrhage: a systematic review. *Lancet Neurol.* 2006;5(12): 1029–32.

NORTRIPTYLINE

THERAPEUTICS

Brands
- Sensoval, Aventyl, Pamelor, Norpress, Allegron, Nortrilen

Generic?
- Yes

Class
- Tricyclic antidepressant (TCA)

Commonly Prescribed for
(FDA approved in bold)
- **Depression**
- Migraine prophylaxis
- Tension-type headache prophylaxis
- Fibromyalgia
- Neuropathic pain
- Post-herpetic neuralgia
- Back or neck pain
- Smoking cessation
- Bulimia nervosa
- Insomnia
- Anxiety
- Nocturnal enuresis
- Pseudobulbar affect

How the Drug Works
- The mechanism of action is probably related to reuptake inhibition of serotonin and norepinephrine at the synaptic clefts of brain and spinal cord
- It also exhibits antagonism on 5-HT$_{2A}$, 5-HT$_{2C}$, 5-HT$_6$, 5-HT$_7$, α_1-adrenergic, muscarinic, H$_1$, and NMDA receptors, and agonism on opioid (σ_1, σ_2) receptors
- Antinociceptive and antidepressive effects are more likely related to adaptive changes in serotonin and norepinephrine receptor systems over time
- Compared to amitriptyline, nortriptyline has less affinity for serotonin transporter (SERT), α_1-adrenergic, muscarinic, H$_1$, and 5-HT$_{2A}$, but higher affinity for norepinephrine transporter (NET)

How Long Until It Works
- Migraines: effective in as little as 2 weeks, but can take up to 3 months on a stable dose to see full effect

- Neuropathic pain: usually some effect within 4 weeks
- Depression: 2 weeks but up to 2 months for full effect
- Insomnia, anxiety, depression: may be effective immediately, but effects often delayed 2–4 weeks

If It Works
- Migraine: goal is a 50% or greater decrease in migraine frequency or severity. Consider tapering or stopping if headaches remit for more than 6 months or if considering pregnancy
- Neuropathic pain: the goal is to reduce pain intensity and symptoms, but usually does not produce remission
- Insomnia: continue to use if tolerated and encourage good sleep hygiene
- Depression: continue to use and monitor for AEs. Usually not first-line treatment for depression

If It Doesn't Work
- Increase to highest tolerated dose
- Migraine: address other issues, such as medication overuse, other coexisting medical disorders, such as anxiety, and consider changing to another agent or adding a second agent
- Chronic pain: either change to another agent or add a second agent
- Insomnia: if no sedation occurs despite adequate dosing, stop and change to another agent

 ### Best Augmenting Combos for Partial Response or Treatment-Resistance
- Migraine: for some patients, low-dose polytherapy with 2 or more drugs may be better tolerated and more effective than high-dose monotherapy. May use in combination with AEDs, antihypertensives, natural products, and non-medication treatments, such as biofeedback, to improve headache control
- Neuropathic pain: TCAs, AEDs (gabapentin, pregabalin, carbamazepine, lamotrigine), SNRIs (duloxetine, venlafaxine, milnacipran, mirtazapine, bupropion), capsaicin, and mexiletine are agents used for neuropathic pain. Opioids (morphine, tramadol) may be appropriate for long-term use in some cases but require careful monitoring

Tests

- Consider checking ECG for QTc prolongation at baseline and when increasing dose, especially in those with a personal or family history of QTc prolongation, cardiac arrhythmia, heart failure, or recent myocardial infarction. In patients on diuretics, measure potassium and magnesium at baseline and periodically

ADVERSE EFFECTS (AEs)

How the Drug Causes AEs

- Anticholineric and antihistaminic properties are causes of most common AEs. Blockade of α_1-adrenergic receptor may cause orthostatic hypotension and sedation

Notable AEs

- Constipation, dry mouth, blurry vision, increased appetite, nausea, diarrhea, heartburn, weight gain, urinary retention, sexual dysfunction, sweating, itching, rash, fatigue, weakness, sedation, nervousness, restlessness

 Life-Threatening or Dangerous AEs

- Orthostatic hypotension, tachycardia, QTc prolongation, and rarely death
- Increased intraocular pressure
- Paralytic ileus, hyperthermia
- Rare activation of mania or suicidal ideation
- Rare worsening of existing seizure disorders

Weight Gain

- Common

unusual · not unusual · common · problematic

Sedation

- Common

unusual · not unusual · common · problematic

What to Do About AEs

- For minor AEs, lower dose or switch to another agent. If tiredness/sedation are bothersome, lower dose or consider desipramine or protriptyline. For serious AEs, lower dose and consider stopping

Best Augmenting Agents to Reduce AEs

- Try magnesium for constipation. For migraine, consider using with agents that cause weight loss as an AE (i.e., topiramate)

DOSING AND USE

Usual Dosage Range

- Migraine/pain: 10–100 mg/day
- Depression, anxiety: 75–150 mg/day
- Smoking cessation: 75–100 mg/day

Dosage Forms

- Capsules: 10, 25, 50, 75 mg
- Liquid solution: 10 mg/5 mL

How to Dose

- Initial dose 10–25 mg/day taken about 1 hour before retiring. For depression, effective range from 10 to 150 mg. For pain, typically 100 mg or less

 Dosing Tips

- Start at a low dose, usually 10 mg, and titrate up every few days as tolerated. Low doses are often effective for pain even though they are below the usual effective antidepressant dose. At doses of 100 mg or greater, monitor plasma levels of drug. Patients may choose to divide doses to 3–4 times daily dosing

Overdose

- Cardiac arrhythmias and ECG changes; death can occur. CNS depression, convulsions, severe hypotension, and coma are not rare. Patients should be hospitalized. Activated charcoal is preferred to emesis or lavage. Sodium bicarbonate can treat arrhythmia and hypotension. Treat shock with vasopressors, oxygen, or corticosteroids. Treat seizure with diazepam or phenytoin. Dialysis and hemoperfusion has no effect

Long-Term Use

- Safe for long-term use

Habit Forming

- No

How to Stop

- Taper slowly to avoid withdrawal symptoms, including rebound insomnia. Withdrawal usually lasts less than 2 weeks. For patients with well-controlled pain disorders, taper very slowly (over months) and monitor for recurrence of symptoms

Pharmacokinetics

- Metabolized primarily by CYP2D6 (7–10% Whites are poor metabolizers). Half-life 13–90 hours. Extensively bound to proteins

 Drug Interactions

- CYP2D6 inhibitors (e.g., duloxetine, paroxetine, fluoxetine, bupropion, cimetidine, quinidine, phenothiazines, propafenone) and valproic acid can prevent its metabolism and increase nortriptyline concentrations
- Phenothiazines (e.g., chlorpromazine, prochlorperazine, promethazine) increase TCA levels
- Enzyme inducers (e.g., rifampin, smoking, dexamethasone) can lower levels
- Secondary amine TCAs (nortriptyline, desipramine) are weak inhibitors of CYP2C19 and CYP2D6
- Use with clonidine has been associated with increases in blood pressure and hypertensive crisis
- Tramadol increases risk of seizures in patients taking TCAs
- May reduce absorption and bioavailability of levodopa
- May alter effects of antihypertensive medications, and prolongation of QTc, especially problematic in patients taking drugs that induce bradycardia
- Quinolones, such as greprafloxacin and sparfloxacin, increase risk of cardiac arrhythmias when used with TCAs
- Use together with anticholinergics can increase AEs (i.e., risk of ileus)
- Methylphenidate may inhibit metabolism and increase AEs
- Use within 2 weeks of MAOIs may risk serotonin syndrome

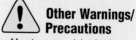 **Other Warnings/ Precautions**

- May increase risk of seizure

Do Not Use

- Proven hypersensitivity to drug or other TCAs
- In acute recovery after myocardial infarction or uncompensated heart failure
- In conjunction with antiarrhythmics that prolong QTc interval
- In conjunction with medications that inhibit CYP2D6

SPECIAL POPULATIONS

Renal Impairment

- Use with caution. May need to lower dose

Hepatic Impairment

- Use with caution. May need to lower dose

Cardiac Impairment

- Do not use in patients with recent myocardial infarction, severe heart failure, history of QTc prolongation, orthostatic hypotension, or electrolyte imbalance (hypocalcemia, hypokalemia, hypomagnesemia)

Elderly

- More sensitive to AEs, such as sedation, hypotension. At risk for anticholinergic crisis. Start with lower doses

 Children and Adolescents

- Not as well studied but similar effectiveness compared with amitriptyline in children. In children less than 12, most commonly used at low dose for treatment of enuresis

 Pregnancy

- Category D. Crosses the placenta and may cause fetal malformations or withdrawal symptoms. Generally not recommended for the treatment of pain or insomnia during pregnancy. For patients with depression or anxiety, SSRIs may be safer than TCA

Breast Feeding

- Some drug is found in breast milk and use while breast feeding is not recommended

THE ART OF NEUROPHARMACOLOGY

Potential Advantages

- Very effective in the treatment of multiple pain disorders. Useful for treatment of depression, anxiety, and insomnia, which are common in chronic pain disorders. Less sedation than tertiary amine TCAs (i.e., amitriptyline)

Potential Disadvantages

- AEs are often greater than SSRIs or SNRIs and many AEDs. Less effective for insomnia than tertiary amine TCAs (i.e., amitriptyline)

Primary Target Symptoms

- Headache frequency and severity
- Neuropathic pain

 Pearls

- In patients with chronic pain, offers relief at doses below usual antidepressant doses
- For patients with significant anxiety or depressive disorders, as effective as newer drugs but many more AEs. Consider treatment of depression or anxiety with another agent and using a low dose of nortriptyline or other TCA for pain
- TCAs can often precipitate mania in patients with bipolar disorder. Use with caution
- Despite interactions, expert psychiatrists may use with MAOIs for refractory depression. Combination with atypical neuroleptics is another option

- For post-stroke depression, may be superior to SSRIs and may even increase survival
- Many patients do not improve. The number needed to treat for moderate pain relief in neuropathic pain is 2–3
- Increases non-REM sleep time and decreases sleep latency. When starting, there is often an activating effect, and insomnia may temporarily worsen
- Nortriptyline and other secondary amines (amoxapine, desipramine, protriptyline) have lower rates of sedation and orthostatic hypotension than tertiary amines (amitriptyline, clomipramine, doxepin, imipramine, trimipramine) and relatively more norepinephrine than serotonin blocking activity
- From a recent Cochrane review on TCA and ADHD, most evidence on TCAs relates to desipramine. Findings suggest that, in the short term, desipramine improves the core symptoms of ADHD, but its effect on the cardiovascular system remains an important clinical concern. Thus, evidence supporting the clinical use of desipramine for the treatment of children with ADHD is low
- Based on a Cochrane review, the likelihood of quitting smoking using bupropion or nortriptyline appears to be similar to that for nicotine replacement therapy, but the likelihood of quitting using bupropion appears to be lower than the likelihood of quitting using varenicline

Suggested Reading

Gillman PK. Tricyclic antidepressant pharmacology and therapeutic drug interactions updated. *Br J Pharmacol.* 2007;151(6):737–48.

Heymann RE, Helfenstein M, Feldman D. A double-blind, randomized, controlled study of amitriptyline, nortriptyline and placebo in patients with fibromyalgia. An analysis of outcome measures. *Clin Exp Rheumatol.* 2001;19(6):697–702.

Hughes JR, Stead LF, Hartmann-Boyce J, Cahill K, Lancaster T. Antidepressants for smoking cessation. *Cochrane Database Syst Rev.* 2014;1: CD000031.

Otasowie J, Castells X, Ehimare UP, Smith CH. Tricyclic antidepressants for attention deficit hyperactivity disorder (ADHD) in children and adolescents. *Cochrane Database Syst Rev.* 2014;9: CD006997.

Silberstein SD, Goadsby PJ. Migraine: preventive treatment. *Cephalalgia.* 2002;22(7): 491–512.

Verdu B, Decosterd I, Buclin T, Stiefel F, Berney A. Antidepressants for the treatment of chronic pain. *Drugs.* 2008;68(18): 2611–32.

Zin CS, Nissen LM, Smith MT, O'Callaghan JP, Moore BJ. An update on the pharmacological management of post-herpetic neuralgia and painful diabetic neuropathy. *CNS Drugs.* 2008;22(5):417–42.

THERAPEUTICS

Brands
- Zyprexa, Zyprexa Zydis, Zyprexa Relprevv, Zyprexa IntraMuscular, Symbyax (olanzapine/fluoxetine)

Generic?
- Yes

Class
- Atypical antipsychotic

Commonly Prescribed for
(FDA approved in bold)
- **Schizophrenia for adolescents or adults**
- **Monotherapy for bipolar I disorder, manic or mixed episode**
- **Adjunct therapy to valproate or lithium for bipolar I disorder, manic or mixed episode**
- **Bipolar I depression (Symbyax only)**
- **Treatment-resistant depression (Symbyax only)**
- **Acute agitation associated with schizophrenia and bipolar I mania (IntraMuscular only)**
- Augmentation for refractory obsessive-compulsive disorder
- Migraine refractory to standard treatment
- Acute psychosis
- Delirium
- Antiemetic

How the Drug Works
- It is a thiobenzodiazepine derivative that binds strongly to $5\text{-HT}_{2A/2B/2C}$, 5-HT_6, D_{1-5}, $H_{1,2}$, and $\alpha_{1,2}$ receptors, and moderately to 5-HT_3 and M_{1-5} receptors. It exerts the action via D_2 antagonism (for positive symptoms), 5-HT_{2A} antagonism (negative symptoms), and 5-HT_3 antagonism (antiemetic)

How Long Until It Works
- Migraine: hours. Often use to initiate sleep
- Schizophrenia/bipolar: may be effective in days, more commonly takes weeks or months to determine best dose and achieve best clinical effect. Usually 4–6 weeks
- Agitation/insomnia: may be effective immediately

If It Works
- Continue to use at lowest required dose. Most patients with schizophrenia see a reduction in psychosis with neuroleptics

If It Doesn't Work
- Increase dose
- Psychosis related to Parkinson's disease (PD) or dementia with Lewy bodies (DLB): clozapine is more efficacious. For acute treatment only
- Insomnia: if no sedation occurs despite adequate dosing, change to another agent

Best Augmenting Combos for Partial Response or Treatment-Resistance
- Patients with affective disorders, such as bipolar disorder, may respond to mood-stabilizing AEDs, lithium, or benzodiazepines. For PD/DLB, treating dementia and psychosis with rivastigmine/donepezil and clozapine, respectively, may be efficacious

Tests
- Prior to starting treatment and periodically during treatment, monitor weight, blood pressure, lipids, and fasting glucose due to risk of metabolic syndrome

ADVERSE EFFECTS (AEs)

How the Drug Causes AEs
- Antagonism on H_1, 5-HT_{2C}, and D_2 receptors may cause weight gain; antagonism on α_1 can cause orthostatic hypotension; antagonism on M_1 may cause anticholinergic effect and M_3 for diabetogenic effect; antagonism on H_1 and 5-HT_{2A} can cause sedation

Notable AEs
- CNS: dizziness, personality disorder, akathisia, sedation, fatigue, asthenia, tremor
- Autonomic: dry mouth, postural hypotension
- Gastrointestinal: constipation, weight gain, increased appetite, abdominal pain

Life-Threatening or Dangerous AEs
- Tardive dyskinesia (lower than conventional neuroleptics)
- Severe weight gain and metabolic syndrome/diabetes

- Neuroleptic malignant syndrome (rare compared with conventional antipsychotics)
- Cognitive and motor impairment
- Agranulocytosis, rare (structure similar to clozapine)
- Seizure
- Post-injection delirium/sedation syndrome (olanzapine pamoate only)

Weight Gain

- Problematic

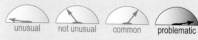
unusual   not unusual   common   problematic

Sedation

- Problematic

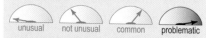
unusual   not unusual   common   problematic

What to Do About AEs

- Take at night: for many disorders there is no need for daytime dosing
- Medical management for obesity, including weight loss and exercise, may help combat weight gain

Best Augmenting Agents to Reduce AEs

- Most AEs cannot be reduced with an augmenting agent

DOSING AND USE

Usual Dosage Range

- Bipolar disorder/schizophrenia: 5–20mg/day

Dosage Forms

- Tablet: 2.5, 5, 7.5, 10, 15, 20mg
- Tablet, oral disintegrating: 5, 10, 15, 20mg
- Injection: 10mg/vial
- Injection, extended release (olanzapine pamoate): 210, 300, 405mg/vial

How to Dose

- Start at 10mg/day. Adjust 5mg per 1 day (bipolar) or per 1 week (schizophrenia). Maintain at 5–20mg/day
- For agitation: maximum 3 doses of 10mg 2–4 hours apart
- Olanzapine pamoate: long-acting for deep IM gluteal injection only. It is only indicated for the treatment of schizophrenia in adults. Dose ranges from 150mg/2 weeks to

405 mg/4 weeks. Suspend in designated diluent prior to use

 Dosing Tips

- For injection, do not administer IV or SC. For oral form, can be taken with food. Use at night if sedation is a problem. Elderly and children often need lower doses

Overdose

- Agitation/aggressiveness, dysarthria, tachycardia, various extrapyramidal symptoms, reduced level of consciousness. Manage with gastric lavage and activated charcoal. No antidote

Long-Term Use

- Safe for long-term use with appropriate monitoring

Habit Forming

- No, although reportedly used to manage stimulant drug withdrawal

How to Stop

- No need to taper, but psychosis or insomnia often recurs

Pharmacokinetics

- T_{max} 6 hours (oral), 15–45 minutes (IM). 93% protein bound. Half-life 21–54 hours. Reach steady state in 1 week. Extensively metabolized by direct glucuronidation and CYP450-mediated oxidation (CYP1A2, 2D6)

 Drug Interactions

- Potent CYP1A2 inhibitors (e.g., fluoroquinolones, fluvoxamine, verapamil) and potent CYP2D6 inhibitors (e.g., fluoxetine, paroxetine, bupropion, quinidine) can increase olanzapine serum level
- Potent CYP1A2 inducers (e.g., carbamazepine, tobacco, rifampin, omeprazole) may lower olanzapine serum level
- Does not exert CYP450 enzyme inducing or inhibiting effect
- Alcohol and diazepam may potentiate orthostatic hypotension

 Other Warnings/ Precautions

- Post-injection delirium/sedation syndrome and increased mortality in elderly patients with dementia-related psychosis

Do Not Use

- Proven hypersensitivity to olanzapine

Renal Impairment

- No dose adjustment needed. Olanzapine not removed by dialysis

Hepatic Impairment

- No clearance difference in patients with mild to moderate cirrhosis (Child-Pugh Classification A or B)

Cardiac Impairment

- May worsen orthostatic hypotension. Low but non-trivial risk for QTc prolongation. Use with caution

Elderly

- Start with lower doses. Half-life 1.5× longer. Associated with greater risk for infection and cardiovascular event in dementia patients

 Children and Adolescents

- Efficacy and safety unknown. May accumulate more due to lower body weight. Monitor for weight gain and other AEs

 Pregnancy

- Category C. Probably safer than AEDs during pregnancy for bipolar disorder. Use only if benefit outweighs risks

Breast Feeding

- Found in breast milk. Use while breast feeding is generally not recommended

Potential Advantages

- May allow sleep in patients with severe migraine. Low risk of tardive dyskinesia. Low QTc prolongation risk

Potential Disadvantages

- Probably less effective than clozapine. Does not usually improve motor symptoms of PD. Risk of weight gain and metabolic syndrome. Risk of blood dyscrasia

Primary Target Symptoms

- Psychosis, depression, mania, and insomnia

 Pearls

- Not recommended for treatment of psychosis in PD or Alzheimer's dementia. Greater risk for mortality and cerebrovascular events in elderly patients with dementia
- Often effective at low doses for insomnia, but not recommended as a first-line option
- For chronic pain treatment, 5 or 10mg of olanzapine has been studied. Olanzapine's antinociceptive effect may be related to its action on α_2-adrenergic receptors and to a lesser extent on involvement of opioid and serotonergic receptors
- Olanzapine showed comparable antinausea effect to aprepitant in preventing chemotherapy-induced nausea and vomiting
- Clozapine and olanzapine can induce significant weight gain
- For treating agitation, olanzapine 10mg IM (number needed to treat 3), aripiprazole 9.75mg IM (number needed to treat 5), ziprasidone 10–20mg IM (number needed to treat 3)
- Inhaled loxapine is a possible alternative to parenteral injections for rapid reduction of agitation
- Risperidone and olanzapine seem as efficacious as haloperidol in the treatment of delirium. However, there remains insufficient evidence to support the use of antipsychotic in delirium
- May be effective for refractory migraine or headache disorders. Can be used as an acute treatment for severe attacks or for chronic use with appropriate monitoring

Suggested Reading

Citrome L. Comparison of intramuscular ziprasidone, olanzapine, or aripiprazole for agitation. *J Clin Psychiatry.* 2007;68 (12):1876–85.

Flaherty JH, Gonzales JP, Dong B. Antipsychotics in the treatment of delirium in older hospitalized adults: a systematic review. *J Am Geriatr Soc.* 2011;59 Suppl 2:S269–76.

Seppi K, Weintraub D, Coelho M, Perez-Lloret S, Fox SH, Katzenschlager R, et al. The Movement Disorder Society Evidence-Based Medicine Review Update: Treatments for the non-motor symptoms of Parkinson's disease. *Mov Disord.* 2011;26 Suppl 3:S42–80.

Silberstein SD, Peres MFP, Hopkins MM, Shechter AL, Young WB, Rozen TD. Olanzapine in the treatment of refractory migraine and chronic daily headache. *Headache.* 2002;42 (6):515–18.

THERAPEUTICS

Brands
- Zofran, Zuplenz

Generic?
- Yes

Class
- Antiemetic

Commonly Prescribed for
(FDA approved in bold)
- **Prevention of nausea and vomiting (chemotherapy, radiotherapy, postoperative)**
- Nausea and vomiting (pregnancy)
- Pruritus (opioid related)
- Acute gastroenteritis vomiting (children)

How the Drug Works
- Selective blocking agent of 5-HT$_3$ receptors on both peripheral vagal nerve terminal and central chemoreceptor trigger zone (area postrema)

How Long Until It Works
- Usually works in less than 30 minutes

If It Works
- Use at lowest effective dose

If It Doesn't Work
- Increase dose, or discontinue and change to another agent

Best Augmenting Combos for Partial Response or Treatment-Resistance
- May try adding D$_2$ antagonist, NK$_1$ antagonist, antihistamine, benzodiazepine, or corticosteroid

Tests
- None required

ADVERSE EFFECTS (AEs)

How the Drug Causes AEs
- Blocking of 5-HT$_3$ receptors

Notable AEs
- Headache, flushing, arrhythmia, urticaria, constipation, fever
- Transient blurred vision, elevated hepatic function tests

 ### Life-Threatening or Dangerous AEs
- Hypersensitivity
- QTc prolongation

Weight Gain
- Unusual

unusual   not unusual   common   problematic

Sedation
- Unusual

unusual   not unusual   common   problematic

What to Do About AEs
- Reduce dose or discontinuation

Best Augmenting Agents to Reduce AEs
- Symptomatic management

DOSING AND USE

Usual Dosage Range
- 8–32 mg

Dosage Forms
- Tablets: 4, 8, 16, 24 mg
- Orally disintegrating tablet: 4, 8 mg
- Film: 4, 8 mg
- Injection: 2 mg/mL, 4 mg/5 mL, 32 mg/50 mL

How to Dose
- For chemotherapy-induced nausea/vomiting: 8–32 mg IV or orally 15–30 minutes before chemotherapy
- Before anesthesia induction: 4 mg IV undiluted over 2–5 minutes

 ### Dosing Tips
- Should be administered 30 minutes before emetogenic cancer chemotherapy; 1–2 hours before radiotherapy;

or 1 hour before induction of anesthesia

Overdose
• Sudden blindness of 2–3 minutes, hypotension, or vasovagal episode has been reported

Long-Term Use
• No long-term side effect

Habit Forming
• No

How to Stop
• No need to taper

Pharmacokinetics
• Metabolized predominantly by CYP3A4. Half-life 3–6 hours

 Drug Interactions
• Increased level by CYP3A4 inhibitor (protease inhibitors, macrolides, azole antifungals, nefazodone, etc.)
• Decreased level by CYP3A4 inducer (carbamazepine, phenytoin, barbiturates, etc.)

Other Warnings/ Precautions
• May mask a progressive ileus or gastric obstruction

Do Not Use
• Concomitant apomorphine or known hypersensitivity to drug

SPECIAL POPULATIONS

Renal Impairment
• No adjustment necessary

Hepatic Impairment
• In severe impairment, 8 mg total daily

Cardiac Impairment
• Avoid in congenital QTc syndrome

Elderly
• Typically needs no adjustment

  Children and Adolescents
• For > 12 years old, same dosage as adults
• For 4–11 years old, use lower dose

 Pregnancy
• Category B. Use for significant migraine or nausea during pregnancy if needed

Breast Feeding
• Found in breast milk. Little information is available. Bottle feed if possible

THE ART OF NEUROPHARMACOLOGY

Potential Advantages
• Quick onset and effective

Potential Disadvantages
• May cause QTc prolongation. Drug interaction with CYP3A4 inhibitor/inducer

Primary Target Symptoms
• Nausea and vomiting

Pearls
• Palonosetron, which has longer half-life and induces prolonged inhibition of receptor function, may be more effective than ondansetron and has less QTc prolongation tendency
• Avoid concomitant use of apomorphine
• Ondansetron taken during pregnancy was not associated with a significantly increased risk of adverse fetal outcomes

Suggested Reading

Pasternak B, Svanström H, Hviid A. Ondansetron in pregnancy and risk of adverse fetal outcomes. *N Engl J Med.* 2013;368(9):814–23.

Schwartzberg L, Barbour SY, Morrow GR, Ballinari G, Thorn MD, Cox D. Pooled analysis of phase III clinical studies of palonosetron versus ondansetron, dolasetron, and granisetron in the prevention of chemotherapy-induced nausea and vomiting (CINV). *Support Care Cancer.* 2014;22(2):469–77.

OXCARBAZEPINE

THERAPEUTICS

Brands
- Trileptal, Oxtellar XR

Generic?
- Yes

 Class
- Antiepileptic drug (AED)

Commonly Prescribed for
(FDA approved in bold)
- **Partial seizures as monotherapy (≥ 4 years old) and adjunctive therapy (≥ 2 years old)**
- Generalized tonic-clonic seizures
- Mixed seizure patterns
- Trigeminal neuralgia
- Temporal lobe epilepsy (children and adults)
- Neuropathic pain
- Alcohol withdrawal

 How the Drug Works
- Primarily inhibits voltage-dependent sodium channel conductance
- Modulates calcium channels (N, P/Q type), potassium conductance, glutamate release, and NMDA receptors

How Long Until It Works
- Seizures: 2 weeks or less
- Trigeminal neuralgia or neuropathic pain: hours to weeks

If It Works
- Seizures: goal is the remission of seizures. Continue as long as effective and well tolerated. Consider tapering and slowly stopping after 2 years without seizures, depending on the type of epilepsy
- Trigeminal neuralgia: should dramatically reduce or eliminate attacks. Periodically attempt to reduce to lowest effective dose or discontinue

If It Doesn't Work
- Increase to highest tolerated dose
- Epilepsy: consider changing to another agent, adding a second agent, using a medical device, or a referral for epilepsy

surgery evaluation. When adding a second agent, keep drug interactions in mind
- Trigeminal neuralgia: try an alternative agent. For truly refractory patients referral to tertiary headache center, consider surgical or other procedures

 Best Augmenting Combos for Partial Response or Treatment-Resistance
- Epilepsy: drug interactions can complicate multi-drug therapy
- Pain: can combine with other AEDs (gabapentin or pregabalin) or TCAs

Tests
- Check sodium levels for symptoms of hyponatremia or in patients susceptible to hyponatremia

ADVERSE EFFECTS (AEs)

How the Drug Causes AEs
- CNS AEs are probably caused by sodium channel blockade effects

Notable AEs
- Sedation, dizziness, ataxia, headache, tremor, emotional lability
- Nausea, vomiting, anorexia, dyspepsia
- Blurry or double vision, upper respiratory tract infection, rhinitis

 Life-Threatening or Dangerous AEs
- Rare blood dyscrasias: leukopenia, thrombocytopenia
- Dermatological reactions uncommon and rarely severe but include erythema multiforme, toxic epidermal necrolysis, and Stevens-Johnson syndrome. Drug reaction with eosinophilia and systemic symptoms (DRESS)/multi-organ hypersensitivity
- Hyponatremia/SIADH (syndrome of inappropriate antidiuretic hormone secretion)
- Suicidal behavior and ideation

Weight Gain
- Not unusual

unusual not unusual common problematic

Sedation

- Not unusual

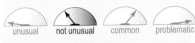

unusual   not unusual   common   problematic

What to Do About AEs

- Use with caution in patients with low sodium at baseline, or those on medications that can lower sodium such as diuretics

Best Augmenting Agents to Reduce AEs

- Most AEs cannot be reduced with an augmenting agent

DOSING AND USE

Usual Dosage Range

- Epilepsy: 900–2400 mg/day
- Pain: Often a low dose is effective. Usually 1200 mg/day or less

Dosage Forms

- Film-coated tablets: 150, 300, 600 mg
- Extended-release tablets: 150, 300, 600 mg
- Oral suspension: 300 mg/5 mL

How to Dose

- Epilepsy: start at 600 mg/day in 2 divided doses. Increase by up to 300 mg/day every 3 days to goal dose. Some increased effectiveness but also more side effects above 1200 mg/day dose
- Trigeminal neuralgia/pain: start at 150–300 mg/day and increase every 3 days by 150–300 mg/day until pain relief
- Adjust dose as needed when using with other AEDs or other drugs that affect levels

 Dosing Tips

- Can dose twice daily or 3 times daily in sensitive patients, titrate slowly
- Levels typically need to be 1/3 higher than carbamazepine dose for a similar effect
- Conversion to monotherapy: concomitant AEDs should be withdrawn over 3–6 weeks

Overdose

- Sedation, ataxia. No reported deaths

Long-Term Use

- Safe for long-term use

Habit Forming

- No

How to Stop

- Taper slowly
- Abrupt withdrawal can lead to seizures in patients with epilepsy

Pharmacokinetics

- Most of the pharmacological activity is through the 10-monohydroxy metabolite (MHD) of oxcarbazepine. Half-life is 2 hours (longer for extended release), but that of its metabolite is 9 hours. Oxcarbazepine is rapidly reduced by liver cytosolic enzymes to MHD and futher metabolized by glucuronic conjugation. About 40% protein bound, mostly renally excreted. Bioavailability is over 95%

 Drug Interactions

- Inhibitor of CYP2C19 and mild inducer of CYP3A4/5 (weaker than carbamazepine), but not other CYP450 enzymes
- Oxcarbazepine increases levels of phenytoin and phenobarbital and lowers levels of lamotrigine, and other CYP3A4 substrates
- Phenytoin, primidone, phenobarbital, carbamazepine decrease levels of oxcarbazepine metabolite. Consider initiating at higher dose
- Valproate and verapamil lower levels to a lesser extent. Dose adjustment may not be needed
- Can decrease concentration of hormonal contraceptives

 Other Warnings/ Precautions

- CNS AEs increase when used with other CNS depressants
- Rare systemic disorders: systemic lupus erythematosus
- May affect bone metabolism with long-term treatment
- Risk of hyponatremia is highest in the first 3 months. Check sodium level for symptoms of hyponatremia (nausea, headache, lethargy, or worsening headache)

Do Not Use

- Patients with a proven allergy to oxcarbazepine. Patients with carbamazepine allergies have a 30% chance of allergy to oxcarbazepine

SPECIAL POPULATIONS

Renal Impairment

- Lower dose for patients with renal insufficiency (CrCl < 30 mL/min). Reduce initial dose by half and titrate slowly. Do not use extended release in patients undergoing dialysis

Hepatic Impairment

- Safe for patients with mild to moderate disease at usual doses. Use with caution in patients with severe disease

Cardiac Impairment

- No known effects

Elderly

- May need lower dose, especially when CrCl is reduced

Children and Adolescents

- 4–16 years: initiate at 8–10 mg/kg. 20–29 kg: titrate to 900 mg/day. 29–39 kg: titrate to 1200 mg/day. > 39 kg: titrate to 1800 mg/day. Maximum 60 mg/kg/day over 2–4 weeks
- Side effects similar to adults

Pregnancy

- Category C. Teratogenicity in animal studies
- Risks of stopping medication must outweigh risk to fetus for patients with epilepsy. Seizures and potential status epilepticus place the woman and fetus at risk and can cause reduced oxygen and blood supply to the womb
- Patients taking for headache, pain, or bipolar disorder should generally stop before considering pregnancy
- Levels may change during pregnancy. Checking levels may ensure therapeutic dose

- Supplementation with 0.4 mg of folic acid before and during pregnancy is recommended

Breast Feeding

- Breast milk levels are 50% of levels in mother's blood
- Generally recommendations are to discontinue drug or bottle feed
- Monitor infant for sedation, poor feeding, or irritability

THE ART OF NEUROPHARMACOLOGY

Potential Advantages

- Proven effectiveness as monotherapy and adjunctive for partial seizures. Generally fewer AEs than carbamazepine and no autoinduction. Probably effective for trigeminal neuralgia

Potential Disadvantages

- Ineffective for absence, atypical absence, and myoclonic seizures. Similar or greater rate of hyponatremia than carbamazepine

Primary Target Symptoms

- Seizure frequency and severity
- Pain

Pearls

- Effective for partial epilepsies but not absence or myoclonic seizures, infantile spasms
- May worsen or improve generalized tonic-clonic seizure control
- To measure levels, check levels of monohydroxy derivative (the metabolite)
- Hyponatremia (less than 125 mEq/L) occurs in about 2.5% of patients
- Consider as an alternative for the treatment of trigeminal neuralgia, often effective in hours or days. Better tolerated than carbamazepine. Benefit may not be sustained
- Recent studies suggest ineffective in migraine
- May be helpful for neuropathic pain, such as painful diabetic neuropathy
- May be beneficial for impulsive aggressive behaviors

- In conversion of oxcarbazepine immediate-release to extended-release, higher doses of extended-release may be necessary

- It is less likely to be withdrawn than phenytoin

Suggested Reading

Arya R, Glauser TA. Pharmacotherapy of focal epilepsy in children: a systematic review of approved agents. *CNS Drugs.* 2013;27:273–86.

Ettinger AB, Argoff CE. Use of antiepileptic drugs for nonepileptic conditions: psychiatric disorders and chronic pain. *Neurotherapeutics.* 2007;4(1):75–83.

Gomez-Arguelles JM, Dorado R, Sepulveda JM, Herrera A, Arrojo FG, Aragón E, et al. Oxcarbazepine monotherapy in carbamazepine-unresponsive trigeminal neuralgia. *J Clin Neurosci.* 2008;15(5):516–19.

Harden CL, Pennell PB, Koppel BS, Hovinga CA, Gidal B, Meador KJ, et al. American Academy of Neurology; American Epilepsy Society. Practice parameter update: management issues for women with epilepsy – focus on pregnancy (an evidence-based review): vitamin K, folic acid, blood levels, and breastfeeding: report of the Quality Standards Subcommittee and

Therapeutics and Technology Assessment Subcommittee of the American Academy of Neurology and American Epilepsy Society. *Neurology.* 2009;73(2):142–9.

Keating GM. Eslicarbazepine acetate: a review of its use as adjunctive therapy in refractory partial-onset seizures. *CNS Drugs.* 2014;28:583–600.

Nolan SJ, Muller M, Tudur Smith C, Marson AG. Oxcarbazepine versus phenytoin monotherapy for epilepsy. *Cochrane Database Syst Rev.* 2013;5:CD003615.

Silberstein SD, Holland S, Freitag F, Dodick DW, Argoff C, Ashman E. evidence-based guideline update: pharmacologic treatment for episodic migraine prevention in adults: report of the Quality Standards Subcommittee of the American Academy of Neurology and the American Headache Society. *Neurology.* 2012;78:1337–45.

PENICILLAMINE

THERAPEUTICS

Brands
- Cuprimine, Depen

Generic?
- Yes

 ### Class
- Chelating agent

Commonly Prescribed for
(FDA approved in bold)
- **Wilson's disease (WD)**
- **Cystinuria**
- **Rheumatoid arthritis (severe, active)**
- Lead poisoning

 ### How the Drug Works
- In WD, copper accumulates in body tissues, causing neurological/psychiatric problems and/or liver failure. Penicillamine is cysteine, doubly substituted with methyl groups. Penicillamine binds to (chelates) copper, allowing it to be excreted in the urine

How Long Until It Works
- Urinary excretion of copper will increase in less than 24 hours. Clinical improvement usually takes 6 months or more; many patients may experience paradoxical worsening after starting treatment

If It Works
- Continue treatment, if tolerated, and aim for 24-hour urine copper excretion of 2mg. Most patients remain on drug for the rest of their life but if all results return to normal (serum copper < 10mcg/dL), consider changing to zinc. Monitor for recurrence of symptoms or changes in urinary copper excretion

If It Doesn't Work
- Increase to as much as 2g daily. Intolerance is more common than ineffectiveness. Change to trientine, and for liver failure or truly refractory patients, liver transplantation is curative

 ### Best Augmenting Combos for Partial Response or Treatment-Resistance
- Change to trientine if ineffective or poorly tolerated. A diet low in copper-containing foods, such as nuts, chocolate, liver, and dried fruit, is recommended

Tests
- Patients with WD have low serum ceruloplasmin and serum copper, but increased urinary excretion of copper is diagnostic. In pediatric patients, a 24-hour urinary copper excretion more than 1600mcg after 500mg dose of penicillamine is considered diagnostic of WD. While on treatment, check CBC and urinalysis, and monitor for skin changes and fever twice weekly for 1 month, then every 2 weeks for the next 5 months, and monthly for the remainder of treatment

ADVERSE EFFECTS (AEs)

How the Drug Causes AEs
- Unknown

Notable AEs
- Fever, pruritus, changes in taste perception, tinnitus, optic neuritis, neuropathies, abdominal pain, anorexia, pancreatitis, proteinuria/hematuria, oral ulcerations, alopecia

 ### Life-Threatening or Dangerous AEs
- Myasthenic syndrome, usually starting with ptosis and diplopia, that can lead to generalized myasthenia if penicillamine is not stopped. Hematological AEs, such as leukopenia, thrombocytopenia. Nephrotic syndrome/renal failure. Drug fever, often with a macular cutaneous eruption and often in 2–3 weeks after starting treatment. Rarely obliterative brochiolitis, with unexplained cough or wheezing

Weight Gain
- Unusual

unusual   not unusual   common   problematic

Sedation
- Unusual

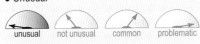

What to Do About AEs
- Leukopenia, neutropenia: discontinue drug
- Patients with moderate proteinuria can continue drug cautiously at lower dose but if renal function worsens or urinary protein is more than 1 g in 24 hours, discontinue drug. Urinary proteinuria can take up to a year to improve
- Give vitamin B6 (pyridoxine) 25 mg weekly, or 50 mg weekly to children, pregnant women, and patients with malnutrition or an intercurrent illness
- For drug fever, temporarily discontinue drug, give corticosteroid therapy, and restart drug at lower dose with a slower titration
- Pulmonary symptoms: check pulmonary function tests
- Patients with significant AEs: change to trientine

Best Augmenting Agents to Reduce AEs
- Most AEs cannot be reduced with the use of an augmenting agent

DOSING AND USE

Usual Dosage Range
- 0.75–2 g/day

Dosage Forms
- Tablets: 125, 250 mg

How to Dose
- Start at 250 mg/day and increase gradually over the next 1–2 weeks to target dose. The usual dose is between 0.75 and 1.5 g daily, although patients will occasionally require as much as 2 g/day. The goal is to achieve a 24-hour copper excretion over 2 mg/day for the first 3 months. After the first few months, the urinary copper excretion decreases to less than 0.5 mg/day and eventually less than 150 mcg/day, with a serum copper less than 10 mcg/dL. Usually the dose will not require adjustment after the first 2 weeks

 Dosing Tips
- Give at least 1 hour before or 2 hours after meals to ensure absorption

Overdose
- Symptoms unknown

Long-Term Use
- Many AEs, such as nephrotoxicity (a lupus erythematosus-like syndrome), bone marrow suppression/thrombocytopenia, can develop after extended use. Can cause skin complications, such as elastosis perforans serpiginosa, aphthous stomatitis, and can affect pyridoxine metabolism

Habit Forming
- No

How to Stop
- No need to taper

Pharmacokinetics
- Bioavailability is 40–70%, and drug is 80% protein bound with peak plasma levels 1–3 hours after ingestion. When stopping, after prolonged usage, there is a slow elimination phase for 4–6 days

 Drug Interactions
- Decreases levels of digoxin
- Increases effects and toxicity of gold therapy, antimalarial or cytotoxic drugs, phenylbutazone, and oxyphenbutazone
- Iron salts and antacids decrease absorption of penicillamine

 Other Warnings/ Precautions
- May cause a positive antinuclear antibody (ANA) test and lupus erythematosus-like syndrome. Some patients allergic to penicillin may have cross-sensitivity to penicillamine

Do Not Use
- Patients with known hypersensitivity to the drug, history of penicillamine-related aplastic anemia, or agranulocytosis

Renal Impairment
- Use with caution in WD due to lack of alternatives. In rheumatoid arthritis, use another agent

Hepatic Impairment
- Usually improves hepatic disease in WD, even if severe

Cardiac Impairment
- No known effects

Elderly
- Use with caution

Children and Adolescents
- WD can occur in children, usually ages 5 or older. Start with lower dose penicillamine, and adjust based on urinary copper excretion

Pregnancy
- Category C. Use only for WD or cystinuria (not rheumatoid arthritis). Reduce dose to 750 mg daily, and reduce to 250 daily for a planned cesarean section 6 weeks before the expected birth date

Breast Feeding
- Patients taking penicillamine should not breast feed

Potential Advantages
- Proven, long-standing treatment for WD, usually effective

Potential Disadvantages
- Multiple AEs, including paradoxical worsening in 20–50% of patients

Primary Target Symptoms
- Monitor urinary copper to determine effectiveness. Treatment should improve neurological symptoms, such as parkinsonism, dystonia, ataxia, depression, and psychosis, over time

 Pearls
- 10–50% WD patients may experience initial neurological worsening at the beginning of treatment
- Trientine is better tolerated with fewer side effects. Zinc is another alternative for maintenance treatment
- Other agents with known effects in WD include tetrathiomolybdate and IM dimercaprol
- In asymptomatic individuals diagnosed by abnormal test results or family screening, it is uncertain if zinc or penicillamine is most appropriate initial treatment
- Urinary copper excretion (> 1600 mcg/ 24 h) upon D-penicillamine (at 0 and 12 hours) is diagnostic of WD
- Can induce anti-MuSK- and anti-AChR-positive myasthenia gravis
- Garlic and penicillamine have similar effect in lowering serum lead level

---

Suggested Reading

Brewer GJ. The risks of free copper in the body and the development of useful anticopper drugs. *Curr Opin Clin Nutr Metab Care.* 2008;11(6): 727–32.

Kianoush S, Balali-Mood M, Mousavi SR, Moradi V, Sadeghi M, Dadpour B, et al. Comparison of therapeutic effects of garlic and d-penicillamine in patients with chronic occupational lead poisoning. *Basic Clin Pharmacol Toxicol.* 2011;110(5):476–81.

Patil M, Sheth KA, Krishnamurthy AC, Devarbhavi H. A review and current perspective on Wilson disease. *J Clin Exp Hepatol.* 2013; 3(4):321–36.

Wiggelinkhuizen M, Tilanus ME, Bollen CW, Houwen RH. Systematic review: clinical efficacy of chelator agents and zinc in the initial treatment of Wilson disease. *Aliment Pharmacol Ther.* 2009;29(9): 947–58.

PERAMPANEL

Brands
- Fycompa

Generic?
- No

 Class
- Antiepileptic drug (AED)

Commonly Prescribed for
(FDA approved in bold)
- **Adjunctive therapy for the treatment of partial-onset seizures with or without secondarily generalized seizures in patients with epilepsy aged 12 years and older**
- Primary generalized tonic-clonic seizures in patients with epilepsy aged 12 years and older. Lennox-Gastaut syndrome

 How the Drug Works
- Perampanel is a non-competitive selective antagonist of the ionotropic α-amino-3-hydroxy-5-methyl-4 isoxazolepropionic acid (AMPA) glutamate receptor on postsynaptic neurons. Its binding stabilizes the resting state of the channel and disrupts channel opening in response to agonist (e.g., glutamate) binding
- The precise mechanism by which perampanel exerts its antiepileptic effects in humans has not been fully elucidated

How Long Until It Works
- Drug steady state is reached in weeks

If It Works
- The goal is seizure remission. Continue as long as effective and well tolerated. Consider tapering and slowly stopping after 2 years without seizures, depending on the type of epilepsy

If It Doesn't Work
- Increase to highest tolerated dose
- Consider changing to another agent, adding a second agent, using a medical device, or a referral for epilepsy surgery evaluation. When adding a second agent, keep drug interactions in mind

 Best Augmenting Combos for Partial Response or Treatment-Resistance
- Drug interactions can complicate multi-drug therapy

Tests
- Not available

How the Drug Causes AEs
- CNS AEs are probably caused by glutamate blockade effects

Notable AEs
- Dizziness, gait disturbance, somnolence, fatigue, falls, nausea, vertigo
- Hostility and aggressive behavior in 10–20% of patients under maximum dosage. They usually appear within the first 6 weeks of treatment

 Life-Threatening or Dangerous AEs
- Suicidal behavior and ideation
- Withdrawal epilepsy, although rare due to its long half-life

Weight Gain
- Not unusual

unusual   not unusual   common   problematic

Sedation
- Not unusual

unusual   not unusual   common   problematic

What to Do About AEs
- Discontinue the drug immediately if symptoms are severe or are worsening

Best Augmenting Agents to Reduce AEs
- Drug discontinuation

Usual Dosage Range
- 8–12 mg daily

Dosage Forms
- Tablets: 2, 4, 6, 8, 10, 12 mg

How to Dose
- Epilepsy: start at 2 mg at bedtime (without enzyme-inducing AEDs) or 4 mg at bedtime (with enzyme-inducing AEDs)
- Increase by 2 mg/week to a dose of 4–12 mg daily

 Dosing Tips
- Titrate slowly to avoid adverse effects
- Close monitor the response and tolerability under concomitant therapy
- Conversion to monotherapy: concomitant AEDs should be withdrawn over 3–6 weeks

Overdose
- Altered mental status and behavioral changes. Most typically recover without sequelae
- The reactions caused by perampanel may be prolonged due to its long half-life

Long-Term Use
- Safe for long-term use

Habit Forming
- Potential of abuse due to euphoria but lower incidence than ketamine. Doses producing euphoria are higher than usually prescribed (24 mg or greater)

How to Stop
- A gradual withdrawal is generally recommended with AEDs, but if withdrawal is a response to AEs, prompt withdrawal can be considered

Pharmacokinetics
- Extensively metabolized via oxidation (CYP3A4 or CYP3A5) and sequential glucuronidation. Half-life 105 hours. Excretion 22% in urine and 48% in feces

 Drug Interactions
- 12 mg/day or greater decreases effectiveness of hormonal contraceptives containing levonorgestrel
- CNS depressants (alcohol, antihistamine, benzodiazepines, narcotics) produce additive effect

- CYP3A4 inducer (carbamazepine, oxcarbazine, phenytoin, rifampin, St. John's wort, dexamethasone) decreases perampanel plasma concentration
- CYP3A4 inhibitor (azoles, macrolides, some antivirals, grapefruit) increases perampanel plasma concentration
- Topiramate decreases perampanel concentration

 Other Warnings/ Precautions
- Potential for abuse at supertherapeutic doses
- CNS AEs increase when used with other CNS depressants

Do Not Use
- No contraindication

Renal Impairment
- Not recommended for patients with severe renal impairment or on hemodialysis

Hepatic Impairment
- Maximum recommended daily dose is 6 mg and 4 mg once daily at bedtime for patients with mild and moderate hepatic impairment, respectively. Increase by 2 mg every 2 weeks. Not recommended for patients with severe hepatic impairment

Cardiac Impairment
- No known effects

Elderly
- Increased risk of dizziness and gait disturbance. Slow increment of 2 mg every 2 weeks

 Children and Adolescents
- It is not known if perampanel is safe and effective in children under 12 years of age

 Pregnancy
- Category C. Teratogenicity in animal studies

- Risks of stopping medication must outweigh risk to fetus for patients with epilepsy. Seizures and potential status epilepticus place the woman and fetus at risk and can cause reduced oxygen and blood supply to the womb
- Supplementation with 0.4 mg of folic acid before and during pregnancy is recommended

Breast Feeding

- It is not known if perampanel passes into breast milk
- Generally recommendations are to discontinue drug or bottle feed
- Monitor infant for sedation, poor feeding, or irritability

THE ART OF NEUROPHARMACOLOGY

Potential Advantages

- Novel mechanism as an add-on therapy, unique mechanism of action. Once-daily dosing

Potential Disadvantages

- Drug interactions, via CYP3A4, and issues in persons with hepatic or renal disease

Primary Target Symptoms

- Seizure frequency and severity

 Pearls

- Effective for partial epilepsies but uncertain for primary generalized seizures
- Based on a recent study on Parkinson's disease, there were no significant changes in dyskinesia or cognitive function in any perampanel group vs. placebo
- NMDA antagonism (felbamate) and AMPA antagonism (lamotrigine, perampanel) both elicit their antiepileptic potentials via GluK1 antagonism, which can be beneficial in combination with other treatments (sodium or calcium channel blocker, potassium, GABA enhancer)
- No study on known effect for neuropathic pain
- Similar chemicals (tezampanel, selurampanel) were effective for acute migraine treatment. In theory perampanel should behave similarly
- Although overactivity of AMPA receptor has been involved in dopa-induced dyskinesia, perampanel (AMPA antagonist) use in Parkinson's disease with motor fluctuation has shown no benefit

 Suggested Reading

Eggert K, Squillacote D, Barone P, Dodel R, Katzenschlager R, Emre M, et al. Safety and efficacy of perampanel in advanced Parkinson's disease: a randomized, placebo-controlled study. *Mov Disord.* 2010;25(7):896–905.

Gomez-Mancilla B, Brand R, Jürgens TP, Göbel H, Sommer C, Straube A, et al. Randomized, multicenter trial to assess the efficacy, safety and tolerability of a single dose of a novel AMPA receptor antagonist BGG492 for the treatment of acute migraine attacks. *Cephalalgia.* 2014;34(2):103–13.

Schmidt D, Schachter SC. Drug treatment of epilepsy in adults. *BMJ.* 2014;348:g254.

Steinhoff BJ. Efficacy of perampanel: a review of pooled data. *Epilepsia.* 2014;55 Suppl 1:9–12.

PHENOBARBITAL

THERAPEUTICS

Brands
- Luminal, Alkabel, Solfoton

Generic?
- Yes

 Class
- Antiepileptic drug (AED)

Commonly Prescribed for
(FDA approved in bold)
- **Generalized tonic-clonic, psychomotor, and partial seizures (monotherapy and adjunctive, children and adults)**
- Sedation
- Status epilepticus
- Seizures resulting from cerebral malaria
- Anxiety
- Alcohol or barbiturate withdrawal

 How the Drug Works
- Phenobarbital raises seizure thresholds or alters seizure patterns in animal models
- The exact mechanism of action is unknown but likely enhances $GABA_A$ receptor activity
- Depresses glutamate excitability, alters sodium, calcium, and potassium channel conductance
- It affects polysynaptic midbrain reticular formation

How Long Until It Works
- Seizure prevention: should decrease by 2 weeks
- Status epilepticus: onset of action is 5 minutes following IV injection. Maximal CNS depression after at least 15 minutes

If It Works
- Seizures: goal is the remission of seizures. Continue as long as effective and well-tolerated. Consider tapering and slowly stopping after 2 years without seizures, depending on the type of epilepsy

If It Doesn't Work
- Increase to highest tolerated dose
- Epilepsy: consider changing to another agent, adding a second agent, or referral for epilepsy surgery evaluation. When adding a second agent, keep in mind drug interactions

 Best Augmenting Combos for Partial Response or Treatment-Resistance
- Epilepsy: drug interactions complicate multi-drug therapy. Phenobarbital is a second-line agent in developed countries due to its AE profile

Tests
- CBC, hepatic and kidney function panels at baseline and every 6 months

ADVERSE EFFECTS (AEs)

How the Drug Causes AEs
- CNS AEs are probably caused by effects of increased GABA activity and alteration of ion channel function
- Vitamin D deficiency is caused by induction of metabolism

Notable AEs
- Sedation, ataxia, vertigo, cognitive dulling, depression, nystagmus, irritability, emotional disturbances
- Nausea, vomiting, hypotension
- Rash, uncommonly Stevens-Johnson syndrome

 Life-Threatening or Dangerous AEs
- Megaloblastic anemia, rarely agranulocytosis
- Hypotension
- Respiratory depression: use with caution in patients with asthma or pulmonary disease

Weight Gain
- Common

Sedation
- Problematic

What to Do About AEs
- A dose decrease may improve CNS AEs
- For megaloblastic anemia, treat with folate

Best Augmenting Agents to Reduce AEs

- No treatment for most AEs other than lowering dose or stopping drug

DOSING AND USE

Usual Dose Range

- Epilepsy: 30–120 mg/day (as monotherapy)

Dosage Forms

- Tablet: 15, 16, 30, 60, 90, and 100 mg
- Capsule: 16 mg
- Elixir: 15 or 20 mg/5 mL
- Injection: 30, 60 or 65, or 130 mg/mL

How to Dose

- Epilepsy as monotherapy: start at 30–50 mg at bedtime. Increase in 5–30 mg increments every week until goal dose (usually 90–180 mg/day). Maximum 400 mg/day
- Status epilepticus: give 20 mg/kg IV at rate no greater than 100 mg/min. Do not substitute oral or IM
- When adding to other AEDs start at 30 mg at bedtime and titrate more slowly
- When changing from another AED, the transition should take at least 2 weeks

Dosing Tips

- May induce its own metabolism
- Most patients can take once daily
- Check a serum level (usual goal 10–40 mcg/mL) for optimal dosage. Required dose may be higher for the control of simple and complex partial, compared with tonic-clonic, seizures

Overdose

- Similar to other barbiturates. Respiratory depression, ataxia, nystagmus, tachycardia, hypotension, hypothermia can all occur

Long-term Use

- Safe for long-term use with periodic laboratory monitoring

Habit Forming

- Tolerance, psychological and physical dependence can occur, especially with long-term use at high doses. Use with caution in patients with depression or history of substance abuse

How to Stop

- Abrupt withdrawal can lead to seizures in patients with epilepsy
- Often requires prolonged taper compared to other AEDs

Pharmacokinetics

- Mostly metabolized by CYP2C19. Mean half-life in adults is 80 hours, in children mean is 65 hours. Peak drug levels at 1–3 hours (oral). 25–50% of drug is excreted unchanged in urine. Bioavailability is 100%. May reduce folate by inhibiting dihydrofolate reductase. About 20–50% protein bound

 Drug Interactions

- Potent inducer of CYP450 (all subtypes). Lowers levels of many medications including warfarin, lamotrigine, TCAs, corticosteroids, methadone, cyclosporine, corticotropin, vitamin D, verapamil, and nifedipine, among many others
- Variable effect on phenytoin metabolism
- Many AEDs inhibit CYP2C9 or CYP2C19 and can increase serum levels of phenobarbital, including phenytoin, valproic acid, carbamazepine, and felbamate
- Acetazolamide, ethosuximide, and antacids can lower levels

 Other Warnings/ Precautions

- CNS AEs can be severe when used with other CNS depressants
- Toxicity magnified with alcohol use
- Folate deficiency and hyperhomocystinemia
- Can diminish systemic effects of exogenous or endogenous corticosteroids
- Bone and mineral loss with long-term use, increases vitamin D requirements
- May cause anesthesia at high doses: use with caution in patients with acute or chronic pain
- Increased tendency to fibrosis, including Dupuytren's contractures
- Reduces effectiveness of hormonal contraceptives

Do Not Use

- Patients with a proven allergy to primidone or phenobarbital, or patients with porphyria

Renal Impairment

- Usually a lower dose is required, but there are no clear guidelines on how much to decrease. For patients with CrCl < 10 mL/min, increase dosing interval by 50–100%. Consider supplemental dose post-dialysis

Hepatic Impairment

- Use with caution in patients with significant disease. Do not use in patients with hepatic encephalopathy

Cardiac Impairment

- No known effects

Elderly

- May need lower dose. More likely to experience CNS AEs and can increase fall risk

Children and Adolescents

- Usual dose 2–6 mg/kg/day in 1–2 doses
- Commonly used for neonatal and febrile seizures
- In status epilepticus can give up to 30 mg/kg at rate no greater than 100 mg/min. Effective brain concentrations within 3 minutes
- May cause paradoxical excitement, aggression, tearfulness, or hyperkinetic states
- Can cause cognitive side effects in children when used to prevent febrile seizures

Pregnancy

- Category D. High rate of fetal malformations, and infants can experience withdrawal symptoms after birth
- Risk of neonatal hemorrhage due to vitamin K deficiency. Supplement with folate and vitamin K 1 month prior to and during delivery. Risks of stopping medication must outweigh risk to fetus
- Supplementation with 0.4 mg of folic acid before and during pregnancy is recommended

Breast Feeding

- Drug is found in mother's breast milk in substantial quantities
- Generally recommendations are to discontinue drug or bottle feed, but may assist in preventing infant withdrawal from drug
- Monitor infant for sedation, poor feeding, or irritability

Potential Advantages

- Effective for multiple types of epilepsy. Useful in refractory epilepsy
- Inexpensive. Long half-life
- Lower abuse potential than other barbiturates

Potential Disadvantages

- Sedation and multiple potential AEs. Difficult to discontinue
- Potent hepatic induction complicates therapy with other AEDs
- Unlike many other AEDs, not useful for mood disorders. May cause depression

Primary Target Symptoms

- Seizure frequency and severity
- Anxiety and alcohol withdrawal symptoms

Pearls

- Commonly used in developing countries due to low cost and ability to treat multiple seizure types
- For patients with epilepsy, even with good seizure control, it may be worth changing to another agent due to frequent AEs such as sedation, bone loss, and cognitive slowing
- In children, more effective than phenytoin in small studies for the prevention of febrile seizures, but cognitive AEs are common
- The efficacy/effectiveness of phenobarbital monotherapy in children with partial-onset seizures was similar to carbamazepine, phenytoin, and valproate in Class III open-label trials
- Less popular than benzodiazepines for alcohol withdrawal. Respiratory depression, especially when combined with alcohol, is a potential problem

- Use with extreme caution in patients with a history of substance abuse, depression, or suicidal tendencies

- Because it may take > 15 minutes before maximal CNS depression, injection until seizure stops may lead to severe barbiturate-induced depression

Suggested Reading

Arya R, Glauser TA. Pharmacotherapy of focal epilepsy in children: a systematic review of approved agents. *CNS Drugs* 2013;27:273–86.

Brophy GM, Bell R, Claassen J, Alldredge B, Bleck TP, Glauser T, et al. Guidelines for the evaluation and management of status epilepticus. *Neurocrit Care* 2012;17:3–23.

PHENYTOIN AND FOSPHENYTOIN

Brands
- Dilantin, Phenytek, Epanutin, Fosphenytoin, Cerebyx

Generic?
- Yes

Class
- Antiepileptic drug (AED)

Commonly Prescribed for
(FDA approved in bold)
- **Generalized tonic-clonic and complex partial seizures (monotherapy or adjunctive in adults and children)**
- **Treatment of seizures during or following neurosurgery**
- **Status epilepticus**
- Trigeminal neuralgia
- Glossopharyngeal neuralgia
- Migraine prophylaxis
- Diabetic neuropathic pain
- Junctional epidermolysis bullosa
- Preeclampsia (alternative to magnesium sulfate)
- Cardiac arrhythmias (especially glycoside-induced)
- Seizure prophylaxis after severe traumatic brain injury
- Myotonia

How the Drug Works
- Primarily through the reduction of hyperexcitability on sodium channels
- May modulate T-type calcium channels, but not in the thalamus (unlike AEDs used for absence seizures)

How Long Until It Works
- Seizures: may decrease by 2–3 weeks
- Trigeminal neuralgia: may start working in hours to weeks

If It Works
- Seizures: goal is the remission of seizures. Continue as long as effective and well tolerated. Consider tapering and slowly stopping after 2 years without seizures, depending on the type of epilepsy
- Pain: goal is the reduction of pain severity and frequency. If trigeminal neuralgia remits on medication, periodically attempt to lower dose or discontinue

If It Doesn't Work
- Increase to highest tolerated dose
- Epilepsy: consider changing to another agent, adding a second agent, using a medical device, or a referral for epilepsy surgery evaluation. When adding a second agent, keep drug interactions in mind. Check level if seizures worsening and compliance is an issue
- Pain: try an alternative agent

 Best Augmenting Combos for Partial Response or Treatment-Resistance
- Epilepsy: keep in mind drug interactions and their effect on levels

Tests
- During IV administration, continuous heart monitoring is required, with frequent blood pressure checks
- Obtain CBC monthly for the first few months due to risk of blood dyscrasias

How the Drug Causes AEs
- CNS side effects are probably caused by sodium channel effects

Notable AEs
- Nystagmus, ataxia, dysarthria, insomnia, nervousness, motor twitching, tremor, dizziness, impaired memory
- Gingival hyperplasia, rash (usually morbilliform), hirsutism, coarsening of facial features
- Pneumonia, sinusitis, rhinitis, asthma
- Tinnitus, diplopia, eye pain, taste loss
- Lymph node hyperplasia, chest pain, edema
- Soft tissue injury with IV use

 Life-Threatening or Dangerous AEs
- Hypotension, cardiac conduction abnormalities with rapid IV administration. Can be fatal. Less likely with fosphenytoin
- May inhibit insulin release and cause hyperglycemia. Rare diabetes insipidus

- Blood dyscrasias (thrombocytopenia or agranulocytosis)
- Rare serious allergic rash (Stevens-Johnson syndrome, lupus erythematosus syndrome, radiation-induced erythema multiforme)
- Rare lymphoma or multiple myeloma
- Toxic hepatitis and liver damage
- May cause cerebellar atrophy with long-term use at high doses
- "Purple glove" syndrome is a rare complication associated with IV use. Extremities become swollen, discolored, and painful. May require amputation

Weight Gain
- Not unusual

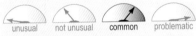

Sedation
- Common

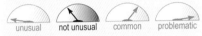

What to Do About AEs
- Side effects may decrease or remit after a longer time on a stable dose
- A small decrease in dose may improve side effects
- Stop drug for any hematological abnormalities
- Recommend good oral hygiene to prevent gingival hyperplasia

Best Augmenting Agents to Reduce AEs
- Take with food to avoid GI AEs
- Most AEs only decrease with stopping drug or lowering dose

DOSING AND USE

Usual Dosage Range
- Epilepsy: 300–600 mg/day for adults
- Trigeminal neuralgia: 300–500 mg/day in divided doses

Dosage Forms
- Chewable tablets: 50 mg
- Capsules: 100 mg, extended release 30, 100, 200, and 300 mg
- Oral suspension: 125 mg/5 mL
- Injection: 50 mg/mL

- As prodrug fosphenytoin: 150 mg in 2 mL or 750 in 10 mL vials. 150 mg fosphenytoin is equivalent to 100 mg phenytoin

How to Dose
- Start at 300 mg/day in 3 divided doses. Can use once daily with extended-release drug once a stable dose is established. Increase up to 600 mg/day
- Follow drug levels to determine effective dose and if compliance is in question
- For patients with hypoalbuminemia, kidney or liver disease, check free drug level
- Status epilepticus: 15–20 mg/kg load, followed by usual maintenance dose of 4–6 mg/kg/day
- Flush the medication with sterile saline after IV administration to avoid local skin irritation

 Dosing Tips
- Adverse events increase with dose
- Usual effective levels are 7–20 mg/L but vary from patient to patient
- Tube feeding can decrease absorption; give 2 hours before or after
- Drug takes 7–10 days to achieve steady state – wait to check levels

Overdose
- At concentrations > 20 mcg/mL: nystagmus
- At concentrations > 30 mcg/mL: ataxia
- At concentrations > 40 mcg/mL: diminished mental capacity, coma, hypotension, lack of pupillary reactivity
- Lethal dose is estimated to be 2–5 g, with death from respiratory and circulatory depression

Long-Term Use
- Safe for long-term use

Habit Forming
- No

How to Stop
- Taper slowly. Abrupt withdrawal can lead to seizures in patients with epilepsy

Pharmacokinetics
- Oral peak plasma levels at 12 hours, IV within 1.5–3 hours. At higher doses, individual patients may not be able to

metabolize drug, leading to high drug levels. This may produce toxic drug levels as half-life increases at higher concentrations. Plasma half-life ranges from 6 to 24 hours. About 90% protein bound. Metabolized in liver; metabolites are excreted in urine

Drug Interactions

- Potent inducer of CYP450 hepatic metabolism, particularly CYP2B6, CYP3A4
- Levels increase due to inhibition of metabolism (valproic acid, acute ethanol, allopurinol, amiodarone, omeprazole, cimetidine, fluconazole, benzodiazepines among others), displacement from protein binding sites (salicylates, TCAs, valproic acid), or unknown mechanisms (ibuprofen and phenothiazines)
- Levels decrease due to drugs that increase metabolism (carbamazepine, barbiturates, chronic ethanol, rifampin), decrease absorption (antacids), or have unknown mechanisms (nitrofurantoin, pyridoxine, and many antineoplastics)
- Can increase metabolism of other drugs, including valproic acid, carbamazepine, amiodarone, mexiletine, theophylline, corticosteroids, cardiac glycosides, estrogens, and corticosteroids. Decreased levels of dopamine, levadopa, phenothiazines, among many others
- Can increase lithium toxicity (even with normal lithium serum levels)
- Decreased effectiveness of meperidine while increasing toxic metabolite
- May displace warfarin, leading to bleeding complications

⚠ Other Warnings/ Precautions

- CNS side effects increase when taken with other CNS depressants
- May decrease serum or free thyroxine concentrations
- Any unusual bleeding or bruising, fever, or mouth sores should raise concern for rare blood dyscrasias
- Use with caution in patients with acute intermittent porphyria

Do Not Use

- Patients with a proven allergy to phenytoin. Do not use in sinus bradycardia,

sino-atrial block, second- or third-degree AV block, or in patients with Adams-Stokes syndrome

Renal Impairment

- Because phenytoin is highly protein bound, it is often easier to use than many other AEDs. No post-dialysis supplement is required

Hepatic Impairment

- Clearance may be decreased in patients with severe liver disease. Reduce dose

Cardiac Impairment

- Use with caution in hypotension or myocardial insufficiency, especially IV
- Fosphenytoin may prolong QTc interval

Elderly

- May be more susceptible to CNS and cardiovascular side effects

Children and Adolescents

- Usual dose is 4–8 mg/kg/day. Maximum 300 mg/day. Checking levels can help determine best dose
- Divide doses equally if possible. If not, give the larger dose at bedtime

Pregnancy

- Category D. Fetal hydantoin syndrome includes craniofacial abnormalities, such as microcephaly and cleft lip and palate, and mild mental retardation. Clinically similar to fetal alcohol syndrome. Potential risk to fetus may be dose related. Perhaps less likely to cause spinal malformations than valproate or carbamazepine
- Risk of neonatal hemorrhage due to vitamin K deficiency. Supplement with 10 mg/day 1 month before expected delivery
- Supplementation with 0.4 mg of folic acid before and during pregnancy is recommended
- Plasma levels may decrease, resulting in increased rate of seizures due to changes in metabolism. Check levels more frequently

- Risks of stopping medication must outweigh risk to fetus for patients with epilepsy. Seizures and potential status epilepticus place the woman and fetus at risk and can cause reduced oxygen and blood supply to the womb
- Patients taking phenytoin for conditions other than epilepsy should generally stop before considering pregnancy

Breast Feeding

- Present in breast milk at 10–60% of serum level
- Generally recommendations are to discontinue drug or bottle feed
- Monitor infant for sedation, poor feeding, or irritability

THE ART OF NEUROPHARMACOLOGY

Potential Advantages

- Highly effective and relatively non-sedating. Low cost and available IV. Ease of monitoring drug levels

Potential Disadvantages:

- Non-linear kinetics, drug interactions, and CNS AEs
- Ineffective for many seizure types, including myoclonic, absence, and atonic seizures, Lennox-Gastaut syndrome, and infantile spasms

Primary Target Symptoms

- Seizure frequency and severity
- Mood stabilization
- Pain

 Pearls

- Useful for many common epilepsy syndromes. Ability to monitor levels is useful in patients with frequent seizures requiring emergency visits
- Reduces risk of epileptic seizures associated with neurosurgery, especially if the doses are therapeutic

- May be used for seizure prophylaxis after severe brain injury
- No significant difference exists between phenytoin and valproate on treatment for partial or generalized tonic-clonic seizure
- Fosphenytoin (20 mg phenytoin equivalent/kg), which is cleaved to phenytoin in 15 minutes, is a preferred first-line IV treatment for status epilepticus (except in patients with a history of primary generalized epilepsy). It may be given 3 times faster or as IM injection without risk of "purple glove" syndrome
- The treatment of generalized tonic-clonic status epilepticus often requires aggressive treatment with simultaneous therapies. In patients with simple or complex partial status epilepticus, overtreatment resulting in intubation may cause more harm than good.
- Fosphenytoin's better tolerability and more rapid IV administration rate make it attractive for drug loading
- AE profile generally better than barbiturates, but worse than most new AEDs
- Persons with variants of CYP2C known to reduce drug clearance are more likely to experience severe cutaneous drug reactions
- In acute trigeminal neuralgia, often effective within days and may be given as IV treatment in an emergency room setting (250 mg over 5 minutes). Effect of drug in chronic facial pain often decreases over time
- Effective in some studies for treatment of diabetic neuropathy (Level of Evidence C)
- Effective treatment for myotonia (delayed relaxation of muscles after activity) in myotonia congenita or myotonic dystrophy patients who require pharmacological treatment of their symptoms. Phenytoin's potential neurotoxicity could outweigh its antimyotonia effects

Suggested Reading

Brophy GM, Bell R, Claassen J, Alldredge B, Bleck TP, Glauser T, et al. Guidelines for the evaluation and management of status epilepticus. *Neurocrit Care.* 2012;17:3–23.

Cheshire WP. Fosphenytoin: an intravenous option for the management of acute trigeminal neuralgia crisis. *J Pain Symptom Manage.* 2001;21(6):506–10.

Chung WH, Chang WC, Lee YS, Wu YY, Yang CH, Ho HC, et al. Genetic variants associated with phenytoin-related severe cutaneous adverse reactions. *JAMA.* 2014;312(5):525–34.

Glauser T, Ben-Menachem E, Bourgeois B, Cnaan A, Guerreiro C, Kälviäinen R, et al. Updated ILAE evidence review of antiepileptic drug efficacy and effectiveness as initial monotherapy for epileptic seizures and syndromes. *Epilepsia.* 2013;54:551–63.

Heatwole CR, Statland JM, Logigian EL. The diagnosis and treatment of myotonic disorders. *Muscle Nerve.* 2013;47:632–48.

Reddy GD, Viswanathan A. Trigeminal and glossopharyngeal neuralgia. *Neurol Clin.* 2014;32:539–52.

Rowe AS, Goodwin H, Brophy GM, Bushwitz J, Castle A, Deen D, et al. Seizure prophylaxis in neurocritical care: a review of evidence-based support. *Pharmacotherapy* 2014;34:396–409.

PIZOTIFEN

THERAPEUTICS

Brands
- Sanomigran

Generic?
- Yes

Class
- Antihistamine

Commonly Prescribed for
- Migraine prophylaxis (children and adults)
- Cluster headache prophylaxis
- Treatment of serotonin syndrome
- Anxiety/social phobia

How the Drug Works
- An antihistamine and 5-HT$_2$ receptor antagonist that is structurally related to TCAs. Has weak anticholinergic effects and may act as a calcium channel blocker at high doses. The relative importance of each action in headache prophylaxis is unclear. Prevention of cortical spreading depression may be one mechanism of action for all migraine preventatives

How Long Until It Works
- Migraines may decrease in as little as 2 weeks, but can take up to 2 months to see full effect

If It Works
- Migraine: goal is a 50% or greater decrease in migraine frequency or severity. Consider tapering or stopping if headaches remit for more than 6 months or if considering pregnancy

If It Doesn't Work
- Increase to highest tolerated dose
- Migraine: address other issues, such as medication overuse, other coexisting medical disorders, such as anxiety, and consider changing to another agent or adding a second agent

Best Augmenting Combos for Partial Response or Treatment-Resistance
- Migraine: for some patients with migraine, low-dose polytherapy with 2 or more drugs

may be better tolerated and more effective than high-dose monotherapy. May use in combination with AEDs, antidepressants, natural products, and non-medication treatments, such as biofeedback, to improve headache control

Tests
- Monitor weight during treatment

ADVERSE EFFECTS (AEs)

How the Drug Causes AEs
- Most are related to antihistamine and anticholinergic activity

Notable AEs
- Weight gain and sedation are most common
- Nausea, weakness, dry mouth, depression, sexual dysfunction, and urinary retention

Life-Threatening or Dangerous AEs
- Increased intraocular pressure
- Rare activation of mania or suicidal ideation
- Rare increase in seizures in patients with epilepsy
- Hypersensitivity reactions

Weight Gain
- Problematic

unusual   not unusual   common   problematic

Sedation
- Common

unusual   not unusual   common   problematic

What to Do About AEs
- Lower dose or switch to another agent. For serious AEs, do not use

Best Augmenting Agents to Reduce AEs
- Try magnesium for constipation. For migraine, consider using with agents that cause weight loss as an AE (e.g., topiramate)

DOSING AND USE

Usual Dosage Range
- 1.5–3 mg/day

Dosage Forms
- Tablets: 0.5, 1.5 mg
- Elixir: 0.25 mg/5 mL

How to Dose
- Migraine/tension-type headache: initial dose is either 0.5 mg 3 times daily or 1.5 mg at night. Increase if needed to 3–4.5 mg daily. At doses above 3 mg/day, divide doses

 Dosing Tips
- Take largest dose at night to minimize drowsiness

Overdose
- CNS depression is most common, but hypotension, tachycardia, and respiratory depression may occur. Anticholinergic effects include fixed pupils, flushing, and hyperthermia

Long-Term Use
- Safe for long-term use

Habit Forming
- No

How to Stop
- No need to taper, but migraine often returns after stopping

Pharmacokinetics
- Rapid absorption with 78% bioavailability. Peak levels at 4–5 hours. Metabolized by glucuronidation. Most drug is excreted as metabolites in urine, but about 18% is excreted in feces. Elimination half-life of metabolite is 23 hours

 Drug Interactions
- Use with MAOIs may increase toxicity and should be avoided
- May lower effectiveness of SSRIs due to serotonin antagonism
- Excess sedation with other CNS depressants (alcohol, barbiturates) can occur

 Other Warnings/ Precautions
- Tablets contain lactose and sucrose

Do Not Use
- Hypersensitivity to drug, angle-closure glaucoma, bladder neck obstruction, patients using MAOIs, symptomatic prostatic hypertrophy

SPECIAL POPULATIONS

Renal Impairment
- No known effects

Hepatic Impairment
- May reduce metabolism. Titrate more slowly

Cardiac Impairment
- Rarely causes arrhythmias and ECG changes. Use with caution

Elderly
- More likely to experience AEs especially anticholinergic

 Children and Adolescents
- Drug has been used in children, usually age 7 and up, but may decrease alertness or produce paradoxical excitation

 Pregnancy
- Category B. Use only if potential benefit outweighs risk to the fetus

Breast Feeding
- Unknown if excreted in breast milk. Do not breast feed on drug

THE ART OF NEUROPHARMACOLOGY

Potential Advantages
- Commonly used migraine preventive, with efficacy in children and adults

Potential Disadvantages
- No large studies that demonstrate effectiveness. Sedation and weight gain

Primary Target Symptoms

- Headache frequency and severity

 Pearls

- Efficacy similar to flunarizine and nimodipine in some studies

- Small studies report effectiveness in preventing recurrent abdominal migraine in children
- Antiserotonin effects make pizotifen a potentially useful drug in the treatment of serotonin syndrome

 Suggested Reading

Barnes N, Millman G. Do pizotifen or propranolol reduce the frequency of migraine headache? *Arch Dis Child.* 2004;89(7):684–5.

Christensen MF. Double blind placebo controlled trial of pizotifen syrup in the treatment of abdominal migraine. *Arch Dis Child.* 1995;73(2):183.

Silberstein SD. Preventive migraine treatment. *Neurol Clin.* 2009;27(2): 429–43.

Victor S, Ryan SW. Drugs for preventing migraine headaches in children. *Cochrane Database Syst Rev.* 2003;4: CD002761.

PRAMIPEXOLE

THERAPEUTICS

Brands
- Mirapex, Mirapex ER, Mirapexin

Generic?
- Yes

Class
- Antiparkinson agent

Commonly Prescribed for
(FDA approved in bold)
- **Parkinson's disease (PD)**
- **Restless legs syndrome (RLS) (not for Mirapex ER)**
- Fibromyalgia

How the Drug Works
- Dopamine agonist, with high affinity for presynaptic and postsynaptic D_2, D_3, D_4 receptors (greater affinity for D_3), inhibiting dopamine synthesis and release. The antiparkinson action is likely due to D_2 agonism within the caudate-putamen. High affinity for D_3 receptors might affect impulse control and dyskinesia. The mechanism of action for RLS is probably related to D_2 or D_3 receptor agonism
- It expresses neuroprotective effects in disease models (e.g., antioxidant, neurotrophic stimulation, attenuates programmed cell death, etc)
- It also has affinity for α_2-adrenergic receptors

How Long Until It Works
- PD: weeks
- RLS: days to weeks

If It Works
- PD: may require dose adjustments over time or augmentation with other agents. Most PD patients will eventually require carbidopa-levodopa to manage their symptoms
- RLS: safe for long-term use with dose adjustments

If It Doesn't Work
- PD: bradykinesia, gait, and tremor should improve. Non-motor symptoms including autonomic symptoms such as postural hypotension, depression, and bladder dysfunction do not improve. If the patient has significantly impaired functioning, add carbidopa-levodopa with or without pramipexole
- RLS: rule out peripheral neuropathy, iron deficiency, thyroid disease. Change to another drug such as a benzodiazepine. Gabapentin enacarbil (not gabapentin) may also be beneficial. In severe cases consider opioids

Best Augmenting Combos for Partial Response or Treatment-Resistance
- For suboptimal effectiveness add carbidopa-levodopa with or without a catechol-*O*-methyltransferase (COMT) inhibitor. Monoamine oxidase (MAO)-B inhibitors may also be beneficial
- For severe motor fluctuations and/or dyskinesias with good "on" time, functional neurosurgery is an option
- For RLS, can change to a different dopamine agonist (ropinirole, carbidopa-levodopa) or add clonazepam. Gabapentin enacarbil may be beneficial. In severe cases consider opioids

Tests
- None required

ADVERSE EFFECTS (AEs)

How the Drug Causes AEs
- Direct effect on dopamine receptors

Notable AEs
- Drowsiness, nausea, dizziness, hallucination, constipation, anorexia, postural hypotension, weakness, edema, urinary frequency. Dyskinesia and hallucinations usually occur only with advanced PD patients

Life-Threatening or Dangerous AEs
- May cause somnolence or sudden-onset sleep, often without warning. Occurs more often than with ergot agonists or carbidopa-levodopa

Weight Gain
- Unusual

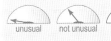

Sedation
- Common

What to Do About AEs
- Nausea can be problematic when initiating drug – titrate slowly
- Hallucinations or delusions may require stopping the medication
- Warn patients about the risks of sleeping while driving

Best Augmenting Agents to Reduce AEs
- Amantadine may help suppress dyskinesias
- Orthostatic hypotension: adjust dose or stop antihypertensives, add supplemental salt, and consider fludrocortisone or midodrine

DOSING AND USE

Usual Dosage Range
- PD: 1.5–4.5 mg daily, divided into 3 daily doses
- RLS: 0.25–0.5 mg daily, 2–3 hours before bedtime

Dosage Forms
- Tablets: 0.125, 0.25, 0.5, 1.0, 1.5 mg
- Tablet (ER): 0.375, 0.75, 1.6, 2.25, 3, 3,75, 4.5 mg

How to Dose
- PD: start at 0.125 mg 3 times daily with or without concomitant levodopa. Each week increase each dose by 0.125 mg until reaching 1.5 mg 3 times daily or desired clinical effect
- RLS: take 2–3 hours before bedtime. Start at 0.125 mg, and increase to 0.25 mg in 4–7 days. After another 4–7 days increase to 0.5 mg if needed. There is no evidence that increasing doses any further is more effective

 Dosing Tips
- Slow titration will minimize nausea and dizziness. Food delays the time to maximum plasma levels by 1 hour

Overdose
- Symptoms include somnolence, agitation, orthostatic hypotension, chest and abdominal pain, nausea, or dyskinesias. For cases of excessive CNS stimulation, neuroleptics can be effective

Long-Term Use
- Safe for long-term use. Effectiveness may decrease over time in PD (years) and RLS (months)

Habit Forming
- No

How to Stop
- Taper and discontinue over a period of 1 week for PD, but no taper is required in RLS patients. PD and RLS symptoms may worsen, but serious AEs from discontinuation are rare

Pharmacokinetics
- 15% protein binding. > 90% bioavailability. Half-life is 8–12 hours. Peak action in 2 hours. Over 90% of drug is excreted unchanged in the urine

 Drug Interactions
- Increases the effect of levodopa
- Drugs that are eliminated by renal secretion (cimetidine, ranitidine, diltiazem, triamterene, verapamil, quinidine, quinine) decrease the clearance of pramipexole
- Dopamine antagonists such as phenothiazines, metoclopramide diminish effectiveness
- Use with caution in patients on antihypertensive medications due to risk of orthostatic hypotension

 Other Warnings/ Precautions
- Dopamine agonists can precipitate impulse control disorders, such as pathological gambling

Do Not Use
- Hypersensitivity to the drug

Renal Impairment
Decrease dose as follows:
- CrCl 35–59 mL/min: start at 0.125 mg twice a day to a maximum of 1.5 twice a day. Severe impairment with CrCl 15–29 mL/min: start at 0.125 mg daily to a maximum of 1.5 mg daily. Use in hemodialysis patients is not recommended

Hepatic Impairment
- No known effects

Cardiac Impairment
- No known effects

Elderly
- There is reduced drug clearance, but no dose adjustment needed as the dose used is the lowest that provides clinical improvement

Children and Adolescents
- Not studied in children (PD is rare in pediatrics)

Pregnancy
- Category C. Use only if benefits of medication outweigh risks

Breast Feeding
- Inhibits prolactin secretion. Unknown if excreted in breast milk

Potential Advantages
- PD: may delay need for carbidopa-levodopa and decreases risk of motor dyskinesias by 30%. This is especially important in younger PD patients. Unlike ergot-based agonists, no known risk of fibrotic complications

- RLS: less risk of dependence compared to opioids or benzodiazepines and less augmentation than levodopa

Potential Disadvantages
- Less effective than carbidopa-levodopa for PD with more AEs such as hallucinations, somnolence, and orthostatic hypotension. Patients with significant motor disability will require carbidopa-levodopa. Risk of impulse control disorders

Primary Target Symptoms
- PD: motor dysfunction including bradykinesia, hand function, gait and rest tremor
- RLS: pain, insomnia

Pearls
- Excellent drug for young patients with early PD. Favorable long-term AEs
- Using pramipexole (over levodopa) as initial treatment for PD has been associated with a lower risk of motor complications and dyskinesias
- AE profile differs from ropinirole. More often associated with postural hypotension, dyskinesia, and edema, but less likely to cause dizziness, syncope, nausea, or respiratory problems
- For patients with mildly symptomatic disease, dopamine agonists are also appropriate for initial therapy, but for patients with significant disability, use carbidopa-levodopa early
- DRD3 Ser9Gly gene polymorphisms are associated with pramipexole efficacy in Chinese Parkinson patients
- For younger patients with bothersome tremor: anticholinergics may help
- Depression is common in PD and may respond to TCAs, pramipexole, or agomelatine
- Cognitive impairment/dementia is common in mid–late stage PD and may improve with acetylcholinesterase inhibitors
- For patients with late-stage PD experiencing hallucinations or delusions, withdraw pramipexole and consider oral atypical neuroleptics (quetiapine, clozapine). Acute psychosis is a medical emergency that may require hospitalization and low-dose haloperidol

- For orthostatic hypotension, droxidopa can be used
- Based on an evidence-based medicine review, pramipexole is efficacious in prevention/delay of motor fluctuation and dyskinesia, as a symptomatic monotherapy or as an adjunct to levodopa; pramipexole ER is efficacious for control of motor symptoms as monotherapy

- First-line treatment for RLS with less augmentation or "rebound" than carbidopa-levodopa. Non-ergot dopamine agonists are probably equally effective in treating RLS
- Increases REM latency and decreases total REM density
- May be an adjunct for drug-resistant bipolar depression

Suggested Reading

Dell'Osso B, Ketter TA. Assessing efficacy/effectiveness and safety/tolerability profiles of adjunctive pramipexole in bipolar depression: acute versus long-term data. *Int Clin Psychopharmacol.* 2013;28(6): 297–304.

Fox SH, Katzenschlager R, Lim S-Y, Ravina B, Seppi K, Coelho M, et al. The Movement Disorder Society Evidence-Based Medicine Review Update: Treatments for the motor symptoms of Parkinson's disease. *Mov Disord.* 2011;26 Suppl 3: S2–41.

Kvernmo T, Houben J, Sylte I. Receptor-binding and pharmacokinetic properties of dopaminergic agonists. *Curr Top Med Chem.* 2008;8(12): 1049–67.

Lang AE. When and how should treatment be started in Parkinson disease? *Neurology.* 2009;72(7 Suppl):S39–43.

Moore TJ, Glenmullen J, Mattison DR. Reports of pathological gambling, hypersexuality, and compulsive shopping associated with dopamine receptor agonist drugs. *JAMA Intern Med.* 2014;174(12):1930–3.

Varga LI, Ako-Agugua N, Colasante J, Hertweck L, Houser T, Smith J, et al. Critical review of ropinirole and pramipexole – putative dopamine D (3)-receptor selective agonists – for the treatment of RLS. *J Clin Pharm Ther.* 2009;34(5):493–505.

Weiner WJ. Early diagnosis of Parkinson's disease and initiation of treatment. *Rev Neurol Dis.* 2008;5(2):46–53; quiz 54–5.

PREDNISONE

THERAPEUTICS

Brands
- Sterapred, Cordrol, Orasone, Prednicot, Panasol, Meticorten, Deltasone, Sterane, Flo-Pred

Generic?
- Yes

Class
- Corticosteroid

Commonly Prescribed for
(FDA approved in bold)
- **Acute exacerbation of multiple sclerosis (MS)**
- **Optic neuritis**
- **Inflammatory myopathies: dermatomyositis (DM) and polymyositis (PM)**
- **Temporal arteritis (TA)**
- **Cerebral edema associated with brain tumor or head injury**
- **Asthma**
- **Chronic obstructive pulmonary disease**
- **Rheumatological disorders: gouty arthritis, rheumatoid arthritis, bursitis (many others)**
- **Systemic lupus erythematosus**
- **Neoplastic disorders: lymphoma and acute leukemia**
- **Hematological disorders: hemolytic anemia, idiopathic thrombocytopenia purpura (many others)**
- **Allergic conditions, such as atopic dermatitis, drug hypersensitivity reactions**
- **Acute episodes in Crohn's disease and ulcerative colitis**
- **Nephrotic syndrome**
- **Tuberculous meningitis**
- Chronic inflammatory demyelinating polyneuropathy (CIDP)
- Myasthenia gravis (MG)
- Duchenne's muscular dystrophy (DMD)
- Migraine headache
- Cluster headache
- Idiopathic intracranial hypertension
- Acute demyelinating encephalomyelitis (ADEM)
- Graves' ophthalmopathy
- Ophthalmoplegic migraine

How the Drug Works
- Glucocorticoids have anti-inflammatory effects, modify immune responses to stimuli, and have numerous metabolic effects. Prednisone is a synthetic steroid with glucocorticoid and mineralcorticoid activity

How Long Until It Works
- MS, migraine, cluster: days
- MG, DM, PM, CIDP: weeks to months
- TA: days

If It Works
- MS: use for acute exacerbation that causes significant disability. In relapsing-remitting form, long-term disease-modifying treatments improve prognosis
- Migraine: usually used for intractable headache or status migrainosus for short periods of time. After resolution, revert to safer preventive and abortive therapy
- Cluster: start preventive therapy and prednisone at the beginning of a cycle
- MG: weakness and fatigability improve. Decrease dose cautiously if clinical remission occurs
- DM/PM: improves strength and mobility. Start a corticosteroid-sparing agent if needed and taper dose cautiously with clinical remission
- CIDP: improves strength and sensory symptoms and prevents disability. Decrease dose cautiously if clinical remission occurs
- TA: monitor clinical response and sedimentation rate

If It Doesn't Work
- MS: if no improvement, confirm the diagnosis of relapsing-remitting MS. Start long-term disease-modifying therapy
- Migraine: start preventive therapy. IV neuroleptics or dihydroergotamine may be needed to treat status migrainosus
- Cluster: start preventive therapy
- MG: start an adjunctive treatment or change to another modifying therapy. For acute exacerbations, consider plasma exchange or immune globulin
- DM/PM: reconsider the diagnosis (inclusion body myositis, muscular dystrophy)

- CIDP: immune globulin or plasma exchange is effective. Consider other immunomodulators
- TA: reconsider diagnosis. Immunomodulatory drugs may be effective

 Best Augmenting Combos for Partial Response or Treatment-Resistance

- MS: use disease-modifying treatments to reduce relapses that require corticosteroids
- Migraine/cluster: antiemetics and migraine-specific agents may be used with prednisone for acute attacks
- MG: use a corticosteroid-sparing agent such as azathioprine, cyclosporine, mycophenolate mofetil, or cyclophosphamide. Treat acute exacerbations, usually with plasma exchange or immune globulin, and continue symptomatic treatment, such as pyridostigmine
- DM/PM: combine with corticosteroid-sparing agents such as methotrexate or azathioprine
- CIDP: combine with corticosteroid-sparing agent, immune globulin, or plasma exchange
- TA: combine with corticosteroid-sparing agent

Tests

- Monitor blood pressure, blood glucose and electrolytes with long-term therapy

ADVERSE EFFECTS (AEs)

How the Drug Causes AEs

- Most AEs are due to immunosuppression, metabolic or endocrine effects

Notable AEs

- Convulsion, vertigo, paresthesias, aggravation of psychiatric conditions, insomnia
- Amenorrhea, cushingoid state, increased sweating, increased insulin requirement in diabetics, hyperglycemia
- Pancreatitis, abdominal distension, esophagitis, bowel perforation, weight gain
- Cataracts, glaucoma
- Impaired wound healing, petechiae, erythema, hirsutism

- Sodium and fluid retention, hypokalemia, metabolic acidosis
- Muscle weakness, myopathy, muscle mass loss, tendon rupture
- Thrombophlebitis, hypertension

 Life-Threatening or Dangerous AEs

- Fractures, aseptic necrosis of femoral or humoral heads
- Hypokalemia may cause cardiac arrhythmias
- Diabetic ketoacidosis, hyperosmolar coma
- May mask symptoms of infection and prevent ability of patient to prevent dissemination. May activate latent amebiasis or tuberculosis. May prolong coma in cerebral malaria
- Adrenal suppression with long-term use
- Psychosis with clouded sensorium, severe depression, personality changes, or insomnia, usually within 15–30 days after starting treatment. Female sex and higher doses are risk factors

Weight Gain

- Problematic

unusual   not unusual   common   problematic

Sedation

- Unusual

unusual   not unusual   common   problematic

What to Do About AEs

- For diseases such as migraine or MS, avoid using for prolonged periods of time and stop for most significant AEs
- In diseases requiring long-term treatment, consider using corticosteroid-sparing agents – often starting these treatments with prednisone to reduce the dose requirement and possibly allow discontinuation as clinical symptoms improve
- Weight-bearing exercises are recommended to promote bone protection and minimize muscle wasting
- Weight gain: avoid other medications that may exacerbate, dietary modification

- Hypertension: convert to a glucocorticoid with less sodium-retaining potency, such as methylprednisolone or dexamethasone

Best Augmenting Agents to Reduce AEs

- With prolonged treatment, use daily calcium and vitamin D supplements and bisphosphonates to prevent osteoporosis and fractures, and H_2-blocker or proton pump inhibitors to prevent peptic ulcers

DOSING AND USE

Usual Dosage Range

- 5–200 mg daily. (The range of doses varies dramatically depending on the disease being treated)

Dosage Forms

- Tablets: 1, 2.5, 5, 10, 20, 50 mg
- Oral solution: 5 mg/5 mL, 15 mg/5 mL
- Injection: 25 mg/mL

How to Dose

- MS: (1) Give 200 mg for 1 week for acute exacerbations, followed by 80 mg every other day for 1 month. (2) Methylprednisolone 500–1000 mg/day × 3–7 days with oral prednisolone 60 mg, taper 10–21 days
- Migraine: no standard regimen. Usually used for less than 1 week for status migrainosus at doses of 10–60 mg daily with rapid taper
- Cluster: often used for 2–3 weeks at a time. Doses of 10–80 mg/day appear effective. Start with a higher dose and taper over 1–3 weeks
- MG: in outpatients, start at 20 mg daily and increase by 5 mg every 3–5 days until reaching target dose of 1.0 mg/kg/day (usually 50–100 mg) over 4–8 weeks. Then after 1 month at goal dose, slowly taper every month as clinical symptoms improve, either by lowering the daily dose or decreasing doses only on alternate days until patients are taking only every other day
- DM/PM: start at 1 mg/kg (up to 80 mg) daily for 4–6 weeks, usually in combination with a corticosteroid-sparing agent. Decrease by 10 mg a week until taking 40 mg, then by 5 mg a week until taking 20 mg. Then decrease by only 2.5 mg a week until at

10 mg and by 1 mg every 2 weeks until at 5 mg/day. Taper very slowly at lower doses and monitor strength during treatment
- CIDP: induction therapy with 1–1.5 mg/kg/day (usually 50–80 mg and not greater than 100 mg) followed by slow tapering to a low maintenance level. Taper by 5–10 mg per month in clinically stable patients. For recurrence of clinical symptoms, a temporary increase to previous dose is often effective. Alternatively a short-term high-dose (0.5–1 g) methylprednisolone repeated monthly could be used
- DMD: give 0.75 mg/kg/day or alternatively 5 mg/kg every other day
- TA: start at 40–80 mg daily. Start tapering every 2–4 weeks as symptoms permit, but taper more slowly at doses of 20 mg or less. Most patients will require 9–12 months of treatment and symptoms often reappear with a too-rapid taper

 ### Dosing Tips

- Give with food to avoid GI upset
- In patients improving on long-term treatment, consider converting to every-other-day dosing to reduce AEs

Overdose

- Large doses often produce cushingoid changes, including moonface, central obesity, hirsutism, acne, hypertension, osteoporosis, sexual dysfunction, diabetes, hyperlipidemia, peptic ulcer, and electrolyte and fluid imbalance

Long-Term Use

- Often used for long periods of time but long-term AEs may be significant and corticosteroid-sparing agents are often used in MG or DM

Habit Forming

- No

How to Stop

- Taper rapidly for exacerbation of acute disorder, such as MS
- Taper very slowly over months and monitor for recurrence of symptoms in chronic disorders, such as MG or DM
- Acute adrenal insufficiency can occur with too rapid withdrawal. Symptoms include nausea, anorexia, hypoglycemia, dizziness,

orthostatic hypotension, fever, and myalgias. Return of normal adrenal and pituitary function may take up to 9 months

Pharmacokinetics

- Half-life 60 minutes. Hepatic metabolism to prednisolone, which has a half-life of 115–212 minutes. Protein binding 70–90%
- Prednisone 5 mg is equal to prednisolone 5 mg, cortisone 25 mg, dexamethasone 0.75 mg, and methylprednisolone 4 mg

 Drug Interactions

- Do not give live vaccines during therapy with high doses
- Estrogens, oral contraceptives, and ketoconazole may decrease clearance and increase levels
- Barbiturates may reduce effects
- Rifampin, ephedrine, and phenytoin may increase clearance and reduce effects
- Prednisone may increase digitalis or cyclosporine toxicity
- May cause severe hypokalemia with potassium-depleting diuretics
- Reduces salicylate levels and effectiveness
- May inhibit growth-promoting effect of somatrem
- May decrease levels of isoniazid
- May alter activity of oral anticoagulants or theophylline

 Other Warnings/ Precautions

- May suppress reactions to skin tests
- Although occasionally used for chronic active hepatitis, may actually be harmful for hepatitis B

Do Not Use

- Hypersensitivity to drug, systemic fungal infection

SPECIAL POPULATIONS

Renal Impairment

- Patients are more likely to develop edema with corticosteroids. Use with caution

Hepatic Impairment

- No known effects

Cardiac Impairment

- Associated with left ventricular free wall rupture after recent myocardial infarction. Use with caution

Elderly

- Consider lower doses due to lower plasma volumes and decreased muscle mass. Monitor blood pressure, glucose, and electrolytes at least every 6 months

 Children and Adolescents

- Appears safe. Frequently used in asthma, DMD, but may cause growth problems with long-term use

 Pregnancy

- Category C. Relatively lower placental transport compared to other corticosteroids. May cause hypoadrenalism in infants

Breast Feeding

- Appears in breast milk and may suppress growth. Avoid breast feeding with high-dose, long-term treatment

THE ART OF NEUROPHARMACOLOGY

Potential Advantages

- Highly effective treatment for acute MS, TA, and migraine and cluster headache. Relatively fast-acting disease-modifying treatment for many neuromuscular conditions

Potential Disadvantages

- Effectiveness varies depending on the disorder. Numerous AEs, especially with long-term use

Primary Target Symptoms

- Depending on disorder: treating and preventing neurological complications in MS, TA, reducing pain in headache disorders, improving weakness in neuromuscular conditions

Pearls

- Although generally effective for improving symptoms and functioning after acute MS exacerbations, does not improve long-term outcome or disease course. Use for serious symptoms such as weakness, inability to ambulate and not for pure sensory symptoms
- MS patients hospitalized with acute symptoms typically will receive IV treatment with methylprednisolone (usually 1 g up to 5 days) or dexamethasone
- High-dose oral corticosteroid (1250 mg/day × 3 days) was non-inferior to IV corticosteroid (methylprednisolone 1000 mg/day × 3 days) in treating MS relapse within 4 weeks of the study period
- In one optic neuritis trial, oral corticosteroids were associated with a higher frequency of relapse. The significance of this finding is unclear, as oral corticosteroids are frequently used successfully to treat MS flares
- Cardiac arrhythmias are most common with rapid IV administration of methylprednisolone (1 g in 10 minutes) rather than with oral prednisone therapy
- In MG, prednisone may produce remission in about 30% of patients and improve symptoms in another 50%. Benefit begins in 2–3 weeks and peaks at 4–6 months. Often combined with other immunotherapies
- About half of MG patients experience worsening after initiating corticosteroid treatment, with a minority requiring intubation. This usually begins within 5–6 days after starting treatment and may persist for another week
- Because of the risk of initial deterioration, initiate treatment with high-dose corticosteroid mainly in inpatients receiving concurrent treatment with immune globulin or plasma exchange. In other patients, start at a lower dose
- Short courses of IV corticosteroids are typically used in cases of ADEM or transverse myelitis
- In TA, initiating treatment with IV corticosteroids for 2–5 days may improve long-term outcome
- TA typically responds dramatically to prednisone and it is important to begin treatment early to avoid visual complications. Still, given the need for long-term treatment, it is important to confirm diagnosis with temporal artery biopsy
- The treatment of CNS vasculitis is similar to that of MG or DM. Usual starting dose is 1 mg/kg/day. Cyclophosphamide is an alternative treatment
- In DMD, daily prednisone or prednisolone therapy appears to have an anabolic effect, improves muscle strength and forced vital capacity, and prevents loss of ambulation for up to 3 years. Non-ambulatory patients are more likely to experience weight gain. Deflazacort, a prednisone derivative, also appears effective and is less likely to cause weight gain. The optimal age for starting prednisone in DMD is unknown
- An alternative treatment for intractable migraine during pregnancy, due to lack of safe preventive or abortive treatment. Use short-term for bouts of status migrainosus
- When effective in migraine, patients usually improve within 24 hours
- May reduce the duration of attacks of ophthalmoplegic migraine, which may be a recurrent demyelinating neuropathy rather than migraine
- Corticosteroids (often dexamethasone) are commonly used in emergency room settings for severe migraine, and may reduce recurrence. However, they may be associated with greater AEs than standard migraine treatment and do not usually resolve medication-overuse headache
- Corticosteroids are effective in the majority of patients with cluster headache. Effective regimens include dexamethasone 4–8 mg/day, and prednisolone. The majority of patients achieve at least some improvement, but due to long AEs, corticosteroids are generally tapered over 2–3 weeks. The majority of patients experience recurrence after completing the taper, so preventive therapy should be started when initiating treatment
- Shorter corticosteroid courses, to reduce AEs, may be appropriate in cluster headache depending on disease severity and frequency of cycles: for patients with frequent cycles (more than 1/year) consider a taper of 10 days or less
- Prednisone and other corticosteroids may be helpful for symptoms of idiopathic

intracranial hypertension, but withdrawal can actually precipitate worsening. Avoid using, especially since weight gain from frequent use may exacerbate the disease

- Dexamethasone is usually used for the treatment of cerebral edema related to primary or metastatic brain tumors or head trauma

Suggested Reading

Burton JM, O'Connor PW, Hohol M, Beyene J. Oral versus intravenous steroids for treatment of relapses in multiple sclerosis. *Cochrane Database Syst Rev.* 2009;3:CD006921.

Campbell C, Jacob P. Deflazacort for the treatment of Duchenne dystrophy: a systematic review. *BMC Neurol.* 2003;3:7.

Diener HC. How to treat medication-overuse headache: prednisolone or no prednisolone? *Neurology.* 2007;69(1):14–15.

Dodick DW, Capobianco DJ. Treatment and management of cluster headache. *Curr Pain Headache Rep.* 2001;5(1):83–91.

Manzur AY, Kuntzer T, Pike M, Swan A. Glucocorticoid corticosteroids for Duchenne muscular dystrophy. *Cochrane Database Syst Rev.* 2008;1:CD003725.

Mazlumzadeh M, Hunder GG, Easley KA, Calamia KT, Matteson EL, Griffing WL, et al. Treatment of giant cell arteritis using induction therapy with high-dose glucocorticoids: a double-blind, placebo-controlled, randomized prospective clinical trial. *Arthritis Rheum.* 2006;54(10): 3310–18.

Merlini L, Cicognani A, Malaspina E, Gennari M, Gnudi S, Talim B, et al. Early prednisone treatment in Duchenne muscular dystrophy. *Muscle Nerve.* 2003;27(2):222–7.

Pageler L, Katsarava Z, Diener HC, Limmroth V. Prednisone vs. placebo in withdrawal therapy following medication overuse headache. *Cephalalgia.* 2008;28(2):152–6.

Ramo-Tello C, Grau-López L, Tintoré M, Rovira A, Ramió i Torrenta L, Brieva L, et al. A randomized clinical trial of oral versus intravenous methylprednisolone for relapse of MS. *Mult Scler.* 2014;20(6): 717–25.

Vincent A, Leite MI. Neuromuscular junction autoimmune disease: muscle specific kinase antibodies and treatments for myasthenia gravis. *Curr Opin Neurol.* 2005;18(5): 519–25.

PREGABALIN

Brands
- Lyrica, Zeegap

Generic?
- No

Class
- Antiepileptic drug (AED)

Commonly Prescribed for
(FDA approved in bold)
- **Partial-onset seizures (adjunctive for adults)**
- **Neuropathic pain associated with post-herpetic neuralgia**
- **Neuropathic pain associated with diabetic peripheral neuropathy**
- **Neuropathic pain associated with spinal cord injury**
- **Fibromyalgia**
- Facial pain
- Panic disorder
- Mania or bipolar disorder
- Generalized anxiety disorder
- Alcohol/benzodiazepine withdrawal

How the Drug Works
- Structural analog of GABA that binds at the $\alpha_2\delta$ subunit of calcium channel (CACNA2D1) and reduces calcium influx. Modulates calcium channel function but not a channel blocker
- Reduces release of excitatory neurotransmitters, such as glutamate, norepinephrine, and substance P
- Inactive at GABA receptors and does not affect GABA uptake or degradation

How Long Until It Works
- Seizures: 2 weeks
- Pain/anxiety: days to weeks
- Fibromyalgia: often in the first week

If It Works
- Seizures: goal is the remission of seizures. Continue as long as effective and well tolerated. Consider tapering and slowly stopping after 2 years without seizures, depending on the type of epilepsy

- Pain: goal is reduction of pain. Usually reduces but does not cure pain and there is recurrence off the medication. Consider tapering for conditions that may improve over time, e.g., post-herpetic neuralgia or fibromyalgia

If It Doesn't Work
- Epilepsy: consider changing to another agent, adding a second agent, using a medical device, or a referral for epilepsy surgery evaluation. When adding a second agent, keep drug interactions in mind
- Pain: if not effective in 2 months, consider stopping or using another agent

 ## Best Augmenting Combos for Partial Response or Treatment-Resistance
- Epilepsy: no major drug interactions with other AEDs. Using in combination may worsen CNS side effects or weight gain
- Neuropathic pain: TCAs, AEDs (gabapentin, pregabalin, carbamazepine, lamotrigine), SNRIs (duloxetine, venlafaxine, milnacipran, mirtazapine, bupropion), capsaicin, and mexiletine are agents used for neuropathic pain. Opioids (morphine, tramadol) may be appropriate for long-term use in some cases but require careful monitoring. Proven to decrease opioid requirements in patients with post-herpetic neuralgia
- Anxiety: usually used as a short-term adjunctive agent with SSRIs, SNRIs, MAOIs, or benzodiazepines

Tests
- No regular blood tests are recommended

How the Drug Causes AEs
- CNS AEs are probably caused by interaction with calcium channel function

Notable AEs
- Sedation, dizziness, fatigue, blurred vision
- Myoclonus, usually mild and does not cause discontinuation
- Weight gain, nausea, constipation, peripheral edema, angioedema, pruritus, elevated creatine kinase

- Decreased libido, erectile dysfunction. May impair fertility in men
- Euphoria and confusion

 Life-Threatening or Dangerous AEs

- Associated with decreased platelet counts, increased creatine kinase, and mild PR interval prolongation in clinical trials, although rarely of clinical significance

Weight Gain

- Common

Sedation

- Common

- May wear off with time

What to Do About AEs

- Decrease dose or take a higher dose at night to avoid sedation
- Switch to another agent

Best Augmenting Agents to Reduce AEs

- Adding a second agent unlikely to decrease AEs

DOSING AND USE

Usual Dosage Range

- Epilepsy: 150–600 mg/day
- Neuropathic pain: 100–600 mg/day, usually 300 mg or less
- Fibromyalgia: 300–450 mg/day

Dosage Forms

- Capsules: 25, 50, 75, 100, 150, 200, 300 mg

How to Dose

- Start at 150 mg in 2–3 divided doses, can double dose every 3–7 days to 300 mg and 600 mg or goal dose

 Dosing Tips

- Slow increase will improve tolerability. Increase evening dose first

---

- Use a slower titration for patients on other medications that can increase CNS AEs
- Most patients take twice daily, but may be better tolerated initially using 3 times a day dosing, especially during titration phase

Overdose

- No reported deaths. Patients taking higher than recommended dose experience no more side effects than patients taking recommended doses

Long-Term Use

- Safe for long-term use

Habit Forming

- Unlikely in most but occasionally in patients with a history of substance abuse

How to Stop

- Taper slowly
- Abrupt withdrawal can lead to seizures in patients with epilepsy

Pharmacokinetics

- Renal excretion without being metabolized. Linear kinetics. Half-life 5–7 hours. Does not bind to plasma proteins

 Drug Interactions

- No significant interactions, may increase CNS side effects of other medications

 Other Warnings/ Precautions

- Sedation and dizziness can increase risk of falls in elderly patients

Do Not Use

- Patients with a proven allergy to pregabalin or gabapentin
- May cause problems in patients with galactose intolerance or Lapp lactase deficiency (due to the capsule containing galactose)

SPECIAL POPULATIONS

Renal Impairment

- Adjust dose based on CrCl: < 15 mL/min: 25–75 mg/day, 15–30 mL/min: 50–150 mg/day, 30–60 mL/min: 75–300 mg/day
- Dose supplement after hemodialysis

Hepatic Impairment
- No known effects

Cardiac Impairment
- Prolonged PR interval. Increased risk of adverse reactions of second- or third-degree AV block

Elderly
- May need lower dose. More likely to experience AEs

Children and Adolescents
- Safety and efficacy unknown

Pregnancy
- Category C. Some teratogenicity in animal studies. Patients taking for pain or anxiety should generally stop before considering pregnancy
- Supplementation with 0.4 mg of folic acid before and during pregnancy is recommended

Breast Feeding
- Found in breast milk
- General recommendations are to discontinue drug or bottle feed
- Monitor infant for sedation, poor feeding, or irritability

THE ART OF NEUROPHARMACOLOGY

Potential Advantages
- Linear kinetics compared to gabapentin and easy to titrate. Proven efficacy for multiple types of pain and anxiety as well as epilepsy. May help sleep. Relatively low AEs

Potential Disadvantages
- Dosing twice daily. Weight gain. May worsen most primary generalized epilepsies

Primary Target Symptoms
- Seizure frequency and severity
- Pain
- Anxiety

Pearls
- Advantages compared to gabapentin include twice daily dosing, and more clinical trials demonstrating its efficacy for neuropathic pain, central pain, fibromyalgia, and anxiety
- Easier to titrate quickly compared to TCAs, gabapentin
- Good evidence for multiple types of neuropathic pain. May avoid opioid use
- No evidence of benefit beyond 300 mg dose and more AEs for post-herpetic neuralgia or diabetic peripheral neuropathy
- Not effective for trigeminal neuralgia nor neurogenic claudication associated with lumbar stenosis
- 50 mg of pregabalin is equivalent to 300 mg of gabapentin, but at higher gabapentin doses, this ratio does not apply
- First drug with FDA approval to treat fibromyalgia. Improved sleep, vitality, and fatigue as well as pain
- Schedule V controlled substance. Recreational drug users report euphoria with high doses similar to diazepam
- No published controlled trial of pregabalin in episodic migraine prophylaxis. Open-label studies suggested a possible preventive role
- A case report on hypnic headache treatment mentioned using 150 mg at bedtime for prophylaxis

Suggested Reading

Attal N, Cruccu G, Baron R, Haanpää M, Hansson P, Jensen TS, et al. EFNS guidelines on the pharmacological treatment of neuropathic pain: 2010 revision. *Eur J Neurol.* 2010;17(9): 1113–88.

Jensen TS, Madsen CS, Finnerup NB. Pharmacology and treatment of neuropathic pains.*Curr Opin Neurol.* 2009;22(5):467–74.

Linde M, Mulleners WM, Chronicle EP, McCrory DC. Gabapentin or pregabalin for the prophylaxis of episodic migraine in adults. *Cochrane Database Syst Rev.* 2013;6:CD010609.

Moore RA, Straube S, Wiffen PJ, Derry S, McQuay HJ. Pregabalin for acute and chronic pain in adults. *Cochrane Database Syst Rev.* 2009;3:CD007076.

Tzellos TG, Toulis KA, Goulis DG, Papazisis G, Zampeli VA, Vakfari A, et al. Gabapentin and pregabalin in the treatment of fibromyalgia: a systematic review and a meta-analysis. *J Clin Pharm Ther.* 2010;35(6):639–56.

Warner G, Figgitt DP. Pregabalin: as adjunctive treatment of partial seizures. *CNS Drugs.* 2005;19(3):265–72; discussion 273–4.

THERAPEUTICS

Brands
- Mysoline

Generic?
- Yes

Class
- Antiepileptic drug (AED)

Commonly Prescribed for
(FDA approved in bold)
- **Generalized tonic-clonic, psychomotor, and partial seizures (monotherapy and adjunctive, children and adults)**
- Essential tremor
- Psychosis

How the Drug Works
- Primidone and its 2 metabolites (phenobarbital and phenylethylmalonamide [PEMA]) raise seizure thresholds or alter seizure patterns
- The exact mechanism of action is unknown but likely enhances $GABA_A$ receptor activity
- Depresses glutamate excitability, alters sodium, calcium, and potassium channel conductance

How Long Until It Works
- Seizures: should decrease by 2 weeks
- Essential tremor: should improve tremors in 1–2 weeks

If It Works
- Seizures: goal is the remission of seizures. Continue as long as effective and well tolerated. Consider tapering and slowly stopping after 2 years without seizures, depending on the type of epilepsy
- Essential tremors: tremors improve but usually do not remit. Use lowest effective dose

If It Doesn't Work
- Increase to highest tolerated dose
- Epilepsy: consider changing to another agent, adding a second agent, using a medical device, or a referral for epilepsy

surgery evaluation. When adding a second agent, keep drug interactions in mind

Best Augmenting Combos for Partial Response or Treatment-Resistance
- Epilepsy: drug interactions complicate multi-drug therapy. Primidone itself is a second-line agent in developed countries due to AE profile

Tests
- CBC, hepatic and kidney function panels at baseline and every 6 months

ADVERSE EFFECTS (AEs)

How the Drug Causes AEs
- CNS AEs are probably caused by effects of increased GABA activity and alteration of ion channel function
- Vitamin D deficiency is caused by induction of metabolism

Notable AEs
- Ataxia, vertigo, sedation, nystagmus, diplopia
- Nausea, vomiting, anorexia
- Irritability, emotional disturbances, confusion, rash
- 20–25% of patients experience an idiosyncratic reaction with nausea and drowsiness and even obtundation – often on the first dose

Life-Threatening or Dangerous AEs
- Megaloblastic anemia, rarely agranulocytosis
- Respiratory depression: use with caution in patients with asthma or pulmonary disease

Weight Gain
- Common

unusual · not unusual · common · problematic

Sedation
- Problematic

unusual · not unusual · common · problematic

What to Do About AEs

- A small dose decrease may improve CNS AEs
- Do not take the first dose of medication alone, due to risk of idiosyncratic reaction
- Megaloblastic anemia: treat with folate

Best Augmenting Agents to Reduce AEs

- No treatment for most AEs other than lowering dose or stopping drug

---

DOSING AND USE

Usual Dosage Range

- Epilepsy: 500–1000mg/day (as monotherapy)
- Essential tremor: 250–750mg/day, in 2–3 divided doses

Dosage Forms

- Tablets: 50 and 250mg

How to Dose

- Epilepsy as monotherapy: start at 100–125 mg at bedtime for 3 days, then increase to 100–125mg twice daily. On day 7 increase to 100–125mg 3 times daily. On day 10, 250mg 3 times daily to maintenance dose
- Essential tremor: titrate slower and with lower doses
- When adding to other AEDs start at 100–125mg at bedtime and titrate more slowly
- When changing from another AED to primidone, the transition should take at least 2 weeks

 Dosing Tips

- Primidone may induce its own metabolism
- Check a serum level (goal 5–12mcg/mL) for optimal dosage

Overdose

- Similar to barbiturates. Respiratory depression, ataxia, nystagmus, tachycardia, hypotension, hypothermia can all occur. It is dialyzable

Long-Term Use

- Safe for long-term use with periodic laboratory monitoring

Habit Forming

- Tolerance, psychological and physical dependence can occur, especially with long-term use at high doses. Use with caution in patients with depression or history of substance abuse

How to Stop

- Taper slowly
- Abrupt withdrawal can lead to seizures in patients with epilepsy

Pharmacokinetics

- T_{max} 3 hours. It is metabolized by CYP2C9/19 to phenobarbital (minor metabolite) and PEMA (major metabolite); the former has AED activity. Half-life of primidone is 5–12 hours, PEMA is 16 hours, and phenobarbital is days. Renal excretion (40% unchanged). Bioavailability 90–100%
- Primidone itself has minimal protein binding, but the phenobarbital metabolite is about 50% protein bound
- It may reduce folate level by inhibiting dihydrofolate reductase

 Drug Interactions

- It is a CYP1A2/3A4 inducer, which lowers levels of many medications including warfarin, lamotrigine, TCAs, corticosteroids, methadone, cyclosporine, corticotropin, vitamin D, verapamil, and nifedipine among many others
- Variable effect on phenytoin metabolism
- Many AEDs (e.g., phenytoin, valproic acid, carbamazepine, and felbamate) inhibit CYP2C9 or CYP2C19 and can increase primidone/phenobarbital levels
- Acetazolamide, ethosuximide, and antacids can lower levels

 Other Warnings/ Precautions

- CNS AEs can be severe when used with other CNS depressants
- Toxicity magnified with alcohol use
- Folate deficiency and hyperhomocystinemia
- Bone and mineral loss with long-term use, increases vitamin D requirements
- May cause anesthesia at high doses: use with caution in patients with chronic pain

- Reduces effectiveness of hormonal contraceptives

Do Not Use

- Patients with a proven allergy to primidone or phenobarbital, or in patients with porphyria

Renal Impairment

- Decrease dosing intervals as follows. CrCl 10–50 mL/min give 2–3 times daily, < 10 mL/min 1–2 times daily, and for patients on hemodialysis give a supplemental dose after each session

Hepatic Impairment

- Can increase gamma glutamyltranspeptidase and alkaline phosphatase levels. Use with caution in patients with moderate to severe disease

Cardiac Impairment

- May shorten QTc interval

Elderly

- May need lower dose. More likely to experience CNS AEs which can limit effectiveness in essential tremor

 Children and Adolescents

- In children under age 8, start with 50 mg at night for 3 days. Then increase to 50 mg twice daily for 3 days, then 100 mg twice daily for 3 days and increase to maintenance dose
- Usual dose 125–250 mg 3 times daily or 10–25 mg/kg/day
- May cause paradoxical excitement, aggression, tearfulness, or hyperkinetic states. Cognitive side effects can limit use

 Pregnancy

- Category D. High rate of fetal malformations, and infants can experience withdrawal symptoms after birth. Risk of neonatal hemorrhage due to vitamin K deficiency. Supplement with folate and vitamin K prior to

and during delivery. Risks of stopping medication must outweigh risk to fetus for patients with epilepsy

- Patients taking for tremor should generally stop before considering pregnancy
- Supplementation with 0.4 mg of folic acid before and during pregnancy is recommended

Breast Feeding

- Level in breast milk is 80% of mother's blood level
- Generally recommendations are to discontinue drug or bottle feed
- Monitor infant for sedation, poor feeding, or irritability

Potential Advantages

- Effective for multiple types of epilepsy. Useful in refractory epilepsy
- Less toxic than phenobarbital
- Proven effectiveness for essential tremor

Potential Disadvantages

- Sedation and multiple potential side effects
- Potent hepatic induction complicates therapy with other AEDs
- Unlike many other AEDs, not useful for mood disorders. May cause depression

Primary Target Symptoms

- Seizure frequency and severity
- Tremor

 Pearls

- Commonly used in developing countries due to low cost and ability to treat multiple seizure types
- Effective in essential tremor (Level of Evidence A), but the AEs limit its use in elderly patients
- May be useful for some patients with primary orthostatic tremor or dystonic tremor
- Primidone may shorten QTc interval in some patients with long QT syndrome. QTc prolongation by AEDs is one suggested mechanism of sudden death in epilepsy but this is not proven

Suggested Reading

Beghi E. Efficacy and tolerability of the new antiepileptic drugs: comparison of two recent guidelines. *Lancet Neurol.* 2004;3(10): 618–21.

Serrano-Dueñas M. Use of primidone in low doses (250 mg/day) versus high doses (750 mg/day) in the management of essential tremor. Double-blind comparative study with one-year follow-up. *Parkinsonism Relat Disord.* 2003;10(1):29–33.

Sun MZ, Deckers CL, Liu YX, Wang W. Comparison of add-on valproate and primidone in carbamazepine-unresponsive patients with partial epilepsy. *Seizure.* 2009;18(2):90–3.

Zesiewicz TA, Elble RJ, Louis ED, Gronseth GS, Ondo WG, Dewey RB, Okun MS, Sullivan KL, Weiner WJ. Evidence-based guideline update: treatment of essential tremor: report of the Quality Standards subcommittee of the American Academy of Neurology. *Neurology.* 2011;77:1752–5.

PROCHLORPERAZINE

THERAPEUTICS

Brands
- Compazine, Stemetil, Buccastem

Generic?
- Yes

Class
- Antipsychotic, antiemetic

Commonly Prescribed for
(FDA approved in bold)
- **Schizophrenia**
- **Non-psychotic anxiety in adults**
- **Severe nausea and vomiting**
- Migraine (acute)
- Vertigo and labyrinthine disorders
- Mania in bipolar disorder

How the Drug Works
- Dopamine receptor antagonist with greater action at D_2 receptors. Also blocks serotonin 5-HT$_{2A}$ receptors, α_1-adrenergic receptors and is an antihistamine

How Long Until It Works
- Injection effective within 10 minutes, oral 1–2 hours

If It Works
- Use at lowest effective dose
- Continue to assess effect of the medication and if it is still needed

If It Doesn't Work
- Increase dose, or discontinue and change to another agent

Best Augmenting Combos for Partial Response or Treatment-Resistance
- Migraine: often combined with NSAIDs and triptans or ergots
- Nausea and vomiting: corticosteroids

Tests
- Monitor weight, blood pressure, lipids, and fasting glucose with frequent chronic use. Obtain blood pressure and pulse before initial IV use and monitor QTc with ECG

ADVERSE EFFECTS (AEs)

How the Drug Causes AEs
- Motor AEs and prolactinemia: blocking of D_2 receptors
- Hypotension: blocking of α_1-adrenergic receptors

Notable AEs
- Most common: dizziness, sedation, dry mouth, constipation, skin changes
- Tachycardia, hypo or hypertension
- Akathisia, parkinsonism
- Interference with thermoregulatory mechanisms

Life-Threatening or Dangerous AEs
- Tardive dyskinesia
- ECG changes including prolongation of QTc. Rarely cardiac arrest

Weight Gain
- Common (with frequent use)]

unusual not unusual common problematic

Sedation
- Common

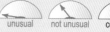

unusual not unusual common problematic

What to Do About AEs
- Rarely causes ECG changes. Use with caution if QTc is above 450 (women) or 440 (men) and do not administer with QTc greater than 500
- If excessive sedation occurs, use only as a rescue agent for inpatients or when patients can lie down or sleep

Best Augmenting Agents to Reduce AEs
- Give fluids to avoid hypotension, tachycardia, and dizziness
- Give anticholinergics (diphenhydramine or benztropine) or benzodiazepines for extrapyramidal reactions

DOSING AND USE

Usual Dosage Range
- Migraine/vertigo: 5–80 mg/day (oral, IM, IV) or 25–100 mg/day (rectal)

Dosage Forms
- Tablets: 5, 10 mg
- Sustained-release capsules: 10 mg
- Syrup: 5 mg/5 mL
- Injection: 5 mg/mL
- Buccal tablets: 3 mg
- Suppositories: 2.5, 5, 25 mg

How to Dose
- Migraine/vertigo: give IV, IM, oral, or suppository. Non-oral routes are useful for severe vomiting. Give 5–10 mg 3–4 times daily as needed for nausea, vertigo, or headache. Alternatively give 25 mg rectally up to 2 times daily

 Dosing Tips
- Migraine/vertigo: effective in hospitalized patients while monitoring blood pressure, pulse, and daily ECG

Overdose
- CNS depression, hypotension, and extrapyramidal reactions are most common. Respiratory suppression or death is rare

Long-Term Use
- Safe for long-term use but may cause irreversible AEs (tardive dyskinesias)

Habit Forming
- No

How to Stop
- No need to taper

Pharmacokinetics
- Hepatic metabolism via CYP2D6 and 3A4. Half-life 4–8 hours depending on route. 91–99% protein bound

 Drug Interactions
- Use with CNS depressants (barbiturates, opiates, general anesthetics) potentiates CNS AEs

- Anticholinergics may decrease effects
- CYP3A4 (ketoconazole, fluoxetine, nefazodone, duloxetine), and 2D6 (duloxetine, paroxetine) inhibitors may increase levels
- May enhance effects of antihypertensives
- Use with alcohol or diuretics may increase hypotension
- May decrease effectiveness of dopaminergic agents or anticoagulants

 Other Warnings/ Precautions
- Use cautiously in patients with Parkinson's disease or Lewy body dementia
- Neuroleptic malignant syndrome is characterized by fever, rigidity, confusion, and autonomic instability, and is more common with IV antipsychotic treatment
- Caution in patients with glaucoma due to anticholinergic effect
- May lower seizure threshold or interfere with phenytoin metabolism

Do Not Use
- Hypersensitivity to drug, CNS depression/ coma, or QTc greater than 500

SPECIAL POPULATIONS

Renal Impairment
- No dose adjustment needed

Hepatic Impairment
- Use with caution

Cardiac Impairment
- May worsen orthostatic hypotension

Elderly
- More likely to experience movement AEs or hypotension. Use lower dose

 Children and Adolescents
- Efficacy and safety unknown for children under age 2. Base dose on weight. 9–13 kg: 2.5 mg up to 3 times daily. 14–17 kg: 2.5 mg 3–4 times daily. 18–38 kg: 2.5–5 mg up to 3 times daily

Pregnancy

- Category C. Extrapyramidal signs have been reported with phenothiazine use during pregnancy. Use only for intractable headache or vomiting

Breast Feeding

- There are no data on the excretion of prochlorperazine into human milk
- Generally recommendations are to discontinue drug or bottle feed
- Monitor infant for sedation, poor feeding, or irritability

THE ART OF NEUROPHARMACOLOGY

Potential Advantages

- Effective short-term medication for intractable migraine, vomiting, or vertigo

Potential Disadvantages

- Not as effective orally. Risk for movement AEs, especially in elderly or with frequent use

Primary Target Symptoms

- Headache, vertigo, and nausea

 Pearls

- In acute migraine, prochlorperazine suppositories are an effective treatment for acute severe headache with nausea
- Pretreat or combine with diphenhydramine, 25–50 mg, to reduce rate of akathisia and dystonic reactions. Benztropine is also useful and may be given orally or IM
- In outpatients with severe or daily headache, may be used daily for short periods of time (3–10 days) as a bridge treatment before preventive medication becomes effective
- May be effective and considered safe in the treatment of migraine in pregnancy
- Slow infusion to avoid hypotensive episode.
- Reported cases of QTc prolongation. Not as common as ondansetron or promethazine

 Suggested Reading

Friedman BW, Esses D, Solorzano C, Dua N, Greenwald P, Radulescu R, Chang E, Hochberg M, Campbell C, Aghera A, Valentin T, Paternoster J, Bijur P, Lipton RB, Gallagher EJ. A randomized controlled trial of prochlorperazine versus metoclopramide for treatment of acute migraine. *Ann Emerg Med.* 2008;52(4):399–406.

Kelley NE, Tepper DE. Rescue therapy for acute migraine, part 2: neuroleptics, antihistamines, and others. *Headache.* 2012;52:292–306.

Khatri R, Hershey AD, Wong B. Prochlorperazine – treatment for acute confusional migraine. *Headache.* 2009;49 (3):477–80.

Marmura MJ, Silberstein SD, Schwedt TJ. The acute treatment of migraine in adults: the American Headache Society evidence assessment of migraine pharmacotherapies. *Headache.* 2015;55:3–20.

Siow HC, Young WB, Silberstein SD. Neuroleptics in headache. *Headache.* 2005;45(4):358–71.

Tanen DA, Miller S, French T, Riffenburgh RH. Intravenous sodium valproate versus prochlorperazine for the emergency department treatment of acute migraine headaches: a prospective, randomized, double-blind trial. *Ann Emerg Med.* 2003;41(6):847–53.

PROMETHAZINE

THERAPEUTICS

Brands
- Phenadoz, Promethagan, Phenergan, Zipan, Remsed

Generic?
- Yes

Class
- Antiemetic, antihistamine

Commonly Prescribed for
(FDA approved in bold)
- **Allergic conditions**
- **Analgesia**
- **Antiemetic**
- **Motion sickness**
- **Induce sedation**
- **Dermatographism**
- Migraine (acute)
- Vertigo
- Nausea and vomiting of pregnancy

How the Drug Works
- It is a phenothiazine derivative acting as a strong histamine (H$_1$) antagonist and moderate muscarinic cholinergic antagonist. In addition, it binds to dopaminergic, serotonergic, α-adrenergic, and NMDA receptors. It acts on voltage-gated ion channels, ATPase, and mitochondrial transition pores. The high lipophilicity allows promethazine to penetrate the BBB and interact with many neural receptors leading to sedation and other CNS effects

How Long Until It Works
- IV: within 5–10 minutes

If It Works
- Use at lowest effective dose
- Continue to assess effect of the medication and if it is still needed

If It Doesn't Work
- Increase dose, or discontinue and change to another agent
- Migraine: change to another antiemetic (prochlorperazine, droperidol, chlorpromazine) or combine with other agents

Best Augmenting Combos for Partial Response or Treatment-Resistance
- Migraine: often combined with NSAIDs, triptans, or ergots

Tests
- ECG prior to drug initiation

ADVERSE EVENTS (AEs)

How the Drug Causes AEs
- Anticholinergic and other CNS effects

Notable AEs
- Sedation, blurred vision, dry mouth, confusion, oculogyric crisis, tardive dyskinesia, tinnitus, akathisia, ataxia, tremor, hallucination, nightmare, agitation, photosensitivity, cholestatic jaundice, and orthostatic hypotension

Life-Threatening or Dangerous AEs
- Respiratory depression
- Neuroleptic malignant syndrome
- Neutropenia, thrombocytopenia
- Delirium
- Seizure
- Narrow-angle glaucoma

Weight Gain
- Common

unusual · not unusual · **common** · problematic

Sedation
- Problematic

unusual · not unusual · common · **problematic**

What to Do About AEs
- Excessive sedation: lower dose or use only as a rescue agent when patient can lie down or sleep
- Movement disorders: lower dose or stop

Best Augmenting Agents to Reduce AEs
- Most AEs do not respond to adding other medications. The most important

intervention is to discontinue promethazine

DOSING AND USE

Usual Dosage Range
- 6.25–25 mg

Dosage Forms
- Tablet: 12.5, 25, 50 mg
- Syrup: 6.25, 25 mg/5 mL
- Suppository: 12.5, 25, 50 mg
- Injection: 25, 50 mg/mL

How to Dose
- Antiemetic: 12.5–25 mg every 4–8 hours
- Migraine: 25 mg orally, IV, or IM

Dosing Tips
- The preferred route is deep IM injection. SC injection is contraindicated
- IV push: 25 mg/min with central line. Over 20 minutes with peripheral line. May cause extravasation and tissue injury

Overdose
- Drowsiness, confusion, and extrapyramidal reactions may occur. The treatment is essentially symptomatic and supportive. Epinephrine should not be used due to partial α blockade and worsening of hypotension

Long-Term Use
- Risk of movement AEs (tardive dyskinesias, parkinsonism) with frequent use. Elevates prolactin levels

Habit Forming
- Physiological or psychological dependence has been observed with promethazine. It is often found in combination with other drugs (e.g., opioid)

How to Stop
- No need to taper for short-term use

Pharmacokinetics
- Bioavailability 25%. 93% protein binding. Metabolized mainly by CYP2D6 in the liver. Half-life 9–19 hours depends on the CYP2D6 genotypes

Drug Interactions
- Decrease dose under strong CYP2D6 inhibitors (e.g., SSRI, bupropion, quinidine, antivirals)
- Increased risk of arrhythmias when concomitant use of other QTc prolonging drugs (e.g., fluoroquinolone, cisapride, antipsychotics)
- Anticholinergics and opioids decrease effects on GI motility
- Increased risk of extrapyramidal effects when combined with MAOI
- Concomitant doses of opioids or barbiturates should be decreased by ¼ to ½ of the usual dose to avoid additive effects. Combination of opioid and promethazine intensifies the sedation effect and increases life-threatening events

Other Warnings/ Precautions
- Promethazine injection contains sulfites

Do Not Use
- Hypersensitivity to drug. Less than 2 years old

SPECIAL POPULATIONS

Renal Impairment
- No adjustment needed

Hepatic Impairment
- Use with caution in patients with moderate or severe hepatic impairment

Cardiac Impairment
- Prolonged QTc

Elderly
- More likely to experience movement AEs

Children and Adolescents
- Risk of fatal respiratory depression in patients < 2 years

Pregnancy

- Category B. Drug of choice for morning sickness. May be used during labor and delivery

Breast Feeding

- It may be found in breast milk. Its use is not recommended

THE ART OF NEUROPHARMACOLOGY

Potential Advantages

- Effective medication for allergy, migraine, and vomiting

Potential Disadvantages

- Risk of somnolence, tissue injury, QTc prolongation, extrapyramidal symptoms, and dependence

Primary Target Symptoms

- Allergy, headache, and nausea

 Pearls

- In acute undifferentiated headache treatment comparing prochlorperazine (10 mg IV) with promethazine (25 mg IV), promethazine group reported more drowsiness, less effect at 30 minutes, but equal effectiveness at 60 minutes
- When combined with meperidine, similar effectiveness to ketorolac for acute migraine treatment
- Oral promethazine (25 mg) plus sumatriptan (50 mg) seemed more effective in acute migraine management than sumatriptan alone (50 mg). Somnolence and extrapyramidal symptoms were more common in the promethazine group
- IV promethazine (12.5 mg) may be as effective as ondansetron (4 mg) or metoclopramide (10 mg) in nausea reduction in emergency department adults

 Suggested Reading

Asadollahi S, Heidari K, Vafaee R, Forouzanfar MM, Amini A, Shahrami A. Promethazine plus sumatriptan in the treatment of migraine: a randomized clinical trial. *Headache*. 2014;54:94–108.

Barrett TW, DiPersio DM, Jenkins CA, Jack M, McCoin NS, Storrow AB, et al. A randomized, placebo-controlled trial of ondansetron, metoclopramide, and promethazine in adults. *Am J Emerg Med*. 2011;29:247–55.

Callan JE, Kostic MA, Bachrach EA, Rieg TS. Prochlorperazine vs. promethazine for headache treatment in the emergency department: a randomized controlled trial. *J Emerg Med*. 2008;35:247–53.

Kelley NE, Tepper DE. Rescue therapy for acute migraine, part 2: neuroleptics, antihistamines, and others. *Headache*. 2012;52:292–306.

THERAPEUTICS

Brands
- Inderal, Inderal-LA, InnoPran XL, Hemangeol

Generic?
- Yes

Class
- β-blocker

Commonly Prescribed for
(FDA approved in bold)
- **Migraine prophylaxis**
- **Essential tremor**
- **Hypertension**
- **Angina pectoris due to coronary atherosclerosis**
- **Cardiac arrhythmias (including supraventricular arrhythmias, ventricular tachycardia, digitalis intoxication)**
- **Myocardial infarction (MI)**
- **Hypertrophic subaortic stenosis**
- **Pheochromocytoma**
- Akathisia (antipsychotic induced)
- Parkinsonian tremor
- Congestive heart failure
- Tetralogy of Fallot
- Hyperthyroidism (adjunctive)
- Generalized anxiety disorder
- Post-traumatic stress disorder
- Prevention of variceal bleeding

How the Drug Works
- Migraine: proposed mechanisms include inhibition of adrenergic pathway, interaction with serotonin system and receptors, inhibition of nitric oxide production, normalization of contingent negative variation, and inhibition of thalamic trigeminovascular neurons. Prevention of cortical spreading depression may be one mechanism of action for all migraine preventives
- Tremor: effectiveness is likely due to peripheral β_2-receptor antagonism

How Long Until It Works
- Migraines: within 2 weeks, but can take up to 3 months on a stable dose to see full effect
- Tremor: within days

If It Works
- Migraine: goal is a 50% or greater decrease in migraine frequency or severity. Consider tapering or stopping if headaches remit for more than 6 months or if considering pregnancy
- Tremor: reduction in the severity of tremor, allowing greater functioning with daily activities and clearer speech

If It Doesn't Work
- Increase to highest tolerated dose
- Migraine: address other issues, such as medication overuse, other coexisting medical disorders, such as anxiety, and consider changing to another drug or adding a second drug
- Tremor: coadministration with primidone up to 250 mg/day can augment response. Second-line medications include benzodiazepines such as clonazepam, gabapentin, topiramate, methazolamide, nadolol, and botulinum toxin (useful for voice and hand tremor). For truly refractory patients, thalamotomy and deep brain stimulation of the ventral intermediate nucleus of the thalamus are options
- Alternatives for tremor include hand weights and eliminating caffeine. Low doses of alcohol reduce tremor, but are not generally recommended

Best Augmenting Combos for Partial Response or Treatment-Resistance
- Migraine: for some patients, low-dose polytherapy with 2 or more drugs may be better tolerated and more effective than high-dose monotherapy. May use in combination with AEDs, antidepressants, natural products, and non-pharmacological treatments, such as biofeedback, to improve headache control
- Tremor: can use in combination with primidone or second-line medications

Tests
- None required

ADVERSE EFFECTS (AEs)

How the Drug Causes AEs
- Antagonism of β-adrenergic receptors

Notable AEs

- Bradycardia, hypotension, hyper or hypoglycemia, weight gain
- Bronchospasm, cold/flu symptoms, sinusitis, pneumonias
- Dizziness, vertigo, fatigue/tiredness, depression, sleep disturbances
- Sexual dysfunction, decreased libido, dysuria, urinary retention, joint pain
- Exacerbation of symptoms in peripheral vascular disease and Raynaud's syndrome

 ### Life-Threatening or Dangerous AEs

- In acute chronic heart failure, may further depress myocardial contractility
- Can blunt premonitory symptoms of hypoglycemia in diabetes and mask clinical signs of hyperthyroidism
- Non-selective β-blockers such as propranolol can inhibit bronchodilation, making them contraindicated in asthma, severe chronic obstructive pulmonary disease
- Do not use in pheochromocytoma unless α-blockers are already being used
- Risk of excessive myocardial depression in general anesthesia

Weight Gain

- Common

unusual   not unusual   common   problematic

Sedation

- Common

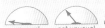
unusual   not unusual   common   problematic

What to Do About AEs

- Lower dose, change to extended-release formulation, or switch to another agent

Best Augmenting Agents to Reduce AEs

- When patients have significant benefit from β-blocker therapy but hypotension limits treatment, consider α-adrenergic agonists (midodrine) or volume expanders (fludrocortisone) for symptomatic relief

DOSING AND USE

Usual Dosage Range

- 40–400 mg/day

Dosage Forms

- Tablets: 10, 20, 40, 60, 80, 90 mg
- Extended-release capsules: 60, 80, 120, 160 mg
- Oral solution: 20 mg/5 mL, 40 mg/5 mL
- Injection: 1 mg/mL

How to Dose

- Migraine: Initial dose 40 mg/day in divided doses or once daily in extended-release preparations for most patients. Gradually increase over days to weeks to usual effective dose: 40–400 mg/day
- Tremor: Start 40 mg twice a day. The dosage may be gradually increased as needed to 120–320 mg/day in 2–3 divided doses

 ### Dosing Tips

- For extended-release capsules, give once daily at bedtime consistently, with or without food. Doses above 120 mg had no additional antihypertensive effect in clinical trials
- Food can enhance bioavailability

Overdose

- Bradycardia, hypotension, low-output heart failure, shock, seizures, coma, hypoglycemia, apnea, cyanosis, respiratory depression, and bronchospasm. Epinephrine and dopamine are used to treat toxicity

Long-Term Use

- Safe for long-term use

Habit Forming

- No

How to Stop

- Do not abruptly discontinue. Gradually reduce dosage over 1–2 weeks. May exacerbate angina, and there are reports of tachyarrhythmias or MI with rapid discontinuation in patients with cardiac disease

Pharmacokinetics

- Half-life 3–5 hours, 8–11 hours in extended-release form. Bioavailability is 30%, 9–18% for long-acting. Hepatic metabolism to hydroxypropranolol (also pharmacologically active). 90% protein binding. Good CNS penetration due to high lipid solubility

 Drug Interactions

- Cimetidine, oral contraceptives, ciprofloxacin, hydralazine, hydroxychloroquine, loop diuretics, certain SSRIs (with CYP2D6 metabolism), and phenothiazines can increase levels and/or effects of propranolol
- Use with calcium channel blockers can be synergistic or additive, use with caution
- Barbiturates, penicillins, rifampin, calcium and aluminum salts, thyroid hormones, and cholestyramine can decrease effects of β-blockers
- NSAIDs, sulfinpyrazone, and salicyclates inhibit prostaglandin synthesis and may inhibit the antihypertensive activity of β-blockers
- Propranolol can increase AEs of clonidine, gabapentin, and benzodiazepines
- Propranolol can increase levels of some triptans and lidocaine, resulting in toxicity, and increase the anticoagulant effect of warfarin
- Increased postural hypotension with prazosin and peripheral ischemia with ergot alkaloids
- Sudden discontinuation of clonidine while on β-blockers or when stopped together can cause life-threatening increases in blood pressure

Other Warnings/Precautions

- May elevate blood urea, serum transaminases, alkaline phosphatase, and lactate dehydrogenase
- Rare development of antinuclear antibodies (ANA)
- May worsen symptoms of myasthenia gravis
- Can lower intraocular pressure, interfering with glaucoma screening test

Do Not Use

- Sinus bradycardia, greater than first-degree heart block, cardiogenic shock
- Bronchial asthma, severe chronic obstructive pulmonary disease
- Proven hypersensitivity to β-blockers

Renal Impairment

- No significant changes in half-life or concentration, even with severe failure. Among β-adrenergic blockers, nadolol, sotalol, and atenolol are eliminated by the kidney and require dose adjustment. Use with caution

Hepatic Impairment

- Hepatic metabolism causes increased drug levels and half-life with significant hepatic disease. Use with caution

Cardiac Impairment

- Do not use in acute shock, MI, hypotension, and greater than first-degree heart block, but indicated in clinically stable patients post-MI to reduce risk of reinfarction starting 1–4 weeks after event. Metoprolol, another β-blocker, is commonly used to reduce mortality and hospitalization for patients with stable chronic heart failure already receiving ACE inhibitors and diuretics

Elderly

- Use with caution. May increase risk of stroke

 Children and Adolescents

- Usual dose in children is 2–4 mg/kg in 2 divided doses. Maximum 16 mg/kg/day. Clinical trials for migraine prophylaxis did not include children. When stopping, taper slowly over 1–2 weeks

 Pregnancy

- Category C. Embryotoxic in animal studies only at doses much higher than maximum recommended human doses. May reduce perfusion of the placenta. Use if potential benefit outweighs risk to the fetus. Most β-blockers are class C, except atenolol, which is D, and acebutolol, pindolol, and sotalol, which are B

Breast Feeding

- Not recommended. Propranolol is found in breast milk, due to high lipid solubility, more than many other β-blockers

THE ART OF NEUROPHARMACOLOGY

Potential Advantages

- Proven effectiveness in migraine and ability to treat coexisting conditions, such as hypertension or anxiety. For tremor, less sedation than primidone and benzodiazepines

Potential Disadvantages

- Multiple potential undesirable AEs, including bradycardia, hypotension, and fatigue

Primary Target Symptoms

- Migraine frequency and severity
- Tremor

 Pearls

- Alternative β-blockers for migraine: metoprolol 100–200 mg/day, timolol

20–60 mg/day (FDA approved), atenolol 50–200 mg/day, nadolol 20–160 mg/day (less sedative)
- β-blockers that are partial agonists, with intrinsic sympathomimetic activity, are not effective in migraine prophylaxis. These include acebutolol, alprenolol, and pindolol
- Often used in combination with other drugs in migraine. Using to treat migraine may allow patients to better tolerate medications that cause tremor, such as valproate
- Adding propranolol to topiramate (long acting) does not add benefit to topiramate when the chronic migraine is inadequately controlled with topiramate alone
- Not effective for cluster headache
- May worsen depression, but helpful for anxiety
- 50–70% of patients with essential tremor receive some relief, usually with about 50% improvement or greater
- β₁-selective antagonists are less effective in essential tremor but metoprolol may be an option in patients with asthma or severe chronic obstructive pulmonary disease
- Recent studies have downgraded β-blockers as a first-line treatment for hypertension compared with other classes due to lack of effectiveness, increased rate of stroke in elderly, and risk of provoking type II diabetes

 Suggested Reading

Law MR, Morris JK, Wald NJ. Use of blood pressure lowering drugs in the prevention of cardiovascular disease: meta-analysis of 147 randomised trials in the context of expectations from prospective epidemiological studies. *BMJ.* 2009;338:b1665.

Lyons KE, Pahwa R. Pharmacotherapy of essential tremor: an overview of existing and upcoming agents. *CNS Drugs.* 2008;22(12): 1037–45.

Ramadan NM. Current trends in migraine prophylaxis. *Headache.* 2007;47 Suppl 1:S52–7.

Silberstein SD, Holland S, Freitag F, Dodick DW, Argoff C, Ashman E. Evidence-based guideline update: pharmacologic treatment for episodic migraine prevention in adults: report of the Quality Standards Subcommittee of the American Academy of Neurology and the American Headache Society. *Neurology.* 2012;78:1337–45.

Taylor FR. Weight change associated with the use of migraine-preventive medications. *Clin Ther.* 2008;30(6):1069–80.

PYRIDOSTIGMINE

THERAPEUTICS

Brands
- Mestinon, Mestinon Timespan, Regonal

Generic?
- Yes

 Class
- Cholinesterase inhibitor

Commonly Prescribed for
(FDA approved in bold)
- **Myasthenia gravis (MG)**
- **Reversal of non-depolarizing muscle relaxants**
- Orthostatic hypotension

 How the Drug Works
- It is a quaternary amine that reversibly inhibits the cholinesterase enzyme and improves the neuromuscular transmission in MG. It is poorly absorbed in the gut and does not cross the BBB

How Long Until It Works
- Orally about 30 minutes, IM form within 15 minutes, IV within 5 minutes

If It Works
- Continue to use to reduce symptoms of MG. Often combined with disease-modifying therapy such as immunosuppression or thymectomy

If It Doesn't Work
- Increase to the maximal dose: if no effect, question the diagnosis of MG. Remove potential offending medications. If not controlled at 240–360 mg daily, consider immunomodulating treatment

 Best Augmenting Combos for Partial Response or Treatment-Resistance
- Generally not combined with other symptomatic treatments. For refractory MG, add immunotherapy

Tests
- None

ADVERSE EFFECTS (AEs)

How the Drug Causes AEs
- Cholinergic properties of the drug

Notable AEs
- Muscarinic AEs include diarrhea, abdominal cramps, nausea, increased salivation, miosis, increased bronchial secretions, rash, worsening of bronchial asthma, and diaphoresis. Nicotinic AEs, including fasciculation and muscle cramping, are less bothersome

 Life-Threatening or Dangerous AEs
- Bradycardia – possibly leading to hypotension – is most common with IV use
- Cholinergic crisis – worsening weakness, usually with overdose of drug and severe cholinergic AEs – is very rare

Weight Gain
- Unusual

unusual not unusual common problematic

Sedation
- Unusual

unusual not unusual common problematic

What to Do About AEs
- Lower to tolerable dose, take with food

Best Augmenting Agents to Reduce AEs
- Treat GI AEs with anticholinergics that do not affect nicotinic receptors (so no weakness): glycopyrrolate 1 mg, propantheline 15 mg, or hyoscyamine sulfate 0.125 mg. Use 3 times a day or take with each pyridostigmine dose. For diarrhea try loperamide or diphenoxylate hydrochloride-atropine. To prevent bradycardia and excessive secretions with IV form, use atropine 0.6–1.2 mg IV immediately prior

DOSING AND USE

Usual Dosage Range

- MG: 180–1500 mg/day in divided doses. The average dose is 600 mg/day
- Reversal of non-depolarizing muscle relaxants: 10–20 mg

Dosage Forms

- Tablets: 60 mg
- Extended-release tablets: 180 mg
- Syrup: 60 mg/5 mL
- Injection: 5 mg/mL in 2 mL ampule

How to Dose

- Start at 30–60 mg every 4–6 hours during daytime. Increase as tolerated each day with 3–6 times daily dosing (up to 120 mg every 2–3 hours) until having significant relief of MG symptoms or until AEs become bothersome. Usual effective dose is 60 mg 3–4 times daily but varies from patient to patient
- Extended-release form is very useful for patients with difficulties on awakening. Use once or twice daily (total 180–1080 mg). Wait at least 6 hours between doses

 Dosing Tips

- Take with food to reduce GI AEs. Do not crush the extended-release tablet

Overdose

- Symptoms may include abdominal pain, diarrhea and vomiting, excessive salivation, cold sweating, pallor, urinary urgency, blurry vision, muscle fasciculations, anxiety or panic, and paralysis. Treat with atropine IV 0.5–1 mg initially and use up to 10 mg

Long-Term Use

- Safe for long-term use

Habit Forming

- No

How to Stop

- No need to taper but MG symptoms will likely worsen

Pharmacokinetics

- Poorly absorbed from GI tract. Onset of action 20–45 minutes orally (T_{max} 1–2 hours) with duration of action 3–6 hours

and half-life about 4 hours. IM/IV forms: duration 2–4 hours, onset of action in < 15 minutes IM and < 5 minutes IV. Drug excreted largely unchanged in urine up to 72 hours after administration

 Drug Interactions

- Do not combine with other cholinesterase inhibitors
- May increase neuromuscular blocking effects of succinylcholine
- Magnesium may depress skeletal muscle effect and reduce drug effectiveness
- Corticosteroids may decrease drug effect, and increase drug effect with discontinuation
- Antiarrhythmics and local/general anesthetics decrease drug effectiveness and can cause generalized MG complications

 Other Warnings/ Precautions

- Pyridostigmine pretreatment offers no benefit against the nerve agent Soman unless the nerve agent antidotes atropine and pralidoxime are administered once symptoms of poisoning appear. Pyridostigmine should be discontinued at the first sign of nerve agent poisoning since it may exacerbate the effects of a sublethal exposure to Soman
- Pyridostigmine should be used with caution in patients with bronchial asthma, chronic obstructive pulmonary disease, bradycardia, cardiac arrhythmias, and people being treated for hypertension with β-adrenergic receptor blockers

Do Not Use

- Known hypersensitivity to the cholinesterase inhibitors. Mechanical intestinal or urinary obstruction

SPECIAL POPULATIONS

Renal Impairment

- No known effects

Hepatic Impairment

- No known effects

Cardiac Impairment
- Use with caution in MG patients with bradycardia, arrhythmias, hypotension, or AV block

Elderly
- May have slower clearance of drug

Children and Adolescents
- Safe for use. Total daily oral dose should not exceed 7mg/kg. Congenital MG usually presents in the first 2 years of life. These patients do not have antibodies (anti-AChR or anti-MuSK) or respond to immunosuppressants. Neonatal MG occurs in 12% of the pregnancies with a mother with MG. Symptoms start in the first 2 days and resolve within a few weeks. Juvenile MG starts in childhood but after the peripartum period

Pregnancy
- Category C. Use only if benefits of medication outweigh risks. However, it has been used to treat MG during pregnancy for more than 50 years

Breast Feeding
- Excreted in breast milk. Do not use

THE ART OF NEUROPHARMACOLOGY

Potential Advantages
- Fewer AEs than other cholinesterase inhibitors for the symptomatic treatment of MG. Serious AEs are rare

Potential Disadvantages
- Does not cure MG. Need for frequent dosing. Eventually loses efficacy

Primary Target Symptoms
- To improve weakness, visual problems, and respiratory symptoms associated with MG

Pearls
- Patients can occasionally develop drug resistance. Monitor symptoms and increase dose as needed

- It may worsen MG caused by anti-MuSK antibodies with frequent muscle cramps and fasciculations
- Most cases of MG crisis are caused by worsening of the disease itself or other factors (e.g., infection, drugs)
- Cholinergic crisis, which can be caused by desensitized receptors, may occur at doses higher than 600mg/day
- In crisis (i.e., when patients are intubated) there is no need to give drug. May prolong intubation due to increased secretions. Usually restart when patients become stronger and prior to extubation
- Oral supplement before or during surgery, during labor or post-partum, or during MG crisis, give 1/30 the usual oral dose either IM or as a slow IV infusion
- Avoid using telithromycin, aminoglycosides, interferon-α, penicillamine, IV magnesium, and IV lidocaine in MG patients. Use β-blockers, fluoroquinolones, and CNS depressants such as opioids or muscle relaxants with caution. Neuromuscular blocking agents can be used for anesthesia but in MG could delay extubation or recovery of muscle strength
- Occasionally used postoperatively for bladder distention or urinary retention
- Pyridostigmine, alone or in combination with midodrine, can be used for orthostatic intolerance (including postural tachycardia syndrome) by potentiating ganglionic sympathetic traffic through muscarinic effects. Long-term data are lacking
- Extended-release form is used at bedtime by patients symptomatic at night or in the early morning. There is no clear evidence to support its daytime use
- In animal studies, combination of stress and pyridostigmine has been associated with cognitive dysfunction probably due to BBB breakdown or other peripheral pathways. Long-term exposure has the potential to induce neuromuscular dysfunction, with or without downregulation of acetylcholine receptors
- May be used for protection from the action of fluorophosphates and organophosphate pesticides

Suggested Reading

Argov Z. Management of myasthenic conditions: nonimmune issues. *Curr Opin Neurol.* 2009; 22(5):493–7.

Engel AG. Why does acetylcholine exacerbate myasthenia caused by anti-MuSK antibodies? *J Physiol (Lond).* 2013;591:2377.

Gales BJ, Gales MA. Pyridostigmine in the treatment of orthostatic

intolerance. *Ann Pharmacother.* 2007; 41(2):314–18.

Maggi L, Mantegazza DR. Treatment of myasthenia gravis. *Clin Drug Investig.* 2011;31:691–701.

Wendell LC, Levine JM. Myasthenic crisis. *Neurohospitalist* 2011;1:16–22.

QUETIAPINE

THERAPEUTICS

Brands
- Seroquel, Ketipinor, Seroquel XR

Generic?
- Yes

Class
- Atypical antipsychotic

Commonly Prescribed for
(FDA approved in bold)
- **Schizophrenia**
- **Bipolar disorder (depression and mania) as monotherapy or adjunct to lithium and divalproex**
- **Adjunctive therapy for major depressive disorder (extended-release only)**
- Psychosis associated with Parkinson's disease (PD) or dementia with Lewy bodies (DLB)
- Augmentation for refractory obsessive-compulsive disorder
- Autism
- Alcoholism
- Gilles de la Tourette syndrome (GTS)
- Insomnia
- Anxiety

How the Drug Works
- A benzothiazepine derivative. At lower dose, quetiapine is $H_{1,2}$ and α_1-adrenergic blocker. At higher dose, quetiapine starts blocking more $D_{2,3}$ (as other neuroleptics) and $5\text{-}HT_{2A}$ receptors
- Lower $D_{2/3}$ binding constant than haloperidol reduces its risk of motor side effects
- Binding to other receptors may improve depression and cognitive problems

How Long Until It Works
- Schizophrenia/bipolar: may be effective in days, more commonly takes weeks or months to determine best dose and achieve best clinical effect. Usually 4–6 weeks
- Insomnia: may be effective immediately

If It Works
- Continue to use at lowest required dose. Most patients with schizophrenia see a reduction in psychosis with quetiapine (and

other neuroleptics), but some patients, including many with PD and DLB, may improve more than 50%

If It Doesn't Work
- Increase dose
- In psychosis related to PD or DLB, reduce dose or eliminate offending medications, such as dopamine agonists or amantadine
- If not effective consider changing to clozapine. In PD and DLB, avoid long-term use of conventional antipsychotics
- Insomnia: if no sedation occurs despite adequate dosing, change to another agent

Best Augmenting Combos for Partial Response or Treatment-Resistance
- Patients with affective disorders, such as bipolar disorder, may respond to mood-stabilizing AEDs, lithium, or benzodiazepines. In PD and DLB, cholinesterase inhibitors may improve symptoms (particularly in DLB)

Tests
- Prior to starting treatment and periodically during treatment, monitor weight, blood pressure, lipids, and fasting glucose due to risk of metabolic syndrome

ADVERSE EFFECTS (AEs)

How the Drug Causes AEs
- Motor AEs: blocking of D_2 receptors
- Sedation, weight gain: blocking of H_1 receptors
- Hypotension: blocking of α_1-adrenergic receptors
- Dry mouth, constipation: blocking of muscarinic receptors

Notable AEs
- Most common: sedation, weight gain, constipation, dry mouth, dizziness
- Less common: tachycardia, nausea, akathisia, elevation of hepatic transaminases. May increase risk of cataracts

Life-Threatening or Dangerous AEs
- Tardive dyskinesias (lower than other neuroleptics)

- Severe weight gain and metabolic syndrome/diabetes
- Neuroleptic malignant syndrome (rare compared with conventional antipsychotics)
- Prolong QTc interval

Weight Gain
- Common

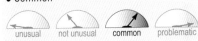

Sedation
- Problematic

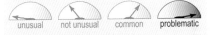

What to Do About AEs
- Take at night: for many disorders there is no need for daytime dosing. Medical management for obesity, including weight loss and exercise, may help combat weight gain

Best Augmenting Agents to Reduce AEs
- Most AEs cannot be reduced with an augmenting agent

DOSING AND USE

Usual Dosage Range
- Bipolar disorder/schizophrenia: 150–800 mg/day
- Psychosis in PD/DLB: 25–200 mg/day

Dosage Forms
- Tablets: 25, 50, 100, 200, 300, 400 mg
- Tablets, extended release: 50, 150, 200, 300, 400 mg

How to Dose
- Start at 25 mg twice a day for acute psychosis or mania. If not tolerated, give larger dose in the evening. Increase by 25–50 mg (twice a day) every 1–2 days until effective dose is reached
- For depression or psychosis with PD or DLB, consider dosing all the medication at night. Start PD and DLB patients with psychosis on 12.5 mg at night and increase by 12.5 mg every 1–2 days until symptoms improve. Most patients respond to a lower dose (average 50–75 mg/day)

- Titrate more rapidly when treating acute mania or schizophrenia: up to 800 mg/day in some cases

 Dosing Tips
- Patients with bipolar disorder (mania or depression) often need a high dose (over 400 mg/day) to achieve best results. Elderly and children often need lower doses

Overdose
- Sedation, hypotension, bradycardia, and dysarthria have been reported. Death is rare

Long-Term Use
- Safe for long-term use with appropriate monitoring

Habit Forming
- No, although may be used by addicts to manage drug withdrawal

How to Stop
- Gradual withdrawal is advised

Pharmacokinetics
- Hepatic metabolism to inactive metabolites via CYP3A4. Half-life 6–7 hours, and steady state reached in 2 days. Protein binding 83%

 Drug Interactions
- Strong CYP3A4 inhibitor (e.g., protease inhibitor, macrolide, azole antifungals, nefazodone) and moderate CYP3A4 inhibitor (e.g., aprepitant, verapamil, grapefruit juice) can increase drug levels; reduce to one-sixth of original dose under concomitant strong CYP3A4 inhibitor
- CYP enzyme inducer (e.g., dexamethasone, rifampin, carbamazepine, phenytoin, barbiturate, St. John's wort) can lower drug level; increase up to 5-fold of the original dose
- Quetiapine may slightly lower levels of valproate and lorazepam

 Other Warnings/ Precautions
- May increase risk of cataracts, aspiration pneumonia, and priapism

- Increased mortality from quetiapine use in dementia-related psychosis

Do Not Use
- Proven hypersensitivity to quetiapine

SPECIAL POPULATIONS

Renal Impairment
- No dose adjustment needed

Hepatic Impairment
- Use with caution. Use lower initiating and titrating doses

Cardiac Impairment
- May worsen orthostatic hypotension. Higher risk of QTc prolongation than most second-generation antipsychotics. Less risk for torsade de pointes than ziprasidone, chlorpromazine, and haloperidol. Use with caution

Elderly
- Start with lower doses. Clearance reduced by about 40%

Children and Adolescents
- Efficacy and safety unknown. Not approved for patients < 10 years old

Pregnancy
- Category C. Probably safer than AEDs during pregnancy for bipolar disorder. PD and DLB are uncommon in women of childbearing age. Use only if benefit outweighs risks

Breast Feeding
- Unknown if found in breast milk. Use while breast feeding is generally not recommended

THE ART OF NEUROPHARMACOLOGY

Potential Advantages
- Useful in controlling psychosis associated with PD at relatively low doses without risk of drug-induced parkinsonism or tardive dyskinesia. No risk of blood dyscrasia

Potential Disadvantages
- Probably less effective than clozapine. Risk of weight gain and metabolic syndrome. Drug interaction by CYP450

Primary Target Symptoms
- Psychosis, depression, mania, and insomnia

 Pearls

- Most commonly used drug for treating psychosis in PD, although investigational (clozapine is efficacious but with risk of agranulocytosis). Use low doses and titrate much more slowly when treating PD or DLB with neuroleptics compared to patients with mania or schizophrenia
- Previous studies suggested usefulness in treating psychosis in patients with Alzheimer's dementia, but subsequently shown to worsen cognitive function with significant AEs, even increased mortality
- Often effective at low doses for insomnia, but not recommended as a first-line option
- In an open pilot study, quetiapine was useful as preventive for migraine refractory to atenolol, nortriptyline, and flunarizine
- Less weight gain than clozapine or olanzapine; more than ziprasidone and aripiprazole
- May cause urinary retention with concomitant use of SNRI (e.g., duloxetine)

Suggested Reading

Keating GM, Robinson DM. Spotlight on quetiapine in bipolar depression. *CNS Drugs.* 2007;21(8):695–7.

Krymchantowski AV, Jevoux C, Moreira PF. An open pilot study assessing the benefits of quetiapine for the prevention of migraine refractory to the combination of atenolol, nortriptyline, and flunarizine. *Pain Med.* 2010; 11(1):48–52.

Kurlan R, Cummings J, Raman R, Thal L; Alzheimer's Disease Cooperative Study Group. Quetiapine for agitation or psychosis in patients with dementia and parkinsonism. *Neurology.* 2007;68(17):1356–63.

Miyasaki JM, Shannon K, Voon V, Ravina B, Kleiner-Fisman G, Anderson K, et al.; Quality Standards Subcommittee of the American Academy of Neurology. Practice Parameter: evaluation and treatment of depression, psychosis, and dementia in Parkinson disease (an evidence-based review): report of the Quality Standards Subcommittee of the American Academy of Neurology. *Neurology.* 2006; 66(7):996–1002.

Poewe W. When a Parkinson's disease patient starts to hallucinate. *Pract Neurol.* 2008;8(4): 238–41.

Rabey JM, Prokhorov T, Miniovitz A, Dobronevsky E, Klein C. Effect of quetiapine in psychotic Parkinson's disease patients: a double-blind labeled study of 3 months' duration. *Mov Disord.* 2007;22(3):313–18.

Seppi K, Weintraub D, Coelho M, Perez-Lloret S, Fox SH, Katzenschlager R, et al. The Movement Disorder Society Evidence-Based Medicine Review Update: Treatments for the non-motor symptoms of Parkinson's disease. *Mov Disord.* 2011;26 Suppl 3:S42–80.

QUININE SULFATE

THERAPEUTICS

Brands
- Formula Q, Legatrin, Qualaquin

Generic?
- Yes

 Class
- Neuromuscular drug

Commonly Prescribed for
(FDA approved in bold)
- **Malaria**
- Symptomatic myotonia (myotonia congenita, myotonic dystrophy)
- Leg cramps
- Congenital myasthenic syndrome

 How the Drug Works
- Quinine has several actions on skeletal muscle. Increases the refractory period by acting on the muscle membrane and sodium channel, decreases motor end-plate excitability, and affects the distribution of calcium within the muscle fiber

How Long Until It Works
- 1–2 hours

If It Works
- Continue to use

If It Doesn't Work
- Change to an alternative agent

 Best Augmenting Combos for Partial Response or Treatment-Resistance
- Myotonia: AEDs, such as phenytoin and carbamazepine, are effective. The antiarrhythmic drug mexiletine (also a sodium channel blocker) is an alternative

Tests
- Obtain baseline ECG due to risk of cardiac arrhythmia (common in myotonic dystrophy)

ADVERSE EFFECTS (AEs)

How the Drug Causes AEs
- Drug effect of blocking sodium channels

Notable AEs
- "Cinchonism" is a common set of AEs seen in most patients; includes headache, flushing, vertigo, hearing difficulties, tinnitus, blurry vision, and nausea. More severe symptoms include vomiting, abdominal pain, deafness, and blindness
- Hypersensitivity reactions include flushing, pruritus, rash, fever, tinnitus, and dyspnea
- Chest pain, orthostatic hypotension, hypoglycemia, anorexia, jaundice, and abnormal liver function tests

 Life-Threatening or Dangerous AEs
- Cardiac arrhythmias, including AV block, atrial fibrillation, QTc prolongation, ventricular fibrillation, ventricular tachycardia, torsade de pointes, and cardiac arrest
- Hemolysis associated with glucose-6-phosphate dehydrogenase deficiency
- Severe hypersensitivity (angioedema)
- Rarely asthma or pulmonary edema

Weight Gain
- Unusual

unusual · not unusual · common · problematic

Sedation
- Unusual

unusual · not unusual · common · problematic

What to Do About AEs
- Lower dose for most AEs, but discontinue for serious AEs

Best Augmenting Agents to Reduce AEs
- Most AEs cannot be reduced by an augmenting agent

DOSING AND USE

Usual dosage range
- 260–2000 mg/day

Dosage Forms
- Tablets: 260 mg
- Capsules: 324 mg

How to Dose
- Take 1–2 tablets or capsules at night and as needed during the day, up to 3 times daily

 Dosing Tips
- Take with food to reduce GI irritation

Overdose
- Tinnitus, dizziness, rash, intestinal cramping, and headache are common. At higher doses fever, vomiting, convulsions, and apprehension occur. Blindness, hearing loss, arrhythmia, and death may occur. Gastric lavage or emesis are indicated and acidification of urine will enhance elimination

Long-Term Use
- Safe for long-term use. Continue to assess need for use

Habit Forming
- No

How to Stop
- No need to taper

Pharmacokinetics
- Peak action 1–3 hours, half-life 4–5 hours. Most drug does not cross BBB. 70–90% protein bound. Mostly hepatic metabolism

 Drug Interactions
- Antacids delay or decrease absorption
- Cimetidine reduces clearance and increases half-life
- Mefloquine coadministration may cause convulsions
- Rifampin increases hepatic clearance and lowers level
- Urinary alkalinizers, such as acetazolamide, sodium bicarbonate, increase levels
- Quinine enhances the action and levels of oral anticoagulants, digoxin, and succinylcholine
- May potentiate the effects of neuromuscular blocking agents

 Other Warnings/ Precautions
- May produce an elevated value for urinary 17-ketogenic steroids

Do Not Use
- Known hypersensitivity, pregnancy, glucose-6-phosphate dehydrogenase deficiency, myasthenia gravis

SPECIAL POPULATIONS

Renal Impairment
- Drug concentrations are increased with severe renal failure. Reduce dose and take twice a day or less. The effect of mild to moderate disease on drug levels is unknown

Hepatic Impairment
- Use with caution. Patients with severe disease may need a lower dose

Cardiac Impairment
- Risk of cardiac arrhythmias. Use with caution and consider alternative treatments

Elderly
- No known effects

 Children and Adolescents
- Appears safe in the treatment of malaria, but not studied for myotonia

 Pregnancy
- Category X with multiple congenital malformations, including deafness. Do not use

Breast Feeding
- Small amounts are excreted in breast milk. Use with caution

THE ART OF NEUROPHARMACOLOGY

Potential Advantages
- Effective treatment for disabling muscle cramps

Potential Disadvantages
- Risk of cardiac arrhythmias

Primary Target Symptoms

- Symptoms of myotonia (muscle pain, stiffness, weakness, dysphagia), pain

 Pearls

- Many patients with myotonia (delayed relaxation of muscles after activity) do not require pharmacological treatment of their symptoms
- Weakness in myotonia is usually in the arms or hands

- Sodium channel blockers, such as phenytoin, mexiletine, or TCAs, are now first-line treatment due to the risk of quinine precipitating cardiac arrhythmias. Benzodiazepines, calcium channel blockers, taurine, and prednisone and physical therapy may be beneficial for some patients
- Quinine sulfate may be a therapeutic option for patient with slow channel congenital myasthenic syndrome

 Suggested Reading

Cleland JC, Griggs RC. Treatment of neuromuscular channelopathies: current concepts and future prospects. *Neurotherapeutics*. 2008;5(4):607–12.

Duff HJ, Mitchell LB, Wyse DG, Gillis AM, Sheldon RS. Mexiletine/quinidine combination therapy: electrophysiologic correlates of anti-arrhythmic efficacy. *Clin Invest Med*. 1991;14(5):476–83.

Meola G, Sansone V. Treatment in myotonia and periodic paralysis. *Rev Neurol (Paris)*. 2004;160 (5 Pt 2):S55–69.

Peyer A-K, Abicht A, Heinimann K, Sinnreich M, Fischer D. Quinine sulfate as a therapeutic option in a patient with slow channel congenital myasthenic syndrome. *Neuromuscul Disord*. 2013;23(7):571–4.

RAMELTEON

THERAPEUTICS

Brands
- Rozerem

Generic?
- No

Class
- Melatonin receptor agonist

Commonly Prescribed for
(FDA approved in bold)
- **Insomnia characterized by difficulties with sleep onset**
- Adjunctive for bipolar disorder
- REM-associated sleep behavior disorder in patients with Parkinson's disease (PD)
- Prevention of delirium

How the Drug Works
- Selectively binds to melatonin receptors (MT$_1$, MT$_2$; similar affinity) in the suprachiasmatic nuclei (SCN). It increases the activity of MT$_1$ receptors (inhibits arousal from SCN) for sleep onset and stimulates MT$_2$ receptors (synchronizes the circadian clock to day–night cycle) for circadian phase shifting
- No affinity for GABA, dopamine, norepinephrine, acetylcholine, opiate receptors

How Long Until It Works
- Onset in less than an hour. Optimum improvement may take days

If It Works
- Continue to use at lowest required dose with appropriate monitoring

If It Doesn't Work
- Increase dose or combine with other anti-insomnia agents. Re-evaluate underlying conditions

Best Augmenting Combos for Partial Response or Treatment-Resistance
- Often depends on the comorbidity. For insomnia, may use low dose of

antihistamine, TCAs, benzodiazepines, or antipsychotics

Tests
- Not available

ADVERSE EFFECTS (AEs)

How the Drug Causes AEs
- CNS depressant

Notable AEs
- Most common: dizziness, daytime somnolence, headache
- Uncommon: hallucination, abnormal thinking, behavioral change

Life-Threatening or Dangerous AEs
- Complex sleep behavior (e.g., sleep-driving)
- Worsening of depression/suicidal ideation
- Respiratory suppression (not fully studied)

Weight Gain
- Unusual

Sedation
- Problematic

What to Do About AEs
- Reduce dose or discontinue

Best Augmenting Agents to Reduce AEs
- Most AEs cannot be reduced by use of augmenting agent

DOSING AND USE

Usual Dosage Range
- 8 mg

Dosage Forms
- Tablet: 8 mg

How to Dose
- Start with 8 mg within 30 minutes of going to bed

 Dosing Tips
- Do not take with high-fat meal, which delays its absorption

Overdose
- Dose-dependent increases in the frequency and duration of somnolence. No antidote available

Long-Term Use
- Safe for long-term use with appropriate monitoring

Habit Forming
- No

How to Stop
- No withdrawal or rebound effect

Pharmacokinetics
- Hepatic metabolism via primarily CYP1A2, but less by CYP3A4 and CYP2C9. 82% protein bound. Half-life 1–2.5 hours. 84% excreted in urine and 4% in feces

 Drug Interactions
- Use with CNS depressants (ethanol, barbiturates, opiates, general anesthetics) potentiates CNS AEs
- Concentration increased by strong CYP3A inhibitor (ketoconazole, protease inhibitors, macrolides, nefazodone, etc.) and strong CYP1A2 inhibitor (fluoroquinolones, fluvoxamine, verapamil)
- Concentration decreased by CYP3A inducer (rifampin, carbamazepine, phenytoin, phenobarbital, dexamethasone, St. John's wort, etc.) or CYP1A2 inducer (tobacco, omeprazole)

⚠ Other Warnings/ Precautions
- Risk of impaired alertness and motor coordination
- Unexplained amenorrhea, galactorrhea

Do Not Use
- Angioedema due to ramelteon

- Concomitant use with strong CYP1A2 inhibitors (fluvoxamine, fluoroquinolones, verapamil)

Renal Impairment
- No dose adjustment needed

Hepatic Impairment
- Not recommended for severe hepatic impairment. Use with caution in patients with moderate hepatic impairment

Cardiac Impairment
- No dose adjustment

Elderly
- May start with lower dose

 Children and Adolescents
- Efficacy and safety unknown

 Pregnancy
- Category C. Use only if benefit outweighs risks

Breast Feeding
- Caution should be exercised when being administered to a nursing woman

Potential Advantages
- Quick onset. Synchronizes circadian rhythm. Lower risk of dependence and abuse (unscheduled). Less rebound insomnia

Potential Disadvantages
- Cost. Drug interaction with CYP1A2 inhibitors. Unusual behavior. Not studied in patients under multiple sleep medications

Primary Target Symptoms
- Insomnia

Pearls

- Short-term use shows improvement in sleep latency and quality, albeit small magnitude
- Compared to melatonin, ramelteon has greater affinity for M_1 and M_2 receptors but less affinity for M_3 receptors. The effectiveness of ramelteon compared with over-the-counter melatonin has not been studied
- Unlike benzodiazepines, which promote sedation, promotes sleep by shortening sleep onset latency and may help maintain sleep during the early part of the sleep

- Therapeutic potential in treating sleep problems in patients with PD. It can alter the sleep/wake rhythm and correct abnormal REM rhythm
- Adjunct use in bipolar patients seems to maintain longer stability
- It may be used to prevent or perhaps control delirium
- No known effect on endocrine functioning
- Agomelatine (not available in US), which exerts melatonergic effect at night and $5\text{-}HT_{2c}$ antagonism at day, may be useful for treating both PD's sleep and depression problem

 Suggested Reading

Giugni JC, Okun MS. Treatment of advanced Parkinson's disease. *Curr Opin Neurol.* 2014;27(4):450–60.

Hatta K, Kishi Y, Wada K, Takeuchi T, Odawara T, Usui C, et al. Preventive effects of ramelteon on delirium: a randomized placebo-controlled trial. *JAMA Psychiatry.* 2014;71(4):397–403.

Kuriyama A, Honda M, Hayashino Y. Ramelteon for the treatment of insomnia in adults: a systematic review and meta-analysis. *Sleep Med.* 2014;15(4): 385–92.

Norris ER, Burke K, Correll JR, Zemanek KJ, Lerman J, Primelo RA, et al. A double-blind, randomized, placebo-controlled trial of adjunctive ramelteon for the treatment of insomnia and mood stability in patients with euthymic bipolar disorder. *J Affect Disord.* 2013;144(1–2):141–7.

Srinivasan V, Cardinali DP, Srinivasan US, Kaur C, Brown GM, Spence DW, et al. Therapeutic potential of melatonin and its analogs in Parkinson's disease: focus on sleep and neuroprotection. *Ther Adv Neurol Disord.* 2011;4(5):297–317.

THERAPEUTICS

Brands
- Azilect

Generic?
- Yes

Class
- Antiparkinson agent

Commonly Prescribed for
(FDA approved in bold)
- **Parkinson's disease (PD)**

How the Drug Works
- Selectively blocks monoamine oxidase type B (MAO-B) and inhibits metabolism of dopamine, increasing its effectiveness. At higher doses, may affect MAO-A as well as MAO-B and inhibit metabolism of norepinephrine, serotonin, and tyramine, as well as dopamine
- It also exerts neuroprotective effects in preclinical studies

How Long Until It Works
- PD: weeks

If It Works
- PD: may require dose adjustments over time or augmentation with other agents. Most PD patients will eventually require carbidopa-levodopa to manage their symptoms

If It Doesn't Work
- Bradykinesia, gait, and tremor should improve. If the patient has significantly impaired functioning, consider adding a dopamine agonist and/or carbidopa-levodopa

Best Augmenting Combos for Partial Response or Treatment-Resistance
- For suboptimal effectiveness consider adding a dopamine agonist and/or carbidopa-levodopa with or without a catechol-*O*-methyl transferase (COMT) inhibitor
- For younger patients with bothersome tremor: anticholinergics may help

- For severe motor fluctuations and/or dyskinesias with good "on" time, functional neurosurgery is an option
- Cognitive impairment/dementia is common in mid- to late-stage PD and may improve with acetylcholinesterase inhibitors
- For patients with late-stage PD experiencing hallucinations or delusions, consider oral atypical neuroleptics (quetiapine, clozapine). Acute psychosis is a medical emergency that may require hospitalization and short-term use of neuroleptics such as low-dose haloperidol

Tests
- Monitor for any changes in blood pressure

ADVERSE EFFECTS (AEs)

How the Drug Causes AEs
- Increases concentration of peripheral and CNS dopamine. At higher doses affects serotonin and norepinephrine levels

Notable AEs
- As monotherapy: flu syndrome, arthralgia, depression, dyspepsia, somnolence, hallucination, psychotic-like behavior, impulse control behaviors
- As adjunctive with levodopa: dyskinesia, accidental injury, weight loss, postural hypotension, vomiting, anorexia, arthralgia, abdominal pain, constipation, dry mouth, abnormal dream, and tenosynovitis

Life-Threatening or Dangerous AEs
- Exacerbation of hypertension
- Serotonin syndrome, with concomitant use of antidepressant or other MAOIs

Weight Gain
- Unusual

unusual | not unusual | common | problematic

Sedation
- Not unusual

unusual | not unusual | common | problematic

What to Do About AEs

- Lower the dose or change to alternative PD medications

Best Augmenting Agents to Reduce AEs

- Orthostatic hypotension: adjust dose or stop antihypertensives, add supplemental salt, and consider fludrocortisone or midodrine

DOSING AND USE

Usual Dosage Range

- PD: 0.5–1 mg daily

Dosage Forms

- Tablets: 0.5, 1 mg

How to Dose

- Regular tablets: start at 0.5 mg daily and increase to 1 mg daily in a few days if tolerated for desired clinical effect. After 3–4 days, may attempt to lower dose of carbidopa-levodopa

 Dosing Tips

- Food has no effect on metabolism

Overdose

- At doses above 1 mg, rasagiline may become less selective and may inhibit MAO-A as well as MAO-B. This increases the risk of hypertensive crisis. Symptoms include dizziness, insomnia, hypotension or hypertension, headache, sedation, respiratory depression, and death. Symptoms of overdose can be delayed up to 12 hours, and maximal worsening may not occur until the next day

Long-Term Use

- Safe for long-term use. Effectiveness may decrease over time in PD

Habit Forming

- No

How to Stop

- No need to taper

Pharmacokinetics

- Hepatic metabolism via CYP1A2, with metabolites excreted in urine. Half-life 0.6–2 hours. Linear pharmacokinetics in 0.5–2 mg dose range. Bioavailability 36% and protein binding 60–70%. Peak plasma levels at about 30–60 minutes

 Drug Interactions

- Increases the effect of levodopa, potentially requiring dose adjustments
- Reduce drug dosage under concomitant use of strong CYP1A2 inhibitors, such as fluoroquinolone, fluvoxamine, and verapamil
- Risk of serotonin syndrome with meperidine. Do not use meperidine within 2 weeks of drug
- Risk of psychosis or bizarre behavior with opioid analgesics, including methadone, tramadol, propoxyphene, and dextromethorphan
- Rasagiline has a warning with respect to possible serotonin syndrome when used in combination with TCAs, SSRIs, and SNRIs. Amitriptyline, citalopram, sertraline, trazodone, paroxetine, and escitalopram were allowed in studies with rasagiline and there were no reports of serotonin syndrome. Physicians should use their clinical judgment when using rasagiline with antidepressants. Do not use within 5 weeks of fluoxetine due to fluoxetine's long half-life
- Dopamine antagonists, such as phenothiazines, metoclopramide, may diminish effectiveness
- Use with caution in patients on antihypertensive medications due to risk of orthostatic hypotension
- At higher doses can potentially interact with sympathomimetics. These include IV dopamine, norepinephrine and epinephrine, methylphenidate, nasal decongestants, sinus medications, asthma inhalers, and some weight loss treatments

 Other Warnings/ Precautions

- Cutaneous melanoma is more common in PD, but it is unclear if this is a medication effect or not

- Discontinue 14 days prior to elective surgery in case sympathomimetic agents are needed during anesthesia

Do Not Use

- Known hypersensitivity to the drug
- Concomitant use of meperidine, tramadol, methadone, propoxyphene, dextromethorphan, St. John's wort, cyclobenzaprine, and other MAOIs
- Patients with pheochromocytoma
- Foods that contain very high amount (> 150 mg) of tyramine

SPECIAL POPULATIONS

Renal Impairment

- No known effects

Hepatic Impairment

- In patients with mild impairment, give up to 0.5 mg daily dose. Do not use in patients with moderate to severe impairment

Cardiac Impairment

- No known effects

Elderly

- Rasagiline is safe in the elderly, with no reports of increased adverse effects

Children and Adolescents

- Not studied in children (PD is rare in pediatrics)

Pregnancy

- Category C. Use only if benefits of medication outweigh risks

Breast Feeding

- Unknown if excreted in breast milk. Do not use

THE ART OF NEUROPHARMACOLOGY

Potential Advantages

- May delay need for carbidopa-levodopa or allow reduction of dose. Good initial treatment. Better tolerated (less nausea, fewer neuropsychiatric adverse events, less somnolence) than dopamine agonists. Potential, but unproven, neuroprotective effect

Potential Disadvantages

- Potentially less effective for motor symptoms than other PD treatments. Patients with significant motor disability or patients older than 75 may require carbidopa-levodopa. Multiple potential drug interactions

Primary Target Symptoms

- PD: motor dysfunction, including bradykinesia, hand function, gait and rest tremor

Pearls

- A well-tolerated monotherapy and adjunctive medication for PD. Favorable long-term AEs. It is efficacious for treating motor fluctuation but not dyskinesia
- MAO-B inhibitors have drawn interest as possible neuroprotective or disease-modifying agents in PD and Alzheimer's dementia (AD). Two large studies of rasagiline have demonstrated possible disease-modifying benefits in PD
- Putative neuroprotective mechanisms of rasagiline include stabilization of mitochondrial membrane potential, reduction of oxidative stress, which leads to apoptosis, increasing activity of antioxidative enzymes superoxide dismutase and catalase, and increasing glial cell-derived neurotrophic factor, nerve growth factor, and brain-derived neurotrophic factor
- Rasagiline appears to facilitate the conversion of amyloid precursor protein into intracellular soluble APPα, which may be neuroprotective in AD. Still, rasagiline is not proven to have neuroprotective properties
- MAOIs may inhibit cholinesterase and be useful for the treatment of AD. There have not been clinical trials to support use to date. It may improve attention in PD patients with cognitive impairment
- Unlike selegiline, rasagiline does not have methamphetamine metabolites

- In clinical trials, patients taking 1 mg/day did not follow dietary restrictions and no AEs related to tyramine occurred. At a dose of 1 mg or less, the drug is selective for MAO-B and dietary restrictions are likely unnecessary

- In a recent trial, rasagiline 1 mg/day did not show significant benefit on multiple system atrophy
- Under investigation for the treatment of restless legs syndrome
- Melanin binding properties may slow melanoma growth

Suggested Reading

Fox SH, Katzenschlager R, Lim S-Y, Ravina B, Seppi K, Coelho M, et al. The Movement Disorder Society Evidence-Based Medicine Review Update: Treatments for the motor symptoms of Parkinson's disease. *Mov Disord.* 2011;26 Suppl 3:S2–S41.

Goldman JG, Holden S. Treatment of psychosis and dementia in Parkinson's disease. *Curr Treat Options Neurol.* 2014;16:281.

Hoy SM, Keating GM. Rasagiline. *Drug.* 2012;72:643–69.

Poewe W, Seppi K, Fitzer-Attas CJ, Wenning GK, Gilman S, Low PA, et al. Efficacy of rasagiline in patients with the parkinsonian variant of multiple system atrophy: a randomised, placebo-controlled trial. *Lancet Neurol.* 2015;14: 145–52.

RESERPINE

THERAPEUTICS

Brands
- Harmonyl

Generic?
- Yes

Class
- Monoamine-depleting agent

Commonly Prescribed for
(FDA approved in bold)
- **Hypertension**
- **Psychotic states**
- Gilles de la Tourette syndrome (GTS) or tics
- Chorea and dyskinesias in Huntington's disease
- Hemiballism
- Dystonia (especially tardive)
- Myoclonus

How the Drug Works
- Depleting agent that depletes stores of catecholamines (dopamine, norepinephrine) and serotonin in the brain and adrenal medulla. Depression of sympathetic nerve function lowers heart rate and blood pressure

How Long Until It Works
- Hypertension: less than a week
- Psychosis, movement disorders: effects can be seen within a few days

If It Works
- In neurological conditions, continue to assess effect of the medication and determine if still needed

If It Doesn't Work
- Chorea: consider benzodiazepines and AEDs (valproate). Neuroleptics are usually effective. Tetrabenazine (another antiadrenergic) is often better tolerated
- Generalized dystonia: anticholinergics, baclofen, or benzodiazepines may be effective. Surgical treatments (including pallidotomy, thalamotomy, deep brain stimulation, myotomy, rhizotomy, or peripheral denervation) are reserved for refractory cases

- GTS/tics: neuroleptics and α₂-adrenergic agonists are often effective

 Best Augmenting Combos for Partial Response or Treatment-Resistance
- AEs, such as CNS depression, often increase when used with other agents, but if tolerated consider combinations with AEDs or benzodiazepines

Tests
- Monitor blood pressure and pulse

ADVERSE EFFECTS (AEs)

How the Drug Causes AEs
- Related to depletion of catecholamines and serotonin

Notable AEs
- Bradycardia, edema, angina-like symptoms
- Drowsiness, dizziness, depression, nightmares
- Nausea, dry mouth, anorexia, impotence, dyspnea, nasal congestion
- Rash, purpura

 Life-Threatening or Dangerous AEs
- Hypersensitivity reactions
- Deafness, optic atrophy
- Parkinsonism and extrapyramidal tract dysfunction (less common than neuroleptics)

Weight Gain
- Common

unusual / not unusual / common / problematic

Sedation
- Problematic

unusual / not unusual / common / problematic

What to Do About AEs
- Stop drug for serious AEs, and use the lowest needed dose

Best Augmenting Agents to Reduce AEs

- Most AEs cannot be reduced by an augmenting agent

DOSING AND USE

Usual Dosage Range

- 0.1–1 mg/day once daily

Dosage Forms

- Tablets: 0.1, 0.25 mg

How to Dose

- Hypertension: start 0.5–1 mg once daily for 1–2 weeks, but many patients are able to lower dose to 0.1–0.25 mg daily
- Psychosis and movement disorders: start 0.5 mg/day and adjust upward or downward based on patient response to anywhere from 0.1 to 1.0 mg/day

 Dosing Tips

- Patients should be aware that drug has slow onset of action and prolonged effects

Overdose

- Severe sedation ranging from drowsiness to coma. Flushing, conjunctival injection, papillary constriction, and hypotension are common. Bradycardia and respiratory depression in severe cases. Treat symptomatically and observe for 72 hours due to long-acting effects

Long-Term Use

- Safe, but patients often discontinue due to AEs

Habit Forming

- No

How to Stop

- No need to taper

Pharmacokinetics

- Half-life is 33 hours with IV administration. Bioavailability is about 50% and protein binding is about 96%. Metabolism of drug is unknown

 Drug Interactions

- Do not use with MAOIs
- TCAs may decrease antihypertensive effect
- Use with digitalis or quinidine may precipitate cardiac arrhythmias
- Use with caution with direct- or indirect-acting sympathomimetics. Reserpine prolongs the action of direct-acting amines (epinephrine, isoproterenol) and inhibits the action of indirect-acting amines (ephedrine, tyramine, amphetamines)

 Other Warnings/ Precautions

- Increases GI motility and secretions. May precipitate biliary colic
- May cause depression that persists for months after use and may be severe enough to result in suicide

Do Not Use

- Proven hypersensitivity, depression or history of suicidal tendencies, active peptic ulcer, ulcerative colitis, patients receiving electroconvulsive therapy

SPECIAL POPULATIONS

Renal Impairment

- Patients with renal insufficiency may adjust poorly to lowered blood pressure

Hepatic Impairment

- No known effects

Cardiac Impairment

- Avoid using in patients with cardiac arrhythmias, especially those taking digitalis or quinidine

Elderly

- No known effects

 Children and Adolescents

- Not recommended for hypertension but occasionally used for the treatment of generalized dystonias. Monitor for parkinsonism and hypotension

Pregnancy

- Category C. Crosses placental barrier. Use only if there is a clear need

Breast Feeding

- Excreted in breast milk and may cause respiratory difficulties and anorexia. Use only if clearly needed

THE ART OF NEUROPHARMACOLOGY

Potential Advantages

- A useful drug for hypertensive patients with psychosis and many movement disorders without risk of tardive dyskinesia

Potential Disadvantages

- More AEs than tetrabenazine and most other treatments

Primary Target Symptoms

- Reduction in severity of psychosis, chorea, dystonia, myoclonus, or tics

 Pearls

- Effective treatment for hyperkinetic movement disorders such as tics, chorea, dyskinesias, and tardive dystonias
- Compared to tetrabenazine, has a longer half-life and greater peripheral effects (GI AEs and hypotension). In refractory dystonia, reserpine with trihexyphenidyl and pimozide may be effective

---

 Suggested Reading

Bhidayasiri R, Fahn S, Weiner WJ, Gronseth GS, Sullivan KL, Zesiewicz TA, et al. Evidence-based guideline: treatment of tardive syndromes: report of the Guideline Development Subcommittee of the American Academy of Neurology. *Neurology.* 2013;81(5):463–9.

Fernandez HH, Friedman JH. Classification and treatment of tardive syndromes. *Neurologist.* 2003;9(1):16–27.

Paleacu D, Giladi N, Moore O, Stern A, Honigman S, Badarny S. Tetrabenazine treatment in movement disorders. *Clin Neuropharmacol.* 2004;27(5): 230–3.

Shamon SD, Perez MI. Blood pressure lowering efficacy of reserpine for primary hypertension. *Cochrane Database Syst Rev.* 2009;4: CD007655.

RILUZOLE

THERAPEUTICS

Brands
- Rilutek

Generic?
- No

Class
- Neuromuscular drug

Commonly Prescribed for
(FDA approved in bold)
- **Amyotrophic lateral sclerosis (ALS)**
- Cerebellar ataxia
- Depression or anxiety disorders

How the Drug Works
- The mode of action is unknown and probably involves multiple mechanisms. It strongly suppresses the persistent Na^+ current in a wide variety of neurons, potentiates calcium-dependent K^+ current, reduces presynaptic transmitter release, inhibits voltage-gated calcium channels, and enhances neuronal survival through production of neurotrophic factors (glial cell-derived neurotrophic factor [GDNF], brain-derived neurotrophic factor [BDNF]) and activation of mitogen-activated protein kinase [MAPK] pathway

How Long Until It Works
- Steady state is reached in 5 days, but it can take months to assess any clinical effect from the drug

If It Works
- ALS is a degenerative disease and deterioration is the general rule. Riluzole can increase survival or time to tracheostomy but is not a cure

If It Doesn't Work
- It is difficult to determine if the treatment is effective, especially because ALS progression varies greatly from patient to patient. Supportive care is the mainstay of current ALS treatment. This may include monitoring and treatment of gait, swallowing, and respiratory difficulties

Best Augmenting Combos for Partial Response or Treatment-Resistance
- No other medication is indicated for the treatment of ALS progression

Tests
- Measure serum transaminases, including ALT levels, at baseline and monthly for 3 months. Then evaluate every 3 months for the first year and periodically after that. Once ALT exceeds 5 times normal, begin checking weekly, and discontinue if ALT exceeds 10 times normal or clinical symptoms, such as jaundice, occur

ADVERSE EFFECTS (AEs)

How the Drug Causes AEs
- Unknown

Notable AEs
- Nausea, weakness, dizziness, diarrhea, abdominal pain, pneumonia, tremor, anorexia, somnolence, and paresthesias. Elevation of hepatic transaminases

Life-Threatening or Dangerous AEs
- Neutropenia and hepatic effects. Neutropenia is uncommon (less than 1/1000 in clinical trials). Hepatic transaminase elevation is common (about 50% of patients will experience 1 elevated level) but usually clinically insignificant

Weight Gain
- Unusual

unusual   not unusual   common   problematic

Sedation
- Unusual

unusual   not unusual   common   problematic

What to Do About AEs
- Check CBC on all patients with febrile illness and treat aggressively

Best Augmenting Agents to Reduce AEs

- AEs cannot be reduced with use of augmenting agents

DOSING AND USE

Usual Dosage Range

- ALS: 50 mg every 12 hours

Dosage Forms

- Tablets: 50 mg

How to Dose

- Start at 50 mg dose twice daily

 Dosing Tips

- Taking with a high-fat meal will reduce absorption. Take > 1 hour before and > 2 hour after meal

Overdose

- Unknown

Long-Term Use

- Safe for long-term use

Habit Forming

- No

How to Stop

- No need to taper

Pharmacokinetics

- Metabolized by CYP1A2 (N-hydroxylation). 60% bioavailability and 96% protein bound. Elimination half-life is about 12 hours. Drug excreted in urine (90%) and feces (5%). Female patients generally metabolize more slowly and Japanese patients appear to have about 50% slower clearance of drug, even when adjusting for body weight

 Drug Interactions

- Strong CYP1A2 inhibitors (e.g., fluvoxamine, fluoroquinolones, verapamil) and moderate CYP1A2 inhibitors (St. John's wort, acyclovir, amiodarone) increase concentration

- CYP1A2 inducers (rifampin, omeprazole, cigarette smoke, and charcoal-broiled food) lower levels
- The effect of riluzole itself on CYP1A2 activity is unknown
- Concomitant use of carbamazepine or phenobarbital with riluzole has greater risk of hepatotoxicity

⚠ **Other Warnings/ Precautions**

- Cases of interstitial lung disease have been reported in patients treated with riluzole, some of them severe
- Patients being treated with riluzole should be discouraged from drinking excessive amounts of alcohol

Do Not Use

- Known hypersensitivity to the drug

SPECIAL POPULATIONS

Renal Impairment

- Severe renal disease may slow drug clearance. Use with caution

Hepatic Impairment

- Use with caution due to known hepatic risks of riluzole. Significant hepatic impairment may increase drug levels

Cardiac Impairment

- No known effects

Elderly

- No known effects. AEs similar to younger patients in those with normal renal and hepatic function

 Children and Adolescents

- Not studied in children (ALS is rare in pediatrics)

 Pregnancy

- Category C. Use only if benefits of medication outweigh risks

Breast Feeding
- Unknown if excreted in breast milk. Do not use

THE ART OF NEUROPHARMACOLOGY

Potential Advantages
- Only medication approved for the treatment of ALS

Potential Disadvantages
- Lack of long-term effectiveness and high cost. Patients or caregivers expecting dramatic improvement from the drug are likely to be disappointed

Primary Target Symptoms
- Survival and delay of need for tracheostomy

 Pearls
- Well tolerated with few major AEs, but does not reverse ALS symptoms or the disease itself
- Do not expect noticeable clinical improvement
- In clinical trials, extended life 3–6 months on average and delayed need for tracheostomy
- Riluzole 100 mg daily probably prolongs median survival by about 2–3 months in patients with ALS
- Studies found no role as add-on for obsessive-compulsive disorder or depression
- Combination of lithium and riluzole does not slow progression more than riluzole alone
- May be useful for slowing the progression of chronic cerebellar ataxia
- Reportedly useful for a few patients with refractory depression

 Suggested Reading

Bellingham MC. A review of the neural mechanisms of action and clinical efficiency of riluzole in treating amyotrophic lateral sclerosis: what have we learned in the last decade? *CNS Neurosci Ther.* 2011;17(1):4–31.

Bensimon G, Doble A. The tolerability of riluzole in the treatment of patients with amyotrophic lateral sclerosis. *Expert Opin Drug Saf.* 2004;3 (6):525–34.

Cheung YK, Gordon PH, Levin B. Selecting promising ALS therapies in clinical trials. *Neurology.* 2006;67(10):1748–51.

Corcia P, Meininger V. Management of amyotrophic lateral sclerosis. *Drugs.* 2008;68 (8):1037–48.

Miller RG, Mitchell JD, Moore DH. Riluzole for amyotrophic lateral sclerosis (ALS)/motor neuron disease (MND). *Cochrane Database Syst Rev.* 2012;3:CD001447.

Ristori G, Romano S, Visconti A, Cannoni S, Spadaro M, Frontali M, et al. Riluzole in cerebellar ataxia: a randomized, double-blind, placebo-controlled pilot trial. *Neurology.* 2010;74(10):839–45.

RITUXIMAB

THERAPEUTICS

Brands
- Rituxan, MabThera, Zytux

Generic?
- No

Class
- Immunosuppressant

Commonly Prescribed for
(FDA approved in bold)
- **CD20-positive chronic lymphocytic leukemia**
- **Wegener's granulomatosis**
- **Microscopic polyangiitis**
- **CD20-positive B-cell non-Hodgkin lymphoma (NHL)**
- **Rheumatoid arthritis**
- Myasthenia gravis (MG)
- Multiple sclerosis (MS) (relapsing-remitting)
- Multifocal motor neuropathy
- Anti-myelin-associated glycoprotein (MAG) neuropathy
- Chronic inflammatory demyelinating polyneuropathy (CIDP)
- Neuromyelitis optica
- Dermatomyositis
- Stiff-person syndrome
- Primary CNS lymphoma
- Anti-NMDA-receptor encephalitis
- Opsoclonus myoclonus
- Sarcoidosis
- Waldenstrom macroglobulinemia
- Immune thrombocytopenic purpura
- Lupus nephritis

How the Drug Works
- Binds to the CD20 antigen on pre-B and mature B lymphocytes, inducing apoptosis. The antigen is expressed in greater than 90% of B-cell NHL but not on stem cells, pro-B cells, plasma cells, or normal tissues. B cells are felt to be important in the pathogenesis of rheumatoid arthritis, MS, MG, and many other autoimmune diseases
- Rituximab may also decrease other biological markers of inflammation, such as C-reactive protein, serum amyloid protein, and rheumatoid factor

How Long Until It Works
- By 2 weeks, but effect on disease may take months

If It Works
- May allow reduction in dose or discontinuation of corticosteroids or other agents in the treatment of MG, MS, or other neurological conditions

If It Doesn't Work
- Usually used as an adjunctive agent in conjunction with corticosteroids or other agents in MG, but other agents such as azathioprine, mycophenolate mofetil, and cyclosporine are often used instead. In MS, used as an alternative to other agents for refractory relapsing-remitting patients

Best Augmenting Combos for Partial Response or Treatment-Resistance
- Often combined with prednisone or other corticosteroids for treatment of MG, allowing eventual decrease in dose. Occasionally combined with other immunosuppressive agents for many autoimmune diseases, but AEs may increase

Tests
- Obtain CBC before beginning and during therapy, more frequently if patient develops cytopenia

ADVERSE EFFECTS (AEs)

How the Drug Causes AEs
- Serious AEs are related to infusion reactions, immunosuppression, and lymphopenia

Notable AEs
- Infusion reactions in 32% usually take place with the first infusion and may include fever, chills, angioedema, bronchospasm, or blood pressure changes. Infection (mostly respiratory tract infections) fever, chills, weakness, itching, headache, and dyspepsia

Life-Threatening or Dangerous AEs

- Not uncommon: severe lymphopenia (mean exposure 4 days to onset; mean duration 11 days) occurs in about 40% of patients. Neutropenia, leukopenia, and anemia are less common. Reactivation of hepatitis B. Severe mucocutaneous reactions, including Stevens-Johnson syndrome. Severe infection or sepsis. Tumor lysis syndrome
- Rare: JC virus infection leading to progressive multifocal leukoencephalopathy. Bowel obstruction and perforation

Weight Gain

- Unusual

unusual   not unusual   common   problematic

Sedation

- Unusual

unusual   not unusual   common   problematic

What to Do About AEs

- Give slowly or stop infusion for serious AEs. Treat infections appropriately

Best Augmenting Agents to Reduce AEs

- For infusion reactions, pretreat with acetaminophen and antihistamines. Pretreatment with IV glucocorticoids may also help

DOSING AND USE

Usual Dosage Range

- 375 mg/m^2 once weekly for 4–8 doses

Dosage Forms

- Injection: 10 mg/mL

How to Dose

- In most cases, given once weekly for 4–8 weeks. Start infusion at a lower rate of 50 mg/h and increase by rate of 50 mg/h every 30 minutes to a maximum of 400 mg/h.

If tolerated, start at 100 mg/h during subsequent treatments

 Dosing Tips

- Do not mix with other drugs. Infusion should be given by staff familiar with potential AEs

Overdose

- Unknown

Long-Term Use

- Usually used on a short-term basis for refractory disorders

Habit Forming

- No

How to Stop

- No need to taper, but monitor for recurrence of neurological disorder

Pharmacokinetics

- B cells rapidly decrease after administration and peripheral B lymphocytes are nearly depleted by 2 weeks. Most patients continue to have B-cell depletion for 6 months, but most have normal B-cell levels 1 year after treatment. Interestingly CSF levels of rituximab are low (about 0.1% of serum) after systemic application

 Drug Interactions

- Combining with cisplatin causes renal toxicity
- Use with immunosuppressant agents requires close monitoring for infection or other AEs

 Other Warnings/ Precautions

- Tumor lysis syndrome: administer aggressive hydration and anti-hyperuricemic agents, monitor renal function
- Do not administer live virus vaccine (e.g. oral polio, varicella, MMR, nasal influenza, rotavirus) prior to or during rituximab

Do Not Use
- Known hypersensitivity to the drug or its components
- Active infection. Reactivation of hepatitis B. Development of progressive multifocal leukoencephalopathy

SPECIAL POPULATIONS

Renal Impairment
- No contraindications, but rituximab can cause renal toxicity. Use with caution in patients with preexisting renal disease

Hepatic Impairment
- No known effects

Cardiac Impairment
- No known effects

Elderly
- Older patients with B-cell lymphomas were more likely to experience supraventricular arrhythmias and pulmonary reactions on rituximab

Children and Adolescents
- Effectiveness and safety are unknown

Pregnancy
- Category C. Do not use in individuals considering pregnancy. Use contraception during and 12 months after treatment

Breast Feeding
- Discontinue until drug levels are not detectable

THE ART OF NEUROPHARMACOLOGY

Potential Advantages
- Mechanism of action different from most immunosuppressive agents for neurological disorders

Potential Disadvantages
- Not a first-line agent in any neurological disorder due to lack of proven efficacy and serious AEs

Primary Target Symptoms
- Preventive treatment of complications from diseases such as MG or MS

Pearls
- Based on a meta-analysis, rituximab may be more effective in MG patients with anti-MuSK antibodies than with anti-AChR antibodies. The effect may be long-lasting
- There are several case reports describing the use of rituximab in refractory MG, including those with anti-MuSK antibodies. Its actions on B cells distinguish rituximab from other agents that act on the cell cycle by inhibiting production of B and T lymphocytes (azathioprine, cyclophosphamide, methotrexate, and mycophenolate mofetil) or immunosuppression of T cells (cyclosporine and tacrolimus). The relative efficacy of rituximab compared to other agents is unknown
- Less proven in MS than natalizumab, another monoclonal antibody. One phase II trial showed that treatment of RRMS with rituximab was associated with decline of contrast-enhancing lesions versus placebo (-91%, $p < 0.001$) as well as significant reduction in risk for relapse (20.3% vs. 40.0%, $p = 0.04$)
- Studies investigating the use of rituximab in the treatment of primary progressive MS have mixed results. One study showed benefit for subjects under 51 years old
- In a small study of 16 children with opsoclonus myoclonus and an increased percentage of CD20 B cells in CSF, 4 infusions of rituximab 375 mg/m^2 were given in combination with corticotropin or immunoglobulins. Treatment allowed reduction in corticotropin dose with few relapses
- Open-label studies demonstrate effectiveness in the treatment of immune-mediated neuropathies, such as multifocal motor and vasculitic neuropathies. In anti-MAG neuropathy treatment improved clinical symptoms, electrophysiological findings, and anti-MAG antibody titers
- Studies of rituximab for the treatment of chronic inflammatory demyelinating polyneuropathy show mixed results

- Case reports indicate usefulness in the treatment of anti-*N*-methyl D aspartate (NMDA) receptor encephalitis, a rare autoimmune, usually paraneoplastic, disease (associated with, e.g., ovarian teratoma)

- A case series reported potential efficacy in primary CNS lymphoma due to high prevalence of CD20 surface marker, despite poor BBB penetration
- The role of intrathecal administration for CNS lymphomas or other CNS disorders is unclear

 Suggested Reading

Batchelor TT, Grossman SA, Mikkelsen T, Ye X, Desideri S, Lesser GJ. Rituximab monotherapy for patients with recurrent primary CNS lymphoma. *Neurology.* 2011;76(10):929–30.

Finsterer J. Treatment of immune-mediated, dysimmune neuropathies. *Acta Neurol Scand.* 2005;112(2):115–25.

Hawker K, O'Connor P, Freedman MS, Calabresi PA, Antel J, et al. Rituximab in patients with primary progressive multiple sclerosis: results of a randomized double-blind placebo-controlled multicenter trial. *Ann Neurol.* 2009;66(4): 460–71.

Iorio R, Damato V, Alboini PE, Evoli A. Efficacy and safety of rituximab for myasthenia gravis: a systematic review and meta-analysis. *J Neurol.* 2015;262:1115–19.

Muraro PA, Bielekova B. Emerging therapies for multiple sclerosis. *Neurotherapeutics.* 2007; 4(4):676–92.

Rizvi SA, Bashir K. Other therapy options and future strategies for treating patients with multiple sclerosis. *Neurology.* 2004; 63(12 Suppl 6):S47–54.

Titulaer MJ, McCracken L, Gabilondo I, Armangué T, Glaser C, Iizuka T, et al. Treatment and prognostic factors for long-term outcome in patients with anti-NMDA receptor encephalitis: an observational cohort study. *Lancet Neurol.* 2013;12(2):157–65.

Zebardast N, Patwa HS, Novella SP, Goldstein JM. Rituximab in the management of refractory myasthenia gravis. *Muscle Nerve.* 2010;41(3): 375–8.

Brands
- Xarelto

Generic?
- No

Class
- Anticoagulant

Commonly Prescribed for
(FDA approved in bold)
- **Reduction in the risk of stroke and systemic embolism in patients with non-valvular atrial fibrillation (NVAF)**
- **Treatment of deep vein thrombosis (DVT), pulmonary embolism (PE), and reduction in the risk of recurrence of DVT and of PE**
- **Prophylaxis of DVT, which may lead to PE in patients undergoing knee or hip replacement surgery**
- Ventricular dysfunction due to hypertrophic cardiomyopathy
- Hypertensive heart disease

How the Drug Works
- Rivaroxaban is a selective reversible inhibitor of both free factor Xa and prothrombinase activity, thereby reducing the conversion of prothrombin to thrombin and thrombus formation. Thrombin-induced platelet aggregation is also inhibited

How Long Until It Works
- Peak concentration in 2–4 hours

If It Works
- Monitor for signs of bleeding. Assess liver and kidney function periodically as clinically indicated

If It Doesn't Work
- Correct the underlying disorder. Use full dose or switch to anticoagulant of different class

Best Augmenting Combos for Partial Response or Treatment-Resistance
- None

Tests
- The degree of anticoagulation does not need to be assessed. Prolonged PT may indicate greater bleeding risk

How the Drug Causes AEs
- Reduced coagulation due to inhibited thrombin formation

Notable AEs
- Bleeding

Life-Threatening or Dangerous AEs
- Fatal bleeding ($< 0.4\%$), major bleeding ($0.3–5.6\%$), anaphylaxis

Weight Gain
- Unusual

Sedation
- Unusual

What to Do About AEs
- Discontinue treatment, supportive care. Prothrombin complex concentrates. Activated charcoal reduces absorption. Not effective: vitamin K, protamine sulfate, hemodialysis

Best Augmenting Agents to Reduce AEs
- Antiplatelet agent, fibrinolytic agent, other anticoagulants, long-term NSAID, CYP3A4/P-glycoprotein (P-gp) inhibitors

Usual Dosage Range
- 10–20 mg

Dosage Forms
- Tablet: 10, 15, 20 mg

How to Dose
Treatment of NVAF:

- For patients with CrCl > 50 mL/min: 20 mg once daily with the evening meal
- For patients with CrCl 15–50 mL/min: 15 mg once daily with the evening meal

Treatment of DVT, PE:
- 15 mg twice daily with food for 21 days then 20 mg once daily with food

Reduction in the risk of recurrence of DVT and of PE:
- 20 mg once daily with food

Prophylaxis of DVT following hip or knee replacement surgery:
- 10 mg once daily for 35 days (total hip replacement [THR]) or 12 days (total knee replacement [TKR])

Conversion between other anticoagulants:
- Converting from warfarin: discontinue warfarin and start rivaroxaban when INR < 3
- Converting to warfarin: discontinue rivaroxaban and bridge with parenteral anticoagulant until INR 2~3
- Converting from heparin/low molecular weight heparin (LMWH): start at the time of discontinuation (heparin) or 2 hours before the next scheduled time (LMWH)
- Converting to heparin/LMWH: add heparin at the time of next dose of rivaroxaban

Dosing Tips
- Crushed or single tablet

Overdose
- May lead to hemorrhagic complications

Long-Term Use
- Safe for long-term use

Habit Forming
- No

How to stop
- A specific antidote for rivaroxaban is not available. It is not dialyzable due to high protein binding. Investigational antidote includes aripazine and andexanet

Pharmacokinetics
- Metabolized by CYP3A4/5, CYP2J2, and hydrolysis. Substrate of P-gp and ATP-binding cassette G2 transporter. Eliminated

in urine (36%) and feces (28%). Half-life 10 hours. Bioavailability increases with food

Drug Interactions
- Anticoagulants such as heparin, vitamin K antagonists increase bleeding risk
- Antiplatelet agents such as aspirin, dipyridamole, clopidogrel, and abciximab may increase bleeding risk
- Concomitant NSAID or aspirin use has higher bleeding risk
- CYP3A4 and P-gp inhibitors (e.g., ketoconazole, clarithromycin, fluoxetine, naproxen, ritonavir, tacrolimus) increase rivaroxaban concentration
- CYP3A4 and P-gp inducers (rifampin, carbamazepine, phenytoin, St. John's wort, phenobarbital) lower rivaroxaban concentration

Other Warnings/ Precautions
- Procedure with minor bleeding risk: stop 1 day before procedure and start 12–24 hours after procedure. If CrCl < 30 mL/min stop 2 days before
- Procedure with major bleeding risk: stop 2 days before procedure and start 2–3 days after procedure. If CrCl < 30 mL/min stop 3 days before
- Extend discontinuation if CrCl < 30 mL/min

Do Not Use
- History of mechanical heart valve replacement
- Hypersensitivity to the drug
- Evidence of major bleeding (e.g., intracranial, intra-abdominal, retroperitoneal, intra-articular, etc.)
- Serious trauma
- Prior to major surgery

Renal Impairment
- AF: do not use if CrCl < 15 mL/min
- DVT, PE, THR, TKR: do not use if CrCl < 30 mL/min

Hepatic Impairment
- Avoid in moderate or severe impairment

Cardiac Impairment

- Safety information is lacking for use in patients with mechanical valve. Use is not recommended

Elderly

- Slight higher serum concentration if > 65 years old. No dose change needed by age alone

 Children and Adolescents

- Not studied in children

 Pregnancy

- Category C. Insufficient safety data. Usage not recommended

Breast Feeding

- Unknown if present in breast milk. Usage not recommended

THE ART OF NEUROPHARMACOLOGY

Potential Advantages

- Proven treatment for stroke and systemic embolism prevention in adults with AF
- Better than aspirin, non-inferior to warfarin in reducing rate of stroke and systemic embolism from AF

Potential Disadvantages

- Increased risk of bleeding. Lack of antidote or monitoring lab test. Not dialyzable

Primary Target Symptoms

- Reduce recurrent attacks of cerebral embolism caused by cardiogenic thrombi due to AF. Reduce venothromboembolism after orthopedic surgeries

 Pearls

- For patients with NVAF with prior stroke, transient ischemic attack (TIA), or a CHA2DS2-VASc score of 2 or greater (Level of Evidence B)
- For patients with NVAF unable to maintain a therapeutic INR level with warfarin (Level of Evidence C)
- The effect and safety of rivaroxaban in patients with AF and mechanical valve are uncertain
- Not for use in AF with end-stage renal disease
- For single venothromboembolism episode, discontinue rivaroxaban after 6 months. For recurrent venothromboembolism, continue anticoagulation for good
- For cerebral venous thrombosis, despite a lack of evidence, it is often recommended to use warfarin for 3–12 months. Longer duration is reserved for those with severe coagulopathies or recurrent venothromboembolism. For newer anticoagulants, although no evidence available, their lower intracranial bleeding rate might offer them a potential role for cerebral venous thrombosis

---

 Suggested Reading

January CT, Wann LS, Alpert JS, Calkins H, Cleveland JC, Cigarroa JE, et al. 2014 AHA/ACC/HRS guideline for the management of patients with atrial fibrillation: a report of the American College of Cardiology/American Heart Association Task Force on practice guidelines and the Heart Rhythm Society. *Circulation.* 2014;130(23):e199–267. Erratum in *Circulation.* 2014;130(23):e272–4.

Patel MR, Mahaffey KW, Garg J, Pan G, Singer DE, Hacke W, et al. Rivaroxaban versus warfarin in nonvalvular atrial fibrillation. *N Engl J Med.* 2011;365(10): 883–91.

Weimar C. Diagnosis and treatment of cerebral venous and sinus thrombosis. *Curr Neurol Neurosci Rep.* 2014;14(1):417.

RIVASTIGMINE

THERAPEUTICS

Brands
- Exelon, Prometax

Generic?
- Yes

Class
- Cholinesterase inhibitor

Commonly Prescribed for
(FDA approved in bold)
- **Alzheimer's dementia (AD) (mild or moderate)**
- **Dementia associated with Parkinson's disease (PD)**
- Dementia with Lewy bodies (DLB)
- Vascular dementia

How the Drug Works
- A dual-enzyme inhibitor. It increases the concentration of acetylcholine through reversible inhibition of acetylcholinesterase, which increases availability of acetylcholine. It also inhibits butyrylcholinesterase, the activity of which progressively increases in AD. A deficiency of cholinergic function is felt to be important in producing the signs and symptoms of AD. May interfere with amyloid deposition
- Although symptoms of AD can improve, rivastigmine does not prevent disease progression

How Long Until It Works
- Typically 2–6 weeks at a given dose, but effect is best observed over a period of months

If It Works
- Continue to use but symptoms of dementia usually continue to worsen

If It Doesn't Work
- Consider adjusting dose
- Change to another cholinesterase inhibitor or NMDA receptor antagonist (memantine)
- Non-pharmacological measures are the basis of dementia treatment. Maintain regular schedules and routines. Avoid prolonged travel, unnecessary medical procedures or emergency room visits, crowds, and large social gatherings
- Limit drugs with sedative properties such as opioids, hypnotics, AEDs, and TCAs
- Treat other disorders that can worsen symptoms, such as hyperglycemia or urinary difficulties

Best Augmenting Combos for Partial Response or Treatment-Resistance
- Addition of the NMDA receptor antagonist memantine may be beneficial
- Treat depression or apathy with SSRIs but be cautious for increased risk of AEs (e.g., QTc prolongation, injurious falls). Avoid TCAs in demented patients due to risk of confusion. In dementia patients with severe depression, electroconvulsive therapy can be an option
- For significant confusion and agitation avoid neuroleptics (especially in DLB) because of the risk of neuroleptic malignant syndrome. Atypical antipsychotics (e.g., risperidone, clozapine, aripiprazole) or SSRIs can be used instead

Tests
- None required

ADVERSE EFFECTS (AEs)

How the Drug Causes AEs
- Acetylcholinesterase and butyrylcholinesterase inhibition in the CNS and PNS

Notable AEs
- GI AEs (nausea/vomiting, diarrhea, anorexia, increased gastric acid secretion, and weight loss) are most common
- Fatigue, depression, dizziness, increased sweating, and headache

Life-Threatening or Dangerous AEs
- Rarely bradycardia or heart block causing syncope
- Generalized convulsions
- Increases gastric acid secretions, which can predispose to GI bleeding

- Exaggerates succinylcholine-type muscle relaxation during anesthesia

Weight Gain

- Unusual

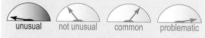

- Weight loss is more common

Sedation

- Unusual

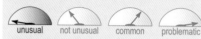

What to Do About AEs

- In patients with dementia, determining if AEs are related to medication or another medical condition can be difficult. For CNS side effects, discontinuation of non-essential centrally acting medications may help. If a bothersome AE is clearly drug-related then lower the dose (especially for GI AEs), titrate more slowly, or discontinue

Best Augmenting Agents to Reduce AEs

- Most AEs do not respond to adding other medications

DOSING AND USE

Usual Dosage Range

- 6–12 mg/day in 2 divided doses for oral formulations, or once 4.6 or 9.5 mg transdermal patch per day

Dosage Forms

- Capsules: 1.5, 3, 4.5, and 6 mg
- Oral solution: 2 mg/mL in a 120 mL bottle
- Patches: 4.6 mg/24 h (5 cm²), 9.5 mg/24 h (10 cm²), 13.3 mg/24 h (15 cm²)

How to Dose

- Start at 1.5 mg twice a day. Increase at a minimum of 2 weeks by 3 mg/day to a maximum of 12 mg/day in 2 divided doses
- Transdermal patch: start 4.6-mg/24-h patch applied once daily. After 4 weeks increase to one 9.5-mg/24-h patch daily if well tolerated

 Dosing Tips

- Slow titration can reduce AEs. Nausea is most common in the titration phase. Food slows absorption

Overdose

- Symptoms of cholinergic crisis can occur: nausea/vomiting, salivation, hypotension, diaphoresis, convulsions, bradycardia/collapse. May cause muscle weakness and respiratory failure. Atropine with an initial dose of 1–2 mg IV is a potential antidote

Long-Term Use

- Safe for long-term use. Effectiveness may decrease over time as the dementing illness progresses

Habit Forming

- No

How to Stop

- Abrupt discontinuation can produce worsening of dementia symptoms, memory and behavioral disturbances. Taper slowly

Pharmacokinetics

- Elimination half-life 1–2 hours. No hepatic metabolism or CYP450 interactions. Metabolites are excreted in urine. Bioavailability 100%. Protein binding 96%

 Drug Interactions

- Increases the effect of anesthetics such as succinylcholine. Stop before surgery
- Anticholinergics interfere with effect of drug
- Other cholinesterase inhibitors and cholinergic agonists (bethanechol) may cause a synergistic effect
- Bradycardia may occur when used with β-blockers
- Nicotine increases drug clearance

 Other Warnings/ Precautions

- Extrapyramidal symptoms may appear or be exacerbated (particularly tremor)
- Weight loss is more common

- Caution is recommended in patients with sick sinus syndrome, conduction defects, gastroduodenal ulcerative conditions, asthma or chronic obstructive pulmonary disease, urinary obstruction, and seizures

Do Not Use

- Known hypersensitivity to the drug or carbamate derivatives

SPECIAL POPULATIONS

Renal Impairment

- Variable changes in clearance with moderate and severe disease. No dose adjustment needed

Hepatic Impairment

- Patients with severe disease have 60% reduced clearance but not clinically significant. No dose adjustment needed

Cardiac Impairment

- Syncope has been reported

Elderly

- No known effects

Children and Adolescents

- Not studied. AD does not occur in children

Pregnancy

- Category B. Use only if benefits of medication outweigh risks

Breast Feeding

- Unknown if excreted in breast milk. Do not use

THE ART OF NEUROPHARMACOLOGY

Potential Advantages

- Proven effectiveness for AD and PD dementia. Low risk of the hepatotoxicity seen with other acetylcholinesterase inhibitors (tacrine) and fewer drug

interactions than donepezil. Available as a transdermal patch. Additional inhibition of butyrylcholinesterase may increase effectiveness

Potential Disadvantages

- Cost and minimal effectiveness. Does not prevent progression of AD or other dementia. GI AEs

Primary Target Symptoms

- Confusion, agitation, memory, performing activities of daily living

Pearls

- May be used in combination with memantine with good effect, but combining with other cholinesterase inhibitors is not recommended
- In most clinical trials, medication treatments for AD patients had a similar rate of benefit
- May be useful for both behavioral problems in AD (delusion, anxiety, and apathy for example) as well as memory disturbance
- When changing from one cholinesterase inhibitor to another, avoid a washout period which could precipitate clinical deterioration
- May delay the need for nursing home placement
- Butyrylcholinesterase inhibition may be more beneficial in later stages of AD when gliosis occurs and acetylcholinesterase decreases
- May be more selective for the form of acetylcholinesterase in the hippocampus (G1)
- Rivastigmine is efficacious for the treatment of dementia in PD (galantamine and donepezil remain investigational). PD patients may benefit from lower doses than in AD (less than 6 mg/day)
- Usually the effect of rivastigmine is not dramatic, but patients with DLB might show more benefit. Effective for the cognitive and behavioral symptoms (agitation, apathy, hallucinations) of DLB, and perhaps REM-sleep behavior disorder
- May help treat dementia in Down's syndrome, which has similar pathology to AD

Suggested Reading

Bentué-Ferrer D, Tribut O, Polard E, Allain H. Clinically significant drug interactions with cholinesterase inhibitors: a guide for neurologists. *CNS Drugs.* 2003;17(13): 947–63.

Chitnis S, Rao J. Rivastigmine in Parkinson's disease dementia. *Expert Opin Drug Metab Toxicol.* 2009;5(8):941–55. Review

Cummings J, Lefèvre G, Small G, Appel-Dingemanse S. Pharmacokinetic rationale for the rivastigmine patch. *Neurology.* 2007; 69(4 Suppl 1):S10–13.

Downey D. Pharmacologic management of Alzheimer disease. *J Neurosci Nurs.* 2008; 40(1):55–9.

Seppi K, Weintraub D, Coelho M, Perez-Lloret S, Fox SH, Katzenschlager R, et al. The Movement Disorder Society Evidence-Based Medicine Review Update: Treatments for the non-motor symptoms of Parkinson's disease. *Mov Disord.* 2011;26 Suppl 3:S42–80.

Stahl SM. The new cholinesterase inhibitors for Alzheimer's disease, Part 1: their similarities are different. *J Clin Psychiatry.* 2000;61(10):710–11.

RIZATRIPTAN

THERAPEUTICS

Brands
• Maxalt, Maxalt MLT

Generic?
• Yes

Class
• Triptan

Commonly Prescribed for
(FDA approved in bold)
• **Acute treatment of migraine in patients with age > 6 years**

 How the Drug Works
• Selective 5-HT$_{1B/1D/1F}$ receptor agonist. In addition to vasoconstriction of meningeal vessels, its antinociceptive effect is likely due to blocking the transmission of pain signals at trigeminal nerve terminals (preventing the release of inflammatory neuropeptides) and synapses of second-order neurons in trigeminal nucleus caudalis

How Long Until It Works
• 1 hour or less

If It Works
• Continue to take as needed. Patients taking acute treatment more than 2 days/week are at risk for medication overuse headache, especially if they have migraine

If It Doesn't Work
• Treat early in the attack – triptans are less likely to work after the headache becomes moderate or severe, regardless of cutaneous allodynia, which is a marker of central sensitization
• Address life style issues (e.g., stress, sleep hygiene), medication use issues (e.g., compliance, overuse), and other underlying medical conditions
• Change to higher dosage, another triptan, another administration route, or combination of other medications. Add preventive medication when needed
• For patients with partial response or reoccurrence, other rescue medications

include NSAIDs (e.g., ketorolac, naproxen), antiemetic (e.g., prochlorperazine, metoclopramide), neuroleptics (e.g., haloperidol, chlorpromazine), ergots, antihistamine, or corticosteroid

 Best Augmenting Combos for Partial Response or Treatment-Resistance
• NSAIDs or neuroleptics are often used to augment response

Tests
• None required

ADVERSE EFFECTS (AEs)

How the Drug Causes AEs
• Direct effect on systemic serotonin receptors (e.g., 5-HT$_{1B}$ agonism on vasoconstriction)

Notable AEs
• Tingling, flushing, sensation of burning, dizziness, sensation of pressure, palpitations, heaviness, nausea

 Life-Threatening or Dangerous AEs
• Serotonin syndrome. Rare cardiac events including acute myocardial infarction, cardiac arrhythmias, and coronary artery vasospasm have been reported with rizatriptan

Weight Gain
• Unusual

unusual · not unusual · common · problematic

Sedation
• Unusual

unusual · not unusual · common · problematic

What to Do About AEs
• In most cases, only reassurance is needed. Lower dose, change to another triptan, or use an alternative headache treatment

Best Augmenting Agents to Reduce AEs

- Treatment of nausea with antiemetics is acceptable. Other AEs decrease with time

DOSING AND USE

Usual Dosage Range

- 5–10 mg, maximum 20 mg/day

Dosage Forms

- Tablets: 5 and 10 mg
- Orally disintegrating tablets: 5 and 10 mg

How to Dose

- Adult: Most patients respond best at 10 mg oral dose (5 mg if taking propranolol). Give 1 pill at the onset of an attack and repeat in 2 hours for a partial response or if the headache returns. Maximum 30 mg/day (3 tablets). Limit 10 days/month
- Adolescent: < 40 kg: 5 mg single dose (do not use with propranolol); ≥ 40 kg: 10 mg single dose (5 mg if taking propranolol)

 Dosing Tips

- Treat early in attack

Overdose

- May cause hypertension, cardiovascular symptoms. Other possible symptoms include seizure, tremor, extremity erythema, cyanosis, or ataxia. For patients with angina, perform ECG and monitor for ischemia for at least 12 hours

Long-Term Use

- Monitor for cardiac risk factors with continued use

Habit Forming

- No

How to Stop

- No need to taper. Patients who overuse triptans often experience withdrawal headaches lasting up to several days

Pharmacokinetics

- Half-life 2 hours. T_{max} 1–2.5 hours, longer with orally disintregrating tablets. Bioavailability is 40%. Metabolism mostly by monoamine oxidase (MAO)-A isoenzyme. 14% protein binding. Food does not affect bioavailability but delays T_{max}

 Drug Interactions

- MAOIs may make it difficult for drug to be metabolized
- Concurrent propranolol use increases peak concentrations – use the 5 mg dose
- Use with sibutramine, a weight loss drug, can cause serotonin syndrome including weakness, irritability, myoclonus, and confusion

 Other Warnings/ Precautions

- For phenylketonurics: tablets contain phenylalanine

Do Not Use

- Within 2 weeks of MAOIs, or 24 hours of ergot containing medications such as dihydroergotamine (DHE)
- Patients with proven hypersensitivity to rizatriptan, known cardiovascular disease, uncontrolled hypertension, or Prinzmetal's angina
- Rizatriptan was not studied in patients with hemiplegic and basilar migraine
- May worsen symptoms in ischemic bowel disease

SPECIAL POPULATIONS

Renal Impairment

- Concentration increases in those with severe renal impairment (CrCl < 2 mL/min). May be at increased cardiovascular risk

Hepatic Impairment

- Drug metabolism decreased with hepatic disease. Do not use with severe hepatic impairment

Cardiac Impairment

- Do not use in patients with known cardiovascular or peripheral vascular disease. May require cardiac stress test or cardiology clearance if tripans are necessary

Elderly

- May be at increased cardiovascular risk

Children and Adolescents

- Safety and efficacy have not been established
- Triptan trials in children were negative, due to higher placebo response

Pregnancy

- Category C. Use only if potential benefit outweighs risk to the fetus. Pregnancy registry studies ongoing. Migraine often improves in pregnancy, and other acute agents (opioids, neuroleptics, prednisone) have more proven safety

Breast Feeding

- Rizatriptan is found in breast milk. Use with caution

THE ART OF NEUROPHARMACOLOGY

Potential Advantages

- Effective and fast acting, even compared to other oral triptans. May be drug of choice for patients with relatively short-lasting migraines. AEs similar to other triptans. Less risk of abuse than opioids or barbiturate-containing treatments. Available as melt formulation

Potential Disadvantages

- Cost, potential for medication-overuse headache. Relatively short half-life, even compared to other triptans

Primary Target Symptoms

- Headache pain, nausea, photo and phonophobia

Pearls

- Early treatment of migraine is most effective
- Compared to other triptans from a meta-analysis, rizatriptan orally disintegrating tablets has the highest 2-hour pain-free response (50%, number needed to treat 3)
- May not be effective when taking during aura, even before headache begins
- In patients with "status migrainosus" (migraine lasting more than 72 hours) neuroleptics and DHE are more effective
- Triptans were not originally studied for use in the treatment of basilar or hemiplegic migraine
- Triptans can be used to treat tension-type headache in migraineurs but not in patients with pure tension-type headache
- Patients taking triptans more than 10 days/month are at increased risk of medication-overuse headache, which is less responsive to treatment
- Chest and throat tightness are usually benign and may be related to esophageal spasm rather than cardiac ischemia. These symptoms occur more commonly in patients without cardiac risk factors
- Combination use of SNRI and triptans usually will not lead to serotonin syndrome, which requires activation of 5-HT_{2A} receptors and a possible limited role of 5-HT_{1A}. However, triptans are agonists at the $5\text{-HT}_{1B/1D/1F}$ receptor subtypes, with weak affinity for 5-HT_{1A} receptors and no activity at the 5-HT_2 receptors. Thus, given the seriousness of serotonin syndrome, caution is certainly warranted and clinicians should be vigilant for serotonin toxicity symptoms and signs to insure prompt treatment
- The site of pharmacological action, whether central or peripheral, remains to be studied. Although triptans generally do not penetrate BBB, it has been postulated that transient BBB breakdown may occur during a migraine attack

Suggested Reading

Dodick D, Lipton RB, Martin V, Papademetriou V, Rosamond W, MaassenVanDenBrink A, et al. Consensus statement: cardiovascular safety profile of triptans (5-HT1B/1D agonists) in the acute treatment of migraine. *Headache*. 2004; 44(5):414–25.

Evans RW, Tepper SJ, Shapiro RE, Sun-Edelstein C, Tietjen GE. The FDA alert on serotonin syndrome with use of triptans combined with selective serotonin reuptake inhibitors or selective serotonin-norepinephrine reuptake inhibitors: American Headache Society position paper. *Headache*. 2010;50(6):1089–99.

Ferrari MD, Roon KI, Lipton RB, Goadsby PJ. Oral triptans (serotonin 5-HT (1B/1D) agonists) in acute migraine treatment: a meta-analysis of 53 trials. *Lancet*. 2001;358(9294):1668–75.

Freitag F, Diamond M, Diamond S, Janssen I, Rodgers A, Skobieranda F. Efficacy and tolerability of coadministration of rizatriptan and acetaminophen vs rizatriptan or acetaminophen alone for acute migraine treatment. *Headache*. 2008;48(6):921–30.

Gladstone JP, Gawel M. Newer formulations of the triptans: advances in migraine management. *Drugs*. 2003;63(21):2285–305.

O'Quinn S, Mansbach H, Salonen R. Comparison of rizatriptan and sumatriptan. *Headache*. 1999;39(1):59–60.

THERAPEUTICS

Brands
- Requip, Requip XL, Adartrel

Generic?
- Yes

Class
- Antiparkinson agent

Commonly Prescribed for
(FDA approved in bold)
- **Parkinson's disease (PD)**
- **Restless legs syndrome (RLS) (except for Requip XL)**

How the Drug Works
- Dopamine agonist, with high affinity for the pre and postsynaptic D_2, D_3, D_4 receptors. The antiparkinson action is likely due to D_2 agonism within the caudate-putamen. High affinity to D_3 receptors might affect impulse control and dyskinesia. The mechanism of action for RLS is probably related to D_2 or D_3 receptor agonism

How Long Until It Works
- PD: weeks
- RLS: days to weeks

If It Works
- PD: may require dose adjustments over time or augmentation with other agents. Most PD patients will eventually require carbidopa-levodopa to manage their symptoms
- RLS: safe for long-term use with dose adjustments

If It Doesn't Work
- PD: bradykinesia, gait, and tremor should improve. Non-motor symptoms including autonomic symptoms such as postural hypotension, depression, and bladder dysfunction do not improve. If the patient has significantly impaired functioning, add carbidopa-levodopa with or without ropinirole
- RLS: rule out peripheral neuropathy, iron deficiency, thyroid disease. Change to another drug such as a benzodiazepine. Gabapentin enacarbil (not gabapentin) may also be beneficial. In severe cases consider opioids

Best Augmenting Combos for Partial Response or Treatment-Resistance
- For suboptimal effectiveness add carbidopa-levodopa with or without a catechol-*O*-methyltransferase (COMT) inhibitor. Monoamine oxidase (MAO)-B inhibitors may also be beneficial
- For severe motor fluctuations and/or dyskinesias with good "on" time, functional neurosurgery is an option
- For RLS, can change to a different dopamine agonist (pramipexole, carbidopa-levodopa) or add another drug such as a clonazepam. Gabapentin enacarbil may be beneficial. In severe cases consider opioids

Tests
- None required

ADVERSE EFFECTS (AEs)

How the Drug Causes AEs
- Direct effect on dopamine receptors

Notable AEs
- Nausea/vomiting, dizziness, hallucination, constipation, somnolence, abdominal pain/discomfort, diaphoresis, anxiety, viral infection, pharyngitis, dyskinesias, and orthostatic hypotension

Life-Threatening or Dangerous AEs
- May cause somnolence or sudden-onset sleep, often without warning. Occurs more often than with ergot agonists or carbidopa-levodopa. Rare syncope or cardiac arrhythmias, most commonly bradycardia

Weight Gain
- Unusual

unusual   not unusual   common   problematic

Sedation
- Common

unusual   not unusual   common   problematic

What to Do About AEs

- Nausea can be problematic when initiating drug – titrate slowly
- Hallucinations or delusions may require stopping the medication
- Warn patients about the risks of sleeping while driving

Best Augmenting Agents to Reduce AEs

- Amantadine may help suppress dyskinesias
- Orthostatic hypotension: adjust dose or stop antihypertensives, add supplemental salt, and consider fludrocortisone or midodrine
- Urinary incontinence: reducing PM fluids, voiding schedules, oxybutynin, desmopressin nasal spray, hyoscyamine sulfate, urological evaluation

DOSING AND USE

Usual Dosage Range

- PD: 3–24 mg daily, divided into 3 daily doses or once daily with XL formulation
- RLS: 4 mg or less 1–3 hours before bedtime

Dosage Forms

- Tablets: 0.25, 0.5, 1, 2, 3, 4, 5 mg
- Extended-release (XL) tablets: 2, 4, 8 mg

How to Dose

- PD (immediate release): start at 0.25 mg 3 times daily. Each week increase each dose by 0.25 mg until reaching 1 mg 3 times daily at week 4. After week 4 increase each dose by 0.5 mg/week if needed until taking 9 mg/day, then by 1 mg each dose until taking a maximum of 24 mg/day in 3 divided doses to reach desired clinical effect
- PD (extended release): start at 2 mg/day for 1–2 weeks, then increase by 2 mg/week until symptomatic relief or maximum of 24 mg/day
- RLS: take 1–3 hours before bedtime. Start at 0.25 mg, and increase to 0.5 mg in 2–3 days. After 1 week increase to 1.0 mg and after that increase by 0.5 mg/week until at 4 mg at bedtime

 Dosing Tips

- Slow titration will minimize nausea and dizziness

Overdose

- Symptoms include somnolence, agitation, orthostatic hypotension, abdominal pain, nausea, or dyskinesias. For cases of excessive CNS stimulation, neuroleptics can be effective

Long-Term Use

- Safe for long-term use. Effectiveness may decrease over time in PD (years) and RLS (months)

Habit Forming

- No

How to Stop

- Taper and discontinue over a period of 1 week. PD and RLS symptoms may worsen, but serious AEs from discontinuation are rare

Pharmacokinetics

- Extensive metabolism in liver by CYP1A2 enzyme. 55% bioavailability. Half-life is 6 hours. It is not a substrate for P-glycoprotein (P-gp) and does not inhibit or induce CYP450

 Drug Interactions

- Increases the effect of levodopa
- Estrogen, especially ethinylestradiol, can reduce clearance of drug
- CYP1A2 inhibitors (ciprofloxacin, cimetidine, diltiazem, erythromycin, mexiletine, fluvoxamine, tacrine) increase ropinirole concentration
- Smoking and omeprazole induce CYP1A2, which decreases ropinirole concentration
- Dopamine antagonists such as phenothiazines, metoclopramide diminish effectiveness
- Use with caution in patients on antihypertensive medications due to risk of orthostatic hypotension

 Other Warnings/ Precautions

- Dopamine agonists can precipitate impulse control disorders, such as pathological gambling, hypersexuality, and compulsive shopping

Do Not Use
- Hypersensitivity to the drug

Renal Impairment
- Dose does not seem to be affected under moderate impairment but not studied in patients with severe disease

Hepatic Impairment
- Drug has hepatic metabolism but impairment does not appear to affect drug clearance. Use with caution

Cardiac Impairment
- Infrequently causes cardiac arrhythmias, rarely ventricular tachycardia. Use with caution

Elderly
- There is reduced drug clearance, but no dose adjustment needed as the dose used is the lowest that provides clinical improvement

 Children and Adolescents
- Not studied in children (PD is rare in pediatrics)

 Pregnancy
- Category C. Teratogenic in some animal studies. Use only if benefits of medication outweigh risks

Breast Feeding
- Inhibits prolactin secretion. Unknown if excreted in breast milk

Potential Advantages
- PD: may delay need for carbidopa-levodopa and decreases risk of motor dyskinesias by 30%. This is especially important in younger PD patients. Available in 1/day dosing. Unlike ergot-based agonists, no known risk of fibrotic complications
- RLS: less risk of dependence compared to opioids or benzodiazepines and less augmentation than levodopa

Potential Disadvantages
- Less effective than carbidopa-levodopa for PD with more AEs such as hallucinations, somnolence, and orthostatic hypotension. Patients with significant motor disability will require carbidopa-levodopa. Risk of impulse control disorders

Primary Target Symptoms
- PD: motor dysfunction including bradykinesia, hand function, gait and rest tremor
- RLS: pain, insomnia

 Pearls
- Excellent drug for young patients with early PD. Favorable long-term AEs
- First-line treatment for RLS with less augmentation or "rebound" than carbidopa-levodopa. Non-ergot dopamine agonists are probably equally effective in treating RLS
- For younger patients with bothersome tremor: anticholinergics may help
- Depression is common in PD and may respond to TCAs, pramipexole, or agomelatine
- Cognitive impairment/dementia is common in mid- to late-stage PD and may improve with acetylcholinesterase inhibitors in short term
- For patients with late-stage PD experiencing hallucinations or delusions, withdraw ropinirole and consider atypical neuroleptics (clozapine, quetiapine). Acute psychosis is a medical emergency that may require hospitalization and low-dose haloperidol
- For orthostatic hypotension, droxidopa can be helpful
- AE profile differs from pramipexole. Less often associated with postural hypotension, dyskinesias, and edema, but more likely to cause dizziness, syncope, nausea, or respiratory problems
- For patients with mildly symptomatic disease, dopamine agonists are also appropriate for initial therapy, but for patients with significant disability, use carbidopa-levodopa early

- Based on a recent evidence-based medicine review: ropinirole is efficacious as symptomatic adjunct to levodopa. Ropinirole XL: likely efficacious in control of motor symptoms (monotherapy), efficacious as adjunct to levodopa, in prevention of dyskinesia, and for treatment of motor fluctuations

Suggested Reading

Chitnis S. Ropinirole treatment for restless legs syndrome. *Expert Opin Drug Metab Toxicol.* 2008;4(5):655–64.

Fox SH, Katzenschlager R, Lim S-Y, Ravina B, Seppi K, Coelho M, et al. The Movement Disorder Society Evidence-Based Medicine Review Update: Treatments for the motor symptoms of Parkinson's disease. *Mov Disord.* 2011;26 Suppl 3:S2–41.

Kvernmo T, Houben J, Sylte I. Receptor-binding and pharmacokinetic properties of dopaminergic agonists. *Curr Top Med Chem.* 2008;8(12): 1049–67.

Lang AE. When and how should treatment be started in Parkinson disease? *Neurology.* 2009;72(7 Suppl):S39–43.

Moore TJ, Glenmullen J, Mattison DR. Reports of pathological gambling, hypersexuality, and compulsive shopping associated with dopamine receptor agonist drugs. *JAMA Intern Med.* 2014;174(12): 1930–3.

Varga LI, Ako-Agugua N, Colasante J, Hertweck L, Houser T, Smith J, et al. Critical review of ropinirole and pramipexole-putative dopamine D(3)-receptor selective agonists-for the treatment of RLS. *J Clin Pharm Ther.* 2009;34(5): 493–505.

Weiner WJ. Early diagnosis of Parkinson's disease and initiation of treatment. *Rev Neurol Dis.* 2008;5(2):46–53; quiz 54–5.

ROTIGOTINE TRANSDERMAL SYSTEM

THERAPEUTICS

Brands
- Neupro

Generic?
- No

Class
- Antiparkinson agent

Commonly Prescribed for
(FDA approved in bold)
- **Symptoms and signs of Parkinson's disease (PD)**
- **Moderate to severe primary restless legs syndrome (RLS)**
- Depression

How the Drug Works
- Dopamine agonist, with high affinity for D_1, D_2, D_3 (ratio 1:12:387) receptors. It binds weakly to α_2-adrenergic receptors. The antiparkinson action is likely due to D_2 agonism within the caudate-putamen. High affinity to D_3 receptors might affect impulse control and dyskinesia. The mechanism of action for RLS is probably related to D_2 or D_3 receptor agonism

How Long Until It Works
- PD: weeks
- RLS: days to weeks

If It Works
- PD: may require dose adjustments over time or augmentation with other agents. Most PD patients will eventually require carbidopa-levodopa to manage their symptoms
- RLS: safe for long-term use with dose adjustments

If It Doesn't Work
- PD: bradykinesia, gait, and tremor should improve. Non-motor symptoms including orthostatic hypotension, depression, and bladder dysfunction do not improve. If the patient has significantly impaired functioning, add carbidopa-levodopa
- RLS: rule out peripheral neuropathy, iron deficiency, thyroid disease. Change to

another drug such as a benzodiazepine. Gabapentin enacarbil (not gabapentin) may also be beneficial. In severe cases consider opioids

Best Augmenting Combos for Partial Response or Treatment-Resistance
- For suboptimal effectiveness add carbidopa-levodopa with or without a catechol-*O*-methyltransferase (COMT) inhibitor. Monoamine oxidase (MAO)-B inhibitors may also be beneficial
- For severe motor fluctuations and/or dyskinesias with good "on" time, functional neurosurgery is an option
- For RLS, can change to a different dopamine agonist (pramipexole, ropinirole, carbidopa-levodopa) or add another drug such as a clonazepam or gabapentin enacarbil. In severe cases consider opioids

Tests
- None required

ADVERSE EFFECTS (AEs)

How the Drug Causes AEs
- Direct effect on systemic dopamine receptors

Notable AEs
- Nausea, vomiting, somnolence, headache, application site reactions, dizziness, anorexia, hyperhidrosis, insomnia, peripheral edema, and dyskinesia

Life-Threatening or Dangerous AEs
- May cause somnolence or sudden-onset sleep, often without warning
- Hallucinations/psychotic-like behavior
- Symptomatic postural hypotension, hypertension, arrhythmia, and syncope
- Impulse control, compulsive behavior

Weight Gain
- Unusual

unusual   not unusual   common   problematic

Sedation
- Common

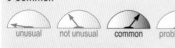

unusual　　not unusual　　**common**　　problematic

What to Do About AEs
- Nausea can be problematic when initiating drug – titrate slowly
- Hallucinations or delusions may require stopping the medication
- Warn patients about the risks of sleeping while driving

Best Augmenting Agents to Reduce AEs
- Amantadine may help suppress dyskinesias
- Orthostatic hypotension: adjust dose or stop antihypertensives, add supplemental salt, and consider fludrocortisone, midodrine, droxidopa
- Urinary incontinence: reducing PM fluids, voiding schedules, oxybutynin, desmopressin nasal spray, hyoscyamine sulfate, urological evaluation

DOSING AND USE

Usual Dosage Range
- PD: 2–8mg/24h
- RLS: 1–3mg/24h

Dosage Forms
- Patch: 1, 2, 3, 4, 6, 8mg/24h

How to Dose
PD:
- Initial: 2mg/24h (early PD), 4mg/24h (advanced PD)
- Titration: 2mg weekly
- Maximum: 6mg/24h (early PD), 8mg/24h (advanced PD)

RLS:
- Initial: 1mg/24h
- Titration 1mg weekly
- Maximum: 3mg/24h

 Dosing Tips
- Slow titration will minimize nausea and dizziness, as well as preventing neuroleptic malignant syndrome. No impact from food

Overdose
- Symptoms include somnolence, agitation, orthostatic hypotension, abdominal pain, nausea, dyskinesias, hallucinations, confusion, convulsions. For cases of excessive CNS stimulation, neuroleptics can be effective

Long-Term Use
- Safe for long-term use. Effectiveness may decrease over time in PD (years) and RLS (months)

Habit Forming
- No

How to Stop
- PD: 2mg/24h every other day
- RLS: 1mg/24h every other day

Pharmacokinetics
- 4% released within 24 hours with shoulder having the higher bioavailability. 90% protein bound. Metabolized extensively via multiple pathways. Half-life 5–7 hours. Excreted in urine (70%) and feces (23%)

 Drug Interactions
- The multiple metabolic pathways render rotigotine less prone to drug interaction

 Other Warnings/ Precautions
- Dopamine agonists can precipitate impulse control disorders, such as pathological gambling, hypersexuality, and compulsive shopping

Do Not Use
- History of hypersensitivity to rotigotine or components of the transdermal patch

SPECIAL POPULATIONS

Renal Impairment
- There were no relevant changes in rotigotine plasma concentrations (up to end-stage renal disease requiring hemodialysis). In subjects with severe renal impairment not on dialysis (CrCl < 30mL/min), exposure to

conjugated rotigotine metabolites was doubled

Hepatic Impairment

- There were no relevant changes in rotigotine plasma concentrations in subjects with moderate hepatic impairment (Child-Pugh Classification B). No information is available on subjects with severe impairment of hepatic function

Cardiac Impairment

- No QTc prolongation

Elderly

- Although not studied, exposures in older subjects (> 80 years) may be higher due to skin changes with aging

Children and Adolescents

- Safety and effectiveness in pediatric patients for any indication have not been established

Pregnancy

- Category C. Teratogenic in some animal studies. Use only if benefits of medication outweigh risks

Breast Feeding

- Inhibits prolactin secretion and may also inhibit lactation. Unknown if excreted in breast milk

THE ART OF NEUROPHARMACOLOGY

Potential Advantages

- PD: may delay need for carbidopa-levodopa and decreases risk of motor dyskinesia due to sustained release. This is especially important in younger PD patients
- RLS: less risk of dependence compared to opioids or benzodiazepines and less augmentation than levodopa

Potential Disadvantages

- Less effective than carbidopa-levodopa for PD with more AEs such as hallucinations, somnolence, and orthostatic hypotension. Patients with significant motor disability will require carbidopa-levodopa. Risk of impulse control disorders

Primary Target Symptoms

- PD: motor dysfunction including bradykinesia, hand function, gait and rest tremor
- RLS: pain, insomnia

Pearls

- Rotigotine shows similar efficacy to dopamine agonists in early or advanced PD
- Efficacious for symptomatic monotherapy, adjunct to levodopa, and treatment of motor fluctuation
- Excellent drug for young patients with early PD. Favorable long-term AEs
- First-line treatment for RLS with less augmentation or "rebound" than carbidopa-levodopa. Non-ergot dopamine agonists are probably equally effective in treating RLS
- For younger patients with bothersome tremor: anticholinergics may help
- Depression is common in PD and may respond to TCAs, pramipexole, or agomelatine
- Dopamine agonists may have antidepressant effects
- Cognitive impairment/dementia is common in mid- to late-stage PD and may improve with acetylcholinesterase inhibitors in short term
- For patients with late-stage PD experiencing hallucinations or delusions, withdraw rotigotine and consider atypical neuroleptics (clozapine, quetiapine). Acute psychosis is a medical emergency that may require hospitalization and low-dose haloperidol
- For orthostatic hypotension, droxidopa can be used
- For patients with mildly symptomatic disease, dopamine agonists are also appropriate for initial therapy, but for patients with significant disability, use carbidopa-levodopa early

Suggested Reading

Fox SH, Katzenschlager R, Lim S-Y, Ravina B, Seppi K, Coelho M, et al. The Movement Disorder Society Evidence-Based Medicine Review Update: Treatments for the motor symptoms of Parkinson's disease. *Mov Disord.* 2011;26 Suppl 3:S2–41.

Giladi N, Boroojerdi B, Korczyn AD, Burn DJ, Clarke CE, Schapira AHV, et al. Rotigotine transdermal patch in early Parkinson's disease: a randomized, double-blind, controlled study versus placebo and ropinirole. *Mov Disord.* 2007;22(16): 2398–404.

Poewe WH, Rascol O, Quinn N, Tolosa E, Oertel WH, Martignoni E, et al. Efficacy of pramipexole and transdermal rotigotine in advanced Parkinson's disease: a double-blind, double-dummy, randomised controlled trial. *Lancet Neurol.* 2007;6(6):513–20.

Reynolds NA, Wellington K, Easthope SE. Rotigotine. *CNS Drugs.* 2005;19(11):973–81.

Trenkwalder C, Beneš H, Poewe W, Oertel WH, Garcia-Borreguero D, de Weerd AW, et al. Efficacy of rotigotine for treatment of moderate-to-severe restless legs syndrome: a randomised, double-blind, placebo-controlled trial. *Lancet Neurol.* 2008;7(7):595–604.

Trenkwalder C, Kies B, Rudzinska M, Fine J, Nikl J, Honczarenko K, et al. Rotigotine effects on early morning motor function and sleep in Parkinson's disease: a double-blind, randomized, placebo-controlled study (RECOVER). *Mov Disord.* 2011;26(1):90–9.

RUFINAMIDE

THERAPEUTICS

Brands
- Banzel, Inovelon

Generic?
- No

Class
- Antiepileptic drug (AED)

Commonly Prescribed for
(FDA approved in bold)
- **Adjunctive therapy for Lennox-Gastaut syndrome (LGS) in patients 4 years and older**
- Tonic or atonic seizure
- Refractory bipolar disorder

How the Drug Works
- The exact mechanism is unknown but likely related to modulation of sodium channel activity and membrane stabilization. Rufinamide prolongs the inactive state of the sodium channel

How Long Until It Works
- Seizures: should decrease by 2 weeks

If It Works
- Seizures: goal is the remission of seizures. Continue as long as effective and well tolerated

If It Doesn't Work
- Increase to highest tolerated dose
- Epilepsy: consider changing to another agent, adding a second agent, using a medical device, or a referral for epilepsy surgery evaluation. When adding a second agent, keep drug interactions in mind

Best Augmenting Combos for Partial Response or Treatment-Resistance
- Generally used adjunctively in combination with other AEDs for refractory epilepsy

Tests
- No regular blood tests are recommended

ADVERSE EFFECTS (AEs)

How the Drug Causes AEs
- CNS AEs are probably caused by effects on sodium channels

Notable AEs
- Somnolence, fatigue, coordination abnormalities, anorexia, nausea/vomiting, headache, dizziness, tremor, nasopharyngitis, influenza

Life-Threatening or Dangerous AEs
- Suicidal ideation
- Blood dyscrasias including leukopenia
- Bundle branch and first-degree AV block infrequently occurred in clinical trials but the relationship of this to rufinamide is unclear
- Multi-organ hypersensitivity syndrome

Weight Gain
- Unusual

unusual   not unusual   common   problematic

Sedation
- Not unusual

unusual   not unusual   common   problematic

What to Do About AEs
- Decrease dose
- Taking drug in *fasting* state will lower absorption and may reduce both AEs and effectiveness

Best Augmenting Agents to Reduce AEs
- Most AEs cannot be reduced by use of augmenting agent

DOSING AND USE

Usual Dosage Range
- Epilepsy: 1600–3200 mg/day in adults

Dosage Forms
- Tablets: 200 or 400 mg

How to Dose

- Start at a daily dose of 400–800 mg/day in 2 divided doses. Increase dose by 400–800 mg/day every 2 days until a maximum of 3200 mg/day in 2 divided doses. Typical dose is 3200 mg

Dosing Tips

- Drug absorption is significantly enhanced by taking with food
- Tablet is easily crushed and given with food

Overdose

- Unknown effect. Use induction of emesis or gastric lavage to remove drug. Hemodialysis will help remove some drug

Long-Term Use

- Safe for long-term use

Habit Forming

- No

How to Stop

- Taper slowly (25% of dose every 2 days)
- Abrupt withdrawal can lead to seizures in patients with epilepsy

Pharmacokinetics

- Extensive hepatic metabolism but not via CYP450 system. Half-life is 6–10 hours and peak levels at 4–6 hours. Food increases absorption. Protein binding is 34%. Renally excreted

Drug Interactions

- Rufinamide has no significant effect on CYP450 enzymes. It is a weak inhibitor of CYP2E1 and a weak inducer of CYP3A4 enzymes but does not typically change concentrations of other medications
- May lower carbamazepine and lamotrigine levels; may increase phenobarbital, phenytoin, and valproic acid levels
- Half-life of drug is lower when using with phenytoin or carbamazepine compared to valproate. Valproate can increase rufinamide concentration up to 70%
- Lowers levels of oral contraceptives by about 20%

Other Warnings/ Precautions

- All patients who develop a rash while taking rufinamide must be closely supervised

Do Not Use

- Patients with a proven allergy to rufinamide or familial short QT syndrome

Renal Impairment

- No dose adjustments needed, but hemodialysis will remove some of the drug

Hepatic Impairment

- No known effects but use with severe disease is not recommended

Cardiac Impairment

- QTc interval shortening. Patients with familial short QT syndrome should not be treated with rufinamide

Elderly

- No known effects

Children and Adolescents

- Approved for use in children 4 and older with LGS
- Start at 10 mg/kg/day in 2 divided doses. Increase by about 10 mg/kg every other day as tolerated to effective dose. Maximum 3200 mg/day or 45 mg/kg/day (whichever is less)

Pregnancy

- Category C. Use only if risks of stopping drug outweigh potential risk to fetus
- Supplementation with 0.4 mg of folic acid before and during pregnancy is recommended

Breast Feeding

- Some drug found in mother's breast milk
- Consider discontinuing drug or bottle feeding

- Monitor infant for sedation, poor feeding, or irritability

THE ART OF NEUROPHARMACOLOGY

Potential Advantages

- Effective in refractory epilepsy, safe to use with other AEDs and wide therapeutic window

Potential Disadvantages

- Few indications and lack of evidence for the treatment of many types of epilepsy, including patients with generalized and complex partial seizures. Unknown effectiveness as monotherapy

Primary Target Symptoms

- Seizure frequency and severity

 Pearls

- Second- or third-line agent in refractory epilepsy. Lack of drug interactions and wide therapeutic index with unique structure (tiazole derivative). Often LGS is not amenable to surgery so multiple AED regimens are common
- In trials of rufinamide in subjects with LGS seizures decreased by over 30% and atonic seizures ("drop attacks") decreased by over 40%. Drop attacks are a major source of injury in LGS
- For LGS treatment, only rufinamide, topiramate, felbamate, lamotrigine are among the alternatives
- In patients with treatment-resistant partial-onset seizures, rufinamide reduced seizure frequency by over 20% from baseline as adjunctive therapy

 Suggested Reading

Coppola G, Besag F, Cusmai R, Dulac O, Kluger G, Moavero R, Nabbout R, Nikanorova M, Pisani F, Verrotti A, et al. Current role of rufinamide in the treatment of childhood epilepsy: literature review and treatment guidelines. *Eur J Paediatr Neurol* 2014;18:685–90.

Ferrie CD, Patel A. Treatment of Lennox-Gastaut Syndrome (LGS). *Eur J Paediatr Neurol.* 2009;13(6):493–504.

Perucca E, Cloyd J, Critchley D, Fuseau E. Rufinamide: clinical pharmacokinetics and concentration-response relationships in patients with epilepsy. *Epilepsia.* 2008;49(7):1123–41.

SELEGILINE

THERAPEUTICS

Brands
- Zelapar, Eldepryl, Emsam

Generic?
- Yes (as oral)

Class
- Antiparkinson agent

Commonly Prescribed for
(FDA approved in bold)
- **Parkinson's disease (PD)**
- **Major depressive disorder, treatment-refractory (patch only)**
- Restless legs syndrome
- Anxiety disorders
- Alzheimer's and other dementias
- Migraine

How the Drug Works
- Selectively and irreversibly blocks monoamine oxidase type B (MAO-B) and increases extrastriatal extracellular dopamine levels. MAO-B is inhibited for at least 24 hours and the activity returns to baseline after 2 weeks. At higher doses, starts to affect MAO-A as well as MAO-B and inhibits metabolism of norepinephrine, serotonin, and tyramine, as well as dopamine

How Long Until It Works
- PD: weeks
- Depression, anxiety: usually months

If It Works
- PD: may require dose adjustments over time or augmentation with other agents. Most PD patients will eventually require carbidopa-levodopa to manage their symptoms

If It Doesn't Work
- Bradykinesia, gait, and tremor should improve. If the patient has significantly impaired functioning, add carbidopa-levodopa with or without a dopamine agonist

Best Augmenting Combos for Partial Response or Treatment-Resistance
- For suboptimal effectiveness, add carbidopa-levodopa with or without a catechol-*O*-methyl transferase (COMT) inhibitor or a dopamine agonist
- For younger patients with bothersome tremor: anticholinergics may help
- For severe motor fluctuations and/or dyskinesias with good "on" time, functional neurosurgery is an option

Tests
- Monitor for any changes in blood pressure

ADVERSE EFFECTS (AEs)

How the Drug Causes AEs
- Increases concentration of peripheral and CNS dopamine. At higher doses affects serotonin and norepinephrine levels

Notable AEs
- Nausea, hallucinations, confusion, lightheadedness, loss of balance, insomnia, orthostatic hypotension, hypertension, weight gain

Life-Threatening or Dangerous AEs
- Hypertensive crisis, especially at higher doses that prevent breakdown of tyramine (via MAO-A mostly). Tyramine-containing foods include aged cheeses, liver, sauerkraut, cured and processed meats, soy, alcohol (especially chianti wine and vermouth), and avocado

Weight Gain
- Common

unusual / not unusual / common / problematic

Sedation
- Unusual

unusual / not unusual / common / problematic

What to Do About AEs
- Lower the dose or change to alternative PD medications

Best Augmenting Agents to Reduce AEs
- Orthostatic hypotension: adjust dose or stop antihypertensives, add supplemental salt, and consider fludrocortisone or midodrine

DOSING AND USE

Usual Dosage Range
- PD: 10mg daily, divided into 2 daily doses taken at breakfast and lunch
- Depression: only the transdermal patch is indicated for the treatment of depression

Dosage Forms
- Tablets: 5mg
- Capsules: 5mg
- Orally disintegrating tablets: 1.25mg
- Transdermal patch: 6, 9, or 12mg/24 h

How to Dose
- Regular tablets: start at 2.5mg (regular tablets) twice daily (usually at breakfast and lunch) and increase to 5mg twice a day in a few days if tolerated. When concomitant therapy with carbidopa-levodopa, after 3–4 days, an attempt may be made to lower dose of carbidopa-levodopa
- Orally disintegrating tablets: start at 1.25mg in the morning before breakfast, and increase to 2.5mg daily if tolerated and desired benefit not achieved
- Transdermal patch: start at 6mg/24 h. Increase every 2 weeks until desired effect achieved in 3mg increments to a maximum of 12mg/day

 Dosing Tips
- Take orally disintegrating tablets before breakfast
- At doses above 10mg, selegiline starts to become less selective and starts to have more MAO-A inhibition. This increases the risk of hypertensive crisis

Overdose
- Symptoms include dizziness, insomnia, hypotension or hypertension, headache, sedation, respiratory depression, and death. Symptoms of overdose can be delayed up to 12 hours, and maximal worsening may not occur until the next day

Long-Term Use
- Safe for long-term use. Effectiveness may decrease over time in PD

Habit Forming
- No

How to Stop
- No need to taper. Drug wears off in 2–3 weeks

Pharmacokinetics
- Orally disintegrating tablets (T_{max} 10–15 minutes) have a more rapid absorption and greater bioavailability than the swallowed tablets (T_{max} 40–90 minutes). The 2.5mg disintegrating tablets have an effect similar to 10mg of the regular tablets. Hepatic metabolism involving CYP2B6 and CYP3A4. Active metabolites include K-desmethylselegiline, L-methamphetamine, and L-amphetamine. 85% of metabolites are then excreted in the urine. Half-life is 1.5–2 hours. 75–79% protein bound

 Drug Interactions
- Increases the effect of levodopa, potentially requiring dose adjustments
- Multiple adverse CNS reactions reported when used with meperidine, including convulsions, coma, and death. Do not use meperidine within 2 weeks of drug
- Other analgesics, including methadone, tramadol, propoxyphene, and dextromethorphan, may also cause reactions
- Do not use within 2 weeks of TCAs, SSRIs, or SNRIs due to risk of serotonin syndrome (hyperthermia, myoclonus, rigidity, autonomic instability, mental status changes, or death). Do not use within 5 weeks of fluoxetine
- Tramadol can increase risk of seizures

- Dopamine antagonists such as phenothiazines, metoclopramide may diminish effectiveness
- Use with caution in patients on antihypertensive medications due to risk of orthostatic hypotension
- At higher, non-selective doses can potentially interact with CNS stimulants due to amphetamine metabolites. These include IV dopamine, norepinephrine and epinephrine, methylphenidate, nasal decongestants, sinus medications, asthma inhalers, diet pills or weight loss treatments, and even levodopa

 Other Warnings/ Precautions

- Orally disintegrating tablets contain phenylalanine

Do Not Use

- Known hypersensitivity to the drug. Patients using meperidine, TCAs, SSRIs, SNRIs, linezolid, and methylene blue

Renal Impairment

- No known effects

Hepatic Impairment

- May require lowering of dose

Cardiac Impairment

- No known effects

Elderly

- Start at a lower dose with careful titration. More likely to experience AEs

 Children and Adolescents

- Not studied in children (PD is rare in pediatrics) and not recommended under age 16

 Pregnancy

- Category C. Use only if benefits of medication outweigh risks

Breast Feeding

- Unknown if excreted in breast milk. Do not use

Potential Advantages

- May delay need for carbidopa-levodopa or allow reduction of dose. Good initial treatment for patients with no cognitive dysfunction and significant disability. Better tolerated (less nausea) than dopamine agonists. May be useful for PD patients with comorbid depression

Potential Disadvantages

- Less effective than most PD treatments, including dopamine agonists, for motor dysfunction. Patients with significant motor disability, cognitive impairment, or patients older than 75 will require carbidopa-levodopa. Multiple drug interactions at doses greater than 10 mg limit titration and effectiveness

Primary Target Symptoms

- PD: motor dysfunction, including bradykinesia, hand function, gait and rest tremor

 Pearls

- Well-tolerated medication for PD with favorable long-term AEs. Selegiline (oral) is effective for controlling motor symptoms as monotherapy or adjunctive to levodopa. It can delay the need for levodopa. There is insufficient evidence for treatment of motor fluctuation
- Orally disintegrating tablet, with reduced presystemic metabolism, provides higher plasma concentration and lower amphetamine metabolites. At this moment, orally disintegrating selegiline remains investigational for symptomatic treatment of PD. It may be more preferable than selegiline tablet in certain patients but clinical difference remains unclear
- It delays the requirement of levodopa treatment, hence delays the development of drug-induced motor complications from levodopa. However, it does not prevent or

delay PD progression. MAOIs have drawn interest as possible neuroprotective agents in PD. Selegiline delays the need for levodopa compared to placebo, but this could be due to the symptomatic benefit of the drug. Newer studies of neuroprotection are evaluating rasagiline, another MAO-B inhibitor, which does not have methamphetamine as a metabolite

- Combination of levodopa and selegiline may improve cognition and affective measures more than levodopa monotherapy. Cognitive impairment/dementia is common in mid- to late-stage PD and may improve with acetylcholinesterase inhibitors
- For patients with late-stage PD experiencing hallucinations or delusions, consider oral atypical neuroleptics (quetiapine, clozapine). Acute psychosis is a medical emergency that may require hospitalization and short-term use of neuroleptics such as low-dose haloperidol
- May be useful in combination with other agents, such as donepezil, for the treatment of Alzheimer's dementia (AD). However, Cochrane review of selegiline found no evidence for its efficacy in AD
- For depression, use the transdermal patch. For PD, use oral selegiline
- At a dose of 10mg or less, the drug is selective for MAO-B and dietary restrictions do not come into play. Selegiline at therapeutic doses does not cause the so-called "cheese effect"
- Insufficient evidence for use in treating tardive dyskinesia

Suggested Reading

Birks J, Flicker L. Selegiline for Alzheimer's disease. *Cochrane Database Syst Rev.* 2003;1: CD000442.

Fabbrini G, Abbruzzese G, Marconi S, Zappia M. Selegiline: a reappraisal of its role in Parkinson disease. *Clin Neuropharmacol.* 2012;35:134–40.

Fox SH, Katzenschlager R, Lim S-Y, Ravina B, Seppi K, Coelho M, et al. The Movement Disorder Society Evidence-Based Medicine Review Update: Treatments for the motor symptoms of Parkinson's disease. *Mov Disord.* 2011;26 Suppl 3:S2–S41.

Krishna R, Ali M, Moustafa AA. Effects of combined MAO-B inhibitors and levodopa vs. monotherapy in Parkinson's disease. *Front Aging Neurosci.* 2014; 6:180.

SODIUM OXYBATE

THERAPEUTICS

Brands
- Xyrem

Generic?
- No (Available only through Xyrem Success Program)

Class
- Psychostimulant

Commonly Prescribed for
(FDA approved in bold)
- **Cataplexy in narcolepsy**
- **Excessive daytime sleepiness (EDS) in narcolepsy**
- Alcohol withdrawal
- Fibromyalgia
- Cluster headache

How the Drug Works
- Sodium oxybate, sodium 4-hydroxybutyrate, is the sodium salt of an endogenous cerebral neurotransmitter gamma-hydroxybutyric acid (GHB). It binds to GHB receptor (excitatory) and weakly to $GABA_B$ receptor (inhibitory). At high concentrations it inhibits noradrenergic, dopaminergic, serotonergic, and cholinergic neurons. At low concentrations it stimulates dopamine release. Its mechanism of action is mediated primarily through $GABA_B$ receptors. It increases slow wave activity during non-REM sleep. It simultaneously alleviates cataplexy, EDS and nocturnal sleep disruption, and consolidates wakefulness

How Long Until It Works
- 5–15 minutes

If It Works
- Continue to use at lowest effective dose. Monitor for risk of altered mental alertness, depression, confusion, and parasomnia

If It Doesn't Work
- Re-evaluate treatment of underlying cause of narcolepsy and cataplexy. Consider adding armodafinil or venlafaxine

Best Augmenting Combos for Partial Response or Treatment-Resistance
- May add armodafinil for excessive sleepiness. May add venlafaxine for cataplexy

Tests
- None required

ADVERSE EFFECTS (AEs)

How the Drug Causes AEs
- Unknown but most AEs are likely related to drug actions on CNS neurotransmitters

Notable AEs
- Nausea, dizziness, vomiting, somnolence, enuresis, confusion, tremor, parasomnia, weight loss, memory impairment

Life-Threatening or Dangerous AEs
- Concomitant use of CNS depressants may increase the risk of respiratory depression
- Suicidality
- Abuse potential (seizure, death)
- Central apnea
- Psychosis and hallucinations have been reported

Weight Gain
- Unusual

unusual   not unusual   common   problematic

Sedation
- Common

unusual   not unusual   common   problematic

What to Do About AEs
- Lower the dose

Best Augmenting Agents to Reduce AEs
- Most AEs do not respond to adding other medications

DOSING AND USE

Usual Dosage Range
- Excessive daytime sleepiness/cataplexy: 6–9 g/night

Dosage Forms
- Oral solution: 0.5 g/mL

How to Dose
- Start at 4.5 g/night in divided doses. One at bedtime and another 2.5–4 hours later
- Titrate 1.5 g/night at weekly interval
- Optimal 6–9 g/night

 Dosing Tips
- Take each dose while in bed and lie down after dosing
- Allow 2 hours after eating before dosing
- Prepare both doses prior to bedtime

Overdose
- Coingestion of alcohol and other drugs is common. Varying degree of CNS depression, apnea, bradycardia, and incontinence. No antidote

Long-Term Use
- Long-term use appears safe. The effect on central apnea is not determined

Habit Forming
- Schedule III substance (active metabolite gamma hydroxybutyric acid is a schedule I substance). Through Xyrem Success Program, only 5 incidents of diversion in approximately 600 000 bottles delivered

How to Stop
- Withdrawal is not problematic. May be associated with anxiety, insomnia

Pharmacokinetics
- Hydrophilic compound. < 1% plasma protein bound. Almost entirely transformed to carbon dioxide. Half-life is 0.5–1 hour

 Drug Interactions
- Divalproex sodium increases its serum concentration
- No CYP450 interaction

 Other Warnings/ Precautions
- Patients should not engage in hazardous occupations or activities requiring complete mental alertness or motor coordination
- Patients should be queried about CNS depression-related events upon initiation of Xyrem therapy and periodically thereafter
- High sodium content that could affect patients with heart failure or impaired renal function

Do Not Use
- Succinic semialdehyde dehydrogenase deficiency (a rare inborn error)
- In combination with sedative hypnotics or alcohol

SPECIAL POPULATIONS

Renal Impairment
- Not studied

Hepatic Impairment
- The starting dose should be reduced by one-half in cirrhotic patients

Cardiac Impairment
- High sodium content may exacerbate heart failure or hypertension

Elderly
- Monitor for impaired motor and/or cognitive function

 Children and Adolescents
- Not studied in children under 18

 Pregnancy
- Category C. Generally not used in pregnancy

Breast Feeding
- Unknown if excreted in breast milk. Do not use

THE ART OF NEUROPHARMACOLOGY

Potential Advantages
- Can be used for both excessive daytime sleepiness and cataplexy

Potential Disadvantages
- Abuse potential

Primary Target Symptoms
- Daytime sleepiness, cataplexy

Pearls
- Short-term use of sodium oxybate does not generate respiratory depression in patients with obstructive sleep apnea

- A randomized trial shows that sodium oxybate significantly decreased alcohol withdrawal symptoms with an efficacy comparable to that of oxazepam
- An international phase III trial demonstrates the association of sleep quality restoration with the multidimensional improvements in fibromyalgia symptoms; restoration of sleep quality should be a therapeutic aim in fibromyalgia
- An open-label trial suggests benefit on myoclonus and essential tremor
- A small open-label study found it to reduce nocturnal and diurnal pain attacks and improve sleep quality in patients with chronic cluster headache

Suggested Reading

Alshaikh MK, Tricco AC, Tashkandi M, Mamdani M, Straus SE, BaHammam AS. Sodium oxybate for narcolepsy with cataplexy: systematic review and meta-analysis. *J Clin Sleep Med.* 2012; 8(4):451–8.

Aran A, Einen M, Lin L, Plazzi G, Nishino S, Mignot E. Clinical and therapeutic aspects of childhood narcolepsy-cataplexy: a retrospective study of 51 children. *Sleep.* 2010;33(11): 1457–64.

Caputo F, Skala K, Mirijello A, Ferrulli A, Walter H, Lesch O, et al. Sodium oxybate in the treatment of alcohol withdrawal syndrome: a randomized double-blind comparative study versus oxazepam. The GATE 1 trial. *CNS Drugs.* 2014;28(8):743–52.

Dauvilliers Y, Arnulf I, Mignot E. Narcolepsy with cataplexy. *Lancet.* 2007;369(9560):499–511.

Frucht SJ, Houghton WC, Bordelon Y, Greene PE, Louis ED. A single-blind, open-label trial of sodium oxybate for myoclonus and essential tremor. *Neurology.* 2005;65(12):1967–9.

Khatami R, Tartarotti S, Siccoli MM, Bassetti CL, Sándor PS. Long-term efficacy of sodium oxybate in 4 patients with chronic cluster headache. *Neurology.* 2011;77(1):67–70.

Spaeth M, Bennett RM, Benson BA, Wang YG, Lai C, Choy EH. Sodium oxybate therapy provides multidimensional improvement in fibromyalgia: results of an international phase 3 trial. *Ann Rheum Dis.* 2012;71(6):935–42.

SUMATRIPTAN, SUMATRIPTAN/NAPROXEN

Brands

- Sumatriptan: Imitrex, Imitrex Statdose, Sumavel DosePro, Imigran, Zecuity, Alsuma
- Sumatriptan/naproxen: Treximet

Generic?

- Yes (depending on formulation)

 Class

- Triptan

Commonly Prescribed for

(FDA approved in bold)
- **Acute treatment of migraine in adults**
- **Cluster headache (injection only)**
- Acute treatment of migraine in adolescents

 How the Drug Works

- Selective 5-HT$_{1B/1D/1F}$ receptor agonist. In addition to vasoconstriction of meningeal vessels, its antinociceptive effect is likely due to blocking the transmission of pain signals at trigeminal nerve terminals (preventing the release of inflammatory neuropeptides) and synapses of second-order neurons in trigeminal nucleus caudalis
- Naproxen is a NSAID (cyclo-oxygenase inhibitor), which inhibits synthesis of prostaglandins, a mediator of inflammation

How Long Until It Works

- Oral or nasal spray: 1 hour or less. SC: within 10–30 minutes

If It Works

- Continue to take as needed. Patients taking acute treatment more than 2 days/week are at risk for medication-overuse headache, especially if they have migraine

If It Doesn't Work

- Treat early in the attack – triptans are less likely to work after the headache becomes moderate or severe, regardless of cutaneous allodynia, which is a marker of central sensitization
- Address life style issues (e.g., stress, sleep hygiene), medication use issues (e.g.,

compliance, overuse), and other underlying medical conditions
- Change to higher dosage, another triptan, another administration route, or combination of other medications. Add preventive medication when needed
- For patients with partial response or reoccurrence, other rescue medications include NSAIDs (e.g., ketorolac, naproxen), antiemetic (e.g., prochlorperazine, metoclopramide), neuroleptics (e.g., haloperidol, chlorpromazine), ergots, antihistamine, or corticosteroid

 Best Augmenting Combos for Partial Response or Treatment-Resistance

- NSAIDs or neuroleptics are often used to augment response
- Use sumatriptan/naproxen combination

Tests

- None required

How the Drug Causes AEs

- Direct effect on systemic serotonin receptors (e.g., 5-HT$_{1B}$ agonism on vasoconstriction)

Notable AEs

- Injection site reaction/pain (SC), bad taste (nasal spray), tingling, flushing, sensation of burning, dizziness, sensation of pressure, heaviness, nausea
- Sumatriptan/naproxen: includes NSAID AEs such as dyspepsia, fluid retention, GI distress

 Life-Threatening or Dangerous AEs

- Serotonin syndrome. Rare cardiac events including acute myocardial infarction, cardiac arrhthymias, and coronary artery vasospasm have been reported with sumatriptan
- Sumatriptan/naproxen: GI bleed, renal insufficiency, inhibition of platelet aggregation

Weight Gain
- Unusual

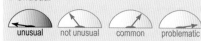

Sedation
- Unusual

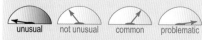

What to Do About AEs
- In most cases, only reassurance is needed. Lower dose, change to the oral form if AE with SC injection, change to another triptan, or use an alternative headache treatment

Best Augmenting Agents to Reduce AEs
- Treatment of nausea with antiemetics is acceptable. Other AEs decrease with time

DOSING AND USE

Usual Dosage Range
- 25–100 mg, maximum 200 mg/day (oral)

Dosage Forms
- Tablets: 25, 50, and 100 mg
- Nasal spray: 5 and 20 mg
- SC injection (Imitrex): 4 and 6 mg per 0.5 mL cartridges for STATdose pen, 6 mg vial
- SC injection (Sumavel DosePro): 4 and 6 mg single-dose, needle-free delivery system
- Iontophoretic transdermal (Zecuity): 6.5 mg 4-hour release
- Sumatriptan/naproxen: 85/550 mg

How to Dose
- Tablets: most patients respond best at 100 mg oral dose. Give 1 pill at the onset of an attack and repeat in 2 hours for a partial response or if the headache returns. Maximum 200 mg/day (2 tablets). Limit 10 days/month
- Nasal spray: one 6.5 mg per 4 hours. Limit 2 in 24 hours
- Transdermal: one 6.5 mg per 2 hours. Limit 2 in 24 hours

- SC injections: 1–6 mg single dose (migraine), 6 mg single dose (cluster headache). May repeat injections in 1 hour. Maximum 12 mg/day

 Dosing Tips
- Treat early in attack. For patients with cluster use SC. For patients with significant nausea/vomiting consider SC or nasal spray

Overdose
- May cause hypertension, cardiovascular symptoms. Other possible symptoms include seizure, tremor, extremity erythema, cyanosis, or ataxia. For patients with angina, perform ECG and monitor for ischemia for at least 10 hours

Long-Term Use
- Monitor for cardiac risk factors with continued use

Habit Forming
- No

How to Stop
- No need to taper. Patients who overuse triptans often experience withdrawal headaches lasting up to several days

Pharmacokinetics
- Half-life 2.5 hours. T_{max} for SC 10–15 minutes, nasal spray 60–90 minutes, orally 60–120 minutes, and sumatriptan/naproxen 60 minutes. Bioavailability is 96% for SC, 14–20% for nasal spray and oral. Metabolism mostly by monoamine oxidase (MAO)-A isoenzyme. 14–21% protein binding

 Drug Interactions
- MAOIs affect the serum concentration of sumatriptan
- Naproxen can inhibit P-glycoprotein, which is an efflux pump, leading to reduced therapeutic threshold and increased toxicity profile

 Other Warnings/ Precautions
- Patients with coronary artery disease should undergo periodic evaluation

- Overuse of triptans may lead to exacerbation of headache

Do Not Use

- Patients with proven hypersensitivity to sumatriptan or naproxen
- Within 2 weeks of MAO-A inhibitors, or within 24 hours of ergot-containing medications such as dihydroergotamine
- History of stroke, transient ischemic attack, hemiplegic/basilar migraine, Wolff-Parkinson-White syndrome, peripheral vascular disease, ischemic heart disease, coronary artery vasospasm, ischemic bowel disease, and uncontrolled hypertension

SPECIAL POPULATIONS

Renal Impairment

- Do not use with severe renal impairment (CrCl < 15mL/min). May be at increased cardiovascular risk

Hepatic Impairment

- Drug metabolism decreased with hepatic disease. Do not use with severe hepatic impairment

Cardiac Impairment

- Do not use in patients with known cardiovascular or peripheral vascular disease. May require cardiac stress test or cardiology clearance if tripans are necessary

Elderly

- May be at increased cardiovascular risk. Half-life is longer. Administer first dose in physician's office if needed

 Children and Adolescents

- Triptan trials in children were negative, due to higher placebo response

 Pregnancy

- Category C. Use only if potential benefit outweighs risk to the fetus. Pregnancy registry studies ongoing. Migraine often improves in pregnancy, and other acute agents (opioids, neuroleptics, prednisone) have more proven safety

Breast Feeding

- Sumatriptan is found in breast milk at low levels. Use with caution

THE ART OF NEUROPHARMACOLOGY

Potential Advantages

- Available as SC. Proven for cluster headache. Most studied triptan. Less risk of abuse than opioids or barbiturate-containing treatments. Added efficacy with naproxen-containing formulation

Potential Disadvantages

- Potential for medication-overuse headache, relatively short half-life

Primary Target Symptoms

- Headache pain, nausea, photo and phonophobia

 Pearls

- Early treatment of migraine is most effective
- Compared to other triptans from a meta-analysis, sumatriptan SC has the highest 2-hour headache relief rate (76%, number needed to treat 3). SC sumatriptan is more effective than other triptans, but has the most AEs
- May not be effective when taking during aura, before headache begins
- In patients with "status migrainosus" (migraine lasting more than 72 hours) neuroleptics and dihydroergotamine are more effective
- Triptans were not originally studied for use in the treatment of basilar or hemiplegic migraine
- Triptans can be used to treat tension-type headache in migraineurs but not in patients with pure tension-type headache
- Patients taking triptans more than 10 days/month are at increased risk of medication-overuse headache, which is less responsive to treatment. Patients with cluster headache who have migraine may also be at risk
- Chest and throat tightness are usually benign and may be related to esophageal spasm rather than cardiac ischemia. These symptoms occur more commonly in patients without cardiac risk factors

- Combination use of SNRI and triptans usually will not lead to serotonin syndrome, which requires activation of 5-HT_{2A} receptors and a possible limited role of 5-HT_{1A}. However, triptans are agonists at the $5\text{-HT}_{1B/1D/1F}$ receptor subtypes, with weak affinity for 5-HT_{1A} receptors and no activity at the 5-HT_2 receptors. Thus, given the seriousness of serotonin syndrome, caution is certainly warranted and clinicians should be vigilant for serotonin toxicity symptoms and signs to insure prompt treatment

- High bioavailability and quick absorption of sumatriptan SC injection might account for its relatively higher pain-relieving efficacy. Although the efficacy of slow-releasing transdermal sumatriptan is not as high as SC injection form, it is still superior to its oral form for migraineurs with disabling nausea
- The site of pharmacological action, whether central or peripheral, remains to be studied. Although triptans generally do not penetrate BBB, it has been postulated that transient BBB breakdown may occur during a migraine attack

Suggested Reading

Brandes JL, Kudrow D, Stark SR, O'Carroll CP, Adelman JU, O'Donnell FJ, Alexander WJ, Spruill SE, Barrett PS, Lener SE. Sumatriptan-naproxen for acute treatment of migraine: a randomized trial. *JAMA.* 2007; 297(13):1443–54.

Evans RW, Tepper SJ, Shapiro RE, Sun-Edelstein C, Tietjen GE. The FDA alert on serotonin syndrome with use of triptans combined with selective serotonin reuptake inhibitors or selective serotonin-norepinephrine reuptake inhibitors: American Headache Society position paper. *Headache.* 2010;50(6):1089–99.

Ferrari MD, Roon KI, Lipton RB, Goadsby PJ. Oral triptans (serotonin 5-HT(1B/1D) agonists)) in acute migraine treatment: a meta-analysis of 53 trials. *Lancet.* 2001;358(9294):1668–75.

Göbel H, Heinze A, Stolze H, Heinze-Kuhn K, Lindner V. Open-labeled long-term study of the efficacy, safety, and tolerability of subcutaneous sumatriptan in acute migraine treatment. *Cephalalgia.* 1999;19(7):676–83; discussion 626.

Scholpp J, Schellenberg R, Moeckesch B, Banik N. Early treatment of a migraine attack while pain is still mild increases the efficacy of sumatriptan. *Cephalalgia.* 2004;24(11):925–33.

SUVOREXANT

THERAPEUTICS

Brands
- Belsomra

Generic?
- No

 Class
- Orexin receptor antagonist

Commonly Prescribed for
(FDA approved in bold)
- **Insomnia characterized by difficulties with sleep onset and/or sleep maintenance**

 How the Drug Works
- Blocks wake-promoting orexin A and orexin B binding to orexin receptor type 1 and type 2 to suppress wake drive. The orexin pathway originates within the lateral hypothalamus and projects to brain nuclei expressing orexin peptide receptors

How Long Until It Works
- Peak concentrations occur around 2 hours

If It Works
- Continue to use at lowest required dose with appropriate monitoring

If It Doesn't Work
- Increase dose or combine with other anti-insomnia agents

 Best Augmenting Combos for Partial Response or Treatment-Resistance
- Often depends on the comorbidity; may use low dose of antihistamine, TCAs, benzodiazepines, or antipsychotics

Tests
- Not available

ADVERSE EFFECTS (AEs)

How the Drug Causes AEs
- CNS depressant

Notable AEs
- Most common: daytime somnolence, abnormal thinking, behavioral change, sleep paralysis, hypnagogic/hypnopompic hallucination, cataplexy-like symptoms

 Life-Threatening or Dangerous AEs
- Complex sleep behavior (e.g., sleep-driving)
- Worsening of depression/suicidal ideation
- Respiratory suppression

Weight Gain
- Unusual

Sedation
- Problematic

What to Do About AEs
- Reduce dose or discontinue

Best Augmenting Agents to Reduce AEs
- Most AEs cannot be reduced by use of augmenting agent

DOSING AND USE

Usual Dosage Range
- Insomnia: 10–20 mg/night

Dosage Forms
- Tablets: 5, 10, 15, 20 mg

How to Dose
- Start with 10 mg within 30 minutes of going to bed, with at least 7 hours remaining before the time of awakening

 Dosing Tips
- Adjust dose to clinical response and AEs. Re-evaluate if insomnia persists after 7–10 days of treatment
- Reduced dose (5 mg) in subjects receiving moderate CYP3A inhibitors (e.g., ciprofloxacin, aprepitant, diltiazem, grapefruit juice, etc.)

Overdose
- Dose-dependent increases in the frequency and duration of somnolence. No antidote available

Long-Term Use
- Safe for long-term use with appropriate monitoring

Habit Forming
- Schedule IV controlled substance. Can become dependent after chronic use but probably less often than benzodiazepines

How to Stop
- No withdrawal or rebound effect

Pharmacokinetics
- Hepatic metabolism via CYP3A and less CYP2C19. > 99% protein bound. Mean half-life 12 hours. 66% excreted in feces and 23% in urine

 ### Drug Interactions
- Use with CNS depressants (ethanol, barbiturates, opiates, general anesthetics) potentiates CNS AEs
- Concentration increased by strong CYP3A inhibitor (ketoconazole, antivirals, clarithromycin, etc.) and moderate CYP3A inhibitors
- Concentration decreased by CYP3A inducer (rifampin, carbamazepine, phenytoin, phenobarbital, dexamethasone, St. John's wort, etc.)
- Slightly increases digoxin level due to inhibition of intestinal P-glycoprotein (P-gp) pump

Other Warnings/ Precautions
- Risk of impaired alertness and motor coordination
- Elevated cholesterol

Do Not Use
- Narcolepsy. Concomitant use of strong CYP3A inhibitor

Renal Impairment
- No dose adjustment needed

Hepatic Impairment
- No dose adjustment needed in mild or moderate hepatic impairment

Cardiac Impairment
- No dose adjustment

Elderly
- No dose adjustment

 ### Children and Adolescents
- Efficacy and safety unknown

 ### Pregnancy
- Category C. Use only if benefit outweighs risks

Breast Feeding
- Caution should be exercised when being administered to a nursing woman

Potential Advantages
- Novel sleep-inducing mechanism involving orexin signaling pathway. Decreases latency to sleep onset and waking after sleep onset without disrupting sleeping architecture. No dose adjustment in moderate hepatic or renal dysfunction

Potential Disadvantages
- Risk of cataplexy. Cost

Primary Target Symptoms
- Insomnia

 ### Pearls
- Use with caution in patients taking concomitant CYP3A inhibitors
- Be aware of the behavioral adverse effects
- Typically it does not produce narcolepsy symptoms
- Theoretically useful for the treatment of compulsive behaviors, anxiety, and panic disorders, although human data are lacking
- Compared with other insomnia agents, it does not promote sleep but rather

inactivates wakefulness. It has lower potential for addiction or dependence. It also has much less amnesia, next-day somnolence, and rebound insomnia
- In a recent study, 40 mg (30 mg for elderly) seems to improve subjective total sleep time

(30 minutes) and sleep onset (10 minutes) than placebo over 3 months
- The actual benefit compared with other insomnia agents remains to be studied
- In a recent study, similar drug (filorexant) failed to show efficacy for migraine prevention

Suggested Reading

Herring WJ, Connor KM, Ivgy-May N, Snyder E, Liu K. Suvorexant in patients with insomnia: results from two 3-month randomized controlled clinical trials. *Biol Psychiatry*. 2014; DOI: 10.1016/j.biopsych.2014.10.003.

Merlo Pich E, Melotto S. Orexin 1 receptor antagonists in compulsive behavior and anxiety:

possible therapeutic use. *Front Neurosci.* 2014;8:26.

Sun H, Kennedy WP, Wilbraham D, Lewis N, Calder N, Li X, et al. Effects of suvorexant, an orexin receptor antagonist, on sleep parameters as measured by polysomnography in healthy men. *Sleep*. 2013;36(2):259–67.

Brands
- Hetlioz

Generic?
- No

Class
- Melatonin receptor agonist

Commonly Prescribed for
(FDA approved in bold)
- **Treatment of non-24-hour sleep–wake disorder (non-24)**
- Circadian rhythm disorders (shift work disorder, jet-lag)
- Sundowning associated with Alzheimer's disease
- Insomnia

How the Drug Works
- Selectively binds to melatonin receptors (MT_1, MT_2) in the suprachiasmatic nuclei (SCN). It increases the activity of MT_1 receptors (inhibits arousal from SCN) for sleep onset and stimulates MT_2 receptors (synchronizes the circadian clock to day–night cycle) for circadian phase shifting. It has greater affinity for MT_2 than MT_1, supporting its use for non-24
- No affinity for GABA, dopamine, norepinephrine, acetylcholine, opiate receptors

How Long Until It Works
- Onset in less than 2 hours. Optimal improvement may take weeks or months

If It Works
- Continue to use

If It Doesn't Work
- Increase dose or combine with other anti-insomnia agents. Re-evaluate underlying conditions

Best Augmenting Combos for Partial Response or Treatment-Resistance
- Non-pharmacological treatment using phototherapy can be beneficial in those with light perception

- For insomnia, may use low dose of antihistamine, TCAs, benzodiazepines, or antipsychotics

Tests
- Not necessary

How the Drug Causes AEs
- CNS depressant

Notable AEs
- Most common: headache, nightmares, increased alanine aminotransferase, upper respiratory or urinary tract infection

Life-Threatening or Dangerous AEs
- Decreased hemoglobin

Weight Gain
- Unusual

unusual — not unusual — common — problematic

Sedation
- Problematic

unusual — not unusual — common — problematic

What to Do About AEs
- Discontinue if severe AEs

Best Augmenting Agents to Reduce AEs
- Most AEs cannot be reduced by use of augmenting agent

Usual Dosage Range
- 20 mg

Dosage Forms
- Capsules: 20 mg

How to Dose
- 20 mg prior to bedtime, at same time every night

Dosing Tips

- Do not take with high-fat meal, which delays its absorption

Overdose

- As with the management of any overdose, general symptomatic and supportive measures should be used, along with immediate gastric lavage where appropriate. IV fluids should be administered as needed. Respiration, pulse, blood pressure, and other appropriate vital signs should be monitored. No antidote available

Long-Term Use

- Safe for long-term use

Habit Forming

- No

How to Stop

- No withdrawal or rebound effect

Pharmacokinetics

- T_{max} 0.5–3 hours. Bioavailability 38%. 90% protein bound. Hepatic metabolism via primarily CYP1A2 and CYP3A4. Half-life 1 hour. 80% excreted in urine and 4% in feces

 Drug Interactions

- Use with CNS depressants (ethanol, barbiturates, opiates, general anesthetics) potentiates CNS AEs
- Strong CYP1A2 inhibitors (e.g., fluoroquinolones, fluvoxamine, verapamil, grapefruit juice, amiodarone) and inducers (e.g., tobacco, omeprazole) affect tasimelteon's concentration
- Strong CYP3A4 inhibitors (e.g., protease inhibitors, macrolides, azole antifungals, nefazodone) and inducers (e.g., carbamazepine, phenytoin, phenobarbital, St. John's wort, glucocorticoid) affect tasimelteon's concentration

⚠️ **Other Warnings/ Precautions**

- Risk of impaired alertness and motor coordination

Do Not Use

- Avoid concomitant use of strong CYP1A2/ 3A4 inhibitors or inducers

SPECIAL POPULATIONS

Renal Impairment

- No dose adjustment needed. 30% lower clearance in subjects with severe renal impairment

Hepatic Impairment

- Not recommended for severe hepatic impairment. Use with caution in patients with moderate hepatic impairment

Cardiac Impairment

- No dose adjustment

Elderly

- At an increased risk of adverse reactions. May start with lower dose

 Children and Adolescents

- Efficacy and safety unknown

 Pregnancy

- Category C. There are no adequate and well-controlled studies of tasimelteon in pregnant women. In animal studies, administration of tasimelteon during pregnancy resulted in developmental toxicity at doses greater than those used clinically. Use only if benefit outweighs risks

Breast Feeding

- It is not known whether this drug is excreted in human milk. Caution should be exercised when administered to a nursing woman

THE ART OF NEUROPHARMACOLOGY

Potential Advantages

- Quick onset. Synchronizes circadian rhythm. No known risk of dependence and abuse (unscheduled). Less rebound insomnia

Potential Disadvantages

- High cost. Drug interaction with CYP1A2/3A4 inhibitor/inducer. Not studied on patients under multiple sleep medications

Primary Target Symptoms

- Circadian rhythm

 Pearls

- Non-24 is defined as difficulty in initiating sleep or in awakening, progressively delayed sleep onset and offset, or inability to maintain stable entrainment to a 24-hour sleep–wake pattern for at least 6 weeks
- Among melatonin-receptor agonists (ramelteon, agomelatine), tasimelteon is the only drug approved by FDA for non-24

 Suggested Reading

Bonacci JM, Venci JV, Gandhi MA. Tasimelteon (Hetlioz TM): a new melatonin receptor agonist for the treatment of non-24-hour sleep-wake disorder. *J Pharm Pract.* 2014; in press.

Johnsa JD, Neville MW. Tasimelteon: a melatonin receptor agonist for non-24-hour sleep-wake disorder. *Ann Pharmacother.* 2014;48(12):1636–41.

TEMOZOLOMIDE

THERAPEUTICS

Brands
- Temodar, Temodal, Temcad, Methazolastone

Generic?
- No

Class
- Antineoplastic agent

Commonly Prescribed for
(FDA approved in bold)
- **Refractory anaplastic astrocytoma**
- **Newly diagnosed glioblastoma multiforme (GBM) combined with radiotherapy**
- **Malignant prolactinoma**
- Oligodendroglioma
- Primary CNS lymphoma
- Melanoma

How the Drug Works
- An alkylating agent prodrug whose clinical actions are due to metabolite methyl triazeno imidazole carboxamide (MTIC). The metabolites methylate DNA guanine bases, resulting in apoptosis of tumor cells. Treatment success is more likely in tumors with silencing of the *O*-6-methylguanine-DNA methyltransferase (*MGMT*) gene, which is important in demethylation

How Long Until It Works
- Used to prolong survival. Clinical benefits may be difficult to determine for weeks to months

If It Works
- May be continued for up to 6 cycles

If It Doesn't Work
- Discontinue treatment, consider alternative salvage chemotherapy such as bevacizumab or dexamethasone depending on clinical situation

Best Augmenting Combos for Partial Response or Treatment-Resistance
- Most patients will receive co-treatment with radiotherapy

- One small study shows potential benefit when combined with chloroquine. Another with the topoisomerase-1 inhibitor irinotecan
- *O*-6-Benzylguanine may be useful in those with treatment-resistant anaplastic glioma, but does not appear to be effective against GBM

Tests
- CBC before and during treatments, especially in elderly patients
- Chest radiographs in those at risk for *Pneumocystis jiroveci* pneumonia (PCP)

ADVERSE EFFECTS (AEs)

How the Drug Causes AEs
- Similar to other alkylating dugs, AEs are related to its effects on rapidly dividing cells

Notable AEs
- Most common: nausea/vomiting, constipation, alopecia, fatigue, anorexia, lymphopenia, thrombocytopenia
- Less common: rash, diarrhea, thrombocytopenia

Life-Threatening or Dangerous AEs
- Severe neutropenia and thrombocytopenia
- Toxic epidermal necrolysis and Stevens-Johnson syndrome have been rarely reported
- Opportunistic infections including PCP
- Rarely may cause respiratory failure

Weight Gain
- Unusual

unusual   not unusual   common   problematic

Sedation
- Unusual

unusual   not unusual   common   problematic

What to Do About AEs
- Lower dose for bothersome AEs and for serious AEs hold drug
- Treatment doses and frequency are based on platelet and neutrophil counts

Best Augmenting Agents to Reduce AEs

- Antiemetics for nausea/vomiting

DOSING AND USE

Usual Dosage Range

- 150–200 mg/m^2/day

Dosage Forms

- Capsules: 5, 20, 100, 140, 180, and 250 mg
- 100-mg powder for injection

How to Dose

For patients with GBM:

- Initial phase: administer 75 mg/m^2 daily for 42 days concomitant with focal radiotherapy up to 49 days provided absolute neutrophil count (ANC) $\geq$ 1500/mm^3 and platelets > 100 000/mm^3. Obtain CBC weekly and give prophylaxis against PCP during this phase
- Maintenance phase: 150 mg/m^2/day for 5 days starting 4 weeks after completing the initial phase followed by 23 days of no treatment. Increase dose to 200 mg/m^2/day for cycles 2–6 provided no serious toxicity, ANC > 1500/mm^3, and platelets > 100 000/mm^3

For patients with refractory anaplastic astrocytoma:

- Give 150–200 mg/m^2/day for 5 days as a starting dose. Measure ANC and platelets on days 22 and 29 (day 1 of the next cycle). Subsequent treatment is based on the lowest count on either day 22 or 29. Each cycle is 5 days and may be continued for up to 2 years if no progression
  - If ANC < 1000/mm^3 or platelets < 50 000/mm^3, postpone therapy and reduce dose by 50 mg/m^2/day after ANC > 1500/mm^3 and platelets > 100 000/mm^3
  - If ANC 1000–1500/mm^3 or platelets 50 000–100 000/mm^3 postpone therapy until after ANC > 1500/mm^3 and platelets > 100 000/mm^3, but do not lower dose
  - If both ANC > 1500/mm^3 and platelets > 100 000/mm^3 either increase dose to 200 mg/m^2/day or maintain 200 mg/m^2/day dose

 Dosing Tips

- Dose 1 hour before a meal

Overdose

- Hematological complications are most common but pyrexia, multi-organ failure, and death have been reported

Long-Term Use

- Regular CBC are essential. Liver function abnormalities are common but generally not serious

Habit Forming

- No

How to Stop

- No need to taper after cycles, but monitor clinical symptoms and neuroimaging to assess response

Pharmacokinetics

- Peak plasma levels occur at a median of 1 hour. Weakly bound to human plasma proteins. Metabolized to methyl triazeno imidazole carboxamide metabolite. About 38% is recovered over 7 days: mostly in urine

 Drug Interactions

- Valproic acid: decreases oral clearance of temozolomide by about 5%

 Other Warnings/ Precautions

- May impair subsequent fertility – in both men and women

Do Not Use

- Hypersensitivity to drug or dacarbazine. Pregnancy

SPECIAL POPULATIONS

Renal Impairment

- Use with caution. Mild impairment does not affect kinetics

Hepatic Impairment

- Use with caution. Mild impairment does not affect clearance

Cardiac Impairment
• No known effects

Elderly
• Side effects in clinical trials in those over 65 were similar to those in younger patients

 Children and Adolescents
• A few open-label studies have evaluated temozolomide for the treatment of various CNS neoplasms such as medulloblastoma/primitive neuroectodermal tumor (PNET), astrocytomas, brainstem gliomas, and ependymomas
• Dose 160–200 mg/m^2 daily for 5 days every 28 days in children aged 3–18
• Toxicity is similar to that in adults, with thrombocytopenia and lymphopenia being most common

 Pregnancy
• Category D. Associated with multiple malformations in animal testing. Do not use

Breast Feeding
• Unknown if present in breast milk. Breast feeding is generally not recommended

THE ART OF NEUROPHARMACOLOGY

Potential Advantages
• One of the few effective agents for glioma treatment. Relatively well tolerated. Improves survival at 2 and 5 years

Potential Disadvantages
• Risk of blood dyscrasias. Survival benefit is relatively modest. Lack of effectiveness for patients with intact *MGMT* gene function

Primary Target Symptoms
• Tumor progression, disability

 Pearls
• First-line treatment with radiotherapy for most malignant gliomas
• Increases progression-free survival from 5 to 7.2 months, and median survival from 12.1 to 14.6 months in GBM. 2- and 5-year survival were 27.2% and 9.8% respectively in those receiving temozolomide and radiotherapy compared to 10% and 1.9% in those receiving only radiotherapy
• Used less commonly (and not FDA approved) for patients with recurrence
• Radiotherapy may cause radiographic worsening after treatment. This is called "pseudoprogression" rather than treatment progression
• May be effective against oligodendrogliomas, and an alternative to the commonly toxic combination of procarbazine/lomustine/vincristine
• As salvage therapy, consider giving low doses for longer periods of time
• Clinical fluctuations are common in those with GBM, but rapid deterioration should raise concern for tumor bleeding, infection, or non-convulsive status epilepticus

Suggested Reading

National Cancer Institute of Canada Clinical Trials Group; Hegi, ME, Mason, WP, Van Den Bent, MJ. Effects of radiotherapy with concomitant and adjuvant temozolomide versus radiotherapy alone on survival in glioblastoma in a randomised phase III study: 5-year analysis of the EORTC-NCIC trial. *Lancet Oncol.* 2009; 10(5):459–66.

Omuro A, DeAngelis LM. Glioblastoma and other malignant gliomas: a clinical review. *JAMA.* 2013;310(17):1842–50.

Osmani AH, Masood N. Temozolomide for relapsed primary CNS lymphoma. *J Coll Physicians Surg Pak.* 2012;22(9):594–5.

Quinn JA, Jiang SX, Reardon DA, et al. Phase II trial of temozolomide plus O6-benzylguanine in adults with recurrent, temozolomide-resistant malignant glioma. *J Clin Oncol.* 2009;27(8):1262–7.

Stupp R, Mason WP, van den Bent MJ, et al. Radiotherapy plus concomitant and adjuvant temozolomide for glioblastoma. *N Engl J Med.* 2005;352(10):987–96.

Zaky W, Wellner M, Brown RJ, et al. Treatment of children with diffuse intrinsic pontine gliomas with chemoradiotherapy followed by a combination of temozolomide, irinotecan, and bevacizumab. *Pediatr Hematol Oncol.* 2013; 30(7):623–32.

TERIFLUNOMIDE

THERAPEUTICS

Brands
- Aubagio

Generic?
- No

Class
- Immunomodulator

Commonly Prescribed for
(FDA approved in bold)
- **Relapsing types of multiple sclerosis (MS)**
- Rheumatoid arthritis

How the Drug Works
- Teriflunomide is the active metabolite of leflunomide. It inhibits dihydro-orotate dehydrogenase, a mitochondrial enzyme involved with pyrimidine biosynthesis, and disrupts interaction of T cells with antigen-presenting cells and reduces activated lymphocytes in the CNS

How Long Until It Works
- Typically takes months to determine clinical effects

If It Works
- May continue as long as needed for relapsing MS. Unclear if effective in progressive forms of MS

If It Doesn't Work
- May change to an alternative agent such as β interferons, glatiramer acetate, natalizumab, or fingolimod

Best Augmenting Combos for Partial Response or Treatment-Resistance
- May be as add-on therapy with β interferon

Tests
- Before starting obtain pregnancy test in all women of childbearing age. Check CBC, liver function tests, and renal function before starting treatment. Screen patients for latent tuberculosis infection with a tuberculin skin test. Perform monthly liver function tests for at least 6 months after starting treatment

ADVERSE EFFECTS (AEs)

How the Drug Causes AEs
- Increased rates of infection are common with all immune-modulating therapies. Hepatoxicity may be related to inhibition of dihydro-orotate dehydrogenase, a mitochondrial enzyme

Notable AEs
- Elevated liver transaminases, alopecia, diarrhea, influenza, nausea, increased blood pressure, hypophosphatemia (mild), and paresthesias

Life-Threatening or Dangerous AEs
- Hepatoxicity (as much as 5%) – fatal liver failure has been reported with leflunomide
- Neutropenia
- Peripheral neuropathy (1–2%, more common in elderly patients)
- Acute renal failure (1%)
- Hyperkalemia
- Stevens-Johnson syndrome and toxic epidermal necrolysis (rare)
- Worsening of preexisting interstitial lung disease

Weight Gain
- Unusual

unusual   not unusual   common   problematic

Sedation
- Unusual

unusual   not unusual   common   problematic

What to Do About AEs
- Severe leukopenia or thrombocytopenia is relatively uncommon but discontinue drug for rare events such as pancytopenia, agranulocytosis, or thrombocytopenia
- If severe infection develops consider discontinuing treatment and undergoing accelerated elimination procedure (outlined in pregnancy section)
- Avoid live vaccines while on treatment

Best Augmenting Agents to Reduce AEs
- Most AEs are not treatable with medications except for hypertension

DOSING AND USE

Usual Dosage Range
- 7 or 14mg/day

Dosage Forms
- Tablets: 7, 14mg

How to Dose
- Take once daily

 Dosing Tips
- May take with or without food

Overdose
- Up to 70mg/day appears to be well tolerated. In case of overdose of significant toxicity use elimination protocol with cholestyramine and/or activated charcoal

Long-Term Use
- May be used as long as indicated and effective

Habit Forming
- No

How to Stop
- No need to taper, but monitor for worsening of MS or other clinical symptoms

Pharmacokinetics
- Maximum plasma concentration is at 1–4 hours
- Extensive plasma protein binding ($> 99\%$)
- Eliminated via direct biliary excretion of drug and renal excretion of metabolites
- Complete drug elimination after discontinuation may take years

 Drug Interactions
- May decrease effects of warfarin with coadministration
- Appears to moderately increase ethinylestradiol and levonorgestrel levels, impacting oral contraceptive choices
- Possible weak inducer of CYP1A2, may decrease levels of substrates such as duloxetine, alosetron, theophylline, and tizanidine

 Other Warnings/ Precautions
- Patients with active acute or chronic infections should not start treatment until the infection is resolved

Do Not Use
- Untreated tuberculosis (treat prior to starting therapy)
- Severe immunodeficiency, bone marrow disease, or severe, uncontrolled infection

SPECIAL POPULATIONS

Renal Impairment
- Appears safe even in those with severe impairment

Hepatic Impairment
- Do not use with severe hepatic impairment. Appears safe in those with mild to moderate impairment but given risk of drug-related hepatoxicity use with caution

Cardiac Impairment
- No known effects. Cardiovascular deaths occurred during extension phases of clinical trials, but the relationship of teriflunomide to these deaths is unclear

Elderly
- No known effects but limited experience in those over 65

 Children and Adolescents
- Effectiveness and safety are unknown

 Pregnancy
- Category X. Significant teratogenicity and embryolethal effects were noted in multiple species during animal testing – even at low doses. If a patient becomes pregnant (or wishes to become pregnant) they should undergo an elimination procedure as follows:
- Cholestyramine 8g every 8 hours for 11 days (may lower to 4mg if not well tolerated)
- Oral activated charcoal powder 50g every 12 hours for 11 days

- Ensure plasma concentrations are less than 0.02 mg/L
- Without elimination procedure, it takes 8 months on average for concentrations to drop below 0.02 mg/L, and may take as long as 2 years

Breast Feeding

- Drug is found in rat milk, but unknown if present in human milk. Breast feeding not recommended while taking teriflunomide

THE ART OF NEUROPHARMACOLOGY

Potential Advantages

- Oral medication which is effective in relapsing MS, even when compared to injectable therapies. Relatively low risk of infections, especially compared to fingolimod

Potential Disadvantages

- Potential serious AEs of hepatotoxicity and significant teratogenicity

Primary Target Symptoms

- Preventing relapses and disability from MS

 Pearls

- Compared to placebo, annual clinical relapses are significantly lower (0.37/year vs. 0.54/year, $p < 0.001$)
- Also superior to placebo in preventing disability
- Clinical effectiveness is not significantly greater with 14 mg vs. 7 mg, but neither are AEs
- Given potential teratogenicity and prolonged elimination, may be better to be used in men or postmenopausal women
- Safety profile (with the exception of potential teratogenicity) and tolerability are fairly good, so may be an option for patients who don't want to use more established injectable therapies
- In a clinical trial in patients on stable doses of interferon-β, both 7 and 14 mg doses significantly decreased rates of new gadolinium-enhancing lesions compared to interferon-β alone. No new serious AEs were observed
- An active metabolite of leflunomide, a drug used for the symptoms of rheumatoid arthritis

 Suggested Reading

Breedveld F, Dayer J. Leflunomide: mode of action in the treatment of rheumatoid arthritis. *Ann Rheum Dis.* 2000; 59(11): 841–9.

Freedman MS, Wolinsky JS, Wamil B, et al. Teriflunomide added to interferon-β in relapsing multiple sclerosis: a randomized phase II trial. *Neurology.* 2012;78(23):1877–85.

O'Connor P, Wolinsky JS, Confavreux C, et al. Randomized trial of oral teriflunomide for relapsing multiple sclerosis. *N Engl J Med.* 2011;365(14):1293–303.

O'Connor PW, Li D, Freedman MS, et al. A Phase II study of the safety and efficacy of teriflunomide in multiple sclerosis with relapses. *Neurology.* 2006;66(6):894–900.

TETRABENAZINE

THERAPEUTICS

Brands
- Nitoman, Xenazine

Generic?
- No

Class
- Monoamine-depleting agent

Commonly Prescribed for
(FDA approved in bold)
- **Chorea in Huntington's disease (HD)**
- Tardive dyskinesia
- Psychosis
- Hemiballism
- Dystonia (especially tardive)
- Myoclonus
- Gilles de la Tourette syndrome (GTS) or tics
- Hypertension

How the Drug Works
- Depleting agent that reversibly inhibits vesicular monoamine transporter type 2 (VMAT2) resulting in depletion of monoamines, primarily dopamine but less effect on others (norepinephrine, serotonin, and histamine), from nerve terminals. It also weakly blocks postsynaptic D_2 receptors. Effectiveness is likely related to dopamine depletion. Sedation and depression are probably due to histamine and serotonin/norepinephrine depletion, respectively

How Long Until It Works
- Rapid onset, lasting 5–6 hours

If It Works
- In neurological conditions, continue to assess effect of the medication, determine if still needed, and adjust to optimal dose

If It Doesn't Work
- Chorea: consider benzodiazepines and AEDs (valproate). Neuroleptics are usually effective. Reserpine is an alternative depleting agent
- Generalized dystonia: anticholinergics, baclofen, or benzodiazepines may be

effective. Surgical treatments (including pallidotomy, thalamotomy, deep brain stimulation, myotomy, rhizotomy, or peripheral denervation) are reserved for refractory cases
- GTS/tics: neuroleptics and α_2-adrenergic agonists are often effective

Best Augmenting Combos for Partial Response or Treatment-Resistance
- Chorea: combine with AEDs, neuroleptics, or benzodiazepines
- Dystonia: combine with anticholinergics or benzodiazepines
- GTS/tics: combine with neuroleptics for refractory cases

Tests
- At doses of 50 mg or greater, test patients for the CYP2D6 gene to determine if they are poor, intermediate, or extensive metabolizers

ADVERSE EFFECTS (AEs)

How the Drug Causes AEs
- Related to monoamine depletion

Notable AEs
- Drowsiness, fatigue, dizziness, depression, anxiety, insomnia
- Parkinsonism, akathisia, orthostatic hypotension, nausea
- Upper respiratory tract infection, dyspnea, dysuria
- Slight increase in liver function tests

Life-Threatening or Dangerous AEs
- Falls and resulting trauma
- Neuroleptic malignant syndrome
- Parkinsonism and extrapyramidal tract dysfunction (less common than neuroleptics)
- QTc prolongation (usually mild)
- Dysphagia

Weight Gain
- Common

unusual   not unusual   common   problematic

Sedation

- Common

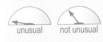

unusual   not unusual   **common**   problematic

What to Do About AEs

- Reducing doses decreases most AEs

Best Augmenting Agents to Reduce AEs

- Most AEs cannot be reduced by an augmenting agent

DOSING AND USE

Usual Dosage Range

- Most respond to 37.5–75mg/day. Some require up to 300mg/day

Dosage Forms

- Tablets: 12.5, 25mg

How to Dose

- Start at 12.5mg daily in the morning and increase to 12.5mg twice a day in 1 week. Increase as needed by 12.5mg/week and dose 3–4 times daily. Avoid single doses over 50mg. Most patients require daily doses of 100mg or less. Titrate dose until satisfactory control or dose-limiting AEs

 Dosing Tips

- Food has no effect on absorption

Overdose

- Reported symptoms include acute dystonia, oculogyric crisis, nausea and vomiting, sweating, sedation, hypotension, confusion, diarrhea, hallucinations, and tremor

Long-Term Use

- Safe, but monitor for long-term AEs

Habit Forming

- No

How to Stop

- No need to taper but symptoms usually reappear

Pharmacokinetics

- The onset is within 30 minutes. It then undergoes rapid metabolism via predominantly CYP2D6 isoenzymes and mostly excreted in urine. Half-life about 10 hours

 Drug Interactions

- Do not use with MAOIs
- Do not use within 20 days of reserpine
- Strong CYP2D6 inhibitors (fluoxetine, paroxetine, quinidine) approximately double levels, requiring reduction in dose. Weaker 2D6 inhibitors (duloxetine, amiodarone, or sertraline) may also increase levels
- CYP2D6 inducers (dexamethasone, rifampin) can reduce levels
- Sedation increases with the use of CNS depressants, such as alcohol

 Other Warnings/ Precautions

- May elevate prolactin levels
- May cause severe depression that may lead to suicide

Do Not Use

- Proven hypersensitivity, active depression or history of suicidal tendencies, or hepatic disease

---

SPECIAL POPULATIONS

Renal Impairment

- Patients with renal insufficiency may adjust poorly to lowered blood pressure

Hepatic Impairment

- Concentrations of drug and metabolites and elimination half-life are dramatically increased. Do not use

Cardiac Impairment

- May increase QTc interval. Avoid in patients with congenital long QT syndrome or in patients on QT-prolonging medications. Patients with recent myocardial infarction or unstable disease were excluded from clinical trials

Elderly

• No known effects

Children and Adolescents

• Not well studied but occasionally used for the treatment of generalized dystonias. Monitor for parkinsonism and hypotension. A trial of levodopa should be considered to rule out dopa-responsive dystonia

Pregnancy

• Category C. Use only if there is a clear need

Breast Feeding

• Unknown if excreted in breast milk. Use only if clearly needed

---

THE ART OF NEUROPHARMACOLOGY

Potential Advantages

• Useful for the treatment of hyperkinetic movement disorders, with fewer AEs than reserpine

Potential Disadvantages

• Not available in many countries. Drowsiness and parkinsonism limit titration. Multiple doses per day needed. Wide individual variability of optimal dose

Primary Target Symptoms

• Reduction in severity of chorea, dystonia, myoclonus, or tics

Pearls

• Most effective in the treatment of tardive dyskinesias, tardive dystonia, HD, and myoclonus
• AAN guideline suggests: if HD chorea requires treatment, clinicians should prescribe tetrabenazine (up to 100 mg/day), amantadine (300–400 mg/day), or riluzole (200 mg/day) (Level of Evidence B). Tetrabenazine likely has very important antichoreic benefits, and riluzole 200 mg/day likely has moderate benefits (Level of Evidence B). The degree of benefit for amantadine is unknown
• Somewhat effective in idiopathic dystonia and GTS
• Dyskinesia related to Parkinson's disease should be treated with lowering levodopa medication doses and using extended-release forms, amantadine, or clozapine. Tetrabenazine may worsen orthostatic hypotension
• Level C evidence for use in treatment of tardive syndrome
• In refractory dystonia, tetrabenazine with trihexyphenidyl and pimozide may be effective
• For the treatment of chorea in HD, aripiprazole often has fewer AEs and is more likely to improve depression rather than worsen symptoms
• Parkinsonism is more common at higher doses (100 mg or greater)
• Although common, weight gain is less common than with neuroleptics in the treatment of GTS
• Compared to reserpine, it has a shorter half-life and has fewer peripheral effects (lower incidence of GI AEs and hypotension)

Suggested Reading

Aia PG, Revuelta GJ, Cloud LJ, Factor SA. Tardive dyskinesia. *Curr Treat Options Neurol.* 2011;13(3):231–41.

Armstrong MJ, Miyasaki JM, American Academy of Neurology. Evidence-based guideline: pharmacologic treatment of chorea in Huntington disease: report of the guideline development subcommittee of the American Academy of Neurology. *Neurology.* 2012;79(6): 597–603.

Bhidayasiri R, Fahn S, Weiner WJ, Gronseth GS, Sullivan KL, Zesiewicz TA, et al. Evidence-based guideline: treatment of tardive syndromes: report of the Guideline Development Subcommittee of the American Academy of Neurology. *Neurology.* 2013;81(5):463–9.

Fernandez HH, Friedman JH. Classification and treatment of tardive syndromes. *Neurologist.* 2003;9(1):16–27.

Kenney C, Hunter C, Jankovic J. Long-term tolerability of tetrabenazine in the treatment of hyperkinetic movement disorders. *Mov Disord.* 2007;22(2):193–7.

Paleacu D, Giladi N, Moore O, Stern A, Honigman S, Badarny S. Tetrabenazine treatment in movement disorders. *Clin Neuropharmacol.* 2004;27(5):230–3.

Setter SM, Neumiller JJ, Dobbins EK, Wood L, Clark J, DuVall CA, et al. Treatment of chorea associated with Huntington's disease: focus on tetrabenazine. *Consult Pharm.* 2009;24(7):524–37.

THERAPEUTICS

Brands
- Gabitril

Generic?
- Yes

Class
- Antiepileptic drug (AED)

Commonly Prescribed for
(FDA approved in bold)
- **Adjunctive for partial seizures in adults and children age 12 or older**
- Temporal lobe epilepsy (children and adults)
- Panic disorder

How the Drug Works
- Enhances activity of GABA by binding to sites associated with GABA uptake into presynaptic neurons, allowing more GABA to be available to bind to receptors on postsynaptic cells

How Long Until It Works
- Seizures: should decrease by 2 weeks

If It Works
- Seizures: goal is the remission of seizures. Continue as long as effective and well tolerated. Consider tapering and slowly stopping after 2 years without seizures

If It Doesn't Work
- Increase to highest tolerated dose
- Epilepsy: consider changing to another agent, adding a second agent, using a medical device, or a referral for epilepsy surgery evaluation. When adding a second agent, keep drug interactions in mind

Best Augmenting Combos for Partial Response or Treatment-Resistance
- Epilepsy: titration and combination regimen depends on whether the patients are on an enzyme-inducing drug or not

Tests
- No regular blood tests are recommended

ADVERSE EFFECTS (AEs)

How the Drug Causes AEs
- CNS AEs are probably caused by excess GABA effect

Notable AEs
- Confusion, stuttering, muscle tremor, dizziness, sedation, paresthesias (usually doses > 8 mg/day), abdominal pain
- Less commonly, behavioral symptoms such as amnesia, extreme confusion, or seizures or seizure-like symptoms

Life-Threatening or Dangerous AEs
- Can precipitate seizure in some patients (rare)
- Severe rash (rare) including Stevens-Johnson syndrome
- Falls producing accidental injury

Weight Gain
- Common

unusual   not unusual   **common**   problematic

Sedation
- Common

unusual   not unusual   **common**   problematic

What to Do About AEs
- Decreasing dose may reduce CNS AEs, especially weakness and sedation
- Titrate more slowly

Best Augmenting Agents to Reduce AEs
- Initially dose at night to avoid sedation

DOSING AND USE

Usual Dosage Range
- Epilepsy: 16–56 mg/day

Dosage Forms
- Tablets: 2, 4, 12, 16 mg

How to Dose
- For adults on enzyme-inducing AEDs (phenytoin, carbamazepine, primidone,

phenobarbital), start at 4 mg. Increase dose by 4–8 mg in 1 week and continue to increase by 4–8 mg/week as needed, to a maximum of 56 mg daily. At final doses give in divided doses 2–4 times daily
• In patients not on enzyme-inducing AEDs, give only half the dose and titrate more slowly

 Dosing Tips

• Food and specifically fats slow absorption rate but not the extent of absorption. Most patients take with food
• Titrate slowly in patients not on enzyme-inducing AEDs

Overdose

• Somnolence, weakness, agitation, confusion, depression, respiratory depression, and myoclonus have been reported. Rarely precipitates non-convulsive status epilepticus

Long-Term Use

• Safe for long-term use

Habit Forming

• No

How to Stop

• Taper slowly
• Abrupt withdrawal can lead to seizures in patients with epilepsy

Pharmacokinetics

• Elimination half-life is 2–5 hours in patients on enzyme-inducing AEDs, but 7–9 hours in others. Most drug is metabolized by CYP450 3A system. Bioavailability is about 90% and drug is 96% protein bound

 Drug Interactions

• Carbamazepine, phenytoin, phenobarbital, and primidone increase clearance of tiagabine by about 60%
• Use with other highly protein-bound drugs may increase free levels and drug effect
• Valproate may slightly increase free tiagabine levels and tiagabine causes a slight decrease in valproate concentrations. Usually not clinically relevant

 Other Warnings/ Precautions

• CNS AEs increase when used with other CNS depressants

Do Not Use

• Hypersensitivity to drug

Renal Impairment

• No known effects

Hepatic Impairment

• Lower dose, as patients with moderate disease have reduced clearance by 60%

Cardiac Impairment

• No known effects

Elderly

• May need lower dose

 Children and Adolescents

• For children age 12–18 on enzyme-inducing AEDs (phenytoin, carbamazepine, primidone, phenobarbital), start at 4 mg. Increase dose to 8 mg in 1 week and continue to increase by 4–8 mg/week as needed, to a maximum of 32 mg daily. At final doses, give in divided doses 2–4 times daily
• In children not on enzyme-inducing AEDs, give only half the dose and titrate more slowly

 Pregnancy

• Category C. Multiple malformations in animals. Use only if benefits of using drug outweigh potential risk to fetus
• Supplementation with 0.4 mg of folic acid before and during pregnancy is recommended

Breast Feeding

• Some drug is found in mother's breast milk
• Generally recommendations are to discontinue drug or bottle feed
• Monitor infant for sedation, poor feeding, or irritability

THE ART OF NEUROPHARMACOLOGY

Potential Advantages
- Useful for partial seizures, especially with coexisting panic disorder

Potential Disadvantages
- Depression and cognitive impairment. Does not treat generalized epilepsies

Primary Target Symptoms
- Seizure frequency and severity

Pearls
- Contraindicated in generalized epilepsy and may precipitate non-convulsive status epilepticus
- There are reports of patients with spike-wave discharges who experience exacerbations of EEG abnormalities that correlate with cognitive or neuropsychological reactions on tiagabine

Suggested Reading

Aikiä M, Jutila L, Salmenperä T, Mervaala E, Kälviäinen R. Comparison of the cognitive effects of tiagabine and carbamazepine as monotherapy in newly diagnosed adult patients with partial epilepsy: pooled analysis of two long-term, randomized, follow-up studies. *Epilepsia.* 2006;47(7):1121–7.

Bauer J, Cooper-Mahkorn D. Tiagabine: efficacy and safety in partial seizures – current status. *Neuropsychiatr Dis Treat.* 2008;4(4):731–6.

Koepp MJ, Edwards M, Collins J, Farrel F, Smith S. Status epilepticus and tiagabine therapy revisited. *Epilepsia.* 2005;46(10):1625–32.

Pulman J, Hutton JL, Marson AG. Tiagabine add-on for drug-resistant partial epilepsy. *Cochrane Database Syst Rev.* 2014;2: CD001908.

Sheehan DV, Sheehan KH, Raj BA, Janavs J. An open-label study of tiagabine in panic disorder. *Psychopharmacol Bull.* 2007;40(3): 32–40.

Vossler DG, Morris GL III, Harden CL, Montouris G, Faught E, Kanner AM, et al.. Tiagabine in clinical practice: effects on seizure control and behavior. *Epilepsy Behav.* 2013; 28(2):211–16.

TIMOLOL

Brands
- Blocadren (oral), Betimol, Betim, Timoptic, Istalol (ocular solution)

Generic?
- Yes

Class
- β-blocker

Commonly Prescribed for
(FDA approved in bold)
- **Migraine prophylaxis**
- **Hypertension**
- **Myocardial infarction (MI)**
- **Chronic open-angle glaucoma or ocular hypertension (ocular solution)**
- Congestive heart failure (stable)
- Angina pectoris due to coronary atherosclerosis
- Prevention of variceal bleeding

How the Drug Works
- Migraine: proposed mechanisms include inhibition of adrenergic pathway, interaction with serotonin system and receptors, inhibition of nitric oxide production, and normalization of contingent negative variation. Prevention of cortical spreading depression may be one mechanism of action for all migraine preventives

How Long Until It Works
- Migraines: within 2 weeks, but can take up to 3 months on a stable dose to see full effect

If It Works
- In migraine, the goal is a 50% or greater decrease in migraine frequency or severity. Consider tapering or stopping if headaches remit for more than 6 months or if considering pregnancy

If It Doesn't Work
- Increase to highest tolerated dose
- Migraine: address other issues, such as medication overuse, other coexisting medical disorders, such as anxiety, and consider changing to another drug or adding a second drug

Best Augmenting Combos for Partial Response or Treatment-Resistance
- Migraine: for some patients, low-dose polytherapy with 2 or more drugs may be better tolerated and more effective than high-dose monotherapy. May use in combination with AEDs, antidepressants, natural products, and non-pharmacological treatments, such as biofeedback, to improve headache control

Tests
- None required

How the Drug Causes AEs
- Antagonism of β receptors

Notable AEs
- Bradycardia, hypotension, hyper or hypoglycemia, weight gain
- Bronchospasm, cold/flu symptoms, sinusitis, pneumonias
- Dizziness, vertigo, fatigue/tiredness, depression, sleep disturbances
- Sexual dysfunction, decreased libido, dysuria, urinary retention, joint pain
- Exacerbation of symptoms in peripheral vascular disease and Raynaud's syndrome

Life-Threatening or Dangerous AEs
- In acute or chronic heart failure, may further depress myocardial contractility
- Can blunt premonitory symptoms of hypoglycemia in diabetes and mask clinical signs of hyperthyroidism
- Non-selective β-blockers, such as timolol, can inhibit bronchodilation, making them contraindicated in asthma and severe chronic obstructive pulmonary disease
- Risk of excessive myocardial depression in general anesthesia

Weight Gain
- Not unusual

unusual · not unusual · common · problematic

Sedation

- Common

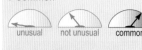

unusual　　not unusual　　**common**　　problematic

What to Do About AEs

- Lower dose, take higher dose in the evening, or switch to another drug

Best Augmenting Agents to Reduce AEs

- When patients have significant benefit from β-blocker therapy but hypotension limits treatment, consider α agonists (midodrine) or volume expanders (fludrocortisone) for symptomatic relief

DOSING AND USE

Dosage Forms

- 10–60 mg/day

Dosage Forms

- Tablets: 5, 10, 20 mg
- Ocular solution: 0.25 or 0.5%

How to Dose

- Migraine: initial dose 10 mg twice daily in migraine. Can gradually increase weekly to usual effective dose: 20–60 mg/day

 Dosing Tips

- Patients on a stable dose of 20 mg/day can take the entire dose once daily, usually in the evening

Overdose

- Bradycardia, hypotension, low-output heart failure, shock, seizures, coma, hypoglycemia, apnea, cyanosis, respiratory depression, and bronchospasm. Epinephrine and dopamine are used to treat toxicity

Long-Term Use

- Safe for long-term use

Habit Forming

- No

How to Stop

- Do not abruptly discontinue. Gradually reduce dosage over 1–2 weeks. Stopping may exacerbate angina, and there are reports of tachyarrhythmias or MI with rapid discontinuation in patients with cardiac disease

Pharmacokinetics

- Half-life 4 hours. Bioavailability is 75%. Hepatic metabolism. Metabolites are excreted by kidney. < 10% protein binding. Lower lipid solubility than propranolol

 Drug Interactions

- Oral contraceptives, ciprofloxacin, and hydroxychloroquine can increase levels and/or effects of timolol and other β-blockers
- Use with calcium channel blockers can be synergistic or additive, use with caution
- Barbiturates, penicillins, rifampin, calcium and aluminum salts, thyroid hormones, and cholestyramine can decrease effects of β-blockers
- NSAIDs, sulfinpyrazone, and salicylates inhibit prostaglandin synthesis and may inhibit the antihypertensive activity of β-blockers
- Timolol can increase levels of lidocaine, resulting in toxicity
- Increased postural hypotension with prazosin and peripheral ischemia with ergot alkaloids
- Sudden discontinuation of clonidine while on β-blockers or when stopping together can cause life-threatening increases in blood pressure

 Other Warnings/ Precautions

- Slight increases in blood urea, serum potassium, and uric acid, with decrease of HDL cholesterol and hematocrit. These alterations are not progressive or clinically significant
- Rare development of antinuclear antibodies (ANA)
- May worsen muscle weakness in myasthenia gravis

Do Not Use

- Sinus bradycardia, greater than first-degree heart block, cardiogenic shock
- Bronchial asthma, severe chronic obstructive pulmonary disease
- Proven hypersensitivity to β-blockers

SPECIAL POPULATIONS

Renal Impairment

• No significant changes in half-life or concentration with moderate failure, but marked hypotensive episodes have occurred in patients undergoing dialysis. Use with caution

Hepatic Impairment

• May need to reduce dose with significant hepatic disease

Cardiac Impairment

• Do not use in acute shock, MI, hypotension, and greater than first-degree heart block, but indicated in clinically stable patients post-MI to reduce risk of reinfarction. Metoprolol, another β-blocker, is commonly used to reduce mortality and hospitalization for patients with stable chronic heart failure already receiving ACE inhibitors and diuretics

Elderly

• Use with caution. May increase risk of stroke

Children and Adolescents

• Not studied in children. The pediatric dose is unknown

Pregnancy

• Category C. Embryotoxic in animal studies only at doses much higher than maximum recommended human doses. May reduce perfusion of the placenta. Use if potential benefit outweighs risk to the fetus. Most β-blockers are class C, except atenolol, which is D and acebutolol, pindolol, and sotalol, which are B

Breast Feeding

• Not recommended. Timolol is found in breast milk

THE ART OF NEUROPHARMACOLOGY

Potential Advantages

• Proven effectiveness in migraine and fewer drug interactions than propranolol. Perhaps fewer CNS side effects

Potential Disadvantages

• Multiple potential AEs including bradycardia, hypotension, and fatigue. Less known efficacy for treating coexisting conditions, such as anxiety and tremor, compared with propranolol

Primary Target Symptoms

• Migraine frequency and severity

Pearls

• Alternative β-blockers for migraine: metoprolol 100–200 mg/day, propranolol 40–400 mg/day (FDA approved), atenolol 50–200 mg/day, nadolol 20–160 mg/day

• β-blockers that are partial agonists, with intrinsic sympathomimetic activity, are not effective in migraine prophylaxis. These include acebutolol, alprenolol, and pindolol

• Often used in combination with other drugs in migraine

• Not effective for cluster headache

• β_1-selective antagonists, such as metoprolol, may be an option for patients with asthma or severe chronic obstructive pulmonary disease

• Recent studies have downgraded β-blockers as a first-line treatment for hypertension compared with other classes due to lack of effectiveness, increased rate of stroke in elderly, and risk of provoking type II diabetes

• Often used in combination with other agents for hypertension, especially thiazide diuretics

Suggested Reading

Law MR, Morris JK, Wald NJ. Use of blood pressure lowering drugs in the prevention of cardiovascular disease: meta-analysis of 147 randomised trials in the context of expectations from prospective epidemiological studies. *BMJ*. 2009;338: b1665.

Ramadan NM. Current trends in migraine prophylaxis. *Headache*. 2007;47 Suppl 1:S52–7.

Silberstein SD. Preventive migraine treatment. *Neurol Clin*. 2009;27(2):429–43.

Taylor FR. Weight change associated with the use of migraine-preventive medications. *Clin Ther*. 2008;30(6):1069–80.

TIZANIDINE

THERAPEUTICS

Brands
- Zanaflex, Sirdalud

Generic?
- Yes

Class
- α₂-adrenergic agonist, muscle relaxant

Commonly Prescribed for
(FDA approved in bold)
- **Acute and intermittent management of increased muscle tone related to spasticity**
- Migraine prophylaxis
- Neck pain/lower back pain
- Myofascial pain
- Trigeminal neuralgia

How the Drug Works
- Central α₂-adrenergic agonist (mostly at α₂ₐ receptors) that also acts at imidazoline receptors. Both α₂ₐ and imidazoline receptors are involved in the supraspinal inhibitory effects on mono- or poly-synaptic reflexes, hence reducing spasticity, which can result from neurological conditions, such as multiple sclerosis (MS), amyotrophic lateral sclerosis (ALS), primary lateral sclerosis, and spinal cord injury. α₂ₐ-agonist also increases presynaptic inhibition in locus coeruleus, periaqueductal gray area, and parabrachial nucleus, hence the anesthetic responses. Both receptors are involved in sympatholytic responses

How Long Until It Works
- Hours to weeks

If It Works
- Slowly titrate to most effective tolerated dose

If It Doesn't Work
- Increase to highest tolerated dose. If ineffective, gradually reduce dose and consider alternative medications

Best Augmenting Combos for Partial Response or Treatment-Resistance
- Botulinum toxin is effective, especially as an adjunct for focal spasticity, e.g., post-stroke or head injury affecting the upper limbs. For conditions with multiple areas of spasticity, i.e., cerebral palsy, this combination can be very useful
- May be used carefully in combination with baclofen, although additive sedation can be problematic
- Use other centrally acting muscle relaxants with caution due to potential additive CNS depressant effect

Tests
- Monitor liver and renal function at baseline and at 1, 2, and 3 months. Monitor hepatic enzymes at 6 months and periodically after that

ADVERSE EFFECTS (AEs)

How the Drug Causes AEs
- Related to α₂ and imidazoline agonist effect, causing hypotension and increased sedation

Notable AEs
- Dry mouth, weakness, and somnolence are most common. Dizziness, hypotension, and elevation of hepatic transaminases. Hallucinations (usually visual) occur in about 3% of patients

Life-Threatening or Dangerous AEs
- Bradycardia and prolongation of QTc interval with higher doses. Tizanidine withdrawal can cause rebound hypertension

Weight Gain
- Not unusual

unusual | not unusual | common | problematic

Sedation
- Common

unusual | not unusual | common | problematic

What to Do About AEs

- Lower the dose and titrate more slowly

Best Augmenting Agents to Reduce AEs

- Most AEs cannot be reduced by an augmenting agent. MS-related fatigue can respond to CNS stimulants such as modafinil but it is easier to temporarily lower the dose until tolerance develops

DOSING AND USE

Usual Dosage Range

- 6–24 mg/day in 3–4 divided doses, maximum 36 mg/day

Dosage Forms

- Tablets: 2, 4 mg
- Capsules: 2, 4, 6 mg
- Nasal spray: 32.73, 16.36 mg/mL

How to Dose

- Start with one 2 or 4 mg tablet daily. Increase by 2–4 mg every 3 days as tolerated to a goal of 24 mg/day – either 8 mg 3 times a day or 6 mg 4 times a day – or until desired clinical effect is met. Some patients may increase to 36 mg/day if tolerated

 Dosing Tips

- Sedation peaks the first week. Slower titration may reduce AEs

Overdose

- One case of profound respiratory depression reported. Ensure adequate airway protection and intubate if needed. Gastric lavage and forced diuresis with furosemide and mannitol may be helpful

Long-Term Use

- Not well studied

Habit Forming

- No

How to Stop

- Taper slowly to avoid rebound tachycardia and hypertension (although much less problematic than clonidine)

Pharmacokinetics

- Bioavailability is 40%, with hepatic metabolism into inactive metabolites. 30% protein bound. Half-life is 20–40 hours and peak effect at 1–1.5 hours. The duration of effect is 3–6 hours. Food has complex effects on its pharmacokinetic profiles

 Drug Interactions

- Strong CYP1A2 inhibitor (e.g., fluvoxamine, fluoroquinolones, verapamil) and moderate CYP1A2 inhibitor (St. John's wort, acyclovir, amiodarone) increase concentration
- Oral contraceptives decrease tizanidine clearance by about 50%
- Alcohol impairs tizanidine clearance and adds to depressant effect
- Tizanidine delays the effect of acetaminophen
- Use with other CNS depressants increases sedation

 Other Warnings/ Precautions

- Decreased spasticity can be problematic for some patients who require tone to maintain upright posture, balance, and ambulation
- In animal studies, dose-related corneal opacities and retinal degeneration occurred

Do Not Use

- Known hypersensitivity. Patients taking potent CYP1A2 inhibitor (e.g., fluvoxamine, ciprofloxacin)

SPECIAL POPULATIONS

Renal Impairment

- Clearance is reduced in patients with CrCl < 25 mL/min. Reduce dose. Monitor for dry mouth, somnolence, asthenia, dizziness

Hepatic Impairment

- Due to potential for elevation of hepatic transaminases, use with caution in any patient with significant hepatic disease

Cardiac Impairment

- QTc prolongation reported. Cautious under concomitant CYP1A2 inhibitor

Elderly

- Drug metabolism is slower in elderly patients. Increased risk of injury. Use with caution

 Children and Adolescents

- Not studied in children

 Pregnancy

- Category C. Use only if there is a clear need

Breast Feeding

- Unknown if excreted in breast milk but likely due to lipid solubility. Do not use

THE ART OF NEUROPHARMACOLOGY

Potential Advantages

- Effective treatment for spasticity with relatively benign AE profile. Effectiveness is similar to diazepam and oral baclofen with fewer AEs and less severe withdrawal symptoms

Potential Disadvantages

- Hypotension can be problematic in some and rebound hypertension from discontinuation may be confused for autonomic dysreflexia. Sedation often limits use

Primary Target Symptoms

- Spasticity, pain

 Pearls

- Recommended by National Institute for Health and Care Excellence (NICE) as second-line drug for the treatment of spasticity in MS
- Generally well-tolerated alternative to other muscle relaxants, such as oral baclofen, dantrolene, and diazepam
- Chemically similar to another α_{2A}-adrenergic agonist, clonidine, but has only a fraction (1/10 to 1/50th) of the blood pressure lowering effect
- In migraine prophylaxis, may be helpful for some patients either as an acute pain medication or as a "bridge" treatment for daily pain. Some studies suggest usefulness as a longer-term prophylactic agent but AEs often outweigh benefit
- A 2002 study showed that tizanidine 18–24 mg may be useful as adjunctive for prophylaxis of chronic daily headache. Headache-related disability was not found to be different
- Effective for some patients with acute myofascial pain, back pain, and neck pain
- Level C evidence for trigeminal neuralgia
- The antinociceptive effect may be attributed to the imidazoline agonism. Similarly, isometheptene (imidazoline I_1 receptor agonist without α activity), which is the active ingredient in the over-the-counter drug Midrin, has been used for acute headache relief
- Tizanidine nasal spray has greater bioavailability and shorter onset than oral counterpart

Suggested Reading

Attal N, Cruccu G, Baron R, Haanpää M, Hansson P, Jensen TS, et al. EFNS guidelines on the pharmacological treatment of neuropathic pain: 2010 revision. *Eur J Neurol.* 2010;17(9): 1113–88.

Delgado MR, Hirtz D, Aisen M, Ashwal S, Fehlings DL, McLaughlin J, et al. Practice parameter: pharmacologic treatment of spasticity in children and adolescents with cerebral palsy (an evidence-based review): report of the Quality Standards Subcommittee of the American Academy of Neurology and the Practice Committee of the Child Neurology Society. *Neurology.* 2010;74: 336–43.

Freitag FG. Preventative treatment for migraine and tension-type headaches: do drugs having effects on muscle spasm and tone have a role? *CNS Drugs.* 2003;17(6):373–81.

Kamen L, Henney HR 3rd, Runyan JD. A practical overview of tizanidine use for spasticity secondary to multiple sclerosis, stroke, and spinal cord injury. *Curr Med Res Opin.* 2008;24(2):425–39.

Marmura MJ, Silberstein SD, Schwedt TJ. The acute treatment of migraine in adults: the American Headache Society evidence assessment of migraine pharmacotherapies. *Headache.* 2015;55:3–20.

Mathew NT. The prophylactic treatment of chronic daily headache. *Headache.* 2006;46(10): 1552–64.

Nair KPS, Marsden J. The management of spasticity in adults. *BMJ.* 2014;349:g4737.

Saulino M, Jacobs BW. The pharmacological management of spasticity. *J Neurosci Nurs.* 2006;38(6):456–9.

Smith H, Elliott J. Alpha(2) receptors and agonists in pain management. *Curr Opin Anaesthesiol.* 2001;14(5):513–18.

TOPIRAMATE

THERAPEUTICS

Brands
- Topamax, Topamax Sprinkle, Trokendi XR, Qudexy XR

Generic?
- Yes

Class
- Antiepileptic drug (AED)

Commonly Prescribed for
(FDA approved in bold)
- **Partial-onset seizures (adjunctive; adults and pediatric patients age 2–16)**
- **Primary generalized tonic-clonic seizures (adjunctive; adults and pediatric patients age 2–16)**
- **Lennox-Gastaut syndrome adjunctive therapy (age > 2)**
- **Migraine prophylaxis (Topamax only)**
- Cluster headache prophylaxis
- Myoclonic epilepsy
- Neuralgia/neuropathic pain
- Drop attacks associated with Lennox-Gastaut syndrome
- Obesity
- Bipolar disorder
- Binge-eating disorder/bulimia
- Idiopathic intracranial hypertension
- Alcohol dependence
- Essential tremor
- Phantom limb pain

How the Drug Works
There are multiple mechanisms of action, and it is uncertain which of these give the drug its effectiveness
- Augments the GABA$_{A1}$ receptor
- Blocks voltage-dependent sodium and calcium (N-type) channels
- Antagonizes the glutamate receptor (AMPA/kainate subtype)
- Inhibits carbonic anhydrase (isoenzymes II and IV)
- May inhibit protein kinase activity
- Possible serotonin activity on 5-HT$_{2C}$ receptor

How Long Until It Works
- Seizures: may decrease by 2 weeks

- Migraines: may decrease in as little as 2 weeks, but can take up to 3 months on a stable dose to see full effect

If It Works
- Seizures: goal is the remission of seizures. Continue as long as effective and well tolerated. Consider tapering slowly, stopping after 2 years without seizures, depending on the type of epilepsy
- Migraine: goal is a 50% or greater reduction in migraine disability. Consider tapering or stopping if headaches remit for more than 6 months or if considering pregnancy

If It Doesn't Work
- Increase to highest tolerated dose
- Epilepsy: consider changing to another agent, adding a second agent, using a medical device, or a referral for epilepsy surgery evaluation. When adding a second agent, keep drug interactions in mind
- Migraine: address other issues, such as medication overuse, other coexisting medical disorders, such as anxiety, and consider changing to another agent or adding a second agent

Best Augmenting Combos for Partial Response or Treatment-Resistance
- For some patients with epilepsy or migraine, low-dose polytherapy with 2 or more drugs may be better tolerated and more effective than high-dose monotherapy
- Epilepsy: keep in mind drug interactions and their effect on levels
- Migraine: consider β-blockers, antidepressants, natural products, other AEDs, and non-medication treatments such as biofeedback to improve headache control

Tests
- Mild to moderate decreases in bicarbonate can occur with topiramate, but are uncommon reasons for discontinuation. Routine screening for metabolic acidosis is not recommended

ADVERSE EFFECTS (AEs)

How the Drug Causes AEs
- CNS AEs may be caused by sodium channel blockade or GABA$_A$ receptor augmentation

- Carbonic anhydrase inhibition causes paresthesia, metabolic acidosis, low urinary citrate excretion, increased urinary pH, and formation of calcium phosphate kidney stones

Notable AEs

- Somnolence, dizziness, cognitive problems, especially word-finding difficulties, mood problems, insomnia
- Anorexia, diarrhea, weight loss
- Palinopsia – a visual disturbance that cause persistence of images (rare and frightening for the patient but benign)

 ## Life-Threatening or Dangerous AEs

- Metabolic acidosis
- Kidney stones (calcium phosphate)
- Narrow angle-closure glaucoma (rare)
- Suicidal ideation and behavior
- Fever, dehydration, and lack of sweating (more common in children)
- Hyperammonemia/encephalopathy, hypothermia with concomitant valproic acid use

Weight Gain

- Unusual

unusual   not unusual   common   problematic

Sedation

- Common

unusual   not unusual   common   problematic

What to Do About AEs

- AEs often decrease or remit after a longer time on a stable dose
- Paresthesia may respond to high-potassium diets or potassium tablets
- Cognitive AEs tend to improve with small decreases in dose
- For patients with kidney stones, check the type of stone. Topiramate usually causes calcium phosphate stones

Best Augmenting Agents to Reduce AEs

- Paresthesias related to topiramate may improve with high-potassium diet or tablets
- Other AEs are more likely to be reduced by lowering dose

Usual Dosage Range

- Epilepsy: 200–400mg/day in adults, with maximum 1600mg/day. 5–9mg/kg/day in pediatric patients. Given as 2 divided doses
- Migraine: 25–200mg/day. Patients can take once daily at bedtime to increase compliance. Can use higher doses as tolerated

Dosage Forms

- Sprinkle capsule (Topamax Sprinkle): 15, 25mg
- Tablet (Topamax, topiramate): 25, 50, 100, 200mg
- Extended-release capsule (Trokendi XR, Qudexy XR): 25, 50, 100, 200mg

How to Dose

- Adults: initial 25–50mg/day
- Epilepsy, monotherapy: increase 50mg weekly for 4 weeks, then 100mg weekly until 400mg/day in 2 divided doses
- Epilepsy, adjunctive: increase 25–50mg weekly until 200–400mg/day in 2 divided doses
- Migraine: increase 25mg weekly until 100mg/day in divided dose
- Pediatrics: see Children and Adolescents

 ### Dosing Tips

- Adverse events increase with dose increases
- Weight loss is often dose related, but patients on lower doses (50mg) still lose weight
- Slow titration minimizes sedation and other AEs
- Some patients need higher doses for migraine or cluster headache prophylaxis

Overdose

- Convulsions, drowsiness, sleep disturbance, blurred vision, diplopia, stupor, hypotension, abdominal pain, agitation, dizziness, lethargy, depression, and metabolic acidosis. No reported deaths except with poly-drug overdoses

Long-Term Use

- Safe for long-term use

Habit Forming
• No

How to Stop
• Taper slowly
• Abrupt withdrawal can lead to seizures in patients with epilepsy. Tremor is also common
• Headaches may return within days to months of stopping, but patients often continue to do well for 6 or more months after stopping

Pharmacokinetics
• Mostly (80%) eliminated unchanged in urine. Peak levels at 2 hours and half-life 21 hours

 Drug Interactions
• Phenytoin, carbamazepine, valproic acid, and pioglitazone can increase topiramate clearance and decrease topiramate levels
• Lamotrigine and hydrochlorothiazide may increase topiramate levels
• Topiramate may increase levels of amitriptyline
• Topiramate can decrease levels of lithium, digoxin, and valproic acid
• Carbonic anhydrase inhibitors such as acetazolamide increase the risk of metabolic acidosis and kidney stones
• Topiramate can interact with CNS depressants and alcohol with neuropsychiatric and cognitive consequences
• Higher-dose topiramate (> 200 mg) can decrease plasma concentrations of estrogens and progestins in patients taking oral contraceptives, perhaps even hormone-releasing intrauterine system as well (1.1 vs. 0.2% normal annual failure rate). Use a higher dose of estrogen or consider alternative methods of contraception in these patients

 Other Warnings/ Precautions
• Patients taking a ketogenic diet for seizures are more likely to experience severe metabolic acidosis on topiramate

Do Not Use
• Patients with a proven allergy to topiramate

Renal Impairment
• Topiramate is renally excreted and removed by hemodialysis. Lower dose and give an extra dose after dialysis sessions

Hepatic Impairment
• May be decreased in patients with significant liver disease

Cardiac Impairment
• No known effects

Elderly
• Elderly patients may be more susceptible to AEs

 Children and Adolescents
• Approved for treatment of children over age 2 for epilepsy management
• Starting dose 1–3 mg/kg/day at night, increasing every 1–2 weeks by 1–3 mg/kg/day until goal dose of 5–9 mg/kg/day in 2 divided doses
• Paresthesias and cognitive AEs are less common in children

 Pregnancy
• Category D. Increases the risk of cleft lip and cleft palate birth defects in babies born to women who use the medication during pregnancy
• Associated with hypospadias in male infants
• Risks of stopping medication must outweigh risk to fetus for patients with epilepsy. Seizures and potential status epilepticus place the woman and fetus at risk and can cause reduced oxygen and blood supply to the womb
• Patients with migraine should generally stop topiramate before considering pregnancy. Migraine usually improves in the last 2 trimesters
• Supplementation with 0.4 mg of folic acid before and during pregnancy is recommended

Breast Feeding

- Found in breast milk
- General recommendations are to discontinue drug or bottle feed
- Monitor infant for sedation, poor feeding, or irritability

THE ART OF NEUROPHARMACOLOGY

Potential Advantages

- Effectively treats both migraine and epilepsy. Usually causes weight loss, unlike many other medications for epilepsy and migraine

Potential Disadvantages

- Cognitive AEs. Weight loss in thin patients can be troublesome. Kidney stones and metabolic acidosis

Primary Target Symptoms

- Seizure frequency and severity
- Migraine frequency and severity

 Pearls

- As initial therapy: partial-onset seizure (Level of Evidence C), generalized tonic-clonic seizure (Level of Evidence C), juvenile myoclonic epilepsy (Level of Evidence D)
- For epilepsy, higher doses may be needed. AEs are more common when using in combination with other drugs that can produce CNS depression
- Broad-spectrum AED effective against almost all seizure types (maybe even infantile spasms)

- Potentially an adjunctive treatment for status epilepticus due to enteral formulation
- For migraine (Level of Evidence A), the individual dose may vary widely. Some patients benefit from doses as low as 25 mg/day but others may require much higher doses than the 100 mg/day approved for migraine prophylaxis. It works for both episodic and chronic migraines
- Animal studies suggest that topiramate may act outside of the trigeminocervical complex for migraine prevention
- Topiramate may be effective in treating idiopathic intracranial hypertension (pseudotumor cerebrii) and is often easier to tolerate, with more weight loss, than acetazolamide
- Topiramate is not a first-line medication for cluster headache
- Case reports on hypnic headache treatment suggest it may be effective
- Topiramate is probably effective for essential tremor (Level of Evidence B), although higher doses are often needed to see an effect
- Topiramate may be used as adjunctive treatment of manic symptoms in bipolar disorder, but its efficacy was not established in clinical trials
- Although it has been associated with negative effect on mood and behavior (depression, aggression, psychosis), it may be effective for depression or augment SSRIs in treatment of resistant major depressive disorder, and anti-impulsive effects
- Combination with phentermine can be used for weight loss

Suggested Reading

Allison DB, Gadde KM, Garvey WT, Peterson CA, Schwiers ML, Najarian T, et al. Controlled-release phentermine/topiramate in severely obese adults: a randomized controlled trial (EQUIP). *Obesity*. 2011;20(2):330–42.

Celebisoy N, Gökçay F, Sirin H, Akyürekli O. Treatment of idiopathic intracranial hypertension: topiramate vs acetazolamide, an open-label study. *Acta Neurol Scand*. 2007; 116(5):322–7.

Glauser T, Ben-Menachem E, Bourgeois B, Cnaan A, Guerreiro C, Kälviäinen R, et al. Updated ILAE evidence review of antiepileptic drug efficacy and effectiveness as initial monotherapy for epileptic seizures and syndromes. *Epilepsia*. 2013;54(3): 551–63.

Silberstein SD, Holland S, Freitag F, Dodick DW, Argoff C, Ashman E. Evidence-based guideline update: pharmacologic treatment for episodic migraine prevention in adults: report of the Quality Standards Subcommittee of the American Academy of Neurology and the American Headache Society. *Neurology*. 2012;78(17):1337–45.

Taylor FR. Weight change associated with the use of migraine-preventive medications. *Clin Ther*. 2008;30(6):1069–80.

van Passel L, Arif H, Hirsch LJ. Topiramate for the treatment of epilepsy and other nervous system disorders. *Expert Rev Neurother*. 2006; 6(1):19–31.

Zesiewicz TA, Elble RJ, Louis ED, Gronseth GS, Ondo WG, Dewey RB, et al. Evidence-based guideline update: treatment of essential tremor: report of the Quality Standards subcommittee of the American Academy of Neurology. *Neurology*. 2011;77(19):1752–5.

TRIENTINE HYDROCHLORIDE

Brands
- Syprine

Generic?
- Yes

 Class
- Chelating agent

Commonly Prescribed for
(FDA approved in bold)
- Wilson's disease (WD) in patients intolerant of penicillamine

 How the Drug Works
- In WD copper accumulates in body tissues (especially the liver and CNS), causing neurological/psychiatric problems and/or liver failure. Trientine binds to (chelates) copper, allowing it to be excreted in the urine

How Long Until It Works
- 6 months or more

If It Works
- Continue treatment, if tolerated. Most patients remain on drug for the rest of their life but if serum copper returns to normal (< 10 mcg/dL) consider changing to elemental zinc or zinc sulfate. Monitor for recurrence of symptoms or changes in urinary copper excretion

If It Doesn't Work
- Increase to as much as 2000 mg daily for poor clinical response or if free serum copper is above 20 mcg/dL. For liver failure or truly refractory patients, liver transplantation is curative

 Best Augmenting Combos for Partial Response or Treatment-Resistance
- Change to penicillamine if ineffective. A diet low in copper-containing foods, such as nuts, chocolate, liver, and dried fruit, is recommended

Tests
- Adequately treated patients should have free serum copper below 10 mcg/dL. Monitor 24-hour urinary copper excretion every 6–12 months (should be between 0.5 and 1 mg)

How the Drug Causes AEs
- Unknown

Notable AEs
- Heartburn, iron deficiency anemia, anorexia, cramps, muscle pain, and epigastric pain have been reported. Rarely muscle spasm or dystonia has occurred. The relationship of these symptoms to trientine is unclear

 Life-Threatening or Dangerous AEs
- Myasthenia gravis and systemic lupus erythematosus have been reported

Weight Gain
- Unusual

unusual | not unusual | common | problematic

Sedation
- Unusual

unusual | not unusual | common | problematic

What to Do About AEs
- Discontinue only for serious AEs

Best Augmenting Agents to Reduce AEs
- Most AEs cannot be reduced with the use of an augmenting agent

Usual Dosage Range
- 1000–2000 mg/day

Dosage Forms
- Tablets: 250 mg

How to Dose
- Start at 750–1250 mg/day in 2–4 divided doses. Increase to as much as 2 g daily in divided doses as needed

 Dosing Tips
- Give at least 1 hour before or 2 hours after meals to ensure absorption

Overdose
- Symptoms unknown

Long-Term Use
- Safe for long-term use

Habit Forming
- No

How to Stop
- No need to taper

Pharmacokinetics
- Not available

 Drug Interactions
- Mineral supplements block the absorption of trientine. Do not give within 2 hours of iron supplements

 Other Warnings/ Precautions
- Capsule contents can cause contact dermatitis

Do Not Use
- Known hypersensitivity

Renal Impairment
- Use with caution

Hepatic Impairment
- Usually improves hepatic disease in WD, even if severe

Cardiac Impairment
- No known effects

Elderly
- Use with caution

 Children and Adolescents
- WD can occur in children, usually ages 5 or older. In children 12 or younger, start at 500–750 mg/day in 2–4 divided doses. Increase to maximum of 1500 mg/day. Dose children over 12 as adults

 Pregnancy
- Category C. Use only if needed

Breast Feeding
- Unknown if excreted in breast milk

THE ART OF NEUROPHARMACOLOGY

Potential Advantages
- Compared to penicillamine, fewer AEs and easier to dose. Small head-to-head studies show effectiveness is similar

Potential Disadvantages
- Penicillamine has been used for a longer period of time with more evidence of effectiveness

Primary Target Symptoms
- Monitor serum and urinary copper to determine effectiveness. Treatment should improve neurological symptoms, including parkinsonism, dystonia, ataxia, depression, and psychosis

 Pearls
- The high incidence of paradoxical worsening and multiple AEs seen with penicillamine have led many to suggest that trientine should be the first-line agent in WD
- Not indicated for rheumatoid arthritis or cystinuria
- Other agents with known effects in WD include tetrathiomolybdate and IM dimercaprol
- In asymptomatic WD individuals diagnosed by abnormal test results or family screening, it is uncertain if zinc, trientine, or penicillamine is most appropriate initial treatment

Suggested Reading

Brewer GJ. Novel therapeutic approaches to the treatment of Wilson's disease. *Expert Opin Pharmacother.* 2006;7(3):317–24.

Brewer GJ. The risks of free copper in the body and the development of useful anticopper drugs. *Curr Opin Clin Nutr Metab Care.* 2008;11(6): 727–32.

Das SK, Ray K. Wilson's disease: an update. *Nat Clin Pract Neurol.* 2006;2(9):482–93.

Wiggelinkhuizen M, Tilanus ME, Bollen CW, Houwen RH. Systematic review: clinical efficacy of chelator agents and zinc in the initial treatment of Wilson disease. *Aliment Pharmacol Ther.* 2009;29(9):947–58.

TRIHEXYPHENIDYL

THERAPEUTICS

Brands
- Artane, Tremin (discontinued)

Generic?
- Yes

Class
- Antiparkinson agent, anticholinergic

Commonly Prescribed for
(FDA approved in bold)
- **Extrapyramidal disorders**
- **Parkinsonism**
- Idiopathic generalized dystonia
- Focal dystonias
- Dopa-responsive dystonia
- Cerebral palsy
- Tardive dyskinesia

How the Drug Works
- Trihexyphenidyl is a synthetic anticholinergic with relatively greater CNS activity than most other anticholinergics
- May also inhibit the reuptake and storage of dopamine at dopamine neurons and transporters, prolonging dopamine action
- In Parkinson's disease (PD), it works presumably by restoration of the striatal dopamine-acetylcholine balance through blockade of postsynaptic muscarinic receptors; this may benefit from denervation hypersensitivity caused by loss of the ascending cholinergic input to that region from the basal forebrain

How Long Until It Works
- PD/extrapyramidal disorders: minutes to hours
- Dystonia: days to weeks

If It Works
- PD: do not abruptly discontinue or change doses of other PD treatments. Usually most effective in combination with other medications

If It Doesn't Work
- PD: generally trihexyphenidyl is an adjunctive medication for common PD symptoms, such as tremor, rigidity, and drooling. Other cardinal PD symptoms, such as bradykinesia and gait difficulties, are most likely to improve with other PD treatments, such as levodopa, dopamine agonists, amantadine, or monoamine oxidase (MAO)-B inhibitors
- Extrapyramidal disorders: increase to highest tolerated dose. Long-standing disorders are less likely to respond to treatment

Best Augmenting Combos for Partial Response or Treatment-Resistance
- For bradykinesia or gait disturbances causing significant functional disturbance, levodopa is most effective. For idiopathic PD patients, especially younger patients with normal cognition and milder disability, dopamine agonists are also a good first choice. Amantadine and MAO-B inhibitors may also be useful
- Depression is common in PD and may respond to low-dose SSRIs

Tests
- None

ADVERSE EFFECTS (AEs)

How the Drug Causes AEs
- Prevents the action of acetylcholine on related receptors

Notable AEs
- Constipation, urinary retention, behavioral, dry mouth, tachycardia, palpitations, hypotension, disorientation, confusion, hallucinations, nausea/vomiting, dilation of colon, rash, blurred vision, diplopia, elevated temperature, decreased sweating, erectile dysfunction

Life-Threatening or Dangerous AEs
- May precipitate narrow-angle glaucoma. Risk of heat stroke, especially in elderly patients. Can precipitate tachycardia, cardiac arrhythmias, and hypotension in susceptible patients. May cause urinary retention in patients with prostate hypertrophy

Weight Gain
- Unusual

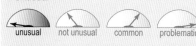

Sedation
- Common

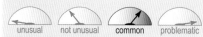

What to Do About AEs
- Confusion, hallucinations: if possible stop trihexyphenidyl and any other anticholinergics
- Sedation: can take entire dose at night or lower dose
- Dry mouth: chewing gum or water can help
- Urinary retention: if drug cannot be discontinued, obtain urological evaluation

Best Augmenting Agents to Reduce AEs
- Most AEs cannot be reduced with the use of an augmenting agent

DOSING AND USE

Usual Dosage Range
- PD: 6–15 mg/day
- Extrapyramidal reactions: 5–15 mg/day

Dosage Forms
- Tablets: 2, 5 mg
- Elixir: 2 mg/5 mL
- Capsule, extended release: 5 mg

How to Dose
- PD: start at 1 mg the first few days. Then increase in 2 mg increments every 3–5 days as tolerated or until clinical effect reached. Divide total dose and give 3 times daily, usually with meals. Patients on very high doses may elect to take 4 doses daily: with meals and at bedtime. Usual dose is 6–10 mg in idiopathic PD but higher on average (12–15 mg) in post-encephalitic PD
- Drug-induced extrapyramidal disorders: wait a few hours to assess effect and increase dose empirically as tolerated. The total daily dose varies from patient to patient. To achieve more rapid relief, temporarily lower dose of the offending agent (phenothiazine, thioxanthene, or butyrophenone) when starting

 Dosing Tips
- Taking with meals may reduce AEs

Overdose
- Complications may include circulatory collapse, cardiac arrest, respiratory depression or arrest, CNS depression or stimulation, psychosis, shock, coma, seizures, ataxia, combativeness, anhidrosis and hyperthermia, fever, dysphagia, decreased bowel sounds, and sluggish pupils. Induce emesis, use gastric lavage or activated charcoal. Oxygen or intubation may be needed for respiratory depression. Catheterize for urinary retention. Treat hyperthermia appropriately with cooling devices, local miotics for mydriasis/cycloplegia. Use physostigmine to reverse cardiac effects and use fluids and vasopressors if needed

Long-Term Use
- Generally safe for long-term use. Effectiveness may decrease over time (years) in PD and AEs. Moreover, in PD, long-term use of anticholinergic is associated with cognitive decline (more cortical plaques or tangles)

Habit Forming
- No

How to Stop
- No need to taper

Pharmacokinetics
- Half-life is 6–10 hours, but the time to peak effect is 1–1.3 hours. Mostly urinary excretion. Bioavailability is about 100% but metabolism not well understood

 Drug Interactions
- Use with amantadine may increase AEs
- Trihexyphenidyl and all other anticholinergics may increase serum levels and effects of digoxin
- Can lower concentration of haloperidol and other phenothiazines, causing worsening of schizophrenia symptoms. Phenothiazines

tend to increase anticholinergic AEs with concurrent use

- Can decrease gastric motility, resulting in increased gastric deactivation of levodopa and reduction in efficacy

 Other Warning/ Precautions

- Use with caution in hot weather: may increase susceptibility to heat stroke
- Anticholinergics have additive effects when used with drugs of abuse, such as cannabinoids, barbiturates, opioids, and alcohol

Do Not Use

- Known hypersensitivity to the drug, glaucoma (especially angle-closure type), pyloric or duodenal obstruction, stenosing peptic ulcers, prostate hypertrophy or bladder neck obstructions, achalasia, or megacolon

SPECIAL POPULATIONS

Renal Impairment

- Use with caution but no known effects

Hepatic Impairment

- Use with caution but no known effects

Cardiac Impairment

- Use with caution in patients with known arrhythmias, especially tachycardia

Elderly

- Use with caution. More susceptible to AEs

 Children and Adolescents

- Do not use in children aged 3 or less. Generalized dystonias may respond to anticholinergic treatment; young patients usually tolerate the medication better than the elderly

 Pregnancy

- Category C. Use only if benefit of medication outweighs risks

Breast Feeding

- Concentration in breast milk unknown. May inhibit lactation. Use only if benefits outweigh risk

THE ART OF NEUROPHARMACOLOGY

Potential Advantages

- Useful adjunctive agent for some PD patients, especially post-encephalitic and younger patients with bothersome tremor. First-line agent for generalized dystonias and well tolerated in the younger age groups

Potential Disadvantages

- Multiple dose-dependent AEs associated with antimuscarinic effects limit use. Not effective in most idiopathic PD patients. Patients with long-standing extrapyramidal disorders may not respond to treatment

Primary Target Symptoms

- Tremor, akinesia, rigidity, drooling, dystonia

 Pearls

- Useful adjunct in younger PD patients with tremor
- Useful in the treatment of post-encephalitic PD
- Constipation and sedation limit use, especially in older patients. Patients with mental impairment do poorly
- Post-encephalitic PD patients usually tolerate higher doses better than idiopathic PD patients
- Generalized dystonias are more likely to benefit from anticholinergic therapy than focal dystonias
- Dystonias related to cerebral palsy, head injuries, and stroke may improve with trihexyphenidyl, especially in younger, cognitively normal patients
- Schizophrenic patients may abuse trihexyphenidyl and other anticholinergic medications to relieve negative symptoms, for a stimulant effect, or to improve symptoms of drug-induced parkinsonism
- In PD, there is significant cholinergic loss and reduced binding capacity to nicotinic receptors. Long-term anticholinergic use in

PD is associated with cognitive decline (cortical plaques or tangles), visual hallucination, gait dysfunction, and falls

- For generalized dystonia, deep brain stimulation is more effective; for focal dystonia, botulinum toxin A is more effective than anticholinergics

Suggested Reading

Batla A, Stamelou M, Bhatia KP. Treatment of focal dystonia. *Curr Treat Options Neurol.* 2012;14(3):213–29.

Brocks DR. Anticholinergic drugs used in Parkinson's disease: An overlooked class of drugs from a pharmacokinetic perspective. *J Pharm Pharm Sci.* 1999;2(2): 39–46.

Carranza-del Rio J, Clegg NJ, Moore A, Delgado MR. Use of trihexyphenidyl in children with cerebral palsy. *Pediatr Neurol.* 2011;44(3): 202–6.

Colosimo C, Gori MC, Inghilleri M. Post-encephalitic tremor and delayed-onset parkinsonism. *Parkinsonism Relat Disord.* 1999;5(3):123–4.

Koy A, Hellmich M, Pauls KAM, Marks W, Lin J-P, Fricke O, et al. Effects of deep brain stimulation in dyskinetic cerebral palsy: a meta-analysis. *Mov Disord.* 2013;28(5):647–54.

Yarnall A, Rochester L, Burn DJ. The interplay of cholinergic function, attention, and falls in Parkinson's disease. *Mov Disord.* 2011;26(14): 2496–503.

Zemishlany Z, Aizenberg D, Weiner Z, Weizman A. Trihexyphenidyl (Artane) abuse in schizophrenic patients. *Int Clin Psychopharmacol.* 1996;11(3):199–202.

VALPROIC ACID

Brands

- Depakote, Depakote ER, Depakene, Depacon, Episenta, Epilim, Epival, Dicorate, Disorate, Divaa, Divalpro, Soval DX, Trend XR, Valna, Stavzor

Generic?

- Yes

Class

- Antiepileptic drug (AED)

Commonly Prescribed for

(FDA approved in bold)

- **Complex partial seizures (monotherapy and adjunctive)**
- **Simple and complex absence seizures (monotherapy and adjunctive)**
- **Adjunctive therapy for multiple seizure types, including absence seizures**
- **Migraine prophylaxis (delayed-release capsule only)**
- **Acute mania in bipolar disorder (delayed-release capsule only)**
- Cluster headache
- Generalized tonic-clonic seizures, including juvenile myoclonic epilepsy
- Lennox-Gastaut syndrome
- Status epilepticus
- Post-hypoxic myoclonus
- Landau-Kleffner syndrome (acquired epileptic aphasia)
- Spinal muscular atrophy
- Acute migraine or status migrainosus
- Schizophrenia/psychosis
- Cyclothymia

How the Drug Works

The mechanisms of action of valproic acid and derivatives (DPX) are probably multiple

- Activates glutamic acid decarboxylase to increase GABA production
- Inhibits GABA transaminase and the catabolism of GABA
- Sodium channel antagonist
- Blocks T-type calcium currents in thalamus
- Suppresses NMDA excitatory neurotransmission

How Long Until It Works

- Seizures: 2 weeks
- Migraines: effective within a few weeks but can take up to 3 months to see full effect
- Mania: usually effective in days

If It Works

- Seizures: goal is the remission of seizures. Continue as long as effective and well tolerated. Consider slowly tapering and stopping after 2 years seizure-free, depending on the type of epilepsy
- Migraine: goal is a 50% or greater reduction in migraine frequency or severity. Consider tapering or stopping if headaches remit for more than 6 months or if patient considering pregnancy

If It Doesn't Work

- Increase to highest tolerated dose. Check a drug level if compliance an issue
- Epilepsy: consider changing to another agent, adding a second agent, using a medical device, or a referral for epilepsy surgery evaluation. When adding a second agent, keep drug interactions in mind
- Migraine: address other issues, such as medication overuse, other coexisting medical disorders, such as anxiety, and consider changing to or adding a second agent

 Best Augmenting Combos for Partial Response or Treatment-Resistance

- Epilepsy: drug interactions complicate multi-drug therapy, especially the older AEDs. Most of the newer drugs, such as gabapentin, topiramate, oxcarbazepine, and zonisamide, are easier to use with DPX
- Migraine: consider β-blockers, antidepressants, natural products, other AEDs, and non-medication treatments, such as biofeedback, to improve headache control

Tests

- Obtain liver function testing and platelet counts before starting, optional to monitor regularly for the first few months and once or twice a year after that. Test urgently if any symptoms of liver disease, new bleeding or easy bruising

- Monitor for weight gain and signs of metabolic syndrome (weight gain, hyperlipidemia, elevated fasting glucose)
- Hyperammonemia may occur, even with normal liver function tests. Often asymptomatic. Check a level for any clinically significant symptoms

ADVERSE EFFECTS (AEs)

How the Drug Causes AEs

- CNS AEs may be caused by sodium or calcium channel effects or GABA effects
- DPX-associated hyperammonemia can cause delirium, tremor
- DPX-associated hepatic toxicity can cause nausea, anorexia, or jaundice

Notable AEs

- Sedation, tremor, dizziness, diplopia, blurred vision, cognitive problems
- Nausea, vomiting, abdominal pain, diarrhea, anorexia, constipation
- Weight gain, peripheral edema, bronchitis, pharyngitis, alopecia, carnitine depletion

 ### Life-Threatening or Dangerous AEs

- Hepatotoxicity and liver disease, especially in children under 2 on multiple antiepilepsy medications. More commonly patients have mild to moderate elevations of serum liver enzymes that are asymptomatic. Patients usually recover
- Rare pancreatitis can occur months to years after starting DPX. Most patients recover but can be fatal
- Thrombocytopenia
- Polycystic ovarian syndrome, including obesity, elevated androgen concentrations, anovulation, and hirsutism
- Significant weight gain and development of insulin resistance/metabolic syndrome (controversial)

Weight Gain

- Problematic

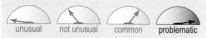

- Usually steady and associated with carbohydrate craving

Sedation

- Common. May wear off with time

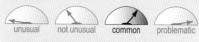

What to Do About AEs

- May be decreased with extended-release formulation
- Decrease dose
- Small elevations in liver enzymes or increased ammonia are common. If there are no symptoms, then the decision to decrease or maintain dose depends on the patient and the severity of the condition treated
- Change to another drug

Best Augmenting Agents to Reduce AEs

- Propranolol for tremor
- Weight gain may improve with augmentation or transition to zonisamide or topiramate
- L-carnitine therapy may reduce symptoms of hyperammonemic encephalopathy
- Zinc and selenium can help alopecia

DOSING AND USE

Usual Dosage Range

- Epilepsy: 10–60 mg/kg/day, may need to increase in some patients
- Migraine: 1000 mg/day, some need a higher dose
- Cluster: 500–2000 mg/day
- Acute mania: usually 1000 mg/day or more

Dosage Forms

- Valproic acid (Depakene): 250 mg capsule or 250 mg/5 mL syrup
- Divalproex sodium (Depakote): 125 mg capsule, or delayed-release pellets. Tablet: 125, 250, 500 mg; extended release: 250, 500 mg
- Valproate sodium (Depacon): 100 mg/mL in 5 mL vials for injection

How to Dose

- Epilepsy: Start at 10–15 mg/kg/day and increase to goal dose
- Migraine: Start at 250–500 mg once daily at bedtime

- As valproic acid: three times a day; as delayed-release divalproex sodium: twice a day. Depakote ER can be taken once daily

Dosing Tips

- Easier to rapidly increase dose than many other AEDs; IV Depacon available for emergency use to treat seizures, status migrainosus, and mania
- When converting to Depakote ER, plasma levels are generally 10–20% lower than immediate release for a given dose
- Oral loading with 20–30 mg/kg/day is an alternative to IV loading
- Depakote ER has fewer GI AEs; avoids peak levels
- For most conditions levels 50–100 mcg/mL are effective, but in some cases higher levels are needed, i.e., cluster headache and mania

Overdose

- Stupor and coma, increased intracranial pressure. Fever. Respiratory insufficiency and supraventricular tachycardia. Supportive care and gastric lavage. Can be fatal

Long-Term Use

- Regular platelet counts and liver function testing. Optional unless patient symptomatic

Habit Forming

- No

How to Stop

- Taper slowly and keep drug interactions in mind
- Abrupt withdrawal can lead to seizures in patients with epilepsy
- Headaches may return within days to months of stopping

Pharmacokinetics

- Metabolized mainly by glucuronidation and β-oxidation but minimally by CYP450 microsomal-mediated oxidation. Plasma half-life is 9–16 hours. 100% bioavailability and 93% protein bound (can replace some protein-bound drugs)

Drug Interactions

Effect from DPX:
- DPX causes interactions by displacing other medications from plasma proteins and inhibiting hepatic metabolism
- Increases levels of carbamazepine, lamotrigine, phenobarbital, ethosuximide, free phenytoin (can cause toxicity even under normal phenytoin serum levels), warfarin, amitriptyline, nortriptyline, zidovudine, diazepam, cimetidine, chlorpromazine, erythromycin, and nimodipine
- Decreases level of topiramate, mycophenolate

Effect on DPX:
- Drugs that affect the expression of hepatic enzymes such as glucuronosyl transferases can alter DPX clearance
- Phenytoin, phenobarbital, primidone, cholestyramine, rifampin, carbamazepine, lamotrigine, topiramate, contraceptives (hepatic inducers) can lower DPX levels
- Addition of salicylates, erythromycin, felbamate, quetiapine, and chlorpromazine can increase DPX levels

⚠️ Other Warnings/Precautions

- CNS AEs increase when taken with other CNS depressants or with most acute or chronic illnesses
- Hepatoxicity: nausea, vomiting, jaundice, edema
- Pancreatitis: abdominal pain, anorexia, nausea
- Teratogenic effects: neural tube defects
- Urea cycle disorders: unexplained delirium in children, mental retardation, vomiting, lethargy, and hyperammonemia
- Risk of hyperammonemia if concomitant use of topiramate

Do Not Use

- Patients with a proven allergy to DPX. Also contraindicated in patients with thrombocytopenia, liver disease, urea cycle disorders, and pancreatitis

Renal Impairment

- No known effects. Highly protein bound, easier to use in patients on dialysis than most other AEDs

Hepatic Impairment

- Do not use

Cardiac Impairment

- No known effects

Elderly

- Use a lower dose and watch for AEs and nutritional intake

 Children and Adolescents

- Approved for use in children and often used in generalized seizures, such as absence and juvenile myoclonic epilepsy
- May help treat infantile spasms related to tuberous sclerosis, especially if corticotropin is ineffective or cannot be used
- For infants with new-onset unexplained seizures, metabolic diseases are not rare. Consider using an alternative agent until ruled out

 Pregnancy

- Category D (epilepsy, bipolar), X (migraine). Increased risk of neural tube defects, cardiac defects, craniofacial abnormalities, and hepatic failure
- Women who continue taking DPX during pregnancy should be considered high-risk and take folate
- In patients that continue taking during pregnancy, consider vitamin K during the last 6 weeks of pregnancy to reduce risk of bleeding
- Patients taking DPX for conditions other than epilepsy should generally stop DPX before considering pregnancy. Migraine usually improves in the last 2 trimesters

Breast Feeding

- Relatively low (1–10%) in breast milk and safer than most other AEDs
- Monitor infant for sedation, poor feeding, or irritability

Potential Advantages

- Highly effective for multiple types of epilepsy due to broad spectrum of action. Treats generalized seizures as well as partial and is approved as monotherapy. Effective for both migraine and cluster headache. Useful for patients with more than one condition, such as migraine and epilepsy or mania

Potential Disadvantages

- Weight gain. Tremor. Risk of polycystic ovarian syndrome and teratogenicity makes it difficult to use in women of childbearing age. Protein binding and enzyme induction cause drug interactions. Liver disease and hepatotoxicity in children under 2

Primary Target Symptoms

- Seizure frequency and severity
- Headache frequency and severity
- Mood stabilizer

 Pearls

- Drug of choice for patients with generalized epilepsies; however, may not be as effective as carbamazepine for focal seizures
- Useful in status epilepticus for patients with contraindications to phenytoin. Loading dose 20–40mg/kg IV and maintenance dose 3–6mg/kg/min IV. Less respiratory depression than other AEDs
- Highly effective for migraine and cluster prophylaxis. For cluster, DPX is more likely to be effective at the upper end of the therapeutic range
- May be useful as an acute headache treatment in the emergency room or infusion setting as IV Depacon (300–1000mg as rapid infusion). For use as a preventive drug after discharge, load the medication (15mg/kg) and then administer 5mg/kg every 8–12 hours. IV Depacon for acute headache is especially useful for patients who cannot tolerate or have contraindications to other medications
- For migraine prophylaxis in non-childbearing migraineurs (level of Evidence A)
- For migraine patients on DPX with tremor and suboptimal headache control, propranolol may improve headaches and treat tremor

- DPX may have neuroprotective properties, such as inhibition of apoptosis and slowing of neurofibrillary tangle formation, suggesting usefulness for treatment of neurodegenerative diseases. However, studies for treatment of Alzheimer's dementia and associated psychosis have been largely negative, with poor tolerability in this population

- Preliminary studies suggest utility in treating spinal muscular atrophy, especially in young children
- Maternal use of valproate during pregnancy was associated with a significantly increased risk of autism spectrum disorder and childhood autism in the offspring, even after adjusting for maternal epilepsy

Suggested Reading

Christensen J, Grønborg TK, Sørensen MJ, Schendel D, Parner ET, Pedersen LH, et al. Prenatal valproate exposure and risk of autism spectrum disorders and childhood autism. *JAMA.* 2013;309(16):1696–703.

Cohen AS, Matharu MS, Goadsby PJ. Trigeminal autonomic cephalalgias: current and future treatments. *Headache.* 2007;47(6):969–80.

Glauser TA, Cnaan A, Shinnar S, Hirtz DG, Dlugos D, Masur D, et al. Ethosuximide, valproic acid, and lamotrigine in childhood absence epilepsy. *N Engl J Med.* 2010;362(9):790–9.

Limdi NA, Knowlton RK, Cofield SS, Ver Hoef LW, Paige AL, Dutta S, et al. Safety of rapid intravenous loading of valproate. *Epilepsia.* 2007;48(3):478–83.

Linde M, Mulleners WM, Chronicle EP, McCrory DC. Valproate (valproic acid or sodium valproate or a combination of the two) for the prophylaxis of episodic migraine in adults. *Cochrane Database Syst Rev.* 2013;6:CD010609.

Mackay MT, Weiss SK, Adams-Webber T, Ashwal S, Stephens D, Ballaban-Gill K, et al.; American Academy of Neurology; Child

Neurology Society. Practice parameter: medical treatment of infantile spasms: report of the American Academy of Neurology and the Child Neurology Society. *Neurology.* 2004;62(10): 1668–81.

Rauchenzauner M, Haberlandt E, Scholl-Bürgi S, Ernst B, Hoppichler F, Karall D, et al. Adiponectin and visfatin concentrations in children treated with valproic acid. *Epilepsia.* 2008;49(2):353–7.

Silberstein SD, Holland S, Freitag F, Dodick DW, Argoff C, Ashman E. Evidence-based guideline update: pharmacologic treatment for episodic migraine prevention in adults: report of the Quality Standards Subcommittee of the American Academy of Neurology and the American Headache Society. *Neurology.* 2012;78(17):1337–45.

Swoboda KJ, Scott CB, Reyna SP, Prior TW, LaSalle B, Sorenson SL, et al. Phase II open label study of valproic acid in spinal muscular atrophy. *PLoS One.* 2009;4(5):e5268.

Trinka E. The use of valproate and new antiepileptic drugs in status epilepticus. *Epilepsia.* 2007;48 Suppl 8:49–51.

Brands
- Effexor, Effexor XR, Effexor XL, Efectin, Efexor, Trevilor, Venla

Generic?
- Yes

 ### Class
- Serotonin and norepinephrine reuptake inhibitor (SNRI)

Commonly Prescribed for
(FDA approved in bold)
- **Major depressive disorder**
- **Generalized anxiety disorder (Effexor XR only)**
- **Panic disorder (Effexor XR only)**
- **Social phobia (Effexor XR only)**
- Migraine or tension-type headache prophylaxis
- Diabetic neuropathy
- Other painful peripheral neuropathies
- Cancer pain (neuropathic)
- Depression secondary to stroke
- Stress urinary incontinence
- Fibromyalgia
- Binge-eating disorder
- Post-traumatic stress disorder (PTSD)
- Attention deficit hyperactivity disorder
- Perimenopausal/menopausal hot flushes
- Cataplexy

 ### How the Drug Works
- Both venlafaxine and its active metabolite (desvenlafaxine) are potent inhibitors of serotonin and norepinephrine reuptake transporters (SERT, NET), increasing serotonin and norepinephrine levels within hours, but antidepressant effects take weeks. Effect is more likely related to adaptive changes in serotonin and norepinephrine receptor systems over time
- Weakly blocks dopamine reuptake pump (dopamine transporter)
- Interacts with μ-opioid receptors and α_2-adrenergic receptor

How Long Until It Works
- Migraines: effective in as little as 2 weeks, but can take up to 10 weeks on a stable dose to see full effect

- Tension-type headache prophylaxis: effective in 4–8 weeks
- Neuropathic pain: usually some effect within 4 weeks
- Diabetic neuropathy: may have significant improvement with high doses within 6 weeks
- Depression: 2 weeks but up to 2 months for full effect

If It Works
- Migraine/tension-type headache: goal is a 50% or greater reduction in headache frequency or severity. Consider tapering or stopping if headaches remit for more than 6 months or if considering pregnancy
- Neuropathic pain: the goal is to reduce pain intensity and symptoms, but usually does not produce remission. Continue to use and monitor for AEs
- Diabetic neuropathy: the goal is to reduce pain intensity and reduce use of analgesics, but usually does not produce remission. Continue to use and maintain strict glycemic control and diabetic management
- Depression: continue to use and monitor for AEs. May continue for 1 year following first depression episode or indefinitely if > 1 episode of depression

If It Doesn't Work
- Increase to highest tolerated dose
- Migraine and tension-type headache: address other issues, such as medication overuse, other coexisting medical disorders, such as anxiety, and consider changing to another agent or adding a second agent
- Neuropathic pain: either change to another agent or add a second agent

 ### Best Augmenting Combos for Partial Response or Treatment-Resistance
- Headache: for some patients, low-dose polytherapy with 2 or more drugs may be better tolerated and more effective than high-dose monotherapy. May use in combination with AEDs, antihypertensives, natural products, and non-medication treatments, such as biofeedback, to improve headache control
- Neuropathic pain: TCAs, AEDs (gabapentin, pregabalin, carbamazepine, lamotrigine), SNRIs (duloxetine, venlafaxine, milnacipran, mirtazapine, bupropion), capsaicin, and

mexiletine are agents used for neuropathic pain. Opioids (morphine, tramadol) may be appropriate for long-term use in some cases but require careful monitoring

Tests

- Check blood pressure at baseline and when increasing dose
- Monitor sodium, intraocular pressure, suicidality, and unusual changes in behavior

ADVERSE EFFECTS (AEs)

How the Drug Causes AEs

- By increasing serotonin and norepinephrine on non-therapeutic responsive receptors throughout the body. Most AEs are dose- and time-dependent

Notable AEs

- Constipation, dry mouth, sweating, blurry vision, mydriasis, anorexia, nausea, weight loss or gain, hypertension, headache, asthenia, dizziness, tremor, dream disorder, insomnia, somnolence, abnormal ejaculation, impotence, orgasm disorder, sweating, itching, sedation, nervousness, restlessness, cholesterol/triglyceride elevation

 Life-Threatening or Dangerous AEs

- Serotonin syndrome
- Rare hepatitis
- Rare activation of mania or suicidal ideation
- Rare worsening of coexisting seizure disorders

Weight Gain

- Not unusual

unusual not unusual common problematic

Sedation

- Not unusual

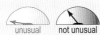
unusual not unusual common problematic

- May cause insomnia in some patients

What to Do About AEs

- For minor AEs, lower dose, titrate more slowly, or switch to another agent. For

serious AEs, lower dose and consider stopping, taper to avoid withdrawal symptoms

Best Augmenting Agents to Reduce AEs

- Try magnesium for constipation
- Cyproheptadine can be used for serotonin syndrome by blocking 5-HT receptors and SERT
- Sexual dysfunction (anorgasmia, impotence) may be reversed by agents with α_2-adrenergic antagonist activity (e.g., buspirone, amantadine, bupropion, mirtazapine, ginkgo biloba, etc.)

DOSING AND USE

Usual Dosage Range

- 37.5–375 mg/day

Dosage Forms

- Tablet (immediate release): 25, 37.5, 50, 75, 100 mg
- Tablet (extended release): 37.5, 75, 150, 225 mg
- Capsule (extended release; insoluble shell): 37.5, 75, 150 mg

How to Dose

- Initial dose 37.5–75 mg taken daily. Increase by 75 mg in 1 week. Titrate as tolerated to effective dose, typically 150–375 mg for pain syndromes. Dose once daily as extended release or divided into 2–3 doses as immediate release

 Dosing Tips

- Higher doses are typically used for pain. Extended-release formulation allows for once-a-day dosing and may be better tolerated. Extended-release capsule/tablet should be swallowed whole and not be crushed or chewed

Overdose

- Signs and symptoms may include cardiac arrhythmias, usually tachycardia, ECG changes (prolonged QTc interval or bundle branch block), sedation, seizures, bowel perforation, serotonin syndrome, fever, rhabdomyolysis, hyponatremia, blood pressure abnormalities, extrapyramidal effects, headache, nervousness, tremor; death can occur

Long-Term Use

- Safe for long-term use with monitoring of blood pressure and suicidality

Habit Forming

- No

How to Stop

- Taper slowly (no more than 50% reduction every 3–4 days until discontinuation) to avoid withdrawal symptoms (agitation, anxiety, confusion, dry mouth, dysphoria, etc.). Pain often worsens shortly after decreasing dose

Pharmacokinetics

- Venlafaxine is metabolized via the CYP2D6 isoenzyme and is a weak inhibitor of this isoenzyme. O-desmethylvenlafaxine is the only major active metabolite of venlafaxine. Half-life 5 hours for venlafaxine and 11 hours for active metabolite O-desmethylvenlafaxine. Venlafaxine extended release provides a slower rate of absorption but the same absorption as immediate-release tablet. For XR capsule, drug release is controlled by diffusion through the coating membrane. Eliminated primarily in urine

 Drug Interactions

- For venlafaxine, the differences between CYP2D6 poor and extensive metabolizers are not clinically important because the sum of venlafaxine and desvenlafaxine is similar in the two groups
- Venlafaxine is a weak inhibitor of CYP2D6. However, venlafaxine XR and desvenlafaxine are less likely to affect CYP2D6 substrates
- For venlafaxine, may reduce dose in the presence of CYP2D6 inhibitors (paroxetine, fluoxetine, bupropion, duloxetine, sertraline, citalopram, methadone, ranitidine, cimetidine) especially in patients with hypertension, hepatic impairment and in elderly
- The release of serotonin by platelets is important for maintaining hemostasis. Combined use of SSRIs or SNRIs (such as venlafaxine) and NSAIDs, and/or drugs that

have anticoagulant effects, has been associated with an increased risk of bleeding

- May decrease effects of antihypertensive medications, such as metoprolol
- May decrease clearance and increase effect of antipsychotics (haloperidol, clozapine)
- May increase the risk of seizure or serotonin syndrome with tramadol
- May cause serotonin syndrome when used within 14 days of MAOIs
- May increase risk of cardiotoxicity and arrhythmia when used with TCAs

 Other Warnings/ Precautions

- May increase risk of seizure
- Patients should be observed closely for clinical worsening, suicidality, and changes in behavior in known or unknown bipolar disorder

Do Not Use

- Proven hypersensitivity to drug
- Concurrently with MAOI; allow at least 14 days between discontinuation of an MAOI and initiation of venlafaxine or at least 7–14 days between discontinuation of venlafaxine and initiation of an MAOI
- Concurrent use of serotonin precursors (e.g., tryptophan)
- In patients with uncontrolled narrow angle-closure glaucoma
- In patients treated with linezolid or methylene blue IV

Renal Impairment

- Use with caution. Decrease usual dose by 25–50%

Hepatic Impairment

- Use with caution. Decrease usual dose by 50%

Cardiac Impairment

- Use with caution. Dose-dependent effect on blood pressure. Venlafaxine may prolong QTc, particularly in the elderly

Elderly

- No adjustments necessary

Children and Adolescents

- Safety and efficacy not established. Use with caution. Observe closely for clinical worsening, suicidality, and changes in behavior in known or unknown bipolar disorder. Parents should be informed and advised of the risks

Pregnancy

- Category C. Generally not recommended for the treatment of headaches or neuropathic pain during pregnancy. Neonates exposed to venlafaxine or other SNRIs or SSRIs late in the third trimester have developed complications necessitating extended hospitalizations, respiratory support, and tube feeding. Respiratory distress, cyanosis, apnea, seizures, temperature instability, feeding difficulty, vomiting, hypoglycemia, hypotonia, hyperreflexia, tremor, jitteriness, irritability, and constant crying consistent with a toxic effect of the drug or drug discontinuation syndrome have been reported

Breast Feeding

- Some drug is found in breast milk and use while breast feeding is not recommended

THE ART OF NEUROPHARMACOLOGY

Potential Advantages

- Very effective in the treatment of multiple pain disorders. Effective for treatment of comorbid depression and anxiety in chronic pain. Less sedation than tertiary amine TCAs (i.e., amitriptyline)

Potential Disadvantages

- May cause or worsen hypertension. Usually higher doses are need for pain disorders than for depression

Primary Target Symptoms

- Reduction in headache frequency, duration, and/or intensity
- Reduction in neuropathic pain
- Reduction in depression, anxiety

Pearls

- At low dose (75 mg/day) venlafaxine works as an SSRI. At higher doses (150–225 mg/day), it exhibits dual activity as SNRI. This may explain why higher doses are needed in pain disorders than depression and anxiety
- In patients with migraine or tension-type headache, best responders were those on dosages of 150 mg (XR formulation) or more, and safety and efficacy have been reported at those doses
- Treat neuropathic pain with effects similar to TCAs but with no antihistamine, fewer anticholinergic AEs (e.g., sedation, orthostatic hypotension, etc.). Venlafaxine (3 studies) has a number needed to treat of 3.1 (2.2–5.1) and a relative risk of 2.2 (95% confidence interval 1.5–3.1) (3 studies)
- Efficacy as well as AEs are usually dose-dependent
- Efficacy and harm risk may not differ much between immediate- and extended-release formulations. The adherence to treatment may differ
- XR formulation allows for once-daily dosing, improves tolerability, and reduces certain AEs (i.e., nausea)
- If high blood pressure is not a major concern, may work well with metoprolol in migraine prophylaxis, as venlafaxine lowers the antihypertensive effect of metoprolol
- Venlafaxine can often precipitate mania in patients with bipolar disorder. Use with caution
- For post-stroke depression, may be superior to SSRIs and may even increase survival
- May be useful as an adjunct for patients with pain and coexisting ADHD
- Treats cataplexy in patients with narcolepsy with cataplexy
- Combination use of SNRI and triptans usually will not lead to serotonin syndrome, which requires activation of 5-HT_{2A} receptors and a possible limited role of 5-HT_{1A}. However, triptans are agonists at the $5\text{-HT}_{1B/1D/1F}$ receptor subtypes, with weak affinity for 5-HT_{1A} receptors and no activity at the 5-HT_2 receptors. Thus, given the seriousness of serotonin syndrome, caution is certainly warranted and clinicians should be vigilant for serotonin toxicity symptoms and signs to insure prompt treatment

- It may reduce PTSD symptoms (re-experiencing, avoidance, and hyperarousal) but not nightmare. Prazosin, which is an

α_1-adrenoceptor blocker that crosses BBB, has been used for PTSD (nightmare, sleep, alcohol dependence, anxiety)

Suggested Reading

Aran A, Einen M, Lin L, Plazzi G, Nishino S, Mignot E. Clinical and therapeutic aspects of childhood narcolepsy-cataplexy: a retrospective study of 51 children. *Sleep.* 2010;33 (11):1457–64.

Evans RW, Tepper SJ, Shapiro RE, Sun-Edelstein C, Tietjen GE. The FDA alert on serotonin syndrome with use of triptans combined with selective serotonin reuptake inhibitors or selective serotonin-norepinephrine reuptake inhibitors: American Headache Society position paper. *Headache.* 2010;50(6):1089–99.

Green B. Prazosin in the treatment of PTSD. *J Psychiatr Pract.* 2014;20(4):253–9.

Ozyalcin SN, Talu GK, Kiziltan E, Yucel B, Ertas M, Disci R. The efficacy and safety of venlafaxine in the prophylaxis of migraine. *Headache.* 2005;45(2):144–52.

Saarto T, Wiffen PJ. Antidepressants for neuropathic pain: a Cochrane review. *J Neurol Neurosurg Psychiatry.* 2010;81(12): 1372–3.

Wellington K, Perry CM. Venlafaxine extended-release: a review of its use in the management of major depression. *CNS Drugs.* 2001;15(8): 643–69.

Zissis NP, Harmoussi S, Vlaikidis N, Mitsikostas D, Thomaidis T, Georgiadis G, Karageorgiou K. A randomized, double-blind, placebo-controlled study of venlafaxine XR in out-patients with tension-type headache. *Cephalalgia.* 2007; 27(4):315–24.

VERAPAMIL

THERAPEUTICS

Brands
- Calan, Cordilox, Securon, Verapress, Vertab, Univer, Covera-HS, Verelan, Isoptin SR

Generic?
- Yes

Class
- Calcium channel blocker

Commonly Prescribed for
(FDA approved in bold)
- **Angina (vasospastic, unstable, or effort associated)**
- **Essential hypertension**
- **Paroxysmal supraventricular tachycardia, atrial fibrillation/flutter (IV formulation, immediate-release tablet)**
- Prophylaxis of hemiplegic migraine or migraine with prolonged aura
- Cluster headache prophylaxis
- Peyronie's disease, plantar fibromatosis, Dupuytren's disease (gel)

How the Drug Works
- Cluster: proposed prior mechanisms included inhibition of smooth muscle contraction preventing arterial spasm and hypoxia, prevention of vasoconstriction or platelet aggregation, and alterations of serotonin release and uptake
- Voltage-gated calcium channels mediate calcium influx and are important in regulating neurotransmitter and hormone release

How Long Until It Works
- Migraines: may decrease in as little as 2 weeks, but can take up to 3 months on a stable dose to see full effect
- Cluster: usually effective in weeks

If It Works
- Migraine: goal is a 50% or greater reduction in migraine frequency or severity. Consider tapering or stopping if headaches remit for more than 6 months or if considering pregnancy

- Cluster: reduction in the severity or frequency of attacks

If It Doesn't Work
- Increase to highest tolerated dose
- Migraine/cluster: address other issues, such as medication overuse, other coexisting medical disorders, such as anxiety, and consider changing to another agent or adding a second agent

Best Augmenting Combos for Partial Response or Treatment-Resistance
- Cluster: at the start of the cycle can use a corticosteroid slam and taper. Lithium, topiramate are effective preventive medications for cluster patients

Tests
- At higher doses, monitor ECG for PR interval

ADVERSE EFFECTS (AEs)

How the Drug Causes AEs
- Direct effects of calcium receptor antagonism, slowing of AV conduction

Notable AEs
- Bradycardia, hypotension, weakness, headache
- Constipation, nausea, myalgia
- Allergic rhinitis, ankle edema, gingival hyperplasia
- First-degree AV block
- Upper respiratory infection, flu-like syndrome

Life-Threatening or Dangerous AEs
- Pulmonary edema, worsening of chronic heart failure in patients with moderate to severe cardiac function
- Rarely produces second- or third-degree AV block
- Rare hypertrophic cardiomyopathy
- Can worsen muscle transmission and cause weakness in patients with muscular dystrophies

Weight Gain

- Unusual

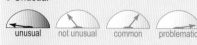

unusual   not unusual   common   problematic

Sedation

- Unusual

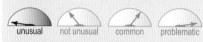

unusual   not unusual   common   problematic

What to Do About AEs

- For common AEs, lower dose, change to extended-release formulation, or switch to another agent. For serious AEs, do not use

Best Augmenting Agents to Reduce AEs

- Constipation can be treated by usual agents, such as magnesium

---

DOSING AND USE

Usual Dosage Range

- 120–480 mg/day

Dosage Forms

- Tablets: 40, 80, 120 mg. Extended release 120, 180, 240 mg
- Extended-release capsules: 100, 180, 240, 300, 360 mg
- Injection: 2.5 mg/mL
- Gel: 15% transdermal

How to Dose

- Migraine: initial dose 40–120 mg/day and effective usually at 120–360 mg/day for most patients. Gradually increase over days to weeks to usual effective dose. Immediate release dose 3 times a day. Sustained or extended release twice or once daily
- Cluster: start at 120–240 mg daily and increase by 40–120 mg/week until attacks are suppressed or a daily dose of 960 mg/day. May use as much as 1200 mg/day with ECG monitoring

 Dosing Tips

- Doses above 360 mg had no additional antihypertensive effect in clinical trials
- Can titrate with immediate release then change to longer acting once at a stable dose

Overdose

- Bradycardia, hypotension, with the possibility of low-output heart failure and shock. Treat with lavage, charcoal, cathartics. For hypotension, use dopamine, IV calcium, β agonists, or norepinephrine. For AV block, atropine is also helpful. For rapid ventricular rate due to anterograde conduction, use DC cardioversion or IV lidocaine

Long-Term Use

- Safe for long-term use

Habit Forming

- No

How to Stop

- Decrease 2 weeks after cessation of cluster attacks. Less risk of rebound tachycardia than β-blockers

Pharmacokinetics

- Metabolized by primarily CYP3A4. Half-life 2.8–7.4 hours with 1 dose but increased with repetitive dosing. SR about 12 hours. T_{max} 1–2 hours, 11 hours extended release, 7–9 hours sustained release. Oral bioavailability 20–35%. 90% protein binding

 Drug Interactions

- Verapamil (CYP3A4 inhibitor) can alter hepatic function, increasing plasma concentrations and effect of anesthetics, digoxin, statins, ethanol, buspirone, imipramine, prazosin, sirolimus, tacrolimus, carbamazepine, theophyllines, some benzodiazepines, and muscle relaxants
- Verapamil can lower lithium levels but increase toxicity
- Phenytoin, rifampin, and calcium salts decrease concentration of verapamil
- Potent CYP3A4 inhibitors such as ketoconazole increase levels
- H_2 antagonists (cimetidine, ranitidine) increase verapamil levels
- Use with β-blockers can be synergistic or additive, use with caution

 Other Warnings/ Precautions

- Increased intracranial pressure with verapamil IV in patients with supratentorial tumors

• Elevated liver enzymes have occurred

Do Not Use

• Sick sinus syndrome, greater than first-degree heart block
• Severe chronic heart failure, cardiogenic shock, severe left ventricular dysfunction
• Hypotension less than 90 mm Hg systolic
• Proven hypersensitivity to verapamil or other calcium channel blockers
• Do not give IV verapamil in close proximity to IV β-blockers

Renal Impairment

• About 70% of verapamil metabolites are excreted by the kidney. Monitor for PR interval prolongation and side effects. Use with caution

Hepatic Impairment

• Verapamil is highly metabolized by the liver. Give about 30% of usual dose to patients with severe dysfunction

Cardiac Impairment

• Do not use in acute shock, severe chronic heart failure, hypotension, and greater than first-degree heart block as above. Not for Wolff-Parkinson-White syndrome

Elderly

• Use with caution and start with lower doses

 Children and Adolescents

• Little is known about efficacy or safety. Use with caution if at all

 Pregnancy

• Category C (all calcium channel blockers). Use only if potential benefit outweighs risk to the fetus

Breast Feeding

• Not recommended. Verapamil is found in breast milk

Potential Advantages

• First-line preventive for cluster headache and better tolerated than most other preventive options, but may need a very high dose

Potential Disadvantages

• Generally not effective for migraine headache. Multiple potential drug interactions

Primary Target Symptoms

• Headache frequency and severity

 Pearls

• Relatively little evidence for effectiveness in migraine, but the first-line agent for cluster headache
• For patients with cycles of cluster headache, taper off starting 2 weeks after last attack
• May help patients with migraine with atypical or prolonged aura (e.g., hemiplegic migraine)
• There is no evidence that verapamil is more effective in the treatment of hypertension beyond 360 mg/day

Suggested Reading

Ashkenazi A, Schwedt T. Cluster headache – acute and prophylactic therapy. *Headache.* 2011;51(2):272–86.

Cohen AS, Matharu MS, Goadsby PJ. Trigeminal autonomic cephalalgias: current and future treatments. *Headache.* 2007;47(6):969–80.

Cohen AS, Matharu MS, Goadsby PJ. Electrocardiographic abnormalities in patients with cluster headache on verapamil therapy. *Neurology.* 2007;69(7):668–75.

Law MR, Morris JK, Wald NJ. Use of blood pressure lowering drugs in the prevention of cardiovascular disease: meta-analysis of 147 randomised trials in the context of expectations from prospective epidemiological studies. *BMJ.* 2009;338:b1665.

Silberstein SD, Holland S, Freitag F, Dodick DW, Argoff C, Ashman E. Evidence-based guideline update: pharmacologic treatment for episodic migraine prevention in adults: report of the Quality Standards Subcommittee of the American Academy of Neurology and the American Headache Society. *Neurology.* 2012; 78(17):1337–45.

VIGABATRIN

Brands
- Sabril

Generic?
- No

Class
- Antiepileptic drug (AED)

Commonly Prescribed for
(FDA approved in bold)
- **Refractory complex partial seizures in patients ≥ 10 years of age, as adjunctive therapy in patients who have responded inadequately to several alternative treatments**
- **Infantile spasms: monotherapy in infants 1 month to 2 years of age**
- Panic disorder
- Cocaine or methamphetamine dependence

 How the Drug Works
- Inhibits catabolism of GABA by inhibiting GABA transaminase (GABA-T). This increases synaptic levels of GABA but does not act directly on GABA receptors. May decrease levels of excitatory neurotransmitters (glutamate, aspartate, glutamine) in the brain

How Long Until It Works
- Seizures: by 2 weeks

If It Works
- Seizures: goal is the remission of seizures. Continue as long as effective and well tolerated
- Monitor vision every 3–6 months

If It Doesn't Work
- Increase to highest tolerated dose
- Epilepsy: consider changing to another agent, adding a second agent, using a medical device, or a referral for epilepsy surgery evaluation. When adding a second agent, keep drug interactions in mind

 Best Augmenting Combos for Partial Response or Treatment-Resistance
- Often used in combination with other AEDs. Lack of significant drug interactions makes it easier to use than many other AEDs

Tests
- No regular blood tests are recommended

How the Drug Causes AEs
- CNS AEs are probably caused by changes in GABA levels

Notable AEs
- Somnolence, fatigue, weight gain, headache, dizziness, anxiety, depression, ataxia, hyperactivity (children), psychosis (adults), upper respiratory tract infection

 Life-Threatening or Dangerous AEs
- Retinal atrophy and visual field defects in about one-third of patients, peaking at 1 year but occurring as soon as a few weeks. Visual field loss may be irreversible

Weight Gain
- Not unusual

unusual | not unusual | common | problematic

Sedation
- Not unusual

unusual | not unusual | common | problematic

What to Do About AEs
- Decrease dose
- Vision loss may require stopping drug

Best Augmenting Agents to Reduce AEs
- Most AEs cannot be reduced by an augmenting agent

DOSING AND USE

Usual Dosage Range
- Epilepsy: 2–4 g/day

Dosage Forms
- Tablets: 500 mg

How to Dose
- In adults, start at 1 or 2 g/day. Increase or decrease by 500 mg depending on clinical response and tolerability. Usual most effective dose is 2–4 g/day in once- or twice-daily doses

Dosing Tips
- Food slows rate but not extent of absorption

Overdose
- Vertigo and tremor have been reported

Long-Term Use
- Safe

Habit Forming
- No

How to Stop
- Taper slowly over 2 weeks or more
- Abrupt withdrawal can lead to seizures in patients with epilepsy

Pharmacokinetics
- Mostly excreted unchanged in urine. No hepatic metabolism. Bioavailability is 80–90%. Peak levels at 2 hours. Half-life is 5–8 hours in young adults but 12–13 hours in the elderly

Drug Interactions
- Vigabatrin lowers phenytoin levels by 20% but there are no other significant interactions with other AEDs

Other Warnings/ Precautions
- It may increase suicidal behavior and ideation
- Patients should not drive or operate heavy machinery

Do Not Use
- Patients with a proven allergy to vigabatrin

SPECIAL POPULATIONS

Renal Impairment
- May require lowering of dose if CrCl < 60 mL/min

Hepatic Impairment
- No known effects

Cardiac Impairment
- No known effects

Elderly
- May need lower dose

Children and Adolescents
- Start at 40 mg/kg/day. Increase to 80–100 mg/kg/day depending on clinical response. Alternatively, start at 500 mg and increase by 500 mg/week to optimal dose. Children over 50 kg will use the adult dose

Pregnancy
- Category C. Use only if risks of stopping drug outweigh potential risk to fetus
- Supplementation with 0.4 mg of folic acid before and during pregnancy is recommended

Breast Feeding
- Some drug is found in mothers' breast milk
- Generally recommendations are to discontinue drug or bottle feed
- Monitor infant for sedation, poor feeding, or irritability

THE ART OF NEUROPHARMACOLOGY

Potential Advantages
- Effective in infantile spasm and low drug interactions

Potential Disadvantages
- Vision loss. May worsen absence, myoclonic, or generalized tonic-clonic seizures

Primary Target Symptoms
- Seizure frequency and severity

 Pearls

- Usually used in combination with other AEDs in refractory epilepsy
- Vigabatrin should be considered a drug of choice for infantile spasms in patients with tuberous sclerosis. Visual changes are minor compared to poor outcomes of untreated infantile spasms. Hormonal therapy (low-dose corticotropin) may be considered for use in preference to vigabatrin in infants with cryptogenic infantile spasms, to possibly improve developmental outcome
- The effect of the drug is related to the resynthesis of GABA-T enzyme molecules rather than vigabatrin plasma levels
- Patients with symptomatic infantile spasms, i.e. related to tuberous sclerosis, may improve more rapidly. Infantile spasms usually remit by age 5, but are often replaced by other types of seizures
- Visual field deficits can be monitored by formal visual field testing. Consider checking electroretinography for monitoring vision loss in infants and children that cannot perform perimetry

 Suggested Reading

Curatolo P, Bombardieri R, Cerminara C. Current management for epilepsy in tuberous sclerosis complex. *Curr Opin Neurol.* 2006;19(2):119–23.

Fechtner RD, Khouri AS, Figueroa E, Ramirez M, Federico M, Dewey SL, Brodie JD. Short-term treatment of cocaine and/or methamphetamine abuse with vigabatrin: ocular safety pilot results. *Arch Ophthalmol.* 2006;124(9):1257–62.

Gaily E, Jonsson H, Lappi M. Visual fields at school-age in children treated with vigabatrin in infancy. *Epilepsia.* 2009;50(2):206–16.

Go CY, Mackay MT, Weiss SK, Stephens D, Adams-Webber T, Ashwal S, Snead OC; Child Neurology Society; American Academy of Neurology. Evidence-based guideline update: medical treatment of infantile spasms. Report of the Guideline Development Subcommittee of the American Academy of Neurology and the Practice Committee of the Child Neurology Society. *Neurology.* 2012;78:1974–80.

Parisi P, Bombardieri R, Curatolo P. Current role of vigabatrin in infantile spasms. *Eur J Paediatr Neurol.* 2007;11(6):331–6.

THERAPEUTICS

Brands
- Viibryd

Generic?
- No

Class
- Selective serotonin reuptake inhibitor (SSRI)

Commonly Prescribed for
(FDA approved in bold)
- **Major depressive disorder**
- Generalized anxiety disorder
- Chronic pain

How the Drug Works
- It blocks the serotonin transporter (SERT) (Ki = 0.1 nM) and is a presynaptic 5-HT$_{1A}$ partial agonist

How Long Until It Works
- 2 weeks to 2 months for full effect

If It Works
- Continue to use and monitor for AEs

If It Doesn't Work
- Increase to highest tolerated dose. Consider adding a second agent or changing to another one

Best Augmenting Combos for Partial Response or Treatment-Resistance
- For some patients, low-dose polytherapy with 2 or more drugs may be better tolerated and more effective than high-dose monotherapy

Tests
- None available

ADVERSE EFFECTS (AEs)

How the Drug Causes AEs
- By increasing serotonin on non-therapeutic responsive receptors throughout the body. Most AEs are dose- and time-dependent

Notable AEs
- Incidence $\geq$ 5%: insomnia, nausea, vomiting, diarrhea

Life-Threatening or Dangerous AEs
- Serotonin syndrome
- Rare activation of mania or suicidal ideation, especially during the initial few months
- Angle-closure glaucoma
- Rare worsening of existing seizure disorders
- Rare hyponatremia and abnormal bleeding

Weight Gain
- Unusual

unusual · not unusual · common · problematic

Sedation
- Not unusual

unusual · not unusual · common · problematic

What to Do About AEs
- For minor AEs, lower dose, titrate more slowly, or switch to another agent. For serious AEs, lower dose and consider stopping, taper to avoid withdrawal

Best Augmenting Agents to Reduce AEs
- Cyproheptadine can be used for serotonin syndrome by blocking 5-HT receptors and SERT

DOSING AND USE

Usual Dosage Range
- 40 mg once daily

Dosage Forms
- Tablet: 10, 20, 40 mg

How to Dose
- Initial 10 mg daily for 7 days, followed by 20 mg daily for 7 days, then increase to 40 mg daily

Dosing Tips

- Should be taken with food (high fat or light meal). Reduce gradually

Overdose

- Often in combination with other drugs. Symptoms include serotonin syndrome, lethargy, restlessness, hallucinations, and disorientation
- Establish and maintain an airway. Gastric lavage with activated charcoal should be considered. Cardiac and vital sign monitoring is recommended, along with general symptomatic and supportive care. Due to the large volume of distribution of vilazodone, forced diuresis, dialysis, hemoperfusion, and exchange transfusion are unlikely to be of benefit. There are no specific antidotes

Long-Term Use

- Safe for long-term use

Habit Forming

- No

How to Stop

- Taper slowly (no more than 50% reduction every 3–4 days until discontinuation) to avoid withdrawal symptoms (agitation, anxiety, confusion, dry mouth, dysphoria, etc.)

Pharmacokinetics

- Metabolized by CYP3A4 (major), CYP2C19/ 2D6 (minor). 1% and 2% eliminated by urine and feces, respectively. Bioavailability 72% with food. Half-life 25 hours. 96–99% protein bound

 Drug Interactions

- Serotonin syndrome may occur with concomitant use of MAOIs or serotonergic drugs
- Reduce dose (20 mg maximum) in the presence of CYP3A4 inhibitors (clarithromycin, ketoconazole, itraconazole)
- Increase dose (80 mg maximum) in the presence of CYP3A4 inducers (carbamazepine, phenobarbital, rifampin, glucocorticoids, St. John's wort)

- Abnormal bleeding: use caution in concomitant use with NSAIDs, aspirin, warfarin, or other drugs that affect coagulation

 Other Warnings/ Precautions

- May increase risk of seizure

Do Not Use

- Concurrently with MAOI; allow at least 14 days between discontinuation of an MAOI and initiation of vilazodone or at least 7–14 days between discontinuation of vilazodone and initiation of an MAOI
- Concurrent use of serotonin precursors (e.g., tryptophan)
- In patients with uncontrolled narrow angle-closure glaucoma
- In patients treated with linezolid or methylene blue IV

SPECIAL POPULATIONS

Renal Impairment

- No dose adjustment

Hepatic Impairment

- No dose adjustment

Cardiac Impairment

- No QTc prolongation

Elderly

- No dose adjustment

 Children and Adolescents

- Safety and effectiveness not established in pediatric patients

 Pregnancy

- Category C. Neonates exposed to SNRIs or SSRIs late in the third trimester have developed complications necessitating extended hospitalizations, respiratory support, and tube feeding. Respiratory distress, cyanosis, apnea, seizures, temperature instability, feeding difficulty, vomiting, hypoglycemia, hypotonia, hyperreflexia, tremor, jitteriness, irritability, and constant crying consistent with a toxic effect of the drug or drug discontinuation syndrome have been reported

Breast Feeding

- Some drug is found in breast milk and use while breast feeding is not recommended

THE ART OF NEUROPHARMACOLOGY

Potential Advantages

- Multimodal (SERT inhibitor plus 5-HT$_{1A}$ partial agonist) antidepressant. Minimal sexual dysfunction

Potential Disadvantages

- Requires gradual titration. CYP3A4 drug interactions

Primary Target Symptoms

- Depression and anxiety

Pearls

- The combination of SSRI with 5-HT$_{1A}$ receptor agonism in theory should achieve greater therapeutic efficacy compared to current antidepression treatment but remains to be determined clinically
- Relatively lower sexual dysfunction than other antidepressants, probably due to 5-HT$_{1A}$ agonist effect
- Probably not effective for migraine prophylaxis; may reduce headache frequency but not intensity
- In theory, it may be useful for managing chronic pain owing to 5-HT$_{1A}$ effect on dorsal horn and raphe nucleus

Suggested Reading

Clayton AH, Kennedy SH, Edwards JB, Gallipoli S, Reed CR. The effect of vilazodone on sexual function during the treatment of major depressive disorder. *J Sex Med.* 2013; 10(10):2465–76.

Dawson LA, Watson JM. Vilazodone: a 5-HT1A receptor agonist/serotonin transporter inhibitor for the treatment of affective disorders. *CNS Neurosci Ther.* 2009;15(2):107–17.

Frampton JE. Vilazodone: in major depressive disorder. *CNS Drugs.* 2011; 25(7):615–27.

Jeong H-J, Mitchell VA, Vaughan CW. Role of 5-HT1 receptor subtypes in the modulation of pain and synaptic transmission in rat spinal superficial dorsal horn. *Br J Pharmacol.* 2012; 165(6):1956–65.

VORTIOXETINE HYDROBROMIDE

Brands
- Brintellix

Generic?
- No

Class
- Atypical antidepressant

Commonly Prescribed for
(FDA approved in bold)
- **Major depressive disorder**

How the Drug Works
- 5-HT$_{1A}$ and 5-HT$_{1B}$ agonist; 5-HT$_3$, 5-HT$_7$, 5-HT$_{1D}$ antagonist; 5-HT transporter inhibitor. May modulate GABA$_A$ transmission

How Long Until It Works
- Few weeks to months

If It Works
- Continue to use and monitor for AEs

If It Doesn't Work
- Increase to highest tolerated dose. Switch to other antidepressant

Best Augmenting Combos for Partial Response or Treatment-Resistance
- Polytherapy might be helpful

Tests
- Serum sodium if SIADH (syndrome of inappropriate antidiuretic hormone secretion)

How the Drug Causes AEs
- By increasing serotonin on non-therapeutic responsive receptors throughout the body. Most AEs are dose- and time-dependent

Notable AEs
- Nausea, constipation, vomiting. Activation of mania/hypomania. Difficulty in sexual desire and performance

Life-Threatening or Dangerous AEs
- Serotonin syndrome
- Angle-closure glaucoma
- SIADH
- Increased risk of bleeding when coadministered with anticoagulants, antiplatelets, or NSAIDs

Weight Gain
- Unusual

Sedation
- Unusual

What to Do About AEs
- For minor AEs, lower dose, titrate more slowly, or switch to another agent. For serious AEs, lower dose and consider stopping, taper to avoid withdrawal symptoms

Best Augmenting Agents to Reduce AEs
- Try magnesium for constipation

Usual Dosage Range
- 10–20 mg/day

Dosage Forms
- Tablet: 5, 10, 15, 20 mg

How to Dose
- Initial dose 10 mg taken daily. Increase to 20 mg if tolerated; 10 mg maximum in known CYP2D6 poor metabolizers

Dosing Tips
- Nausea commonly occurs within the first week. Patients should be monitored appropriately and observed closely for clinical worsening, suicidality, and unusual changes in behavior during the initial few months or upon dose changes

Overdose

- Increased rate of nausea, vomiting, diarrhea, abdominal discomfort, pruritus, somnolence, flushing. No specific antidote. Standard overdose management

Long-Term Use

- Probably safe for long-term use with monitoring of adverse effect. Still need more data

Habit Forming

- No

How to Stop

- Can be discontinued abruptly. For patients taking 15–20 mg/day, recommend reducing to 10 mg/day for a week then full stop

Pharmacokinetics

- Metabolized by CYP450 enzymes, primarily via the CYP2D6 isoenzyme. 59% excreted in feces, 26% in urine. Bioavailability 75% with no effect on food. 98% protein bound. Half-life 66 hours. Steady state reached in 2 weeks

 Drug Interactions

- Lower brintellix dose: CYP2D6 inhibitors (paroxetine, fluoxetine, bupropion, duloxetine, sertraline, citalopram, methadone, ranitidine, cimetidine)
- Increase brintellix dose: Strong CYP2D6 inducer (phenytoin, rifampin, carbamazepine, dexamethasone)
- No dose adjustment for the comedications is needed when brintellix is coadministered with a substrate of CYP450

 Other Warnings/ Precautions

- Monitor closely for worsening, and for emergence of suicidal thoughts and behaviors
- Patients should be observed closely for clinical worsening and changes in behavior in known or unknown bipolar disorder

Do Not Use

- Proven hypersensitivity to drug
- Concurrently with MAOI (selegiline, resagiline, isoniazid, linezolid, methylene blue); do not use MAOIs within 21 days of stopping brintellix; allow at least 14 days after stopping MAOIs before brintellix

Renal Impairment

- No adjustment needed

Hepatic Impairment

- No adjustment needed in moderate impairment

Cardiac Impairment

- No QTc effect

Elderly

- No adjustments necessary. Caution on hyponatremia

 Children and Adolescents

- Safety and efficacy not established

 Pregnancy

- Category C. Brintellix should be used during pregnancy only if the potential benefit justifies the potential risk to the fetus. Neonates exposed to SSRIs or SNRIs late in the third trimester have developed complications requiring prolonged hospitalization, respiratory support, and tube feeding. They may have an increased risk for persistent pulmonary hypertension of the newborn

Breast Feeding

- It is not known whether brintellix is present in human milk

Potential Advantages

- Multimodal benefits on mood, cognitive function, anxiety. No insomnia and weight neutral

Potential Disadvantages

- CYP2D6 substrate

Primary Target Symptoms

• Improve mood and anxiety

 Pearls

• In a recent trial, brintellix significantly improved objective and subjective measures of cognitive function in adults with recurrent MDD and these effects were largely independent of its

effect on improving depressive symptoms
• Lower GI adverse effect (nausea, vomiting) due to its own 5-HT$_3$ antagonism
• Relatively lower sexual dysfunction (1–3%) and sleep disruption (2–5%) than most other antidepressants
• Enhances contextual and episodic memory in rats. In theory may have a role in managing dementia
• May be ineffective for generalized anxiety disorder

 Suggested Reading

Berhan A, Barker A. Vortioxetine in the treatment of adult patients with major depressive disorder: a meta-analysis of randomized double-blind controlled trials. *BMC Psychiatry.* 2014;14:276.

Mahableshwarkar AR, Jacobsen PL, Serenko M, Chen Y. A randomized, double-blind, fixed-dose study comparing the efficacy and tolerability of vortioxetine 2.5 and 10 mg in acute treatment of adults with generalized anxiety disorder. *Hum Psychopharmacol.* 2014;29(1):64–72.

McIntyre RS, Lophaven S, Olsen CK. A randomized, double-blind, placebo-controlled study of vortioxetine on cognitive function in depressed adults. *Int J Neuropsychopharm.* 2014;17(10):1557–67.

Mørk A, Montezinho LP, Miller S, Trippodi-Murphy C, Plath N, Li Y, et al. Vortioxetine (Lu AA21004), a novel multimodal antidepressant, enhances memory in rats. *Pharmacol Biochem Behav.* 2013;105:41–50.

WARFARIN

THERAPEUTICS

Brands
- Coumadin, Jantoven, Carfin, Marevan, Panwarfin, Warx

Generic?
- Yes

Class
- Anticoagulant

Commonly Prescribed for
(FDA approved in bold)
- **Prophylaxis and treatment of venous thrombosis and pulmonary embolism**
- **Prophylaxis and treatment of thromboembolic complications associated with atrial fibrillation (AF) and/or cardiac valve replacement**
- **Reduction in the risk of death, recurrent myocardial infarction (MI), and thromboembolic events such as stroke or systemic embolization after MI**
- Cerebral venous sinus thrombosis
- Arterial dissection

How the Drug Works
- Interferes with the synthesis of vitamin K-dependent clotting factors II, VII, IX, X and anticoagulant proteins C and S as well as vitamin K epoxide reductase (VKORC1) enzyme complex. It decreases risk of thromboembolism

How Long Until It Works
- Anticoagulant effect is delayed for up to 5–7 days due to the long half-lives of factors II, IX, and X. Heparin is preferred for rapid anticoagulation

If It Works
- Continue to use with appropriate monitoring of PT/INR. Early elevation of PT does not reflect anticoagulation

If It Doesn't Work
- Patients can still have stroke despite treatment. Warfarin is only superior to antiplatelet agents for cardiogenic stroke, i.e., related to AF or ventricular thrombus.

Control all stroke risk factors, such as smoking, hyperlipidemia, and hypertension. For acute events, admit patients for treatment and diagnostic testing. Check INR to determine drug effectiveness

Best Augmenting Combos for Partial Response or Treatment-Resistance
- The combination of oral anticoagulants and antiplatelets is not recommended for recent stroke/transient ischemic attack (TIA) but reasonable in acute coronary syndrome or stent placement (Class IIb, Level of Evidence C)
- For patients with rheumatic mitral valve disease who have stroke/TIA while being treated with adequate warfarin, the addition of aspirin might be considered (Class IIb; Level of Evidence C)
- For patients with a mechanical mitral or aortic valve who have a history of ischemic stroke or TIA before its insertion and who are at low risk for bleeding, the addition of aspirin 75–100 mg/day to warfarin is recommended (Class I; Level of Evidence B)

Tests
- Monitor PT/INR to determine effectiveness

ADVERSE EFFECTS (AEs)

How the Drug Causes AEs
- Anticoagulation increases bleeding risk

Notable AEs
- Abdominal pain/cramping, elevated liver enzymes/jaundice, hypotension, weakness, paresthesias, diarrhea, nausea, pruritus, and alopecia

Life-Threatening or Dangerous AEs
- Bleeding complications, especially with elevated INRs. Hemorrhage in organs or tissues can cause death
- Tissue necrosis (especially in protein C deficiency) occurs during warfarin initiation
- Patients with venous thrombosis and heparin-induced thrombocytopenia have

risk of limb ischemia, necrosis, and gangrene when stopping heparin and starting warfarin
• May increase risk of cholesterol plaque emboli, typically 3–10 weeks after starting therapy
• "Purple toes syndrome" is a dark, mottled, often purple discoloration on the sides and plantar surface of toes; may be reversible or may lead to necrosis or gangrene

Weight Gain
• Unusual

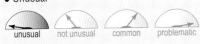

Sedation
• Unusual

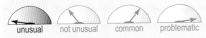

What to Do About AEs
• When major bleeding, stop warfarin. Use rapid reversal with prothrombin complex concentrate and vitamin K 5–10mg IV
• If INR 4–10 without bleeding, no vitamin K needed. If INR > 10 without bleeding, oral vitamin K

Best Augmenting Agents to Reduce AEs
• Most AEs cannot be reduced by an augmenting agent

DOSING AND USE

Usual Dosage Range
• 2–10mg daily

Dosage Forms
• Tablets: 1, 2, 2.5, 3, 4, 5, 6, 7.5, and 10mg
• Injection: 5.4mg (2mg/mL)

How to Dose
• Initiation: 5–10mg once daily for 1–2 days followed by INR-guided dose
• Lower initiation and maintaining dose: elderly, debilitated, genetic variations in CYP2C9 or VKORC1 enzymes
• IV warfarin dosing is the same as oral. Use in patients without the ability to take oral drugs

INR goals
• 2–3 for most conditions, including AF, anterior MI with left ventricular (LV) thrombus, deep vein thrombosis (DVT)/ pulmonary embolism (PE), tissue heart valve, valvular heart disease
• 2.5–3.5 for patients with mechanical heart valves in aortic or mitral positions
• Bridge with heparin until therapeutic INR reached

Warfarin duration
• Indefinite: AF, ≥ 2 DVT/PE
• 3 months: tissue heart valve, first DVT/PE, anterior MI with LV thrombus

 Dosing Tips
• Food decreases rate of absorption. If a dose is missed, do not double the next dose
• Asian patients may also require lower initiation and maintenance doses

Overdose
• Bleeding complications, such as blood in stools or urine, excessive menstrual bleeding, petechiae, or oozing from superficial injuries. Check INR and treat by holding warfarin therapy and giving vitamin K if indicated

Long-Term Use
• Safe for long-term use

Habit Forming
• No

How to Stop
• No need to taper, but patients will be at increased risk of thromboembolic complications soon after

Pharmacokinetics
• Warfarin is a racemic mixture of the R and S stereoisomers. S-warfarin is 3–5 times more potent VKORC1 inhibitor than R-warfarin. While S-warfarin is metabolized primarily by CYP2C9, R-warfarin is metabolized by mainly CYP3A4 with involvement of many other CYP isoenzymes. Once metabolized, they are excreted in urine (92%) and bile. Half-life ranges from 20 to 60 hours (mean 40 hours). Drug 99% protein bound. Polymorphism in VKORC1, CYP2C9, and CYP4F2 influences the response to warfarin

Drug Interactions

- Increased anticoagulant effect due to inhibition of hepatic metabolism: proton pump inhibitors, statins, allopurinol, azole antifungals, quinidine, quinine, sulfonamides
- Increased anticoagulant effect due to reduced clearance: macrolide antibiotics (azithromycin, erythromycin)
- Increased anticoagulant effect due to displacement from binding sites: loop diuretics (furosemide), valproate, nalidixic acid
- Increased anticoagulant effect due to interference with vitamin K: aminoglycosides, tetracyclines, vitamin E
- Increased anticoagulant effect due to GI irritation and effects on platelet function: NSAIDs, penicillins, salicylates, diflunisal
- Increased anticoagulant effect due to unclear reasons: SSRIs, COX-2 inhibitors, cephalosporins, β-blockers, heparin, isoniazid, influenza vaccine, quinolones (ciprofloxacin), ropinirole, tamoxifen, thyroid hormones, tramadol, zafirlukast, methylphenidate
- Decreased anticoagulant effect due to hepatic induction: barbiturates, nafcillin, carbamazepine, rifampin, cigarette smoking
- Decreased anticoagulant effect due to decreased absorption or increased elimination: spironolactone, thiazide diuretics, azathioprine
- Decreased anticoagulant effect due to unclear reasons: clozapine, haloperidol, estrogens, griseofulvin, protease inhibitors, trazodone, ribavirin, isoretinoin, cyclosporine, chlordiazepoxide, oral contraceptives
- May increase or decrease anticoagulant effect: alcohol, corticosteroids, phenytoin, pravastatin, chloral hydrate, ranitidine, propylthiouracil
- Many herbal medications can reportedly increase (ginkgo, dong quai, garlic, among others) or decrease (coenzyme Q10 and St. John's wort) the effect of warfarin
- Vitamin-K-rich vegetables such as broccoli, spinach, seaweed, and turnips decrease warfarin effects

 Other Warnings/ Precautions

- Use warfarin with great caution in patients at risk for trauma, infections of intestinal flora, indwelling catheters, known or suspected protein C or S deficiency (tissue necrosis), enhanced release of atheromatous emboli, moderate to severe hepatic/renal insufficiency, exposed raw surfaces, severe hypertension, or risk of vitamin K deficiency (diarrhea, hepatic disorder, poor nutrition, steatorrhea)

Do Not Use

- Hypersensitivity to the drug; pregnancy; recent or impending surgery or procedure such as lumbar puncture or lumbar anesthesia; bleeding tendencies with active ulceration or overt bleeding of GI, GU, or respiratory tracts; malignant hypertension; eclampsia or preeclampsia; aortic dissection; cerebral aneurysm; bacterial endocarditis; CNS hemorrhage; and unsupervised patients with senility, substance abuse, or psychosis

SPECIAL POPULATIONS

Renal Impairment

- Patients with renal dysfunction are more likely to experience bleeding complications, perhaps due to increase in the unbound fraction of the drug. Use with caution

Hepatic Impairment

- Use with much caution. Patients with moderate to severe disease have an increased risk of bleeding complications due to decreased metabolism and decreased synthesis of clotting factors

Cardiac Impairment

- No known effects

Elderly

- Lower initiation and maintenance doses needed

 Children and Adolescents

- Not well studied in children but appears effective for prevention of thromboembolic complications. May require more frequent monitoring

Pregnancy

- Category D for women with mechanical heart valves. Category X for others. Associated with multiple serious birth malformations, including CNS, and spontaneous abortions. Do not use. Low molecular weight heparin (LMWH) instead of heparin or warfarin is preferred for DVT/ PE prevention in pregnant patients

Breast Feeding

- Compatible. Monitor for bruising or bleeding

THE ART OF NEUROPHARMACOLOGY

Potential Advantages

- Drug of choice for ischemic stroke prevention in patients with mechanical heart valves, cardiac thrombus, and cerebral venous thrombosis

Potential Disadvantages

- Not as useful for non-cardiac ischemic stroke. No role in intracranial stenosis. More bleeding risk than newer anticoagulants. Higher risk of infratentorial microbleeds. Numerous drug interactions

Primary Target Symptoms

- Prevention of the neurological complications that result from ischemic stroke

Pearls

- There is no evidence to suggest that warfarin is superior to antiplatelet medications for secondary stroke prevention unless there is a clear cardiac source (i.e., AF, cardiac thrombus or venous embolism with patent foramen ovale)
- Generally not started acutely (along with heparin) except in particular clinical situations such as cerebral venous sinus thrombosis, high-risk cases with potential early cardiogenic reembolization,

symptomatic dissection, and proven hypercoagulable states
- Combining antiplatelets and warfarin monotherapy in treating AF increases bleeding risk but adds no benefit in ischemic stroke prevention
- Goal INR may be increased in patients with recurrent embolism (to 3 or 3.5) despite therapeutic INR, but INR of 4 or greater does not appear more effective and is associated with more bleeding AEs
- Multiple drug interactions due mostly to hepatic metabolism, often unpredictable, require frequent monitoring with the addition or change of any medication – even those only for short-term use (i.e., antibiotics)
- Warfarin probably should not be interrupted during AF ablation. The COMPARE trial showed that bridging AF patients with heparin or enoxaparin during AF ablation has > 10-fold increased odds of stroke or TIA than uninterrupted warfarin in the 48 hours after ablation
- For most patients with a stroke or TIA in the setting of AF, it is reasonable to initiate oral anticoagulation within 14 days after the onset of neurological symptoms (Class IIa; Level of Evidence B)
- For patients with ischemic stroke or TIA and evidence of aortic arch atheroma, the effectiveness of anticoagulation with warfarin, compared with antiplatelet therapy, is unknown (Class IIb; Level of Evidence C)
- For patients with an ischemic stroke or TIA and both a patent foramen ovale and a venous source of embolism, anticoagulation is indicated, depending on stroke characteristics (Class I; Level of Evidence A)
- For hemorrhagic stroke in the setting of AF, the optimal timing of anticoagulation is uncertain. For most patients, however, it might be reasonable to wait ≥ 1 week (Class IIb; Level of Evidence B)
- For cerebral venous thrombosis, despite a lack of evidence, it is often recommended to use warfarin for 3–12 months. Longer duration is reserved for those with severe coagulopathies or recurrent venous thromboembolism. For newer anticoagulants, their lower intracranial bleeding rate might offer them a potential role for cerebral venous thrombosis

- Although not generally recommended for ischemic stroke without a proven cardiac cause, high levels of amino terminal pro-B-type natriuretic peptide may predict a benefit for anticoagulation in these patients

Suggested Reading

Guyatt GH, Akl EA, Crowther M, Gutterman DD, Schuünemann HJ; American College of Chest Physicians Antithrombotic Therapy and Prevention of Thrombosis Panel. Executive summary: Antithrombotic Therapy and Prevention of Thrombosis, 9th ed: American College of Chest Physicians Evidence-Based Clinical Practice Guidelines. *Chest.* 2012; 141(2 Suppl):7S–47S.

Hansen ML, Sørensen R, Clausen MT, Fog-Petersen ML, Raunsø J, Gadsbøll N, et al. Risk of bleeding with single, dual, or triple therapy with warfarin, aspirin, and clopidogrel in patients with atrial fibrillation. *Arch Intern Med.* 2010;170(16):1433–41.

Kernan WN, Ovbiagele B, Black HR, Bravata DM, Chimowitz MI, Ezekowitz MD, et al. Guidelines for the prevention of stroke in patients with stroke and transient ischemic attack: a guideline for healthcare professionals from the American Heart Association/American Stroke Association. *Stroke.* 2014;45(7):2160–236.

Weimar C. Diagnosis and treatment of cerebral venous and sinus thrombosis. *Curr Neurol Neurosci Rep.* 2014;14(1):417.

ZOLMITRIPTAN

THERAPEUTICS

Brands
- Zomig, Zomig MLT

Generic?
- Yes

Class
- Triptan

Commonly Prescribed for
(FDA approved in bold)
- **Acute treatment of migraine with or without aura in adults**
- Acute treatment of migraine with or without aura in adolescents (nasal spray)
- Cluster headache (nasal spray)

How the Drug Works
- Selective 5-HT$_{1B/1D/1F}$ receptor agonist. In addition to vasoconstriction on meningeal vessels, its antinociceptive effect is likely due to blocking the transmission of pain signals at trigeminal nerve terminals (preventing the release of inflammatory neuropeptides) and synapses of second-order neurons in trigeminal nucleus caudalis

How Long Until It Works
- 1 hour or less

If It Works
- Continue to take as needed. Patients taking acute treatment more than 2 days/week are at risk for medication-overuse headache, especially if they have migraine

If It Doesn't Work
- Treat early in the attack – triptans are less likely to work after the headache become severe, regardless of cutaneous allodynia, which is a marker of central sensitization
- For patients with partial response or reoccurrence, other rescue medications include NSAIDs (e.g., ketorolac, naproxen), antiemetics (e.g., prochlorperazine, metoclopramide), neuroleptics (e.g., haloperidol, chlorpromazine), or corticosteroids

- Change to another triptan or another administration route

Best Augmenting Combos for Partial Response or Treatment-Resistance
- NSAIDs or antiemetics/neuroleptics are often used to augment response

Tests
- None required

ADVERSE EFFECTS (AEs)

How the Drug Causes AEs
- Direct effect on systemic serotonin receptors (e.g., 5-HT$_{1B}$ agonism on vasoconstriction)

Notable AEs
- Paresthesias, dizziness, sensation of pressure (chest or jaw), palpitation

Life-Threatening or Dangerous AEs
- Serotonin syndrome. Rare cardiac events including acute myocardial infarction, cardiac arrhythmias, and coronary artery vasospasm have been reported with zolmitriptan

Weight Gain
- Unusual

unusual   not unusual   common   problematic

Sedation
- Unusual

unusual   not unusual   common   problematic

What to Do About AEs
- In most cases, only reassurance is needed. Lower dose, change to another triptan, or use an alternative headache treatment

Best Augmenting Agents to Reduce AEs
- Treatment of nausea with antiemetics is acceptable. Other AEs decrease with time

DOSING AND USE

Usual Dosage Range
- 2.5–5mg, maximum 10mg/day

Dosage Forms
- Tablets: 2.5 and 5mg
- Orally disintegrating tablets: 2.5, 5mg
- Nasal spray 2.5, 5mg/spray

How to Dose
- Tablets: 1 pill (either 2.5 or 5mg) at the onset of an attack and repeat in 2 hours for a partial response or if the headache returns
- Nasal spray: 1 spray (2.5–5mg) and repeat in 2 hours if needed. 5mg has similar efficacy to but greater adverse reactions than 2.5mg
- Maximum 10mg/day. Limit 10 days/month

Dosing Tips
- Treat early in the attack. Side effects are greater with more than 5mg dose

Overdose
- May cause hypertension, cardiovascular symptoms. Other possible symptoms include seizure, tremor, extremity erythema, cyanosis or ataxia. For patients with angina, perform ECG and monitor for ischemia for at least 15 hours

Long-Term Use
- Monitor for cardiac risk factors with continued use

Habit Forming
- No

How to Stop
- No need to taper. Patients who overuse triptans often experience withdrawal headaches lasting up to several days

Pharmacokinetics
- Half-life 2–3 hours for tablet and orally disintegrating tablets; 3–4 hours for nasal spray. T_{max} oral (2–4 hours), and nasal (3–4 hours). Bioavailability is 40% (tablet) and 102% (nasal spray). Metabolism mostly by CYP1A2 isoenzyme to active N-desmethyl metabolite, which is further metabolized by monoamine oxidase (MAO)-A. 25% protein binding

Drug Interactions
- CYP1A2 inhibitors (fluoroquinolones, fluvoxamine, verapamil, St. John's wort, cimetidine) can increase concentration
- MAOIs can affect the metabolism of zolmitriptan
- Propranolol can increase zolmitriptan concentration but with no interactive effect on blood pressure or pulse rate
- Use with sibutramine, a weight loss drug, may cause a serotonin syndrome including weakness, irritability, myoclonus, and confusion

Other Warnings/ Precautions
- For phenylketonurics: orally disintegrating tablets contain phenylalanine
- Discontinue if any ischemic or hemorrhagic event occurs

Do Not Use
- Patients with proven hypersensitivity
- Within 2 weeks of MAO-A inhibitors, or within 24 hours of ergot-containing medications such as dihydroergotamine
- History of stroke, transient ischemic attack, hemiplegic/basilar migraine, Wolff-Parkinson-White syndrome, peripheral vascular disease, ischemic heart disease, coronary artery vasospasm, ischemic bowel disease, and uncontrolled hypertension

SPECIAL POPULATIONS

Renal Impairment
- Concentration increases in those with severe renal impairment (CrCl < 25mL/min). May be at increased cardiovascular risk

Hepatic Impairment
- Drug metabolism significantly decreased with hepatic disease. Use lower doses and do not use with moderate or severe hepatic impairment

Cardiac Impairment
- Do not use in patients with known cardiovascular or peripheral vascular disease. May have increased risk for vascular event

Elderly

- At an increased risk for cardiovascular incident. Most studies were done in patients < 65 years old. In elderly with no other coronary artery disease risk factors beside age (male > 45, female > 55), it is generally safe

Children and Adolescents

- Safety and efficacy have not been established. A single trial found effectiveness of zolmitriptan (5mg) nasal spray in treating adolescent (> 12 years old) migraine. Many other triptan trials in children have been negative, due to higher placebo response

Pregnancy

- Category C. Use only if potential benefit outweighs risk to the fetus. Migraine often improves in pregnancy, and other acute agents (opioids, neuroleptics, prednisone) have more proven safety

Breast Feeding

- Zolmitriptan is found in breast milk. Use with caution

THE ART OF NEUROPHARMACOLOGY

Potential Advantages

- Effectiveness equal to other triptans. Available as orally disintegrating formulation and nasal spray. Better taste than sumatriptan nasal spray. Less risk of overuse than opioids or barbiturate-containing treatments

Potential Disadvantages

- Cost, potential for medication-overuse headache. Relatively greater rate of CNS AEs than other triptans

Primary Target Symptoms

- Headache pain, nausea, photo and phonophobia

Pearls

- Early treatment of migraine is most effective
- Compared to other triptans, zolmitriptan has the highest 2-hour pain-free responses
- May not be effective when taking during aura, before headache begins
- In patients with "status migrainosus" (migraine lasting more than 72 hours) neuroleptics and dihydroergotamine are more effective
- Triptans were not originally studied for use in the treatment of basilar or hemiplegic migraine
- Triptans can be used to treat tension-type headache in migraineurs but not in patients with pure tension-type headache
- Patients taking triptans more than 10 days/month are at increased risk of medication-overuse headache, which is less responsive to treatment
- Chest and throat tightness are usually benign and may be related to esophageal spasm rather than cardiac ischemia. These symptoms occur more commonly in patients without cardiac risk factors
- Recent studies suggest zolmitriptan nasal spray is useful for acute management of cluster headache
- Combination use of SNRI and triptans usually will not lead to serotonin syndrome, which requires activation of 5-HT$_{2A}$ receptors and a possible limited role of 5-HT$_{1A}$. However, triptans are agonists at the 5-HT$_{1B/1D/1F}$ receptor subtypes, with weak affinity for 5-HT$_{1A}$ receptors and no activity at the 5-HT$_2$ receptors. Thus, given the seriousness of serotonin syndrome, caution is certainly warranted and clinicians should be vigilant for serotonin toxicity symptoms and signs to insure prompt treatment
- Zolmitriptan may synergize with propranolol in lowering portal pressure
- The site of pharmacological action, whether central or peripheral, remains to be studied. Although triptan generally does not penetrate BBB, it has been postulated that transient BBB breakdown may occur during a migraine attack

Suggested Reading

Ashkenazi A, Schwedt T. Cluster headache – acute and prophylactic therapy. *Headache.* 2011;51(2):272–86.

Dodick D, Lipton RB, Martin V, Papademetriou V, Rosamond W, MaassenVanDenBrink A, et al. Consensus statement: cardiovascular safety profile of triptans (5-HT agonists) in the acute treatment of migraine. *Headache.* 2004; 44(5):414–25.

Evans RW, Tepper SJ, Shapiro RE, Sun-Edelstein C, Tietjen GE. The FDA alert on serotonin syndrome with use of triptans combined with selective serotonin reuptake inhibitors or selective serotonin-norepinephrine reuptake inhibitors: American Headache Society position paper. *Headache.* 2010;50(6):1089–99.

Ferrari MD, Roon KI, Lipton RB, Goadsby PJ. Oral triptans (serotonin 5-HT(1B/1D) agonists) in acute migraine treatment: a meta-analysis of 53 trials. *Lancet.* 2001;358(9294):1668–75.

Gladstone JP, Gawel M. Newer formulations of the triptans: advances in migraine management. *Drugs.* 2003;63(21):2285–305.

Lewis DW, Winner P, Hershey AD, Wasiewski WW; Adolescent Migraine Steering Committee. Efficacy of zolmitriptan nasal spray in adolescent migraine. *Pediatrics.* 2007;120(2):390–6.

Rapoport AM, Mathew NT, Silberstein SD, Dodick D, Tepper SJ, Sheftell FD, et al. Zolmitriptan nasal spray in the acute treatment of cluster headache: a double-blind study. *Neurology.* 2007;69(9):821–6.

Tepper SJ, Chen S, Reidenbach F, Rapoport AM. Intranasal zolmitriptan for the treatment of acute migraine. *Headache.* 2013;53 Suppl 2:62–71.

Brands
- Zonegran

Generic?
- Yes

Class
- Antiepileptic drug (AED), structurally a sulfonamide

Commonly Prescribed for
(FDA approved in bold)
- **Partial-onset seizures (adjunctive in adults)**
- Partial-onset seizures (adjunctive in pediatric patients)
- Primary generalized tonic-clonic seizures (adjunctive; adults and pediatric patients age 2–16)
- Myoclonic epilepsy, Lennox-Gastaut syndrome, absence seizure
- Infantile spasms (West syndrome)
- Idiopathic intracranial hypertension
- Migraine prophylaxis
- Adjunct to levodopa for Parkinson's disease
- Obesity
- Binge-eating disorder/bulimia
- Tardive dyskinesias
- Neuropathic pain

How the Drug Works
Unknown but there are multiple mechanisms of action that may be important
- Sodium channel antagonist
- Modulates N-, P-, and T-type calcium channels
- Binds to GABA receptors
- Weak carbonic anhydrase inhibitor
- Monoamine oxidase (MAO)-B inhibition
- May help facilitate dopamine and serotonin neurotransmission

How Long Until It Works
- Seizures: by 2–3 weeks
- Migraines: can take up to 3 months on a stable dose to see full effect

If It Works
- Seizures: goal is the remission of seizures. Continue as long as effective and well tolerated. Consider tapering and slowly stopping after 2 years seizure-free, depending on the type of epilepsy
- Migraine: goal is a 50% or greater reduction in migraine frequency or severity. Consider tapering or stopping if headaches remit for more than 6 months or if patient considering pregnancy

If It Doesn't Work
- Increase to highest tolerated dose
- Epilepsy: consider changing to another agent, adding a second agent, using a medical device, or a referral for epilepsy surgery evaluation. When adding a second agent, keep drug interactions in mind
- Migraine: address other issues such as medication overuse, other coexisting medical disorders, such as anxiety, and consider changing to another agent or adding a second agent

Best Augmenting Combos for Partial Response or Treatment-Resistance
- For some patients with epilepsy or migraine, low-dose polytherapy with 2 or more drugs may be better tolerated and more effective than high-dose monotherapy
- Epilepsy: keep in mind drug interactions and their effect on levels
- Migraine: consider β-blockers, antidepressants, natural products, other AEDs, and non-medication treatments, such as biofeedback, to improve headache control

Tests
- Mild to moderate decreases in bicarbonate can occur with zonisamide, but are uncommon reasons for discontinuation. Routine screening for metabolic acidosis is not recommended

How the Drug Causes AEs
- CNS AEs may be caused by sodium or calcium channel effects or GABA effects
- Carbonic anhydrase inhibition causes metabolic acidosis and may lead to kidney stones

Notable AEs

- Sedation, depression, irritability, fatigue, ataxia
- Anorexia, abdominal pain, nausea
- Kidney stones

 Life-Threatening or Dangerous AEs

- Metabolic acidosis
- Increased blood urea nitrogen and creatinine (non-progressive)
- Kidney stones (calcium or urate)
- Blood dyscrasias (aplastic anemia or agranulocytosis)
- Rare serious allergic rash (Stevens-Johnson syndrome)
- Fever, dehydration, and oligohidrosis (more common in children)

Weight Gain

- Unusual

unusual   not unusual   common   problematic

Sedation

- Common

unusual   not unusual   common   problematic

What to Do About AEs

- May decrease or remit after a longer time on a stable dose
- Paresthesias may respond to high-potassium diets or potassium tablets
- A small decrease in dose may reduce AEs

Best Augmenting Agents to Reduce AEs

- Paresthesias may improve with high-potassium diet or tablets
- Other AEs are more likely to be reduced by lowering dose

DOSING AND USE

Usual Dosage Range

- Epilepsy: 100–600 mg/day in adults. Most patients do best at 400 mg or less. Once/day dosing is fine
- Migraine: 100–600 mg/day. Most studies use 400 mg

- Parkinson's disease: used as low-dose adjunctive medication, typically 25–100 mg/day

Dosage Forms

- 25, 50, 100 mg

How to Dose

- In adults, start at low dose (100 mg/day for epilepsy, or 50 mg/day for migraine). After 1 week, increase to 200 mg/day. Wait at least 2 weeks before increasing to 300 mg and for each new increase
- For children, most often start at 2–4 mg/kg/day, dosed once or twice daily, and increase by 2 mg/kg/day every 1–2 weeks until at maintenance dose of 4–8 mg/kg/day. Maximum pediatric dose 12 mg/kg/day

 Dosing Tips

- AEs increase with dose increases but can be delayed due to the long half-life of the drug
- Weight loss is often dose related
- Slow titration can help minimize sedation and other AEs

Overdose

- Nystagmus, drowsiness, slurred speech, blurred vision, diplopia, stupor, hypotension, and bradycardia, respiratory depression, and metabolic acidosis. No reported deaths except with poly-drug overdoses

Long-Term Use

- Safe for long-term use

Habit Forming

- No

How to Stop

- Taper slowly
- Abrupt withdrawal can lead to seizures in patients with epilepsy. Tremor is also common
- Headaches may return within days to months of stopping

Pharmacokinetics

- Majority is renally excreted. Metabolized in part by CYP450 3A4 system. Plasma half-life is 63 hours

Drug Interactions

- Any drug that affects hepatic CYP3A4 can affect zonisamide levels
- CYP3A4 inhibitors such as nefazodone, fluoxetine, fluvoxamine, ketoconazole, clarithromycin, and many antivirals increase zonisamide levels
- CYP3A4 inducers such as phenytoin, phenobarbital, primidone, and especially carbamazepine decrease zonisamide levels
- May interact with carbonic anhydrase inhibitors, increasing risk of kidney stones

⚠ Other Warnings/ Precautions

- CNS AEs increase when taken with other CNS depressants
- Patients taking a ketogenic diet for seizures are more likely to experience severe metabolic acidosis on zonisamide
- Can be associated with severe rash – new-onset rash may be sign of hypersensitivity syndrome
- Any unusual bleeding or bruising, fever, or mouth sores should raise concern for rare blood dyscrasias that can occur with zonisamide

Do Not Use

- Proven allergy to zonisamide. Because zonisamide contains a sulfa moiety, it may cause allergy in patients with proven sulfa allergy

Children and Adolescents

- Approved for children aged 16 and up; few data about its use in younger patients but is used off-label for epilepsy and migraine
- May help treat infantile spasms related to tuberous sclerosis, especially if corticotropin is ineffective or cannot be used

Pregnancy

- Category C. Teratogenic in animal studies but no studies in humans
- Risks of stopping medication must outweigh risk to fetus for patients with epilepsy. Seizures and potential status epilepticus place the woman and fetus at risk and can cause reduced oxygen and blood supply to the womb
- Supplementation with 0.4 mg of folic acid before and during pregnancy is recommended
- Patients taking for conditions other than epilepsy should generally stop zonisamide before considering pregnancy. Migraine usually improves in the last 2 trimesters

Breast Feeding

- 90% of mother's blood drug level in breast milk
- Generally recommendations are to discontinue drug or bottle feed
- Monitor infant for sedation, poor feeding, or irritability

SPECIAL POPULATIONS

Renal Impairment

- Zonisamide is primarily renally excreted and patients with severe renal disease may require a slower titration

Hepatic Impairment

- Clearance may be decreased in patients with severe liver disease

Cardiac Impairment

- No known effects

Elderly

- May be more susceptible to CNS AEs

THE ART OF NEUROPHARMACOLOGY

Potential Advantages

- Highly effective for epilepsy, possibly effective for migraine. Usually causes weight loss, unlike many other medications. Ability to use once daily due to long half-life can increase compliance

Potential Disadvantages

- Weight loss in thin patients can be troublesome. Kidney stones. Fatigue and other CNS AEs

Primary Target Symptoms

- Seizure frequency and severity
- Migraine frequency and severity

Pearls

- For epilepsy, higher doses may be needed. AEs are more common when using in combination with other drugs that can produce CNS symptoms
- For migraine or idiopathic intracranial hypertension, zonisamide can be an alternative when topiramate is not well tolerated
- Zonisamide can be considered for patients who cannot tolerate topiramate for migraine prevention. In patients who simply did not improve on topiramate despite adequate doses and tolerability, consider a drug in a different class
- Low-dose zonisamide (25–100 mg) as adjunct to levodopa can effectively control motor symptoms in Parkinson's disease and decrease "off" time, perhaps by facilitation of dopamine synthesis, MAO-B inhibition, and glutamate release inhibition
- Zonisamide is used for treatment of essential tremor, but in clinical trials was only of modest benefit
- Insufficient data on diabetic neuropathic pain
- No proven effectiveness in bipolar disorder, and not a first-line treatment
- Occasionally used to offset weight gain seen with psychotropic agents or to treat binge-eating disorder
- In an open-label study, zonisamide plus bupropion resulted in more weight loss than zonisamide alone

Suggested Reading

Ashkenazi A, Benlifer A, Korenblit J, Silberstein SD. Zonisamide for migraine prophylaxis in refractory patients. *Cephalalgia*. 2006;26(10): 1199–202.

Bigal ME, Krymchantowski AV, Rapoport AM. Prophylactic migraine therapy: emerging treatment options. *Curr Pain Headache Rep.* 2004;8(3):178–84.

Fox SH, Katzenschlager R, Lim S-Y, Ravina B, Seppi K, Coelho M, et al. The Movement Disorder Society Evidence-Based Medicine Review Update: Treatments for the motor symptoms of Parkinson's disease. *Mov Disord.* 2011;26 Suppl 3:S2–41.

Jain KK. An assessment of zonisamide as an anti-epileptic drug. *Expert Opin Pharmacother.* 2000;1(6):1245–60.

Leppik IE. Zonisamide: chemistry, mechanism of action, and pharmacokinetics. *Seizure.* 2004;13 Suppl 1:S5–9; discussion S10.

Mohammadianinejad SE, Abbasi V, Sajedi SA, Majdinasab N, Abdollahi F, Hajmanouchehri R, et al. Zonisamide versus topiramate in migraine prophylaxis: a double-blind randomized clinical trial. *Clin Neuropharmacol.* 2011; 34(4):174–7.

Powell AG, Apovian CM, Aronne LJ. New drug targets for the treatment of obesity. *Clin Pharmacol Ther.* 2011;90(1): 40–51.

Yang LP, Perry CM. Zonisamide: in Parkinson's disease. *CNS Drugs.* 2009; 23(8):703–11.

List of abbreviations

5-HT	serotonin
AAN	American Academy of Neurology
ACE	angiotensin-converting enzyme
AChR	acetylcholine receptor
ADHD	attention deficit hyperactivity disorder
AED	antiepileptic drug
ALT	alanine aminotransferase
AMPA	α-amino-3-hydroxy-5-methyl-4 isoxazolepropionic acid
ANA	antinuclear antibodies
aPPT	activated partial thromboplastin time
AV	atrioventricular
BBB	blood–brain barrier
BMI	body mass index
BUN	blood urea nitrogen
CBC	complete blood cell count
C_{max}	peak concentration
CNS	central nervous system
Cr C2	creatinine clearance
CSF	cerebrospinal fluid
CYP450	cytochrome P450
dL	deciliter
ECG	electrocardiogram
EEG	electroencephalogram
EMG	electromyography
FDA	Food and Drug Administration
GABA	gamma-aminobutyric acid
GAD	generalized anxiety disorder
GFR	glomerular filtration rate
GI	gastrointestinal
GU	genitourinary
H_1	histamine 1
HDL	high-density lipoprotein
HLA	human leukocyte antigen
HMG CoA	beta-hydroxy-beta-methylglutaryl coenzyme A
IM	intramuscular
INR	international normalized ratio
IV	intravenous
MAOI	monoamine oxidase jnhibitor
MDD	major depressive disorder

mcg	microgram
mg	milligram
mL	milliliter
mm Hg	millimeters of mercury
MRI	magnetic resonance imaging
MuSK	muscle-specific kinase
NET	norepinephrine transporter
NMDA	N-methyl-D-aspartate
PNS	peripheral nervous system
PT	prothrombin time
QTc	QT corrected
REM	rapid eye movement
SC	subcutaneous
SERT	serotonin transporter
SNRI	dual serotonin and norepinephrine reuptake inhibitor
SSRI	selective serotonin reuptake inhibitor
TCA	tricyclic antidepressant
T_{max}	time of maximum concentration
USP	United States Pharmacopeia
WBC	white blood cell count

Index by Drug Name for
Essential Neuropharmacology:
A Prescriber's Guide

Index by Neurological Use for *Essential Neuropharmacology: A Prescriber's Guide*

Drug names in **bold** are FDA approved

Index by Class for *Essential Neuropharmacology: A Prescriber's Guide*